SALMONELLA – DISTRIBUTION, ADAPTATION, CONTROL MEASURES AND MOLECULAR TECHNOLOGIES

Edited by **Bassam A. Annous** and **Joshua B. Gurtler**

Salmonella – Distribution, Adaptation, Control Measures and Molecular Technologies
Edited by Bassam A. Annous and Joshua B. Gurtler

Published by InTech
Janeza Trdine 9, 51000 Rijeka, Croatia

Publishing Process Manager Adriana Pecar

Technical Editor Teodora Smiljanic

Cover Designer InTech Design Team

Additional hard copies can be obtained from orders@intechopen.com

Salmonella – Distribution, Adaptation, Control Measures and Molecular Technologies,
Edited by Bassam A. Annous and Joshua B. Gurtler
p. cm.
ISBN 978-953-51-0661-6

For EU product safety concerns:
IN TECH d.o.o., Prolaz Marije Krucifikse Kozulić 3, 51000 Rijeka, Croatia,
info@intechopen.com or visit our website at intechopen.com.

Meet the editors

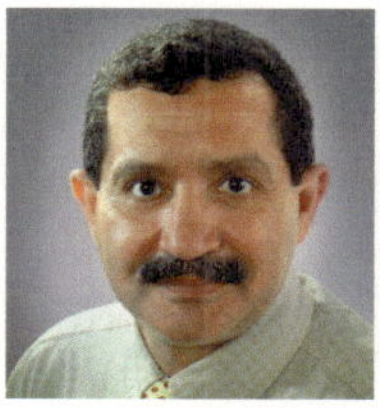

Dr Bassam A. Annous is a Research Microbiologist at the USDA – ARS – Eastern Regional Research Center, in Wyndmoor, PA. He earned a B.S. and a M.S. from the American University of Beirut, and a Ph.D. from the University of Illinois. His research experience has been in the areas of microbial food safety, food science, food engineering and microbial biotechnology. He has designed and validated novel thermal and non-thermal surface pasteurization technologies capable of reaching and inactivating human pathogens attached to inaccessible sites within biofilms on produce surfaces. He has authored 60+ peer-reviewed publications, review articles, and book chapters. He presented 40+ invited talks at scientific meetings and universities in USA, Japan, Canada, Australia, and Mexico. He served by invitation as an expert on three Food Safety and Security panels convened by FAO and WHO of the United Nations.

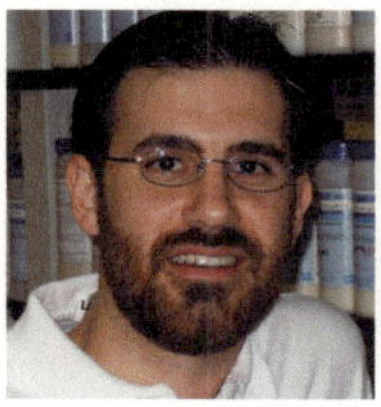

Dr Joshua B. Gurtler is a research scientist at the Eastern Regional Research Center of the USDA Agricultural Research Service in Wyndmoor, PA. He conducted his undergraduate and M.S. work at Auburn University, and completed his Ph.D. and post-doctoral work in food microbiology at the University of Georgia. Dr Gurtler's current work involves innovative interventions for the inactivation of Salmonella, enteric viruses and other foodborne pathogens in fresh produce, crops and soil, and he is currently developing new antimicrobial washes for fresh fruits and vegetables. Previous work evaluated the behavior and elimination of Salmonella, E. coli O157:H7, Yersinia, Cronobacter sakazakii, and spoilage microorganisms in products such as liquid and shell eggs, infant formulas and cereals, and fruit juices. He feels honored to work on this project with Dr Annous.

Contents

Preface

Salmonella has been a microbiological scourge on mankind for untold centuries. USDA researcher Daniel Salmon's discovery of this bacterial pathogen in swine in 1885 marked the beginning of intense efforts to control salmonellae that have continued for the past 127 years. Although progress has been made on many fronts, salmonellosis has yet to be eliminated in either developed nations (gastrointestinal salmonellosis) or in developing nations (gastrointestinal and typhoidal salmonellosis).

Chapters in this book address a wide array of topics related to understanding and controlling the pathogen. This book includes *Salmonella* as studied in the environment, air and in food products; genetic feedback mechanisms and molecular regulation; *Salmonella* virulence and pathogenicity, control by use of bacteriophage, antimicrobial peptides and other antimicrobials; control during animal production; epidemiology; bacterial adaptation; novel and rapid molecular and serological detection methods; antimicrobial resistance patterns; molecular diagnostics for typhoidal illness; proteomics; and survival mechanisms.

This work represents the collective contributions of authors from all around the world. Authors and co-authors hail from a multiplicity of institutions including Oxford University in the U.K., Colleges of Veterinary and Human Medicine, the Egyptian National Research Center, the U.K. Health Protection Agency, the Japanese National Institute of Health Science, and numerous University Departments including departments of Animal Health, Animal Production, Biology, Biology & Medical Parasitology, Bioscience, Botany, Biotechnology & Bioengineering, Chemistry, Genetics & Biotechnology, Genetics & Microbiology, Marine Science, Medicine, Microbial Chemistry, Microbiology, Microbiology & Immunology, Molecular Bioscience, Pharmaceutical Science, and Physics.

As editors of this book, we have done our best to ensure that the chapters represent original material by the authors and we have excluded any work that has either been previously published elsewhere or manuscripts that have taken too much liberty in citing from other published materials. We hope you find this book as intriguing, insightful and thought-provoking as we have.

Bassam A. Annous and Joshua B. Gurtler
U.S. Department of Agriculture – ARS
Eastern Regional Research Center
Wyndmoor, USA

Note: Drs. Annous and Gurtler wish to make clear that while they hold the scientific integrity of the authors in this book in the highest of esteem, any allusion to spontaneous generation of life, self-assembly, initial origins and macroevolutionary hypotheses do not necessarily reflect their own philosophical beliefs.

1

Elucidating the Epidemiology of Human Salmonellosis: The Value of Systematic Laboratory Characterisation of Isolates

P. McKeown[1], P. Garvey[1] and M. Cormican[2]
[1]*Health Protection Surveillance Centre, Dublin*
[2]*National Salmonella Reference Laboratory, Bacteriology Department*
Galway University Hospital
Ireland

1. Introduction

Infection with non-typhoidal *Salmonella enterica* (NTS) represents a significant burden of gastroenteric illness upon the world's population. Most enteric *Salmonella* infection is zoonotic, transmitted from healthy vertebrate animals to humans, largely by means of contaminated food. The reported incidence of enteric salmonellosis increased rapidly after the Second World War in association with progressive industrialisation of the food supply, at a time when the incidence of typhoid was declining, consequent upon the extensive development of water treatment and waste disposal systems, coupled with the pasteurization of milk.[1] As a result, infection with NTS displaced typhoid in the developed world as the major threat to human health from *Salmonella* during the 20th century.

Salmonellae have evolved into a diverse genus of *Enterobacteriaceae;* some members being adapted to specific hosts with others having a broad host range. In addition to their wide spectrum of zoonotic hosts, salmonellae vary greatly in age (*S.* Typhi having emerged more recently than *S.* Typhimurium), in lineage and in clonality. Accordingly, a variety of genome-based methods must be used in order to provide appropriate methods for characterisation of different variants

One hundred million cases of salmonellosis are estimated to occur globally each year. Estimates of incidence range from 32 cases/100,000 population in high income areas of the Asia Pacific region to 3,600/100,000 population in Southeast Asia.[2] Annually, this results in 155,000 deaths worldwide. Mortality rates from salmonellosis are highest in East and Southeast Asia and lowest in the developed countries of Europe, North America and Oceania.

About 80% of all salmonellosis cases are estimated to be foodborne (rising to 94% in the United States).[3] Reported incidence varies widely, not least in developed countries, reflecting both real differences in incidence (driven by variations in farming/food production practices, the existence of *Salmonella* Control Programs and food consumption patterns), and the effects of variability in surveillance parameters, and health care and diagnostic systems. In Western Europe and in high-income regions of North America, total incidence (which includes confirmed NTS cases combined with projections based upon population models) is estimated to be 220/100,000 and 495/100,000 respectively.[2]

These figures do not, however, paint the full picture. Although there is marked regional variation, there has been a steady decrease in the total confirmed notification rates for salmonellosis in the European Union over the last six years from 196,000 cases in 2004 to 108,000 cases in 2009 (or 21.6 cases /100 000 population), representing an average 12% fall per year.[4] The incidence has remained static in Ireland (at 10 cases/100,000 between 2006 and 2008) but has fallen in the UK (from 23 to 19/100,000 cases) over the same period. Certain countries, however, have seen marked increases in reported incidence between 2006 and 2008 (from from 31 to 67 cases/100,000 in Denmark and from 16 to 39 cases/100,000 in Malta) while others report steep declines in incidence (such as the Czech Republic falling from 236 to 103 cases/100,000 and from 64 to 52 cases/100,000 in Germany).[5]

In the United States, approximately 40,000 laboratory-confirmed cases of *Salmonella* infection are reported annually to the National *Salmonella* Surveillance System in the United States, giving an annualised incidence rate, in 2006 of 13.3 cases per 100,000 population (CDC, 2011).[6]

Under-ascertainment of enteric salmonellosis is a significant concern. In the UK, the ratio of *Salmonella* isolates reported nationally to cases occurring in the community has been estimated as being 4.7, i.e. 3.7 undetected community cases for each laboratory confirmed case included in national statistics.[7]

Salmonellosis underascertainment has been estimated in a range of European countries using an intriguing method by Swedish researchers.[8] Investigators calculated the incidence of salmonellosis acquired overseas among returning Swedish travellers on a country-specific basis and compared this derived incidence against nationally reported incidence in the country in which the case had acquired their infection. As a result, they estimated that there was significant variation in the ratio of underdetection by the national reporting systems of the countries involved, ranging from less than one in the case of Finnish and Icelandic systems (i.e. these systems were more sensitive at detecting salmonellosis than the Swedish travel-based system) to 98 and 270 in the case of Greek and Bulgarian systems, suggesting that these systems were considerably less sensitive at detecting salmonellosis than the Swedish travel-based system. Interestingly, the underdetection index for Ireland was 4.3 - precisely the same as that found for the UK.[8] The authors note that the behaviours and risks of Swedish travellers may not be fully representative for those of the native population; nevertheless, it provides an interesting comparative snapshot of potential *Salmonella* underascertainment in Europe.

The Centers for Disease Control and Prevention (CDC) has recently estimated that the true annual incidence of salmonellosis in the US to be 1,027,561 non travel-associated domestic cases,[3] highlighting the perennial issue of infectious intestinal disease underascertainment. Using CDC's estimates, it can be calculated that for every laboratory confirmed case of domestically acquired salmonellosis, there are approximately 25 clinical cases that are not laboratory confirmed.

Salmonellae are effective outbreak organisms and extensive outbreaks of salmonella occur frequently, ranging in size from a couple of cases, to tens of thousands of cases. A significant number of these outbreaks are international in distribution and have involved a wide range of food products including chocolate,[9,10,11] imported eggs,[12] infant formula,[13] fresh basil,[14] raw milk cheese,[15] pork,[16] rucola lettuce,[17] sprouts,[18] pre-cooked meat products,[19] lasagne,[20] pet products,[21] sesame seeds,[22] raw almonds,[23] peanuts,[24] peanut butter,[25] and ready-to-eat vegetables.[26] In addition, in 2008, the European Food Safety Authority reported 490 confirmed foodborne outbreaks of salmonellosis resulting in 7,724 cases, 1,363 hospitalisations and 118 deaths.[27]

In considering the relative and absolute burden of human salmonellosis based on data from the developed world, it is perhaps striking that NTS infection remains a potent public health and clinical challenge, although the majority of developed nations have both well-developed surveillance systems to detect human salmonellosis (and the outbreaks that result), and farm-based and food hygiene surveillance systems specifically designed to control food-borne NTS infection. There is however, some comfort in the static or falling incidence of salmonellosis in many developed countries.

A range of emerging factors facilitate the rapid distribution of all foodborne microbes, including *Salmonella:* globalization of the food supply, an aging and highly mobile population able to distribute an increasingly diversified intestinal flora more widely, a growing proportion of the population at special risk due to immunosuppressive diseases such as cancer, or consuming pharmaceutical agents that inhibit either the immune system (such as cytotoxic agents) or protective gastric acid secretion (such as proton pump inhibitors), changing dietary preferences for raw or lightly cooked food, intensification in farming practice, environmental encroachment with greater exposure to novel pathogens, climate change and international travel and trade between countries.[28]

This importance of increased movement of populations and food is partly reflected in the growing proportion of NTS infection attributed either to international travel or to the consumption of imported food. Up to half of Irish *Salmonella* infections are reported as being acquired outside Ireland.[29] More than 60% of cases of human salmonellosis in Denmark in 2007 were associated with consumption of imported meat or with international travel.[30] The Smittskyddsinstitutet, the Swedish government agency with responsibility to monitor the epidemiology of communicable diseases, estimates that more that 74% of reported NTS infections identified in Sweden are acquired on trips outside that country.[31]

The incidence of salmonellosis increased markedly during the 1970s and 1980s. Between 1976 and 1986, reported infections due to *S.* Enteritidis (a commensal primarily of poultry, particularly chickens) increased more than six-fold in the north-eastern United States,[32] while the incidence of infections due to *S.* Typhimurium remained static.[33] This led investigators to wonder if they were witnessing the onset of a novel pandemic.[34] A number of theories as to the underlying explanation of this increase were considered, including clonal expansion of a single, more virulent variant of S. Enteritidis. It was concluded, however, that this upsurge was most likely triggered by *S.* Enteritidis occupying the ecological niche left vacant by the established avian *Salmonella* pathogens, *S.* Pullorum and S. Gallinarum, when those subtypes had been largely eliminated from poultry flocks,[34] with transmission of human disease being amplified by the progressive intensification of poultry farming.

2. Identification and linking of cases

In Ireland, as is common in most other developed countries, the appearance of a clinical case of salmonellosis will prompt a number of public health and microbiological responses. The management of the individual patient may not require either detailed characterisation or antimicrobial susceptibility testing since *Salmonella* gastroenteritis is generally self-limiting. From a public health perspective however, detailed characterisation of the isolate may help to determine the extent of linkages, and potential sources. Preliminary interviewing of the case seeks to determine if there is epidemiological evidence of linkage (to other cases or a possible source) and to determine if the case is in a high risk category (in this case, high risk means that they are at increased risk of spread of the *Salmonella* strain; for example, if the case were a food handler and confirmed as having salmonellosis s/he would pose a risk of onward transmission). If there is laboratory evidence of linkage, each potentially linked case is administered an extensive national *Salmonella* Trawling Questionnaire, designed to question the case in close detail to determine if there are exposures common to other, similar cases.[35]

It is the knitting together of in-depth clinical public health interviews and definitive characterisation of isolates from clinical (and frequently food and animal) specimens, that facilitate the identification of common sources of infection, therefore close collaboration between public health microbiologists and epidemiologists is essential to effective prevention and control.

2.1 Microbiological identification

Almost all human cases of NTS infection are associated with a single species; *Salmonella enterica*. However, the highly developed system of sub-classification within the species is valuable in linking isolates from different human and non-human sources.

Confirmation of the diagnosis of human salmonellosis and further characterisation of the isolate entails, initially, the bacteriological isolation of the organism from a clinical specimen. Clinical samples are typically stool specimens but blood, urine, spinal fluid, joint fluid, pus and tissues may be examined. The isolation of *Salmonella* from faeces requires the use of media that allows for the preferential growth of *Salmonella* from among the complex mixture of bacteria that comprise the normal gastrointestinal flora. This is achieved by direct culture on selective agar media such as Xylose-Lysine-Desoxycholate agar (XLD) or chromogenic agars. To enhance detection of low numbers of *Salmonella,* stool samples are also, generally inoculated into a selective enrichment broth (often Selenite F broth), which is plated to selective media after overnight incubation. This two-step process means that, although a preliminary indication that a culture is negative on primary plating is typically available at 24 hours, a definitive "Not Detected" report is typically not available for 48 hours. Specimens from normally sterile body sites are typically cultured on non-selective agar media (for example blood agar) or broth because there is no requirement to suppress competing normal flora. Urine samples are a special case because many clinical laboratories do not characterise all significant urine isolates beyond the level of *Enterobacteriaceae* (coliforms). As a result, *Salmonella* urinary tract infections may go unrecognised.

It is important that the limitations of the methods used for detection are understood by practitioners. The reliability of the result is critically dependent upon the quality management systems in place in the clinical laboratory and, ideally, such laboratories should be accredited to the ISO-15189 standard. Even with rigorous control of quality, microbiologists should report samples as "*Salmonella* not detected" (or words of similar meaning), avoiding such terms as "*Salmonella* negative" or "*Salmonella* absent". For epidemiologists and food safety agencies it is important to understand that even if a laboratory uses the term "negative" or "absent" in informal communication, failure to detect *Salmonella* on culture does not entirely exclude the possibility of infection.

Provisional positive results may be available within 24 hours (from the primary plate) or within 48 hours if cultured only from subculture of enrichment broth. Definitive confirmation of the isolate and antimicrobial susceptibility testing may require an additional working day although a provisional positive report from a laboratory with skilled scientists and effective quality systems generally has a very high degree of reliability. Confirmation of a suspect colony as being due to *Salmonella* may be achieved by biochemical and serological characterisation or by molecular methods (the latter may allow for more rapid confirmation).

The extent to which clinical laboratories characterise isolates in their own laboratory before submission to a reference laboratory, and the frequency with which isolates are submitted to reference laboratories, may depend on experience, skills sets, resources and funding/reimbursement systems, and ease of access to reference laboratory services. Although antimicrobial agents are not required in most patients with *Salmonella* gastroenteritis, this can represent useful preliminary characterisation and is essential to guide therapy in those with invasive disease. Antimicrobial susceptibility testing should be performed by standardized methods [European Committee on Antimicrobial Susceptibility Testing EUCAST), or Clinical Laboratory Standards Institute (CLSI) I or International Standards Organization (ISO 20776-1) or by commercial systems validated against these standards. Measurements (diameter of zone of inhibition or minimum inhibitory concentration; MIC) should be interpreted with reference to EUCAST or CLSI interpretive criteria. The use of non-standardised methods for performance or interpretation does not form a sound basis for clinical or public health decision-making. The use of national standards may provide effective clinical guidance but may limit comparability of data with other countries.

Antimicrobial resistance patterns can provide useful supplementary information about the degree of relatedness of members within a particular serotype. Phage typing of serotypes such as *S.* Typhimurium, *S.* Enteritidis and *S.* Agona has been used extensively for epidemiological purposes. Phage typing is a rapid and discriminatory phenotypic method. Interpretation is somewhat subjective; standardization is difficult and phages are not generally available from commercial sources.[36] However, external quality assessment programmes in Europe have confirmed, with a common stock of phage (provided through HPA Colindale) coupled with, common methods and training, that national reference laboratories can produce comparable phage-typing results for *S.* Enteritidis and *S.* Typhimurium. In the past, plasmid profiling was used extensively in identifying outbreak strains and may still be useful in certain settings.

Further typing and subtyping by genome-based methods including pulsed field gel electrophoresis (PFGE),[37] multiple locus variable number tandem repeat (VNTR) analysis

(MLVA), multilocus sequence typing (MLST) can add value, however the discriminatory power of each molecular method may vary based on the serotype under consideration. In the not-too-distant future, single nucleotide polymorphisms (SNPs) and indeed whole genome sequencing may be employed to aid in investigating certain outbreaks.[38]

2.2 Case linkage

Linking of cases of salmonellosis (a necessary first step in the identification of outbreaks) has, by convention, been undertaken using the traditional epidemiological process of describing cases in terms of time, place and person whilst looking for potential linkages between cases that might give a clue as to a possible common source for infection.[39,40] At an early stage, this epidemiological information should be combined with information on characterisation of the isolates, as a first step in determining which cases should be included (and excluded) as being considered part of a particular cluster or outbreak. Serotype and antimicrobial-resistance patterns are generally available at an early stage and may provide pointers that isolates might belong to a homogenous group supporting the possibility of a common source.

In countries with smaller populations and/or low reported incidence of infection, the appearance of a cluster of isolates of an unusual serotype may be readily detected and prompt an investigative response. Countries with larger populations and higher incidence may have greater difficulty in identifying a cluster among the background levels and may have a higher threshold for response. Advanced systems of triggering exist in some countries, and are based on mathematical models to produce an automated alert once an expected threshold is exceeded.

Serotyping and antimicrobial-resistance patterns are of limited value however, in relation to serotypes that are very common and widely distributed. In Ireland, in 2008, the five commonest *Salmonella* serotypes (*S.* Typhimurium, *S.* Enteritidis, *S.* Agona, *S.* Virchow and *S.* Java) accounted for 70% of all isolates (see Figure 1).[41] Isolation of such a common serotype from two sources (i.e. from two cases or from a case and a food item) may well be a chance finding and does not represent persuasive evidence of an epidemiological link. Furthermore, isolates of *S.* Enteritidis are often susceptible to all or most antimicrobial agents tested routinely so that most reference laboratories receive a large number of fully susceptible *S.* Enteritidis isolates.. However, thisdegree of identification will not be adequate to support public health decision making regarding the degree of relatedness of strains and hence the extent of linking that might exist between isolates. It is in this situation that the molecular typing methods briefly outlined above add most value.

There are a number of key principles that must be considered in interpreting laboratory data. First, the extent of characterisation performed should be appropriate to address the epidemiological and public health issues of concern. Serotyping may be sufficient in some cases (especially for rare serotypes) but may be quite inadequate in others. Second, data generated by laboratory typing must always be interpreted in the context of: (1) the current epidemiological situation, (2) decades of accumulated published experience about routes of transmission and (3) an understanding of limitations of the methods used. It is rarely, if ever, appropriate to make a determination that isolates are linked or unlinked based solely on laboratory typing data. It is important to remember that regardless of the sophistication of the typing methods used, the best that can be achieved is the demonstration of evidence of a link between isolates. It is not possible, based on typing methods alone, to determine the pathway of transmission (and hence to establish causality), that is to say typing does not allow one to determine if the person was infected from the food or if the infected person contaminated the food.

Epidemiologists should be aware of the potential for pseudo-infection and pseudo-outbreaks related to laboratory cross-contamination of samples. This can be a particular issue when a laboratory external quality assessment/proficiency programme has recently included a *Salmonella* isolate in a round of testing. It may be helpful to clarify if the isolate was detected on primary agar plate culture, or only following enrichment. In our experience, growth of multiple colonies of *Salmonella* on the primary agar plate is unlikely to be due to laboratory cross contamination. However, when there is no growth on the primary agar plate but *Salmonella* is isolated from the Selenite F broth, it is important to consider the possibility of cross contamination, in particular if the laboratory has cultured a similar isolate from a clinical sample or external quality assessment sample in the previous few days.

3. Irish data on *Salmonella* isolates

Data from Irish national sources give a clear illustration of the degree of variability among and within *Salmonella* serotypes. In Ireland, all *Salmonella* isolates received at the National *Salmonella, Shigella* and *Listeria* Reference Laboratory (NSSLRL) at Galway (this includes all human clinical, and a number of veterinary and environmental isolates) are serotyped, susceptibility to a suite of antimicrobial agents is assessed and all isolates of *S.* Typhimurium and *S.* Enteritis are differentiated by phage typing. Since 2009, MLVA has also been applied routinely to *S.* Typhimurium isolates providing an additional level of discrimination. Additional molecular methods such PFGE are applied selectively during cluster/outbreak investigations.

In all, about 175 different *Salmonella* serotypes were reported to the NSSLRL between 2000 and 2010 among Irish clinical isolates. However, the current epidemiology of *Salmonella* in Ireland is dominated by two serotypes, *S.* Enteritidis and *S.* Typhimurium (including monophasic Typhimurium). These two serotypes accounted for 20% and 38% respectively, of human clinical isolates identified in Ireland in 2010, while other serotypes made up the remaining 42% of isolates (Figure 1). This represents a change in the relative importance of these serotypes since earlier in the decade when *S.* Enteritidis was consistently the most common serotype among Irish clinical isolates.

Within *S.* Typhimurium, approximately 90 definitive types have been detected since 2000, the 10 most common of which are depicted in Table 1. Overall, DT104 and DT104b have been the most common phage types detected. Antimicrobial susceptibility patterns and molecular typing (MLVA and PFGE) indicate significant diversity within these phage types.

Within *S.* Enteritidis, although PT4 and PT1 have been the most common phage types since 2000, the number and proportion of both have declined markedly in recent years; in 2010, PT14b was the most common type (Table 2). MLVA provides increased discrimination within common *S.* Enteritidis phage types; however, unlike S. Typhimurium, there is not at present a clear consensus on a standardized approach to MLVA for this serotype.

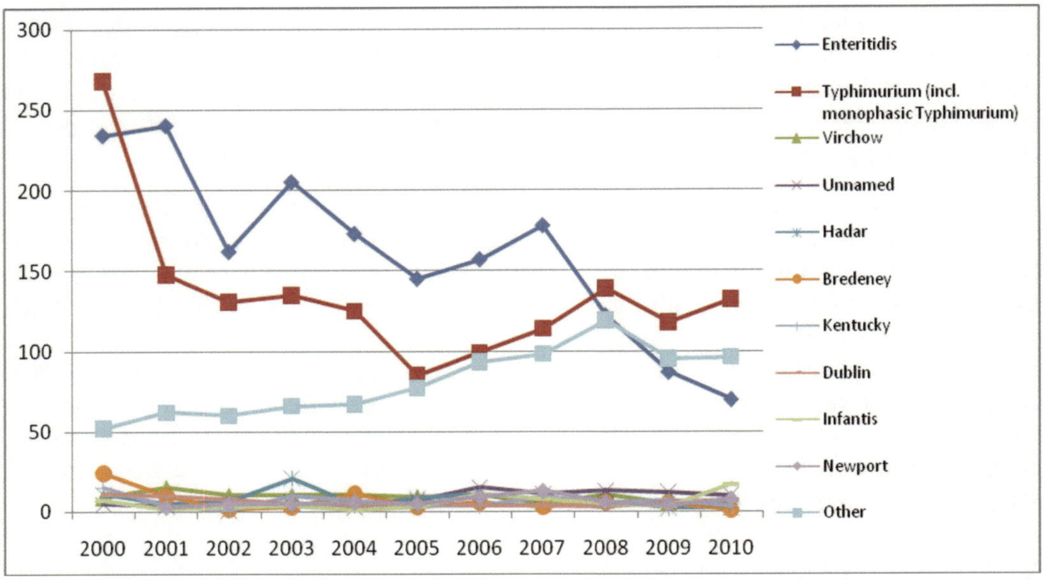

[Data source: NSSLRL, Unpublished data]

Fig. 1. Annual number clinical Salmonella isolates by serotype, Ireland 2000-2010 – [Top ten individually represented with all others combined]

Phage type	2000	2001	2002	2003	2004	2005	2006	2007	2008	2009	2010	Total (%)
DT104	194	39	25	22	48	37	24	21	28	24	26	**488 (33%)**
DT104b	23	48	49	67	23	13	29	14	27	14	14	**321 (21%)**
DT193	11	11	16	4	2	5	11	13	18	27	18	**136 (9%)**
U302	8	6	9	8	2	1	7	4	9	3	1	**58 (4%)**
Untypable	1	2	0	1	0	7	0	9	7	10	15	**52 (3%)**
DT120	1	6	0	0	3	0	1	19	6	6	6	**48 (3%)**
DT8	1				1			1		5	28	**36 (2%)**
DT12	4	1	6	8	1	3		2	4			**29 (2%)**
U311	0	3	3	3	1	0	0	0	0	6	6	**22 (1%)**
Other	25	32	23	22	44	19	27	31	40	23	18	**304 (20%)**
Total	**268**	**148**	**131**	**135**	**125**	**85**	**99**	**114**	**139**	**118**	**132**	**1494 (100%)**

[Data source: NSSLRL, Unpublished data]

Table 1. Annual Number S Typhimurium by Definitive Type, Ireland 2000-2010 [Top nine individually represented with all others combined]

Phage type	2000	2001	2002	2003	2004	2005	2006	2007	2008	2009	2010	Total
PT4	162	86	36	58	43	19	33	70	22	7	9	**545 (31%)**
PT1	26	74	51	53	48	44	29	13	23	9	14	**384 (22%)**
PT21	5	10	5	21	18	12	26	13	22	11	6	**149 (8%)**
PT14b	8	6	8	7	11	22	19	17	11	20	17	**146 (8%)**
PT8	4	7	12	10	10	20	17	35	14	13	4	**146 (8%)**
PT6	3	3	16	13	10	3	4	12	8	4	2	**78 (4%)**
PT6a	8	12	9	11	11	3	1	2	1	4	1	**63 (4%)**
PT13a		6	3	5	1	1	1	1	2	2	1	**23 (1%)**
Untypable	2	1	2	1		2	2	3	1	1	5	**20 (1%)**
Other	16	35	20	26	21	19	25	12	18	16	11	**219 (12%)**
Total	**234**	**240**	**162**	**205**	**173**	**145**	**157**	**178**	**122**	**87**	**70**	**1773 (100%)**

[Data source: NSSLRL, Unpublished data]

Table 2. Annual Number S Enteritidis by Phage Type, Ireland 2000-2010 [Top nine individually represented with all others combined]

4. Outbreaks

Salmonellae are relatively hardy microorganisms, surviving prolonged periods in frozen storage,[42] and in manure and manure-soil mixtures;[43] food at room temperature or slightly above, provides very favourable conditions for their multiplication. A relatively small inoculum (<1000 cells) is generally sufficient to produce clinical illness or colonisation.[44] Many serotypes of NTS have a particularly broad host range and may persist in the gastrointestinal tract of animal hosts for extended periods. These characteristics, coupled with the steady globalisation of the human food supply and global travel, contribute to the potential of *Salmonella* to cause both well-demarcated local and global outbreaks as well as periodic emergence of clonal groups which disseminate in a more diffuse manner (for example, as monophasic *Salmonella* Typhimurium has done in recent years).

Salmonellae spread readily by means of food, from zoonotic hosts and directly from person to person. The progressive intensification and mechanisation of production, and globalisation of distribution of our food supply, has meant that outbreaks of *Salmonella* can be very extensive, and their sources, deeply embedded. In the United States during 2008-9, a multistate outbreak of *Salmonella* Typhimurium - linked to peanut butter – resulted in more than 700 cases of illness.[45] Its final cost was expected to exceed $1Bn.[46] In 2008, an outbreak of *Salmonella* Agona associated with a food production facility in Ireland led to the recognition of 163 associated cases of illness across Europe including two deaths; the implicated facility exported 800 tonnes of cooked food product across the world each week (for a fuller description of this outbreak, see below).[19] An important facet of *Salmonella* outbreaks (in common with many other outbreak pathogens) is that the number of cases detected by investigation almost invariably represents a significant underestimate of the true burden of illness resulting from a particular source. It is also important to note that although enteric salmonellosis is a self-limiting illness in most people, in most substantial outbreaks, a number of associated deaths (particularly among the vulnerable and elderly) is not uncommon.

Outbreaks of salmonellosis are frequent events in developed countries, but show a definite decrease in the EU from 2,201 outbreaks in 2007 to 1,722 in 2009.[47]

5. Examples where molecular microbiology was influential in hypothesis generation or source implication during outbreak investigations in Ireland

The consistent and standardised application of *Salmonella* typing methods has enabled a detailed understanding of the baseline or expected incidence of specific *Salmonella* subtypes in Ireland (as is the case in almost all developed countries). This has been of critical importance in the detection of potential clusters based on deviation from the expected incidence. Close collaboration between epidemiologists and microbiologists is essential in forming a judgement as to which clusters are appropriate for epidemiological investigation. Many of the laboratory techniques are applied in reference laboratories across the developed world using standardised protocols. Communication of laboratory results (including results of genotyping studies) in standardised formats through channels such as those of the European Centre for Disease Prevention and Control (ECDC) and bilaterally between National Reference Laboratories and National Epidemiological Institutes can be vital in both detection and management of international outbreaks.

A large outbreak of *Salmonella* Agona originating in Ireland, involving a number of European countries and linked to an Irish Food manufacturer in 2008 neatly illustrates the concept of hypothesis generation.[19] In this outbreak, six cases of *Salmonella* Agona, each having the same unique PFGE profile (SAGOXB.0066) were identified within a two week period (prior to this outbreak, six cases would be a typical annual total for *Salmonella* Agona isolates in Ireland). Within two weeks of the first cases having been identified, a review of *Salmonella* Trawling Questionnaires, coupled with emerging microbiological evidence of the outbreak strain (displaying the PFGE profile of the clinical isolates) being identified on the premises of an Irish food manufacturer, and in food outlets supplied by this same company, led investigators to hypothesise that a number of food items produced by the Irish Food manufacturer were the vehicles of infection via these food outlets. From data provided through the *Salmonella* Trawling Questionnaires, three quarters of cases reported consuming food from take-away chains and eating sandwiches containing chicken or pork/ham.

Together, epidemiological and microbiological evidence augmented one another in this outbreak. The epidemiological evidence pointed to the commonality of exposure to particular types of retail food outlets (take away chains), to particular food types (sandwiches) and to particular ingredients (chicken ham or pork). The microbiological information consisted of evidence of a common serotype (*Salmonella* Agona), having a particular genotypic profile (PFGE Profile SAGOXB.0066) which was found in a large number of cases across Europe, in the production plant of the Irish Food manufacturer and in food outlets across Europe supplied by this manufacturer (at food outlet level, the outbreak clonal group was eventually identified in unopened packs of food produced by the parent company). Taken together, this evidence was used to form a hypothesis that contamination due to this strain (possibly at the level of the parent company) was distributed by means of particular food items through a supply chain to end user food outlets. It was in this way that the infection was transmitted, and the outbreak propagated.

In investigating the root cause of the outbreak, the investigators noted that food was cooked in the plant in a process that involved chicken, bacon, pork and other food types being placed in "continuous cook" ovens on the "low-risk" side. Cooking would take place and the food was then conveyed to the "high-risk" side. The investigators noted that, *"a number of Salmonella isolates identified in the low risk area on product and in the environment between April and July 2008 were forwarded for definitive typing and found to be the unique pulsed field profile SAGOXB.0066/PT39. It appears that there was a high load of S. Agona in the low risk area and to such an extent that it overcame the existing control mechanisms designed to protect the high risk area from material in the low risk area. Such an amount of a single serovar indicated a hygiene failure sufficiently to propagate such an outbreak."*

When remediation measures were put in place in the affected production plant, the outbreak was controlled.

Without PFGE methods it would have been much more difficult to separate out the outbreak *Salmonella* Agona isolates from non travel-associated endemic isolates across multiple countries. Use of PFGE was instrumental in focussing the investigation towards the likelihood that the outbreak was caused by an internationally distributed commodity, in this case, a food product. PFGE was also used to distinguish between at least one other contemporaneous background Irish *S.* Agona case and the outbreak strain, thus enabling this case to be eliminated from the descriptive and analytical epidemiological investigations. Ensuring that unrelated cases are not included as outbreak cases in analytical studies is particularly important as their exclusion reduces the risk of misclassification (a form of bias), which could alter estimation of the effect size.

The authors of the Outbreak Report say as much when they note that "The detection of the source identified would not have been possible without the use of molecular typing techniques and the sharing of data and co-operation between numerous agencies." [48]

Similarly, a cluster of seven cases diagnosed with *S.* Heidelberg (an uncommon serotype in Ireland) was identified in 2011.[49] In investigating this outbreak, the identification of isolates in reference laboratories in Europe and North America with PFGE profiles indistinguishable from those of the Irish *S.* Heidelberg isolates permitted the recognition of cases which were investigated for possible epidemiological links to the Irish cases. Travel to Tanzania was identified as a common risk factor among cases. Accumulated evidence over a number of years of an association between this serotype and East Africa (among other regions) provided useful circumstantial evidence supporting the hypothesis that the infection was associated with the travel destination. PFGE was important in focussing this investigation towards specific exposures, as the Irish cases had travelled as a group and had shared many exposures throughout their trip making it difficult to establish which was the likely source of infection. In the absence of formal standardisation of molecular typing methods, it would not have been possible to establish the potential links between these international cases, which might otherwise have been considered to be unlinked.

Unusually in 2010, DT8 was the most common *S.* Typhimurium definitive type detected in Ireland. This was due to the occurrence of an outbreak which was associated with exposure to duck eggs.[50] Prior to 2009, there had only been three cases of this definitive type detected over an eight-year period. The detection initially of a cluster of three *S.* Typhimurium DT8 isolates by the reference laboratory within a one-month period in the latter half of 2009, followed by a further cluster of four cases five months later led to the recognition of a temporally diffuse outbreak of 35 cases which occurred over an 18 month period. In this outbreak, hypothesis generation was based primarily on the classical descriptive epidemiological method of administering a trawling questionnaire; however, particularly strong evidence pointing towards the association between the human cases and duck egg exposure was provided through comparison of molecular profiles of *S.* Typhimurium isolates from implicated duck egg farms with isolates from human cases using both MLVA and PFGE. The work of national veterinary reference laboratory and effective liaison between human and veterinary reference laboratory services was also indispensable in defining the source of this outbreak.

This evidence was key in enabling control measures to be introduced, including the signing into Irish law of new legislation (S.I. No. 565 of 2010), the 'Diseases of Animals Act 1966 (Control of *Salmonella* in Ducks) Order 2010', which now sets down a legal basis for the control of salmonellosis in egg-laying duck flocks in Ireland.

Unfortunately, the identification of clusters by microbiological methods does not guarantee a successful outcome to the subsequent epidemiological investigation. On a number of occasions, outbreak control teams have been established to investigate clusters identified in this manner, but for which no definitive epidemiological link could be established between cases and no source of infection was identified. For example, a temporally-defined but geographically diffuse cluster of *S.* Typhimurium DT193 was investigated in 2009. MLVA was used to define those DT193 isolates occurring that year which were included in the investigation. And in 2009, an outbreak control team was established to investigate a rise in the incidence of *S* Enteritidis PT14b. In neither instance could a definitive epidemiological link be established between the cases and no sources of infection were identified.

Known associations between particular reservoirs and *Salmonella* serotypes has been exploited in source attribution studies.[51] This kind of information is also useful in outbreak investigation as it can give an early pointer of likely vehicles for particular strains for hypothesis generation.

6. Emerging factors

In Ireland, it has become apparent in recent years that overseas travel plays an important role in *Salmonella* epidemiology. It is now estimated that up to half of all notified cases may be travel associated (Table 3). This is broadly similar to the proportions in Finland, Sweden and Norway, all of whom report that more than 70% of their salmonellosis cases are travel-associated and is in contrast to the majority of countries in central and southern Europe who report this to be a largely indigenous disease.[4]

	Number of cases	% of total number of cases	% of cases with known travel history
Indigenous	351	31%	51%
Travel-associated	342	30%	49%
Unknown/not specified	445	39%	-
Total	**1138**	**100%**	**100%**

[Data source: CIDR]

Table 3. Number and percentage Salmonella notifications by Travel history, Ireland 2008-2010

Combining epidemiological information on case travel histories with microbiological information enabled confirmation that *S.* Enteritidis is uncommon among indigenous salmonellosis cases in Ireland, with a high proportion being associated with overseas exposure,[29] while *S.* Typhimurium is clearly the dominant serotype among indigenous cases. This is supported by outbreak surveillance data (Table 4). These combined data have also been exploited in studies such as a recent EFSA source attribution study which suggested that after the risk factor 'travel', pigs may be the most important contributor to human *Salmonella* infections in Ireland.[49]

Serotype	Number travel-associated Salmonella outbreaks	Number indigenous Salmonella outbreaks	Total
S Enteritidis	13	13	26
S Typhimurium	3	37	40
Other Salmonella serotypes	5	24	29
Salmonella serotype not reported	4	10	14
Total	**25**	**84**	**109**

[Data source: CIDR]

Table 4. Number Salmonella outbreaks (family and general) by serotype and travel association, Ireland 2004-2010

7. Conclusion

Salmonellosis continues to be an important global cause of infectious intestinal disease and in developed countries maintains its dominant position as one of the top three commonest causes of bacterial gastroenteritis. Enteric salmonellae are potent outbreak organisms and linking of cases that are part of the same outbreak has been facilitated by the recent increased application of molecular methods of characterisation that allow increasingly reliable differentiation and discrimination between and within serotypes. The progressive refinement of discriminatory methods permits the ready inclusion (and exclusion) of isolates within outbreaks in such a way that reduces wasteful investigation of unrelated isolates of the same serotype, while identifying more accurately the true extent of outbreaks. This has been assisted by the increasingly rapid turnaround time for identification of such isolates. Long lead-in time of such methods in the past made them more suited to research purposes but the rapidity with which microbiologists can provide results to epidemiologists makes this a real-time method that facilitates investigation and allows more rapid implementation of control measures. However, the most fundamental requirement in the application of laboratory characterisation of isolates to the protection of public health is not the sophistication of the laboratory methods, but open, effective and timely communication between those delivering the laboratory services and those in the public health and food safety domains charged with surveillance and intervention.

8. References

[1] Tauxe R. Centers for Disease Control and Prevention, National Notifiable Diseases Surveillance Data. 2004.

[2] Majowicz SE, Musto J, Scallan E, Angulo FJ, Kirk M, O'Brien SJ, Jones TF, Fazil A, Hoekstra RM; International Collaboration on Enteric Disease 'Burden of Illness' Studies. The global burden of non-typhoidal *Salmonella* gastroenteritis. *Clin Infect Dis*. 2010 Mar 15;50(6):882-9.)

[3] Scallan E, Hoekstra RM, Angulo FJ, Tauxe RV, Widdowson M-A, Roy SL, et al. Foodborne illness acquired in the United States—major pathogens. *Emerg Infect Dis*. 2011 Jan;17(1):7-15.

[4] European Food Safety Authority. *The European Union Summary Report on Trends and Sources of Zoonoses, Zoonotic Agents and Food-borne Outbreaks in 2009*. EFSA Journal 2011; 9(3):2090. [378pp.] doi:10.2903/j.efsa.2011.2090. Available online: www.efsa.europa.eu/efsajournal.

[5] The European Centre for Disease Prevention and Control. *Annual Epidemiological Report on Communicable Diseases in Europe*, 2010. Stockholm: 2010.

[6] Centers for Disease Control and Prevention (CDC). Vital signs: incidence and trends of infection with pathogens transmitted commonly through food--foodborne diseases active surveillance network, 10 U.S. sites, 1996-2010. *MMWR Morb Mortal Wkly Rep*. 2011 Jun 10;60(22):749-55.

[7] Tam CT, Rodrigues L, Viviani L, *et al.* 2011. Longitudinal study of infectious intestinal disease in the UK (IID2 study): incidence in the community and presenting to general practice. Gut doi:10.1136/gut.2011.238386

[8] De Jong B, Ekdahl K. The comparative burden of salmonellosis in the European Union member states, associated and candidate countries. BMC Public Health. 2006 Jan 10;6:4.K.

[9] Elson R; Outbreak Control Team. UK Health Protection Agency view on food alert announcing the recall of a number of confectionery products. Euro Surveill. 2006 Jun 29;11(6):E060629.2.

[10] Werber D, Dreesman J, Feil F, van Treeck U, Fell G, Ethelberg S, Hauri AM, Roggentin P, Prager R, Fisher IS, Behnke SC, Bartelt E, Weise E, Ellis A, Siitonen A, Andersson Y, Tschäpe H, Kramer MH, Ammon A. International outbreak of Salmonella Oranienburg due to German chocolate. BMC Infect Dis. 2005 Feb 3;5:7.

[11] Craven PC, Mackel DC, Baine WB, Barker WH, Gangarosa EJ. International outbreak of Salmonella Eastbourne infection traced to contaminated chocolate. Lancet. 1975 Apr 5;1(7910):788-92.

[12] Gillespie IA, Elson R. Successful reduction of human Salmonella Enteritidis infection in England and Wales. Euro Surveill. 2005;10(46):pii=2834.

[13] Threlfall EJ, Ward LR, Hampton MD, Ridley AM, Rowe B, Roberts D, Gilbert RJ, Van Someren P, Wall PG, Grimont P. Molecular fingerprinting defines a strain of Salmonella enterica serotype Anatum responsible for an international outbreak associated with formula-dried milk. Epidemiol Infect. 1998 Oct;121(2):289-93.

[14] Pezzoli L, Elson R, Little CL, Yip H, Fisher I, Yishai R, Anis E, Valinsky L, Biggerstaff M, Patel N, Mather H, Brown DJ, Coia JE, van Pelt W, Nielsen EM, Ethelberg S, de Pinna E, Hampton MD, Peters T, Threlfall. Packed with Salmonella--investigation of an international outbreak of Salmonella Senftenberg infection linked to contamination of prepacked basil in 2007. *J.Foodborne Pathog Dis.* 2008 Oct;5(5):661-8.

[15] Van Duynhoven YT, Isken LD, Borgen K, Besselse M, Soethoudt K, Haitsma O, Mulder B, Notermans DW, De Jonge R, Kock P, Van Pelt W, Stenvers O, Van Steenbergen J; Outbreak Investigation Team. A prolonged outbreak of Salmonella Typhimurium infection related to an uncommon vehicle: hard cheese made from raw milk. *Epidemiol Infect.* 2009 Nov;137(11):1548-57.

[16] Bruun T, Sørensen G, Forshell LP, Jensen T, Nygard K, Kapperud G, Lindstedt BA, Berglund T, Wingstrand A, Petersen RF, Müller L, Kjelsø C, Ivarsson S, Hjertqvist M, Löfdahl S, Ethelberg S. An outbreak of Salmonella Typhimurium infections in Denmark, Norway and Sweden, 2008. Euro Surveill. 2009 Mar 12;14(10).

[17] Nygård K, Lassen J, Vold L, Andersson Y, Fisher I, Löfdahl S, Threlfall J, Luzzi I, Peters T, Hampton M, Torpdahl M, Kapperud G, Aavitsland P. Outbreak of Salmonella Thompson infections linked to imported rucola lettuce. Foodborne Pathog Dis. 2008 Apr;5(2):165-73.

[18] Puohiniemi R, Heiskanen T, Siitonen A. Molecular epidemiology of two international sprout-borne Salmonella outbreaks. J Clin Microbiol. 1997 Oct;35(10):2487-91.

[19] Nicolay N, Thornton L, Cotter S, Garvey P, Bannon O, McKeown P, Cormican M *et al.* *Salmonella enterica* serovar Agona European outbreak associated with a food company. *Epidemiol Infect.* 2010 18:1-9.

[20] Nylen G, Fielder HM, Palmer SR. An international outbreak of Salmonella enteritidis associated with lasagne; lessons on the need for cross-national co-operation in investigating food-borne outbreaks. Epidemiol Infect. 1999 Aug;123(1):31-5.

[21] Anon. An international outbreak of human salmonellosis associated with animal-derived pet treats--Canada and Washington state, 2005. *Can Commun Dis Rep.* 2006 Jul 1;32(13):150-5.

[22] Unicomb LE, Simmons G, Merritt T, Gregory J, Nicol C, Jelfs P, Kirk M, Tan A, Thomson R, Adamopoulos J, Little CL, Currie A, Dalton CB. Sesame seed products contaminated with Salmonella: three outbreaks associated with tahini. Epidemiol Infect. 2005 Dec;133(6):1065-72.

[23] Isaacs S, Aramini J, Ciebin B, Farrar JA, Ahmed R, Middleton D, Chandran AU, Harris LJ, Howes M, Chan E, Pichette AS, Campbell K, Gupta A, Lior LY, Pearce M, Clark C, Rodgers F, Jamieson F, Brophy I, Ellis A; Salmonella Enteritidis PT30 Outbreak Investigation Working Group. An international outbreak of salmonellosis associated with raw almonds contaminated with a rare phage type of Salmonella enteritidis. J Food Prot. 2005 Jan;68(1):191-8.

[24] Kirk MD, Little CL, Lem M, Fyfe M, Genobile D, Tan A, Threlfall J, Paccagnella A, Lightfoot D, Lyi H, McIntyre L, Ward L, Brown DJ, Surnam S, Fisher IS. An outbreak due to peanuts in their shell caused by Salmonella enterica serotypes Stanley and Newport--sharing molecular information to solve international outbreaks. *Epidemiol Infect.* 2004 Aug;132(4):571-7.

[25] Sheth AN, Hoekstra M, Patel N, Ewald G, Lord C, Clarke C, Villamil E, Niksich K, Bopp C, Nguyen TA, Zink D, Lynch M. A national outbreak of salmonella serotype tennessee infections from contaminated peanut butter: a new food vehicle for salmonellosis in the United States. *Clin Infect Dis.* 2011 Aug;53(4):356-62.

[26] Ward LR, Maguire C, Hampton MD, de Pinna E, Smith HR, Little CL, Gillespie IA, O'Brien SJ, Mitchell RT, Sharp C, Swann RA, Doyle O, Threlfall EJ. Collaborative investigation of an outbreak of Salmonella enterica serotype Newport in England and Wales in 2001 associated with ready-to-eat salad vegetables. .Commun Dis Public Health. 2002 Dec;5(4):301-4.

[27] European Food Safety Authority. The Community Summary Report on trends and sources of zoonoses, zoonotic agents and food-borne outbreaks in the European Union in 2008. European Food Safety Authority (EFSA), Parma: 2010.

[28] Newell DG, Koopmans M, Verhoef L, Duizer E, Aidara-Kane A, Sprong H, Opsteegh M, Langelaar M, Threfall J, Scheutz F, van der Giessen J, Kruse H. Food-borne diseases - the challenges of 20 years ago still persist while new ones continue to emerge. *Int J Food Microbiol.* 2010 May 30;139 Suppl 1:S3-15.

[29] Garvey P, Scally M, McKeown P, de Lappe N, Doran G, Ward J, Cormican M. Indigenous salmonellosis low in Ireland. Epi-Insight. 2010 March; 11(3). Available at http://ndsc.newsweaver.ie/epiinsight/hkybj5cdjbb1l6t6mifk6p. Accessed 14/9/2011.

[30] Hendriksen R. *Global epidemiology of non-typhoidal Salmonella infections in humans.* PhD Thesis. National Food Institute, Copenhagen. Print

[31] SMI. Swedish national surveillance data, , available at http://www.smittskyddsinstitutet.se/in-english/statistics/salmonellosis/?t=c#statistics-nav, accessed 22/8/2011)

[32] St Louis ME, Morse DL, Potter ME, DeMelfi TM, Guzewich JJ, Tauxe RV, Blake PA. The emergence of grade A eggs as a major source of Salmonella enteritidis

infections. New implications for the control of salmonellosis. *JAMA*. 1988 Apr 8;259(14):2103-7.

[33] Bäumler AJ, Hargis BM, Tsolis RM. Tracing the origins of Salmonella outbreaks. *Science*. 2000 Jan 7;287(5450):50-2.

[34] Rodrigue DC, Tauxe RV, Rowe B. International increase in Salmonella enteritidis: a new pandemic? *Epidemiol Infect*. 1990 Aug;105(1):21-7.

[35] HPSC's national Salmonella Trawling Questionnaire. Available at http://www.hpsc.ie/hpsc/A-Z/Gastroenteric/Salmonellosis/SurveillanceForms. Accessed on 25/8/2011.

[36] Lan R, Reeves PR, Octavia S. Population structure, origins and evolution of major *Salmonella enterica* clones. *Infect Genet Evol*. 2009; 9(5):996-1005.

[37] Gerner-Smidt P, Hise K, Kincaid J, Hunter S, Rolando S, Hyytiä-Trees E, Ribot EM, Swaminathan B; Pulsenet Taskforce. PulseNet USA: a five-year update. *Foodborne Pathog Dis*. 2006;3(1):9-19. Review.

[38] Petersen RF, Litrup E, Larsson JT, Torpdahl M, Sørensen G, Müller L, Nielsen EM. Molecular Characterisation of *Salmonella* Typhimurium Highly Successful Outbreak Strains. *Foodborne Pathog Dis*. 2011 Mar 7. [Epub ahead-of-print].

[39] Gregg M. Field Epidemiology. Oxford University Press, Oxford: 1996.

[40] Hadjinicolaou AV, Demetriou VL, Emmanuel MA, Kakoyiannis CK, Kostrikis LG. Molecular beacon-based real-time PCR detection of primary isolates of *Salmonella* Typhimurium and *Salmonella* Enteritidis in environmental and clinical samples. *BMC Microbiol*. 2009 19;9:97.

[41] The Health Protection Surveillance Centre. Salmonella In the *Annual Report of the Health Protection Surveillance Centre*, 2008. HPSC, Dublin: 2009.

[42] Dominguez SA, Schaffner DW. Survival of salmonella in processed chicken products during frozen storage. *J Food Prot*. 2009 Oct;72(10):2088-92.

[43] You Y, Rankin SC, Aceto HW, Benson CE, Toth JD, Dou Z. Survival of Salmonella enterica serovar Newport in manure and manure-amended soils. *Appl Environ Microbiol*. 2006 Sep;72(9):5777-83.

[44] Blaser MJ, Newman LS. A review of human salmonellosis: I. Infective dose. Rev Infect Dis. 1982 Nov-Dec;4(6):1096-106.

[45] Centers for Disease Control and Prevention. Multistate outbreak of *Salmonella* infections associated with peanut butter and peanut butter-containing products--United States, 2008-2009. *MMWR Morb Mortal Wkly Rep*. 2009 Feb 6;58(4):85-90.

[46] Peanut recall having big impact on small firms. Reuters. March 11, 2009. Available at http://www.reuters.com/article/2009/03/11/us-salmonella-peanuts-idUSTRE52A4AT20090311. Accessed 22/9/2011.

[47] European Food Safety Authority. The Community Summary Report on Trends and Sources of Zoonoses, Zoonotic Agents and Food-borne Outbreaks in the European Union in 2008. EFSA Journal; 2010 8(1):1496.

[48] Report of an International Outbreak Investigation into a Multi-country Outbreak of Salmonella Agona, Europe, 2008. Available at http://www.hpsc.ie/hpsc/A-Z/Gastroenteric/Salmonellosis/Outbreaks/File,12549,en.pdf. Accessed 13/9/2011.

[49] Rebolledo J *et al.* Outbreak of Salmonella Heidelberg Associated with an Aircraft Flight from Tanzania, July 2011. *In preparation.*

[50] Garvey P, McKeown P. Two new cases linked with nationwide 'duck egg' outbreak of Salmonella Typhimurium DT8. Epi-Insight. 2011 April. 12(4). Available at http://ndsc.newsweaver.ie/epiinsight/3zg0ibihqqw87nh5ab6w5b. Accessed 17/9/2011.

[51] European Food Safety Authority. *Estimation of the relative contribution of different food and animal sources to human Salmonella infections in the European Union.* July 2011. EFSA, Parma: 2011. Available at http://www.efsa.europa.eu/en/supporting/pub/184e.htm. Accessed 14/10/2011.

2

Salmonellae in the Environment

Hussein H. Abulreesh
Department of Biology, Faculty of Applied Science, Umm Al-Qura University, Makkah
Saudi Arabia

1. Introduction

Diarrhea due to *Salmonella* infections has been recognised since the late 19th century. Typhoid diseases were, in the early part of the 20th century, the commonest known waterborne diseases in both the United Kingdom and the United States of America (Hunter, 1997; Pui et al., 2011). In addition non-typhoid salmonellae have been recognised as a leading cause of bacterial enteritis in the UK and worldwide (Timbury et al., 2002; Pui et al., 2011). *Salmonella* infections in animals are common and have been well documented in the UK since 1958, with around 10,000 recorded incidences of bovine salmonellosis per year (Linton & Hinton, 1988).

Salmonella species are members of the family *Enterobacteriaceae*, being facultatively anaerobic, non-spore forming, Gram-negative rods (Group five of Bergey's Manual of Determinative Bacteriology) (Holt et al., 1994). Generally they are 2-5 μm long and 0.8-1.5 μm wide, straight rods, being motile by peritrichous flagella. As they are facultatively anaerobic, they have both respiratory and fermentative metabolism. Optimal growth temperature is 37 °C. D-Glucose and other carbohydrates are catabolised with the production of acid and usually gas. They are oxidase negative, catalase positive, indole and Voges-Proskauer negative, and methyl red and Simmons citrate positive. H_2S is produced; urea is not hydrolysed (Holt et al., 1994; Lightfoot, 2004; Percival et al., 2004). The genus *Salmonella* consists of two species: (1) *Salmonella enterica*, which is divided into six subspecies – *S. enterica* subsp. *enterica* (I), *S. enterica* subsp. *salamae* (II), *S. enterica* subsp. *arizonae* (IIIa), *S. enterica* subsp. *diarizonae* (IIIb), *S. enterica* subsp. *houtenae* (IV), *S. enterica* subsp. *indica* (VI); and (2) *Salmonella bongori* (formerly subsp. V). There are around 2541 serovars/serotypes in the genus *Salmonella* (Table 1). This new nomenclature reflects recent advances in *Salmonella* taxonomy which are based on DNA-hybridization studies. For simplicity, serotypes can be abbreviated, for example *S. enterica* subsp. *enterica* serovar Enteritidis to *S. enteritidis* (Bopp et al., 1999; Timbury et al., 2002; Lightfoot, 2004; Percival et al., 2004; Lin-Hui & Cheng-Hsun, 2007; Pui et al., 2011).

Most of the serotypes pathogenic to humans and animals belong to *Salmonella enterica* subsp. *enterica* (i.e. subsp. I). Some serovars have a habitat limited to a particular host species, such as humans (serovars Typhi, Paratyphi A), sheep (serovars Abortusovis), or fowls (serovar Gallinarum). In general, subspecies I strains are usually isolated from humans and warm-blooded animals, whereas subspecies II, IIIa, IIIb, IV, VI and *S. bongori* are usually isolated from cold-blooded animals and the environment (rarely from humans) (Pui et al., 2011). Biochemical reactions of *S. enterica* serovars and differential characteristics of *Salmonella* species and subspecies are given in Tables 2 and 3.

Species / subspecies	Number of serovars
Salmonella enterica subsp.	
enterica	1504
salamae	502
arizonae	95
diarizonae	333
houtenae	72
indica	13
Salmonella bongori	22
Total	2541

Adapted from Lightfoot (2004); Lin-Hui and Cheng-Hsun (2007)

Table 1. Number of serovars in each species and subspecies of *Salmonella*

There are four clinically distinguishable forms of *Salmonella* infection in humans. These are gastroenteritis, enteric fever, bacteremia and other complications of non-typhoidal salmonellosis as well as chronic carrier state (Hunter, 1997; Percival et al., 2004; Pui et al., 2011). Gastroenteritis is caused by at least 150 *Salmonella* serotypes, *Salmonella enteritidis* being the most common serotype. Symptoms include watery, sometimes bloody diarrhea, fever and abdominal pain, and usually occur 18-48 hours after ingestion of the bacterium. The infection generally lasts 2-5 days. After recovery, faecal carriage may persist for up to 12 weeks. Less than 10 % of patients are reported as carriers for a longer period (Hunter, 1997; Percival et al., 2004; Pui et al., 2001).

	Typical *Salmonella*	*S. choleraesuis*	*S. pullorum*	*S. gallinarum*	*S. typhi*	*S. typhisuis*	*S. paratyphi* A
H_2S	+	-	±	±	+ (weak)	+	-
Citrate	+	+*	+	+	-	-	-
Gas from glucose	+	+	+	±	-	+	+
Dulcitol	+	-	-	+	-	+	+
Mucate	+	-	-	+	-	-	-
Maltose	+	+	-	+	+	+	+
Trehalose	+	-	+	+	+	+	+

* Simmon's citrate-negative, Christensen citrate-positive.
Adapted from Jones, et al. (2000)

Table 2. Biochemical reactions of *Salmonella enterica* serovars

Enteric fever is most often caused by *Salmonella typhi* (typhoid fever) and *S. paratyphi* A, B and C (paratyphoid fever). Enteric fever from *S. typhi* is more prolonged and has a higher mortality rate than paratyphoid fever. Symptoms for typhoid fever include sustained fever, diarrhea, abdominal pain and may involve fatal liver, spleen, respiratory and neurological damage. Paratyphoid fever has similar, but less severe symptoms. The incubation period for typhoid fever is 7-14 days and for paratyphoid fever 1-10 days. Between 1 and 3 % of patients become chronic carriers (Hunter, 1997; Percival et al., 2004; Pui et al., 2011).

Salmonella bacteremia is characterised by chills, high remittent fever, anorexia and bacteraemia. The bacterium may localize in any organ in the body and produce focal lesions resulting in meningitis, endocarditis and pneumonia (Percival et al., 2004). Studies aimed at the determination of the infectious dose for salmonellosis suggests that infectious doses are certainly below10^3 and can be <10 organisms (Blaser & Newman, 1982; Hunter, 1997; Pui et al., 2011). Non-typhoidal serotypes may persist in the intestinal tract from 6 weeks to 3 months, with only 0.1 % of non-typhoidal *Salmonella* cases are shed in faeces for periods excceding 12 months. Up to 5 % of untreaed typhoid infections may result in chronic carrier state. Factors contributing to the chronic carrier state are not clearly understood, nonetheless, salmonellosis can be spread by chronic carriers who can infect other individual, particularly those who work in food industries (Pui et al., 2011).

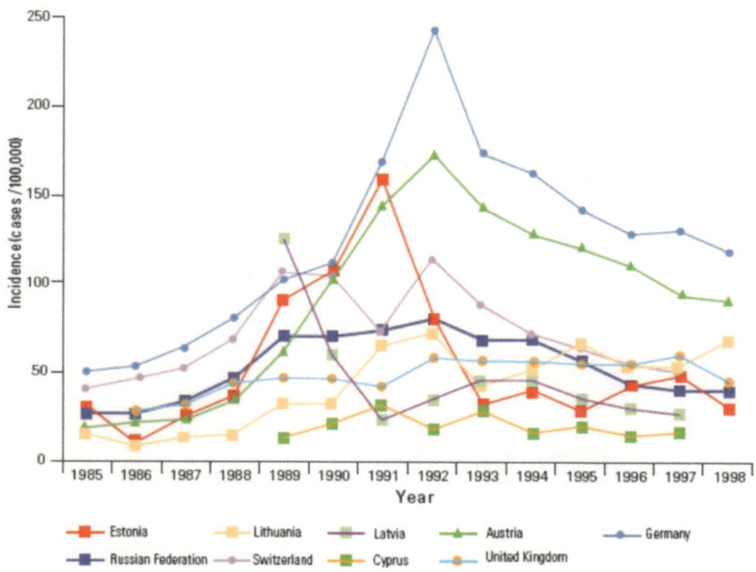

Fig. 1. The reported incidence of salmonellosis in nine European countries between 1985 and 1998 (from Schlundt et al. 2004)

Cases of typhoid (*Salmonella typhi*) and paratyphoid fevers (*S. paratyphi* A and B) have been reported since 1897. In England and Wales between 1911 and 1960 there were about 17 waterborne outbreaks of typhoid and paratyphoid fevers causing about 155 deaths (Galbraith, 1994). In the United States, more than 30 people out of every 100,000 died of typhoid in 1890 (Rusin et al., 2000). Although infections attributed to typhoid and paratyphoid salmonellae have declined in the UK and USA since 1960 (Galbraith, 1994; Leclerc et al., 2004), cases of waterborne typhoid and paratyphoid are still reported regularly from other parts of the world, mainly underdeveloped and poor countries in Asia and Africa, affecting 12.5 million people every year (Hunter, 1997). Waterborne and foodborne salmonellosis (non-typhoidal species) are now the second leading cause of gastroenteritis around the world (Fig. 1), and according to the US Centre for Disease Control and Prevention, 1.4 million cases of salmonellosis occur annually in the USA (Hunter, 1997; Lightfoot, 2004; Percival et al., 2004). Global surveillance data has suggested that increased salmonellosis is associated with the consumption of raw or undercooked eggs, poultry meat or dairy products, and salads prepared with mayonnaise

(Khakhria et al., 1997; Guard-Petter, 2001; Costalunga & Tondo, 2002). Contaminated drinking water is also an important vehicle of *Salmonella* infection (Hunter, 1997; Percival et al., 2004). Handling of pets, such as snakes and lizards, may also lead to infection (Schröter et al., 2004). By and large, salmonellosis is associated with poor hygiene and sanitation during food production (Lightfoot, 2004).

Character	*S. enterica*						
	Subsp. *enterica*	Subsp. *salamae*	Subsp. *arizonae*	Subsp. *diarizonae*	Subsp. *houtenae*	Subsp. *indica*	*S. bongori*
Dulcitol	+	+	-	-	-	d	+
OPNG (2h)	-	-	+	+	-	d	+
Malonate	-	+	+	+	-	-	-
Gelatinase	-	+	+	+	+	+	-
Sorbitol	+	+	+	+	+	-	+
Culture with KCN	-	-	-	-	+	-	+
L(+)-tatrate	+	-	-	-	-	-	-
Galacturonate	-	+	-	+	+	+	+
γ-Glutamyltransferase	+	+	-	+	+	+	+
β-Glucuronidase	_	D	-	+	-	d	-
Mucate	+	+	+	- (70 %)	-	+	+
Salicin	-	-	-	-	+	-	-
Lactose	-	-	- (75 %)	+ (75 %)	-	d	-
Lysis by phage 01	+	+	-	+	-	+	d
Natural habitat	Warm blooded animals		Cold-blooded animals and the environment				

OPNG, *o*-nitropenyl-β-D-galactopyranoside; KCN, potassium cyanide, d, different reactions given by different serovars.
Adapted from: Bopp, et al. (1999); Jones, et al. (2000).

Table 3. Differential characteristics of *Salmonella* species and subspecies

2. Incidence and biodiversity of salmonellae in the environment

The transmission of *Salmonella* species takes the oral-faecal route, by means of contaminated food, primarily poultry and milk products and contaminated water, it is also believed that warm-blooded animals are an asymptomatic carriers of the organism in their gut (Guard-Petter, 2001; Costalunga & Tondo, 2002; Percival et al., 2004; Abulreesh et al., 2007). There is strong evidence to suggest that the organism is ubiquitous and widely distributed in the environment, where particular serovar may be associated with specific ecological niches (Murray, 2000).

2.1 Aquatic environments

Salmonellae are exogenous to aquatic habitats. Their presence in water, therefore, indicates faecal contamination. Sewage effluents, agricultural run-off and direct deposit of faecal materials from wild animals and birds are the major sources of the bacteria in aquatic environments (Alcaide et al., 1984; Baudart et al., 2000; Johnson et al., 2003; Abulreesh et al., 2005). *Salmonella* species have been found in almost all types of aquatic environments that receive faecal contamination, that include drinking water (Bhatta et al., 2007), rivers (Pianetti et al., 1998; Polo et al., 1998; Polo et al., 1999; Dionisio et al., 2000; Lemarchand & Lebaron, 2003; Arvanitidou et al., 2005; Haley et al., 2009), lakes (Claudon et al., 1971; Arvanitidou et al., 1995; Sharma & Rajput, 1996), ponds (Shellenbarger et al., 2008), marine waters (Matinez-Urtaza et al., 2004a; Martinez-Urtaza et al., 2004b; Martinez-Urtaza & Liebana, 2005; Harakeh et al., 2006), run-off water (Claudon et al., 1971), treated and untreated wastewater (Ho & Tam, 2000; Melloul et al., 2002; Espigares et al., 2006, Mafu et al., 2009) worldwide. Abulreesh et al. (2004) were unable to detect salmonellae in water samples from a village pond that receives direct faecal contamination from waterfowl, nevertheless, they managed to isolate the bacterium from bottom sediments of the same pond. This might be attributed, in part, to concentration through sedimentation and also to greater survivability of *Salmonella* spp. in bottom sediments than in water (Burton et al., 1987; Fish & Pettibone, 1995; Winfield & Groisman, 2003). Higher salmonellae recovery rates from bottom sediment than from water in diverse aquatic environments were also observed by Hendricks (1971) and Van Donzel & Geldreich (1971).

It is expected that the diversity of salmonellae population in aquatic environments may depend on sources of contamination. However, salmonellae serotypes that prevail in aquatic environments do not often coinside with the common zoonotic or human serotypes identified in the areas surrounding these aquatic environments (Polo et al., 1999; Dionisio et al., 2000; Matinez-Urtaza et al., 2004; Setti et al., 2009). For instance, Setti et al. (2009) isolated about 57 strains along 122 Km coastline in Morocco, where only three serotypes were identified. Interestingly, these serotypes were Kentucky, Blockey and Senftenberg, were not included among those frequently reported serotypes from human infections or animal origin in Morocco. Likewise, the results obtained by Haley et al. (2009) showed that serotypes Enteritidis, Typhimurium and Heidelberg were not among the serotypes isolated from freshwater environments in U.S.A, even though common sources of these serotypes were present in the watersheds that were examined. The explanation of this discrepancy may be attributed, in part, to different survival rates of different salmonellae serotypes. Other environmental factors such as rainfall and temperature may also play a major role in the diversity and dynamics of salmonellae serotypes in aquatic environments (Martinez-Urtaza et al., 2004a; Simental & Martinez-Urtaza, 2008; Haley et al., 2009; Setti et al., 2009).

The use of faecal indicators (faecal coliforms, *Escherichia coli*, faecal streptococci and *Clostridium perfringens*) aims to evaluate water sources intended for water supply or recreation, by predicting the presence of waterborne pathogens. Significant correlations have been found between total coliforms, faecal coliforms and faecal streptococci and *Salmonella* in marine bathing sites in Portugal (Polo et al., 1998). Similarly, Arvanitidou et al. (2005) noted a close relationship between the presence of *Salmonella* serovars and total coliforms in Greek rivers. Lake Jabalpure in India was found to receive sufficient pollution of organic matter, where high significant correlation was found between the abundance of *Salmonella* and the abundance of total coliforms, faecal coliforms and faecal streptococci (Sharma & Rajput, 1996). Morinigo et al. (1993) found significant correlation between densities of faecal indicators and the presence of *Salmonella* spp. in Spanish fresh and marine natural waters that received faecal discharge.

Together, these and other studies suggest that faecal indicators are potentially a useful warning of the potential presence of salmonellae in aquatic environments (Geldreich, 1996). However, relationships are not always found between faecal indicators and salmonellae in aquatic environments; an observation that may be related to various reasons such as different survival rates between salmonellae and faecal indicators, also the possibility that salmonellae being in a viable but nonculturable state. Lemarchand and Lebaron (2003) found no correlations between salmonellae and any given faecal indicator in French rivers. Detection of *Salmonella* spp. was achieved in water samples from coastal areas in Portugal in the presence of low counts of faecal indicators (Dionisio et al., 2000). No close relationships between the presence of salmonellae and counts of faecal indicators were also noted in fresh and marine waters that receive industrial and domestic effluents in Spain (Morinigo et al., 1993). Furthermore, *Salmonella* spp. were successfully detected in Spanish fresh and marine water that received faecal pollution in the absence of faecal indicators, as well as in aquatic environments with low degree of pollution (Pianetti et al., 1998; Morinigo et al., 1990; Baudart et al., 2000; Dionisio et al., 2000). Thus, the ability of faecal indicators to predict the presence of salmonellae in polluted environmental waters remains questionable, and the absence of faecal indicators is not always a reliable indication of the absence of *Salmonella* spp.

2.2 Domestic and agricultural waste

Sewage effluents serve as frequent source of environmental contamination with *Salmonella* serovars. Obviously, infected individuals are the source of salmonellae in sewage effluents (Sahlström et al., 2004, 2006). In Spain, the most frequently identified serovars in clinical samples from human origin were Enteritidis, Hadar and Typhimurium, these serovars were also noted to be the most frequently encountered in sewage effluents, particularly Hadar (38.1%), followed by Enteritidis (23.8%) (Espigares et al., 2006). Discharge from agricultural waste may, in part, play a role in the presence of different serovars in sewage effluents (Berge et al., 2006), however some salmonellae serovars may present in sewage effluents but could not be traced to a human or animal source (Danielsson, 1977).

It is well-established that waste treatment aims to stabilize sewage sludge, accordingly pathogens may be activated rather than removed (Godfree, 2003). This has been clearly noticed with different *Salmonella* serovars. In Poland a study showed that serovar Virchow was detected in raw and treated sewage. The same serovar was also detected in primary and excess sludge (Olańczuk-Neyman et al., 2003). Similar observation was noted in Sweden, were *Salmonella* spp. were detected in 55% of treated sludge samples, with serovar Hadar being the most frequently isolated from treated and raw sludge (Sahlström et al., 2004). Salmonellae can grow in sewage sludge and effluents after treatment, particularly at low temperatures (Danielsson, 1977), consequently, the application of treated sludge on agricultural land and/or irrigation with treated wastewater, and the discharge of treated effluents in aquatic environments may constitute potential public health hazard (Hutchinson et al., 2008). *Salmonella* was detected in 68.75% of vegetable samples in agricultural land irrigated with wastewater in Morocco (Melloul et al., 2001), moreover, high infection rate with salmonellae was noted in children living in an area with sewage water irrigation practices (Melloul and Hassani, 1999; Melloul et al., 2002).

Livestock manure may disposed on agricultural land and/or widely used as fertilizer, which often contains high concentrations of different types of human pathogens, including

Salmonella. The presence and the levels of any given pathogen in livestock manure depends on (i) source animal, (ii) animal's health state and (iii) the storage and treatment methods of the manure (Venglovsky et al., 2006). Unfortunately, treatment of animal waste does not receive the required attention by public health authorities as in the case of human waste (Murray, 2000), thus the direct disposal of manure or slurry to agricultural lands or discharge to aquatic environments may constitute potential risk for the spread of salmonellae infections to human and animals. In this respect, special attention should be paid to the disinfection of contaminated waste of livestock to prevent the spread of infective agents (e.g. *Salmonella*) in the environment (Venglovsky et al., 2006).

2.3 Free-living wild birds

The intestinal carriage of various salmonellae serovars, including multidrug-resistant strains, by free-living wild birds and their role in the spread of the bacterium in the environment is well documented. These birds include, ducks and geese, pigeons, sea gulls and other species belonging to a wide range of different genera (Kapperud & Rosef, 1983; Palmgren et al., 1997; Hernandez et al., 2003; Tsai & Hsiang, 2005; Kobayashi et al., 2007; Čížek et al., 2007; Abulreesh, 2011) (Table 4). The majority of these birds seem to carry *Salmonella* spp. without obvious symptoms of infection, which suggests that salmonellae inhibiting the intestinal tract of free-living wild birds are commensal (Tizard, 2004; Abulreesh et al. 2005, 2007). Nonetheless, *Salmonella* spp. are also common cause of salmonellosis and other various serious infections in wild birds (Henry, 2000; Poppe, 2000; Tizard, 2004). Although various salmonellae serovars have been isolated from apparently healthy free-living birds, the incidence of the bacterium tends to be low (Table 4). Indeed Fallacara et al. (2001) found only one *Salmonella* isolate in 82 faecal droppings of mallard, while the bacterium was completely absent from 375 faceal samples of Canadian geese. Low incidence or complete absence of salmonellae carriage was also observed in other wild birds such as gulls, passerines, owls, pigeons, thrushes and eagles (Brittingham et al., 1988; Palmgren et al., 1997; Kirk et al., 2002; Hernandez et al., 2003; Reche et al., 2003; Dovč et al., 2004; Abulreesh, 2011).

Healthy free-living wild birds that live well away from pollution may not harbour *Salmonella* serovars (Čížek et al., 1994; Tizard, 2004). Indeed, when Hernandez et al. (2003) sampled Palearctic birds migrating southwards and which were likely to have had no recent experience of areas with domestic animals, they found only one *Salmonella*-positive bird, a mistle thrush (*Turdus viscivorus*), amongst 2,377 samples from 110 bird species. In the same way, a total of 233 faecal samples from eight penguins were all *Salmonella*-negative, suggesting that tourism has not yet introduced human-associated enteric pathogens to the Antarctic (Bonnedahl et al., 2005). Results obtained from different studies suggest that free-living wild birds may acquire salmonellae after exposure to human-contaminated environments or after scavenging on refuse tips and sewage sludge (Fricker, 1984; Ferns & Mudge, 2000; Tizard, 2004; Abulreesh et al., 2005).

Free-living and migratory wild birds are recognized as a potential reservoir for the transmission of human-associated *Salmonella* spp., including multidrug-resistant strains, through the contamination of water, farms and other environments. Therefore, it was concluded that free-living wild birds may play a significant role in the epidemiology of human salmonellosis (Tizard, 2004; Abulreesh et al., 2007; Literák et al., 2007; Tsiodras et al., 2008).

Bird species	Location	p:n (%)	*Salmonella* serovar	Reference
Black-headed Gull (*Larus ridibundus*)	Czech Republic Sweden	38:154 (25) 28:1047 (3)	Typhimurium, Enteritidis, Panama, Anatum Typhimurium	Hubálek et al. (1995) Palmgren et al. (2006)
Waterfowl (ducks and geese)	USA Taiwan	8:450 (2) 91:2000 (5)	Typhimurium ND	Fallacara et al. (2004) Tsai & Hsiang (2005)
Pigeon (*Columba livia*)	Japan Norway Croatia Saudi Arabia	17:436 (4) 3:72 (4) 2:14 (14) 8:400 (2)	ND Typhimurium Typhimurium ND	Tanaka et al. (2005) Refsum et al. (2002) Vlahović et al. (2004) Abulreesh (2011)
Coot (*Fulica atra*)	Czech Republic	1:3 (33)	Typhimurium	Hubálek et al. (1995)
House Sparrow (*Passer domesticus*)	USA Norway	14:451 (3) 7:31 (23)	Montevideo, Meleagridis Typhimurium	Kirk et al. (2002) Refsum et al. (2002)
Starling (*Sturnus vulgaris*)	USA Czech Republic	1:80 (1) 4 isolates	Typhimurium ND	Kirk et al. (2002) Čížek et al. (1994)
Magpie (*Pica pica*)	Norway	1:40 (3)	Typhimurium	Refsum et al. (2002)
Great Tit (*Parus major*)	Norway Czech Republic	6:87 (7) 1 isolate	Typhimurium ND	Refsum et al. (2002) Čížek et al. (1994)
Brown-headed Cowbird (*Molothrus ater*)	USA	3:95 (3)	Meleagiridis, Muenster	Kirk et al. (2002)
Rook (*Corvus frugilegus*)	Croatia	2:13 (15)	Typhimurium, Enteriditis	Vlahović et al. (2004)
Crow (*Corvus corone*)	Norway	1:52 (2)	Paratyphi B	Refsum et al. (2002)

Bird species	Location	p:n (%)	*Salmonella* serovar	Reference
Peregrine Falcon (*Falco peregtinus*)	Sweden	2:69 (3)	Amager	Palmgren et al. (2004)
Long-eared Owl (*Asio otus*) Kestrel (*Falco naumanni*) Buzzard (*Buteo buteo*)	Spain	1:7 (14) 3:59 (5) 1:17 (6)	Typhimurium DT104 Enteritidis Typhimurium DT104	Reche et al. (2003)

p = number of positive samples, n = number of samples tested, (%) percentage of positive samples
ND = not determined

Table 4. Examples of the incidence of *Salmonella* spp. in fresh faeces or cloacal swabs of various free-living wild birds.

2.4 Domestic and wild animals

Salmonellae serovar have long been associated with diseases in animals, and there are reports suggested that salmonellae are wide spread in the intestinal tract of domestic and wild animals of different taxa (Simpsons, 2002; Angulo et al., 2004; Schlundt et al., 2004). Domestic pets such as dogs and cats that live in close proximity to humans have been responsible for a wide range of bacterial and parasitic zoonoses. For instance, Brucellosis (*Brucella canis*) and septic animal bite (*Pasteurella multocida*) were associated with dogs, whereas, cat-scratch disease (*Bartonella henselae*) and abortion and stillbirth (*Toxoplasma gondii*) were linked with cats (Timbury et al., 2002). These animals have also been found to carry different *Salmonella* serovars in their guts; both healthy and diseased individuals (Carter & Quinn, 2000; Sato et al., 2000; Van Immerseel et al., 2004). In Japan, a 4-month-old infant manifested with diarrhea and *Salmonella* Virchow was detected in his stool. The same serovar (Virchow), was also detected in faecal samples from two out of three household dogs that were living in close proximity with the infected infant. This finding lead to the conclusion that *Salmonella* Virchow infection in the infant was transmitted by the household dogs (Sato et al., 2000). In order to determine whether cats can present a potential risk for the transmission of salmonellae to humans, rectal swabs were taken from 278 healthy house cats, 58 dead cats, and 35 group-house cats were examined in Belgium (Van Immerseel et al., 2004). The results showed that 51.4% of the group-housed cats, 8.6% of diseased cats, and 0.36% of the healthy house cats excreted *Salmonella*. Most of the serovars recovered were human-pathogenic and resistant to multiple antibiotics, such as Typhimurium, Enteritidis. Thus, it was concluded that cats that shed salmonellae can pose health hazards to highly susceptible individuals, such as children, the elderly and immunocompromised people (Van Immerseel et al., 2004). Dog and cats can easily acquire *Salmonella* spp., either directly or indirectly via the faecal-oral route. Dogs and cats are allowed to roam, and hunt and thus have access to diverse sources of *Salmonella* serovars. Salmonellae can be transmitted to cats and dogs via contaminated dry pet's food, uncooked offal and bones, raw chicken and unchlorinated water. Scavenging on wildlife carcasses, households rubbish and/or hunting rodents or wild birds are also potential routes of transmission of salmonellae serovars to cats and dogs (Carter & Quinn, 2000).

Cold-blooded animals harbour a wide range of *Salmonella* serovars in their intestinal tract. *S. bongori* and *enterica* subsp. II, IIIa, IIIb, IV and VI are commonly isolated from reptiles, however, isolation of *S. enterica* subsp. I from captive or free-living reptiles is common (Briones et al., 2004). *S. enterica* subsp. I is common in warm-blooded animals, the presence of this subsp. in the faeces of reptiles is probably due to the fact that reptiles usually fed on rodents, rats or mice and other small warm-blooded animals that seem to carry salmonellae (Pfleger et al., 2003). It seems that there is no specific serovar associated with specific reptilian species, yet subsp. III was observed to be predominant in snakes, while subsp. IV was found to be common in iguana lizards (de Sá & Solari, 2001; Pfleger et al., 2003). Serovar Typhimurium and Enteritidis were rarely detected from reptiles (Warwick et al., 2001; Seepersadsingh & Adesiyun, 2003), nevertheless, the carriage of other human-associated salmonellae serovars, particularly multidrug-resistant strains usually occur without obvious symptoms of diarrhea, thus salmonellae seem to be essentially normal component of reptilian intestinal flora (Warwick et al., 2001; Ebani et al., 2005). Cases of reptile-associated human salmonellosis were reported in the United States, Canada and Europe since the 1960's (Weinstein et al., 1995; Woodward et al., 1997; Olsen et al., 2001; Warwick et al., 2001). Transmission of salmonellae from pet reptiles to humans may occur directly (i.e. faecal contamination of food and water) or indirectly (i.e. contamination of hands and other body parts, or households fomites). A number of formal recommendations from the UK Communicable Disease Surveillance Centre and the Department of Health in the USA were issued to advise pet store owners and pet keepers of good code of practice to prevent, or at least minimize, reptiles-related salmonellosis (Warwick et al., 2001). Some of these recommendations include; informing pet owners to wash their hands after handling pet reptiles or their cages, pet reptiles should not be allowed to roam freely throughout the house or living area and other measures (Warwick et al., 2001). Unlike reptiles, the incidence of salmonellae in amphibians seems to be very low (Pfleger et al., 2003) and sometimes totally absent (Briones et al., 2004). *Salmonella* Abidjan and Wandsworth were detected, with low numbers, in the faeces of horned frog (*Ceratophrys cranwelli*). These serovars have not been implicated in human salmonellosis. Apparently, amphibians may not represent an important reservoir of *Salmonella* spp. in nature and may not have potential implications for public health (Briones et al. 2004).

Rodents, rats and mice are common commensal pests and usually regarded as an indicator of unsatisfactory sanitation (Murray, 2000). They are responsible for considerable damage to various stored products and buildings, as well as they can be a source of serious bacterial zoonosis (Healing, 1991; Timbury et al., 2002). Rats and mice are regarded as a potential reservoir of different salmonellae serovars, accordingly, they are considered as a major public health hazard (Murray, 2000). *Salmonella enterica* serovar Typhimurium definitive phage type 104 (DT 104) was recovered from the faeces of house rats (*Rattus rattus* and *Rattus norvegicus*) in Japan. This finding highlights the important role of mice and rats in the dissemination of serovar Typhimurium (DT104), which regarded as one of the emerging zoonotic agent in Europe and the United States because this strain has acquired multiple drug resistance (Yokoyama et al., 2007). In the UK, a total of 100 faecal samples, 50 recatal swabs and 25 swabs taken from the fur, paws and tail of wild urban brown rats (*Rattus norvegicus*) were examined for the presence of *Salmonella* spp (Hilton et al., 2002). The results showed that *Salmonella enterica* was recovered from 8% of the faecal droppings, and 10% of the rectal swabs. No salmonellae were recovered from the fur, paws and tail of the rats. These data suggest that physical spread of *Salmonella* from the body of the animal may not be possible and rat faeces are still the most likely source of *Salmonella* contamination (Hilton et al., 2002). The meat of the African great cane rat (*Thryonomys swinderianus*) is a valued and expensive food delicacy in Nigeria (Oboegbulem

& Okoronkwo, 1990). Almost ten salmonellae serovar were detected from liver and spleen samples of great cane rat that were caught and/or purchased from restaurant in Nsukka, Nigeria. These serovars were Agama, Poona and Ajiobo. Incidentally, these serovars have been isolated from the stool of diarrhea patients in Nigeria. Although no incidence of human salmonellosis attributed to eating cane rat has yet been reported, the consumption of undercooked rat meat and/or eating sugar cane that are contaminated with excretion of carrier rats may constitute potential health hazards (Oboegbulem & Okoronkwo, 1990).

Human-associated *salmonella* serovars such as Typhimurium and Enteritidis were found to be predominant in clinically and subclinically infected hedgehogs. The intestinal tract of hedgehogs seem to be the natural habitat of serovar Enteritidis phage type 11, which may infect humans and dogs, but not livestock. *Salmonella* Agama usually causes infection in cattle; it was detected in the faeces of badgers, which may be the natural reservoir of that serovar (Murray, 2000; Simpson, 2002).

2.5 Farm animals and farm environment

The incidence of salmonellosis in the community is related to the consumption of contaminated food and water. There is significant historical evidence suggesting that poultry products serve as a major source of *Salmonella* infections in humans. At the beginning of this century, *Salmonella pullorum* was one of the most recognized species as it was responsible for pullorum disease, which infects poultry intended for human consumption. Later, fowl typhoid (*S. gallinarum*) was noticed in almost all poultry-producing areas worldwide. With regard to human-associated salmonellae infection that are traced back to the consumption of poultry products, typhoid fever (*S. typhi*) was highly prevalent in the first five to six decades of the 1900's. This serovar was sharply declined in Europe and North America during the late 1940's and was replaced with *S. typhimurium*, which was declined in the last 20 years, particularly with the emergence of *S. enteritidis* as the commenst serovar in poultry in many countries around the world (Poppe, 2000).

The incidence of various salmonellae serovars in the intestinal tract of chickens is well documented; serovars Infantis, Thompson, Agona and Enteritidis were frequently detected from the faces of chickens in Japan (Ahmed et al., 2009). A total of 550 faecal samples were collected from healthy (500) and diseased (50) chicken from different farms in Shanghai, China. The occurrence of salmonellae was (3.8%) from healthy chickens and (12%) from diseased ones (Liu et al., 2010). Among the serovars that were identified from the faeces of healthy chickens; *S. pullorum* and *S. typhimurium* were prevalent, whereas *S. paratyphi* B and *S. senftenberg* were most commonly recovered from the faeces of diseased chickens (Liu et al., 2010). *Salmonella* spp. are not one of the normal common components of the intestinal flora of chickens (Guard-Petter, 2001). Accordingly, colonization of chicken by salmonellae is most likely due to contamination of broiler houses (Guard-Petter, 2001) (Table 5). Contamination of broilers was noted to take horizontal routs that include; contaminated water and feed, fluff, dust, insects, equipments and other fomites inside broilers environment. Transmission by direct contact with other chicks, rodents, wild and domestic birds and animals and personnel contaminated by salmonella serovar is also common (Al-Nakhli et al., 1999; Poppe, 2000; Guard-Petter, 2001; Garber et al., 2003; Skov et al., 2004; Kinde et al., 2005; Padungtod & Kaneene, 2006). On the other hand, vertical transmission of salmonellae in chicken is also common, it occurs when follicles in the ovary are infected or the developing of eggs become infected in the oviduct (Poppe, 2000; Guard-Petter, 2001).

Production	Box liners	Litter	Drag swab	Faecal droppings	Mice	Feed
Broilers	Enteritidis	Java Chester Virchow	Java Sofia Livingstone Concord Mbandaka Virchow Albany Enteritidis PT4	Java Eppendorf Sofia Livingstone Virchow Stockholm		Java Livingstone Concord Mbandaka Virchow
Layers			Enteritidis PT4	Livingstone		
Broilers breeders	Enteritidis PT4	Enteritidis PT4				
Layers breeders					Enteritidis PT4 Java	

Table 5. Isolation of *Salmoenlla* serovars from poultry farm environments in Saudi Arabia, 1998-1997. (Adapted from Al-Nakhli et al., 1999).

Chicken carcasses obtained from slaughterhouses, broilers, retail shops and supermarkets were found to be highly contaminated with various salmonellae serovars (Cogan & Humphrey, 2003; Humphrey & Jørgensen, 2006). Capita et al. (2003) examined the incidence of salmonellae on chicken carcasses, chicken parts (wings, legs, livers and hearts) and processed chicken products (sausage and hamburgers) in Spain. The study revealed that higher detection rates of salmonellae serovars were obtained from carcasses (55%) compared to hamburgers (20%), in addition, chicken carcasses sold in supermarkets were more contamined (75%) than those from poulterers shops (25%). The most frequent serovars encountered were Enteritidis, Poona and Paratyphi B. Likewise, in Portugal chicken carcasses available for consumers in local butcher shops were found to be heavily contaminated with 10 different multidrug-resistant *Salmonella* serovars. Again serovar Enteritidis was predominant together with serovar Hadar (Antunes et al., 2003). Serovar Enteritidis was also reported as the most commonly isolated salmonellae serovar from chicken carcasses and eggs in Brazil, Europe and the United States (Guard-Petter, 2001; de Oliveira et al., 2005; Capita et al., 2007). By contrast, serovar Thompson followed by serovar Enteritidis were the most frequently isolated salmonellae in chicken meat in Iran (Dalla et al., 2010). While in Japan, serovars Infantis, Typhimurium and Haifa were frequently present on chicken carcasses, yet serovar Enteritidis was frequently encountered in unpasteurized liquid eggs (Murakami et al., 2001). In general, serovar Enteritidis has received a considerable attention by public health authorities, as for the last two decades there has been a pandemic of *Salmonella enteritidis* infection worldwide, and this has been largely associated with the consumption of contaminated eggs and undercooked chicken meat (Cogan & Humphrey, 2003; Humphrey & Jørgensen, 2006). Apparently, the sources of carcasses contamination is the intestinal tract of the birds, nevertheless, processing and packing at slaughterhouses and other equipments in broilers could be another major source of contamination. Improved competitive exclusion measures and vaccination of flocks were found to play an important role in the prevention of *Salmonella* serovars to colonize the intestinal tract of chickens and their products (e.g. eggs). Improved processing procedures at slaughterhouses may minimize the rate of contamination on carcasses; refrigeration and reducing the available water on carcasses by drying may also reduce the rate of contamination (Plummer et al., 1995; Poppe, 2000; Cogan & Humphrey, 2003; Humphrey & Jørgensen, 2006).

As mentioned earlier, salmonellae is strongly linked with infection in livestock; species of veterinary significance include *S. typhimurium* and *S. dublin* that are responsible for acute salmonellosis in cattle and calves (Wray & Davies, 2000); serovars Typhimurium and Choleraesuis are predominant in porcine salmonellosis, other serovars such as Enteritidis and Dublin may also cause diseases in pigs (Fedorka-Cray et al., 2000); *S. typhimurium* and *S. abortusovis* are the commonest cause of various salmonellae infections in sheep (Wray & Linklater, 2000). It can be noted that some of the above-mentioned serovars are also commonly involved in human-associated salmonellae infections, in this respect, it is of great importance to ascertain whether or not livestock serve as a reservoir of salmonellae of clinical importance and therefore play a role in their transmission in the community. Several investigations were carried out worldwide, and reported the carriage of various human-associated, multiple drug-resistant *Salmonella* serovars in the intestinal tract of healthy livestock (Bywater et al., 2004; Guerin et al., 2005). Moreover, livestock meat at salughterhouses and retail shops was also found to be contaminated with various salmonellae serovars worldwide (Davies et al., 2004; Mølbak, 2004; Dallal et al., 2010). Livestock may acquire salmonellae through contaminated water and feed, aerosol and poor farm management practices were also identified as risk factors for the transmission of the bacterium to livestock (Wray & Davies, 2000; Suk-Kyung et al., 2011). Reports of salmonellae outbreaks in the community associated with the consumption of unpasteurized milk, undercooked red meat are well documented. An outbreak of multidrug-reisistant *S. typhimurium* in Denmark was traced back to a Danish pig farm; in the UK, outbreak of *S. typhimurium* DT104 was associated with contaminated milk from dairy farm (Mølbak, 2004), between 1993 and 1997, there were 13 reported outbreaks of salmonellosis associated with the consumption of undercooked beef, 16 outbreaks associated with the consumption of pork and 10 outbreaks related to ice cream made of unpasteurized milk in the United States (Schlundt et al., 2004). These reports suggest that livestock represent a potiental source of human salmonellosis (Khakhria et al., 1997; Fedorka-Cray et al., 2000; Wray & Davies, 2000; Wray & Linklater, 2000; Bywater et al., 2004; Mølbak, 2004; Guerin et al., 2005).

3. Environmental factors associated with *Salmonella* infections

Salmonella serovars are ubiquitos and widely distributed in the environment. Climate and other environmental factors play a significant role in the incidence of salmonellae in various ecological niches. Environmental conditions may significantly affect the ability of salmonellae to persist in nature, in particular when these serovars are subject to hostile conditions and their ability to acquire multidrug-resistance.

3.1 Seasonal variation

The presence of *Salmonella* spp. in polluted aquatic environemtns is marked with strong seasonal trend. Various serovars were readily isolated from contaminated rivers in Italy during summer and autumn (Pianetti et al., 1998). In freshwater lakes in India, high density of *Salmonella* spp. was recorded during summer season over a two-year study. The apparent high levels of salmonellae recovered during summer seasons was influenced by discharges of human and animals excreta, and the ability of salmonellae to persist in contaminated fresh waters. Water temperature, Biochemical Oxygen Demand (BOD) and Chemical Oxygen Demand (COD) had influential roles in the presence of salmonellae in high numbers during warmer months in fresh water lakes (Sharma & Rajput, 1996). Similarly, Statistically significant high densities of salmonellae serovars were detected in Salmon River, British Columbia in Canada during the warm seasons (spring and summer) (Jokinen et al., 2010). Positive correlations were found between high rainfall and temperature with the presence of high densities of various salmonellae serovars in August in River Little, Georgia, USA (Haley et al., 2009). Conflicting reports on salmonellae seasonality in natural waters have, however, come from Spain, where various salmonellae serovars were detected in coastal water during warmer (July-September), but were present in even higher densities during colder (October-December) months (Martinez-Urtaza et al., 2004a). Interestingly, serovar Senftenberg and other serovars were found to peak during winter season, by contrast serovar Typhimurium was always present in high densities during summer seasons in marine environments in Spain (Martinez-Urtaza et al., 2004a, b). In general, the seasonal presence of salmonellae serovars in aquatic environments is associated with storm-generated flow, torrential rains and monsoon seasons in temperate and tropical regions, highlighting the washing effect of torrential rainfall as one of the principal environmental drivers of *Salmonella* contamination in aquatic environments (Martinez-Urtaza et al., 2004a, b; Semintal & Martinez-Urtaza, 2008; Haley et al., 2009; Setti et al., 2009).

In faecally contaminated village ponds, salmonellae can be readily detected in bottom sediments during warm months (June-August) but was not detected in colder months (Abulreesh et al., 2004). Seasonal incidence of salmonellae serovars in the faecal droppings of small passerines in Norway (e.g. *Salmonella typhymurium)* were found to peak in Feburary and March (cold months). Interstingly, the incidence of the same serovar (Typhimurium) in other bird species (e.g. gulls, ducks, crows and other species) in Norway was recorded without any apparent seasonality (Refsum et al., 2002). No statistical significant seasonal trends were recorded in the carriage of salmonellae by apparently healthy rock pigeons in Saudi Arabia (Abulreesh, 2011). In the United States, Pedersen et al. (2006) did not find any seasonal patterns with regards to the presence of salmonellae in the faeces of pigeons. Likewise, a temporal study of various salmonellae serovars in animals (chickens, turkeys, cattle and pigs) in Alberta, Canada between 1990 and 2001, showed that a seasonal pattern was not apparent, as the months with highest number of isolates differed from year to year (Guerin et al., 2005).

The incidence of salmonellosis in humans was found to show strong seasonal patterns worldwide. The peak of nontyphoidal salmonellae infection in the community was recorded during summer months (June-September) in the majority of Eropean, Mediterranean countries and North America. The summer seasonality was more marked in northern/western Europe than in the Mediterranean region (Ekdahl et al., 2005; Naumova et al., 2007). Similarly, in Korea the highst peak of nontyphidal salmonellae infection in the community was recorded during the summer (June-August) (Cho et al., 2008). Seasonal trends of human nontyphoidal salmonellosis (Enteritidis) in East Asia and (Typhimurium) in India and nighboring countries were found to peak in colder months (November-December) (Ekdahl et al., 2005). In the case of typhoid infection in the Indian community (serovar Typhi), the maximum number of cases occurred during April-June (dry season) followed by July-September (monsoon season) (Mohanty et al., 2006). Although these cases were coincided with the peak of annual temperature and rainfall, it is not clearly understood which factor drives this seasonality regionally, or how this pattern might relate to the overall presence of salmonellae in the environment (Haley et al., 2009).

3.2 Survival in nature

Salmonella spp. are exclusively of faecal origin, they are therefore, allochthonous to aquatic environments. Once the bacteria are released into the environment (aquatic and terrestrial), they confront a wide range of drastic, stressful conditions, that make their persistence rather difficult and they may die rapidly. Thus, one would expect that salmonellae may not survive for long periods in the environment. This assumption started to change when Pokorný (1988) showed that *Salmonella enteritidis* survived for up to 30 days in seeded pollution-free drinking water microcosms held at 4 °C. In laboratory experiments using sterile water, seeded cells of serovar Typhi was found to remain viable for up to 65 days when microcosms were incubated in the refrigerator (4-6 °C). When microcosms were incubated at room temperature (18-24 °C) and at 37 °C, survival of serovar Typhi was decreased to 25 and 5 days respectively (Uyanik et al., 2008). The apparent long survival of enteric bacteria (e.g. *Campylobacter* and *Salmonella*) at low temperature perhaps explained by increased metabolism and more rapid substrate utilization at higher temperature at the expense of culturability (Abulreesh et al., 2006; Uyanik et al., 2008). In addition, light (particularly U. V. radiation) is potentially lethal to salmonellae in aquatic environments. In laboratory experiments, culturable populations of *Salmonella Typhimurium* in seawater microcosms were decreased rapidly after exposure to direct natural sunlight (Davies & Evison, 1991). The lethat effect of sunlight is probably aggravated by the high salinity of seawater, therefore, the U. V. component of sunlight and the high salinity may act synergistically in causing decrease in the numbers of culturable *S. Typhimurium* (Davies & Evison, 1991). The same conclusion was drawn with regard to the combined effect of sunlight and salinity on the survival of *Salmonella enterica* in seeded *in situ* seawater chambers (Sinton et al., 2007). In freshwaters however, the survival of salmonellae may be extended for periods longer than in seawater, as a result of the presence of humic materials that may absrobe U. V. radiation, therefore, protecting the cells from possible damage to the DNA by radiation (Davies & Evison, 1991). Generally, natural light affects the uptake of nutrients and inhibits active transport and biosynthesis in *Escherichia coli* (Barcina et al., 1990); its effect on salmonellae serovars may require further investigation (Sinton et al., 2007).

Nutrient availability and predation are also important factors in the survival of enteric bacteria, in aquatic environments (Flint, 1987). Using *in situ* membrane diffusion chambers, serovar Typhimurium remained viable for 5 days in tropical rainforest watershed (Jiménez et al., 1989). Thus, it was concluded that salmonellae may not survive for long period in oligotrophic natural waters (Domingo et al., 2000). The densities of viable salmonellae serovars were decreased rapidly, as measured by plate counts, in spiked filtered river and seawater. Filtration may removes valuable biological agents, while filterable substances such as heavy metals, antibiotics and small preadtors (e.g. protozoa) may then be responsible for the rapid decrease of bacteria in filtered natural waters (Cornax et al., 1990; Domingo et al., 2000). High densities of salmonellae were found to survive for as long as 50 days in sediment-containing microcosms compared with the overlying water (Fish & Pettibone, 1995). Aquatic sediments were culture-positive of serovar Typhimurium up to 119 days, while this serovar was viable in water column in the same microcosm for only 54 days (Moore et al., 2003). The observed extended survival of salmonellae in aquatic sediments is probably due concentration of these bacteria by sedimentation of bacteria-bound particles. Sediments may protect enteric bacteria from certain stressful conditions associated with aquatic environments; it also provides enteric bacteria with nutrients and protection against grazing protozoans, thus supports the growth of these bacteria (Lim & Flint, 1989; Fish & Pettibone, 1995).

In terristerial ecosystems, salmonellae were found to multiply and survive in soil for up to 12 months, as soil ecosystems were believed to act as microecological niches where enteric bacteria can survive and even grow. The ability of salmonellae to attach to soil particles was related to cell surface hydrophobicity by which the bacteria can undergo morphological changes in order to adapt to this new environment (Stenstrom, 1989; Davies & Wray, 1996). The ability of salmonellae to survive and grow in soil environments may explain, in part, the detection of *Salmonella* spp. from pasture 2 months, and from soil 8 months after the application of contaminated pig slurry, and highlight the need of proper sanitation of contaminated animal waste before its disposal on agricultural land (Venglovsky et al., 2006). Virtually, *Salmonella* serovars can persist in different environments. On clean laminated surfaces (i.e. utensils), salmonellae was found to survive for less than 4 hours, however when these utensils (stainless steel bowl) were covered with soil, *Salmonella* spp. survived for up to 4 hours (Scott & Bloomfield, 1990). Survival of serovars Enteritidis, Heidelberg and Enteritidis phage type 4 on surfaces was extended to up to 24 hours under dark conditions, but when these surfaces exposed to direct sunlight, the numbers of salmonellae serovars decreased rapidly (Nyeleti et al., 2004). Thus it is not surprising that *Salmonella* spp. can persist and survive in domestic kitechens for a year or even longer (Humphrey, 2001). *Salmonella* spp. persisted in the biofilm material found under the recess of the toilet bowl rim which was difficult to remove with household toilet cleaner. Serovar Enteritidis remained in toilet bowl for up to 4 weeks despite the use of cleaning fluids. Flushing the toilet may contaminate the toilet seat and its lid with salmonellae that were found in biofilm formation in toilet bowl (Barker & Bloomfield, 2000). In conclusion, it was suggested that the ubiquitous nature of *Salmonella* may facilitate a cyclic lifestyle consisting of passage through a host into the environment and back into a new host (e.g. from human intestine to the water then to birds), therefore, the long-term survival of *Salmonella* in the secondary habitat (i.e. water, soil) ensures its passage to the next host (Winfield & Groisman, 2003).

The viable but nonculturable (VBNC) state in the context of enteric bacteria refers to the ability of bacterial cells to remain viable (i.e. retaining basal metabolic activities) yet unable to grow in artificial media in the laboratory (Barer et al., 1993; Oliver, 2005, 2010). This state is believed to be a survival strategy of enteric bacteria that are released into the environment and suffer prolonged exposure to environmental stressors such as suboptimal temperature; U. V. irradiation; nutrient deprivation and biological interactions (McKay, 1992; Barer & Harwood, 1999). Xu et al. (1982) were the first to address the VBNC phenomenon in enteric bacteria when they examined the survival of *Vibrio cholerae* and *Escherichia coli* in estuarine and marine water microcosms. It was found later on that the VBNC state is exhibited by other enteric bacterial species such as *Campylobacter, Shigella, Ligeonella* and *Salmonella* (McKay, 1992; Barer et al., 1993). Nonculturability in salmonellae has been attributed, in part, to nutrient depletion. As a result of nutrient limitations viable cells of serovar Enteritidis lost culturablity within 48 hours at 25 °C when they were incubated in sterile river water (Roszak et al., 1984). Other relevance factors for the possible VBNC state in salmonellae may include exposure to elevated temperatures, U. V. irradiation, salinity, exposure to antibiotics and chlorination (Caro et al., 1999; Oliver, 2000; Smith et al., 2002; Oliver et al., 2005). VBNC forms of salmonellae may undergo morphological transition in response to stress, as they form a shorter rods shape (Roszak et al., 1984). Resuscetation of VBNC *Salmonella* cells may be possible (Roszak et al., 1984; Smith et al., 2002; Dhiaf et al., 2010), yet these resuscitated cells may lose their virulence or ability to cause infection (Caro et al., 1999) as serovar Typhimurium in VBNC forms and active but nonculturable (ABNC) (i.e. resuscitated cells) were unable to infect, nor colonize laboratory animals (Smith et al., 2002).

In contrast, other studies have rejected the whole VBNC concept. It is suggested that VBNC cells are actually dead and that apparent resuscitation represents the growth of surviving culturable cells (Morgan et al., 1991; Weichart et al., 1992; Bogosian et al., 1998). This suggestion was supported by failure of nonresuscitated forms of VBNC *Salmonella typhimurium* to colonize mouse model (Caro et al., 1999). Although the VBNC phenomenon is not fully elucidated, it has a major relevance to public health authorities in two areas: (i) the ability to cause infection, and (ii) the monitoring of enteric pathogens in the environment using conventional culture methods (McKay, 1992; Barer et al., 1993).

3.3 Antibiotic resistance

The emergence of anitmicrbial resistance in pathogenic bacteria, particularly in enteric bacteria is a major public health issue. The over use of antibiotics in food-producing animals, mass treatment and long-term administration of antimicrobial growth promoters may lead to the emergence of multidrug-resistant strains of enteric bacteria, including *Salmonella* spp. These bacteria may become reservoirs of highly transferable drug-resistance genes, and as they spread widely in the environment, they may cause serious infections as they spread within the food chain. Consequently, therapeutic failure of these infections may occur and complications due to these infections may result in increase in morbidity and mortality (Mølbak 2004, 2005).

The implications of infections caused by drug-resistant *Salmonella typhimurium* DT29 was addressed by Anderson (1968). Infections in calves in the UK due to this serovar were proven difficult to treat even after using a range of antibiotics. Instead, this use of multidrug resulted in the acquisition of serovar Typhimurium DT29 transferable multiple drug-resistance, that later caused many infections in humans (Anderson, 1968). In his report Anderson (1968) suggested that infections due multidrug-resistant salmonellae can be eliminated not by the massive use of antibiotics, but by improvement in conditions of animal husbandry and reduction in the opportunities for the initiation and spread of the disease. Unfortunately, these suggestions were not taken well into consideration in many parts of the world and as a result, different serovars of salmonellae have acquired multiple-drug resistance and became ubiquitous in the environment. Various salmonellae serovars resistant to wide range of antimicrobial drugs were isolated from the faeces of diseased and apparently healthy livestock and poultry (Ahmed et al., 2009), food (dairy products; meat; poultry products) (Antunes et al., 2003; Zhao et al., 2003; Dallal et al., 2010), free-living wild animals and birds (Palmgren et al., 1997; Čížek et al., 2007; Abulreesh, 2011), domesticated animals (Seepersadsingh & Adesiyun, 2003; Van Immerseel et al., 2004; Ebani et al., 2005), natural waters (fresh and marine) (Morinigo et al., 1990; Harakeh et al., 2006), sewage effluents and sludge (Berge et al., 2006; Espigares et al., 2006) and from diarrhea patients (Ling et al., 1998; Graziani et al., 2008) worldwide. In general, a well established link between the use of antibiotics in food-producing animals and drug-resistant salmonellae is described and well understood for food-borne nontyphoidal salmonellae (Mølbak, 2004).

Salmonella spp. can acquire resistance to antimicrobial drugs via different mechanisms such as (i) transferable resistance genes; (ii) excessive use of antibiotics in treatment "selective pressure"; and (iii) as a response to exposure to environmental drastic conditions. The resistance of aminoglycosides, β-lactams, chloramphenicol, macrolides, quaternary ammonium and trimethoprime in salmonellae serovars is attributed to the acquisition of foreign genes that encoded enzymes to destroy, chemically inactive, or "pump" the noxious drug out of the bacterial cell or provide an alternative pathway to the one targeted by the antibiotic (D'Aoust & Maurer, 2007). These antibiotic-resistance genes usually reside on mobile genetic elements such as plasmids; transposons and integrons that can potentially transfer resistance from commensal to pathogenic bacteria (Mølbak, 2005; D'Aoust & Maurer, 2007). Integron in particular, described as a genetic material that is capable of capturing, combining, or swapping a large assortment of antibiotic-resistance genes, then integrating the captured genes into a resident integration site. This genetic element (i.e. integron) can create tandem antibiotic-resistant genes. In salmonellae serovars, tetracycline resistance genes are the only resistance genes that have not identified among the integron gene cassettes, nonetheless they are carried on plasmids (Ling et al., 1998; D'Aoust & Maurer, 2007).

Overuse of antibiotics in the treatment clinical or veterinary cases together with environmental stresses (e.g. detergents, dyes, food components, preservatives) can induce the *mar* (multiple antibiotic resistance) operon. This operon regulates the expression of a large number of genes, including those coding for at least one broad-specificity efflux pump (i.e. *arcAB* efflux pump), which are more strongly expressed under drastic conditions of environmental stress (McMahon et al., 2007). There seem to be a role of antimicrobial drug intake for acquiring infections with drug-resistant pathogenic bacteria (Threlfall, 2002; Mølbak, 2004). This was confirmed by Glynn et al. (2004) where patients infected with serovar Typhimurium resistant to ampicillin, chloramphenicol, streptomycin, sulphonamides and tetracycline were most likely to have treated by antibiotics to which that serovar was resistant. This may shed some light on the reasons why outbreaks of drug-resistant pathogens are particularly frequent in hospitals and other environments where antibiotics are commonly used, furthermore, it may explains the fact that drug-resistant bacteria may be more virulent than susceptible ones (Threlfall, 2002; Mølbak, 2004, 2005). In addition, it was found that food preservation processes (e.g. low pH, high NaCl) can lead to the development of populations or subpopulation of salmonellae with decreased susceptibility to a range of currently used antibiotics (e.g. amikacin, ceftriaxone, trimethoprim). Such decreases in antibiotic susceptibility are maintained as long as the food preservation stress is maintained, and in some cases, even after the food preservation stress is removed (McMahon et al., 2007). In general, it is well established that the likelihood that pathogenic bacteria could develop resistance, persist and spread involves more than selective pressure for antibiotics use alone (overuse of antibiotics in treatment of human and animal infections), and could also result from a complex of interactions of genes, ecosystems, and the environment (D'Aoust & Maurer, 2007).

4. Concluding remarks

Despite the decline of typhoidal salmonellae infections in major parts of the world, nontyphoidal salmonellae is the second leading cause of water-and food-borne infections worldwide. *Salmonella* serovars are ubiquitous in natural waters and sediments. The presence of salmonellae in aquatic environments is related to one or a combination of sewage effluents; agricultural run-off and direct faecal contamination from natural fauna. *Salmonella* serovars cause major infections in domestic and wild animals, nonetheless, a wide range of domesticated and free-living animals appears to carry salmonellae without obvious symptoms. *Salmonella* seovars have unique seasonal trends. In the environment, generally they peak during wet seasons and are more associated with rainfall and monsoon seasons. Some serovars peak in aquatic environments during warmer months, while other peak in colder months. Although no seasonal trends were found in the carriage of salmonellae by domestic and wild animals, the presence of salmonellae infection in the community is season-dependent. Untreated water, contaminated raw milk, poultry products and undercooked meat are the major sources of infection. Handling of doestic animals and wild fauna may also poses a risk for acquiring salmonellosis. Salmonellae serovars may survive and remain virulent for long periods in the environment, they may undergo a viable but nonculturable stage as a survival strategy, their ability to cause infection in the VBNC state, however, remains questionable. *Salmonella* spp. can easily acquire drug-resistance genes via transferable genetic elements. In addition, overuse of antibiotics in the treatment of human and veterinary diseases is another mechanism in which salmonellae serovars can aquire resistance to antimicrobial drugs. The ability of faecal indicators to predict the presence of salmonellae in polluted environmental waters remains questionable, and the absence of faecal indicators is not always a reliable indication of the absence of *Salmonella* spp.

5. References

Abulreesh, H. H. (2011). Free living rock pigeon (*Columba livia*) as an environmental reservoir of enteric bacterial pathogens resistant to antimicrobial drugs in Saudi Arabia. *Current Research in Bacteriology*, Vol. 4, pp. 28-33, ISSN 1994-5426.

Abulreesh, H. H.; Paget, T. A. & Goulder, R. (2004). Waterfowl and the bacteriological quality of amenity ponds. *Journal of Water and Health*, Vol. 2, pp. 183-189, ISSN 1477-8920.

Abulreesh, H. H.; Paget, T. A. & Goulder, R. (2005). Waterfowl and human-pathogenic bacteria at amenity sites: a review. Proceedings of the 3rd World Waterfowl Conference, 3-7

November, Guangzhou, China. Pp. 356-362. Published by World's Poultry Sciences Association (WPSA), China Branch, South China Agricultural University.

Abulreesh, H. H.; Goulder, R. & Scott, G. W. (2007). Wild Birds and human pathogens in the context of ringing and migration. *Ringing and Migration*, Vol. 23, 193-200, ISSN 0307-8698.

Ahmed, A. M.; Ishida, Y. & Shimamoto, T. (2009). Molecular characterization of antimicrobial resistance of *Salmonella* isolated from animals in Japan. *Journal of Applied Microbiology*, Vol. 106, pp. 402-409, ISSN 1364-5072.

Al-Nakhli, H. M.; Al-Ogaily, Z. H. & Nassar, T. J. (1999). Representitive *Salmonella* serovars isolated from poultry and poultry environments in Saudi Arabia. *Revue Scientifique et Technique Office International des Epizooties*, Vol. 18, pp. 700-709, ISSN 0253-1933.

Alcaide, E.; Martinez, J. P. & Garay, E. (1984). Comparative study on *Salmonella* isolation from sewage-contaminated natural waters. *Journal of Applied Bacteriology*, Vol. 56, pp. 365-371, ISSN 0021-8847.

Anderson, E. S. (1968). Drug resistance in *Salmonella typhimurium* and its implications. *British Medical Journal*, Vol. 3, pp. 333-339, ISSN 0959-8138.

Angulo, F. J.; Nunnery, J. A. & Bair, H. D. (2004). Antimicrobial resistance in zoonotic enteric pathogens. *Revue Scientifique et Technique Office International des Epizooties*, Vol. 23, pp. 485-496, ISSN 0253-1933.

Antunes, P.; Réu, C., Sousa, J. C., Peixe, L. & Pestana, N. (2003). Incidence of *Salmonella* from poultry products and their susceptibility to antimicrobial agents. *International Journal of Food Microbiology*, Vol. 82, pp. 97-103, ISSN 0168-1605.

Arvanitidou, M.; Stathopoulos, G. A., Constantinidis, T. C. & Katsouyannopoulos, V. (1995). The occurrence of *Salmonella, Campylobacter* and *Yersinia* spp. in river and lake waters. *Microbiological Research*, Vol. 150, pp. 153-158, ISSN 0944-5013.

Arvanitidou, M.; Kanellou, K. & Vagiona, D. G. (2005). Diversity of *Salmonella* spp. and fungi in northern Greek rivers and their correlation to fecal pollution indicators. *Environmental Research*, Vol. 99, pp. 278-284, ISSN 0013-9351.

Barcina, I.; Gonzales, J. M., Iriberri, J. & Egea, L. (1990). Survival strategy of *Escherichia coli* and *Enterococcus faecalis* in illuminated fresh and marine systems. *Journal of Applied Bacteriology*, Vol. 68, pp. 189-198, ISSN 0021-8847.

Barer, M. R.; Gribbon, L. T., Harwood, C. R. & Nwoguh, C. E. (1993). The viable but non-culturable hypothesis and medical bacteriology. *Reviews in Medical Microbiology*, Vol. 4, pp. 183-191, ISSN 0954-139X.

Barer, M. R. & Harwood, C. R. (1999). Bacterial viability and culturability. *Advances in Microbial Physiology*, Vol. 41, pp. 93-137, ISBN 0-12-027741-7.

Barker, J. & Bloomfield, S. F. (2000). Survival of *Salmonella* in bathrooms and toilets in domestic homes following salmonellosis. *Journal of Applied Microbiology*, Vol. 89, pp. 137-144, ISSN 1364-5072

Baudart, J.; Grabulos, J., Barusseau, J. -P. & Lebaron, P. (2000). *Salmonella* spp. and fecal coliform loads in coastal waters from a point vs. nonpoint source of pollution. *Journal of Environmental Quality*, Vol. 29, pp. 241-250, ISSN 0047-2425.

Berge, A. C. B; Dueger, E. L. & Sischo, W. M. (2006). Comparison of *Salmonella enterica* serovar distribution and antibiotic resistance patterns in wastewater at municipal water treatment plants in two California cities. *Journal of Applied Microbiology*, Vol. 101, pp. 1309-1316, ISSN 1364-5072.

Bhatta, D. R.; Bangtrakulnonth, A., Tishyadhigama, P., Saroj, S. D., Bandekar, J. R., Hendriksen, R. S. & Kapadnis, B. P. (2007). Serotyping, PCR, phage-typing and antibiotic sensitivity testing of *Salmonella* serovar isolated from urban drinking water supply systems of Nepal. *Letters in Applied Microbiology*, Vol. 44, pp. 588-594, ISSN 0266-8254.

Blaser, M. & Newman L. (1982). A review of human salmonellosis: 1. Infective dose. *Review of Infectious Diseases*, Vol. 4, pp. 1096-1106, ISSN 0162-0886.

Bogosian, G.; Morris, P. J.L & O'Neil, J. P. (1998). A mixed culture recovery method indicates that enteric bacteria do not enter the viable but noculturable state. *Applied and Environmental Microbiology*, Vol. 64, pp. 1736-1742, ISSN 0099-2240.

Bonnedahl, J.; Broman, T., Waldenström, J., Palmgren, H., Niskanen, T. & Olsen, B. (2005). In search of human-associated bacterial pathogens in Antarctic wildlife: report from six penguin colonies regularly visited by tourists. *Ambio*, Vol. 34, pp. 430-432, ISSN 0044-7447.

Bopp, C. A.; Brenner, F. W., Wells, J. G. & Strockbine, N. A. (1999). *Escherichia, Shigella* and *Salmonella*, In: *Manual of Clinical Microbiology 7th edition*, Murray, P. R., Baron, E. J., Pfaller, M. A., Tenover, F. C. & Yolken, R. H. (Eds), pp. 459-474, ASM Press, ISBN 1555811264, Washington D. C., USA.

Briones, V.; Téllez, S., Goyache, J., Ballesteros, C., Lanzarot, M. d. P., Domínguez, L. & Fernández-Garayzábal, J. F. (2004). *Salmonella* diversity associated with wild reptiles and amphibians in Spain. *Environmental Microbiology*, Vol. 6, pp. 868-871, ISSN 1462-2912.

Bywater, R.; Deluyker, H., Deroover, E., de jong, A., Marion, H., McConville, M., Rowan, T., Shryock, T., Shuster, D., Thomas, V., Vallé, M. & Walters, J. (2004). A European survey of antimicrobial susceptibility among zoonotic and commensal bacteria isolated from food-producing animals. *Journal of Antimicrobial Chemotherapy*, Vol. 54, pp. 744-754, ISSN 0305-7453.

Capita, R.; Álvarez-Astorga, M., Alonso-Calleja, C., Moreno, B. & García-Fernández, M. d. C. (2003). Occurrence of salmonellae in retail chicken carcasses and their products in Spain. *International Journal of Food Microbiology*, Vol. 81, pp. 169-173, ISSN 0168-1605.

Capita, R.; Alonso-Calleja, C. & Prieto, M. (2007). Prevalence of *Salmonella enterica* serovars and genovars from chicken carcasses in slaughterhouses in Spain. *Journal of Applied Microbiology*, Vol. 103, pp. 1366-1375, ISSN 1364-5072.

Caro, A.; Got, P., Lesne, J., Binard, S. & Baleux, B. (1999). Viability and virulence of experimentally stressed nonculturable *Salmonella typhimurium*. *Applied and Environmental Microbiology*, Vol. 65, pp. 3229-3232, ISSN 0099-2240.

Carter, M. E. & Quinn, P. J. (2000). *Salmonella* in dogs and cats. In : Salmonella *in Domestic Animals*, Wray, C. & Wray A. (Eds), pp. 231-244, CAB International Publishing, ISBN 0851992617, Oxon, UK.

Cho, S. -H.; Shin, H. -H., Choi, Y. -H., Park, M. -S. & Lee, B. -K. (2008). Enteric bacteria isolated from acute diarrheal patients in the Republic of Korea between the year 2004 and 2006. *The Journal of Microbiology*, Vol. 46, pp. 325-330, ISSN 1225-8873.

Čížek, A.; Literák, I., Hejlíček, K., Treml, F. & Smola J. (1994). *Salmonella* contamination of the environment and its incidence in wild birds. *Journal of Veterinary Medicine B*. Vol. 41, pp. 320-327, ISSN 0931-1793.

Čížek, A.; Dolejská, M., Karpíšková, D. & Literák, I. (2007). Wild black-headed gulls (*Larus ridibundus*) as an environmental reservoir of *Salmonella* strains resistant to antimicrobial drugs. *European Journal of Wildlife Research*, Vol. 53, pp.55-60, ISSN 1612-4642.

Claudon, D. G.; Thompson, D. I., Christenson, E. H., Lawton, G. W. & Dick, E. C. (1971) Prolonged *Salmonella* contamination of a recreational lake by runoff water. *Applied Microbiology*, Vol. 21, pp. 875-877, ISSN 0099-2240.

Cogan, T. A. & Humphrey, T. J. (2003). The rise and fall of *Salmonella* Enteritidis in the UK. *Journal of Applied Microbiology*, Vol. 94, pp. 114S-119S, ISSN 1364-5072.

Cornax, R.; Morinigo, M. A., Romero, P. & Borrego, J. J. (1990). Survival of pathogenic microorganisms in sea water. *Current Microbiology*, Vol. 20, pp. 293-298, ISSN 0343-8651.

Costalunga, S. & Tondo, E. C. (2002). Salmonellosis in Rio Grande do Sul, Brazil, 1997 to 1999. *Brazillian Journal of Microbiology*, Vol. 33, pp. 342-346, ISSN 1517-8382.

Dallal, M. M. S.; Doyle, M. P., Rezadehbashi, M., Dabiri, H., Sanaei, M., Modarresi, S., Bakhtiari, R., Sharifiy, K., Taremi, M., Zali, M. R. & Sharifi-Yazdi, M. K. (2010). Prevalence and antimicrobial resistance profiles of *Salmonella* serotypes, *Campylobacter* and *Yersinia* spp. isolated from retail chicken and beef, Tehran, Iran. *Food Control*, Vol. 21, pp. 388-392, ISSN 0956-7135.

Danielsson, M. L. (1977). *Salmonella* in sewage and sludge. Serological profiles of isolates, their removal and/or survival in relation to potential health hazards to man and animals. *Acta Veterinaria Scandinavica Supplementum*, Vol. 65, pp. 1-126, ISSN 0044-605X.

D'Aoust, J. -Y. & Maurer, J. (2007). *Salmonella* species. In: *Food Microbiology : Fundamentals and Frontiers 3rd ed*, Doyle, M. P. & Beuchat, L. R. (Eds.), pp. 187-236, ASM Press, ISBN 1-55581-407-7, Washington D.C., USA.

Davies, C. M. & Evison, L. M. (1991). Sunlight and the survival of enteric bacteria in natural waters. *Journal of Applied Bacteriology*, Vol. 70, pp. 265-274, ISSN 0021-8847.

Davies, R. H.; Dalziel, R., Gibbens, J. C., Wilesmith, J. W., Ryan, J. M. B., Evans, S. J., Byrne, C., Paiba, G. A., Pascoe, S. J. S. & Teale, C. J. (2004). National survey for *Salmonella* in pigs, cattle and sheep at slaughter in Great Britian (1999-2000). *Journal of Applied Microbiology*, Vol. 96, pp. 750-760, ISSN 1364-5072.

Davies, R. H. & Wray, C. (1996). Seasonal variations in the isolation of *Salmonella typhimurium*, *Salmonella enteritidis*, *Bacillus cereus* and *Clostridium perfringens* from environmental samples. *Journal of Veterinary Medicine B*, Vol. 43, pp. 119-127, ISSN 0931-1793.

de Oliveira, S. D.; Flores, F. S., dos Santos, L. R. & Brandelli, A. (2005). Antimicrobial resistance in *Salmonella eteritidis* strains isolated from broiler carcasses, food, human and poultry-related samples. *International Journal of Food Microbiology*, Vol. 97, pp. 297-305, ISSN 0168-1605.

de Sá, I. V. A. & Solari, C. A. (2001). *Salmonella* in Brazillian and imported pet reptiles. *Brazilian Journal of Microbiology*, Vol. 32, pp. 293-297, ISSN 1517-8382.

Dhiaf, A.; Ben Abdallah, F. & Bakhrouf, A. (2010). Resuscitation of 20-year starved *Salmonella* in seawater and soil. *Annals of Microbiology*, Vol. 60, pp. 157-160, ISSN 1590-4261.

Dionisio, L. P. C.; Joao, M., Ferreiro, V. S., Fidalgo, M. L., Rosado, M. E. G. & Borrego, J. J. (2000). Occurrence of *Salmonella* spp. in estuarine and costal waters of Portugal. *Antonie van Leeuwenhoek*, Vol. 78, pp. 99-106, ISSN 0003-6072.

Domingo, J. W. S.; Harmon, S. & Bennett, J. (2000). Survival of *Salmonella* species in river water. *Current Microbiology,* Vol. 40, pp. 409-417, ISSN 0343-8651.

Dovč, A.; Zorman-Rojs, O., Rataj, A. V., Bole-Hribovšek, V., Karpež, U. & Dobeic, M. (2004). Health status of free-living pigeons (*Columba livia domestica*) in the city of Ljubljana. *Acta Veterinaria Hungarica,* Vol. 52, pp. 219-226, ISSN 0236-6290.

Ebani, V. V.; Cerri, D., Fratini, F., Meille, N., Valentini, P. & Andreani, E. (2005). *Salmonella enterica* isolates from faeces of domestic reptiles and a study of their antimicrobial in vitro sensitivity. *Research in Veterinary Sciences,* Vol. 78, pp. 117-121, ISSN 0034-5288.

Ekdahl, K.; deJong, B., Wollin, R. & Andersson, Y. (2005). Travel-associated non-typhoidal salmonellosis: geographical and seasonal difference and serotype distribution. *Clinical Microbiology and Infection,* Vol. 11, pp. 138-144, ISSN 1198-743X.

Espigares, E.; Bueno, A., Espigares, M. & Gálvez, R. (2006). Isolation of *Salmonella* serotypes in wastewater and effluent: effect of treatment and potential risk. *International Journal of Hygiene and Environmental Health,* Vol. 209, pp. 103-107, ISSN 1438-4639.

Fallacara, D. M.; Monahan, C. M., Morishita, T. Y. & Wack, R. E. (2001). Fecal shedding and antimicrobial susceptibility of selected bacterial pathogens and a survey of intestinal parasites in free-living waterfowl. *Avian Diseases,* Vol. 45, pp. 128-135, ISSN 0005-2086.

Fallacara, D. M., Monahan, C. M., Morishita, T. Y., Bremer, C. A. & Wack R. F. (2004). Survey of parasites and bacterial pathogenss from free-living waterfowl in zoological settings. *Avian Diseases,* Vol. 48, pp. 759-767, ISSN 0005-2086.

Fedorka-Cray, P. J.; Gray, J. T. & Wray, C. (2000). *Salmonella* infections in pigs. In: Salmonella *in Domestic Animals,* Wray, C. & Wray A. (Eds), pp. 191-207, CAB International Publishing, ISBN 0851992617, Oxon, UK.

Ferns, P. N. & Mudge, G. P. (2000). Abundance, diet and *Salmonella* contamination of gulls feeding at sewage outfalls. *Water Research,* Vol. 34, pp. 2653-2660, ISSN 0043-1354.

Fish, J. T. & Pettibone, G. W. (1995). Influence of freshwater sediment on the survival of *Escherichia coli* and *Salmonella* sp. as measured by three methods of enumeration. *Letters in Applied Microbiology,* Vol. 20, pp. 277-281, ISSN 0266-8254.

Flint, K. P. (1987). The long-term survival of *Escherichia coli* in river water. *Journal of Applied Bacteriology,* Vol. 63, pp. 261-270, ISSN 0021-8847.

Fricker, C. R. (1984). A note on *Salmonella* excretion in the black headed gull (*Larus ribibundus*) feeding at sewage treatment works. *Journal of Applied Bacteriology,* Vol. 56, pp. 499-502, ISSN 0021-8847.

Garber, L.; Smeltzer, M., Fedorka-Cray, P., Ladley, S. & Ferris, K. (2003). *Salmonella enterica* serotype *enteritidis* in table egg layer house environments and in mice in U.S. layer houses and associated risk factors. *Avian Diseases,* Vol. 47, pp. 134-142, ISSN 0005-2086.

Galbraith, N. S. (1994). Historical review of microbial diseases spread by water in England and Wales. In: *Water and Public Health,* Golding, A. M. B., Noah, N. & Stanwell-Smith, R. (Eds), pp. 15-37, Smith Gordon and Company, ISBN 1-85463-018-0, London, UK.

Geldreich, E. E. (1996). Pathogenic agents in freshwater resources. *Hydrological Processes,* Vol. 10, pp. 315-333, ISSN 0885-6087.

Glynn, M. K.; Reddy, V., Hutwagner, L., Rabatsky-Ehr, T., Shiferaw, B., Vugia, D. J., Segler, S., Bender, J., Barrett, T. J. & Angulo, F. J. (2004). Prior antimicrobial agent use increases the risk of sporadic infections with multidrug-resistant *Salmonella enterica* serotype Typhimurium: a FoodNet case-control study, 1996-1997. *Clinical Infectious Diseases*, Vol. 38, pp. S227-S236, ISSN 1058-4838.

Godfree, A. (2003). Health constraints on the agricultural recycling of wastewater sludge. In: *The Handbook of Water and Wastewater Microbiology*, Mara, D. & Horan, N. (Eds), pp. 281-298, Academic Press, ISBN 0-12-470100-0, San Diego, USA.

Guard-Petter, J. (2001). The chicken, the egg and *Salmonella enteritidis*. *Environmental Microbiology*, Vol. 3, pp. 421-430, ISSN 1462-2912.

Guerin, M. T.; Martin, S. W., Darlington, G. A. & Rajic, A. (2005). A temporal study of *Salmonella* serovars in animals in Alberta between 1990 and 2001. *The Canadian Journal of Veterinary Research*, Vol. 69, pp. 88-99, ISSN 0830-9000.

Graziani, C.; Busani, L., Dionisi, A. M., Lucarelli, C., Owczarek, S., Ricci, A., Caprioli, A. & Luzzi, I. (2008). Antimicrobial resistence in *Salmonella enterica* serovar Typhimurium from human and animal sources in Italy. *Veterinary Microbiology*, Vol. 128, pp. 414-418, ISSN 0378-1135.

Haley, B. J.; Cole, D. J. & Lipp, E. K. (2009). Distribution, diversity and seasonality of waterborne samonellae in a rural watershed. *Applied and Environmental Microbiology*, Vol. 75, pp. 1248-1255, ISSN 1098-5336.

Harakeh, S.; Yassine, H. & El-Fadel, M. (2006). Antimicrobial-resistant patterns of *Escherichia coli* and *Salmonella* strains in the aquatic Lebanese environments. *Environmental Pollution*, Vol. 143, pp. 269-277, ISSN 0269-7491.

Healing, T. D. (1991). *Salmonella* in rodents: a risk to man? *Communicable Disease Report Reviewe*, Vol. 1, pp. 114-116, ISSN

Hendricks, C. W. (1971). Increased recovery rate of salmonellae from stream bottom sediments versus surface water. *Applied Microbiology*, Vol. 21, pp. 379-380, ISSN 0099-2240.

Henry, R. R. (2000). *Salmonella* infection in ducks. In: Salmonella *in Domestic Animals*, Wray, C. & Wray A. (Eds), pp. 157-167, CAB International Publishing, ISBN 0851992617, Oxon, UK.

Hernandez, J.; Bonnedahl, J., Waldenström, J., Palmgren, H. & Olsen, B. (2003). *Salmonella* in birds migrating through Sweden. *Emerging Infectious Diseases*, Vol. 9, pp. 753-755, ISSN 1080-6059.

Hilton, A. C.; Willis R. J. & Hickie, S. J. (2002). Isolation of *Salmonella* from urban wild brown rats (*Rattus norvegicus*) in the West Midlands, UK. *International Journal of Environmental Health Research*, Vol. 12, pp. 163-168, ISSN 0960-3123.

Ho, B. S. W. & Tam, T. -Y. (2000). Rapid enumeration of *Salmonella* in environmental waters and wastewater. *Water Research*, Vol. 34, pp. 2397-2399, ISSN 0043-1354.

Holt, J. G.; Krieg, N. R., Sneath, P. H. A., Staley, J. T. & Williams, S. T. (1994). *Bergey's Manual of Determinative Bacteriology* 9th Edition, Williams and Wilkins, ISBN 0-68300-6032, Baltimore, Maryland, USA.

Hubálek, Z.; Sixl, W., Mikuláškova, M., Sixl-Voigt, B., Thiel, W., Halouzka, J., Juřicová, Z., Rosický, B., Mátlova, L., Honza, M., Hájek, V. & Sitko, J. (1995). Salmonellae in gulls and other free-living birds in the Czech Republic. *Central European Journal of Public Health*, Vol. 3, pp. 21-24, ISSN 1210-7778.

Humphrey, T. (2001). The spread and persistence of *Campylobacter* and *Salmonella* in the domestic kitchen. *Journal of Infection*, Vol. 43, pp. 50-53, ISSN 0163-4453.

Humphrey, T. & Jørgensen, F. (2006). Pathogens on meat and infection in animals - Establishing a relationship using *Campyloacter* and *Salmonella* as examples. *Meat Science*, Vol. 74, pp. 89-97, ISSN 0309-1740.

Hunter, P. R. (1997). *Waterborne Diseases: Epidemiology and Ecology*, John Wiley & Sons, ISBN 9780471966463, Chichester, UK.

Hutchinson, M. L.; Avery S. M. & Monaghan, J. M. (2008). The air-borne distribution of zoonotic agents from livestock waste spreading and microbiological risk to fresh produce from contaminated irrigation sources. *Journal of Applied Microbiology*, Vol. 105, pp. 848-857, ISSN 1364-5072.

Jiménez, L.; Muniz, I., Toranzos, G. A. & Hazen, T. C. (1989). Survival and activity of *Salmonella typhimurium* and *Escherichia coli* in tropical freshwater. *Journal of Applied Bacteriology*, Vol. 67, pp. 61-69, ISSN 0021-8847.

Johnson, J. Y. M.; Thomas, J. E., Graham, T. A., Townshend, I., Byrne, J., Selinger, L. B. & Gannon, V. P. J. (2003). Prevalence of *Escherichia coli* O157 :H7 and *Salmonella* spp. in surface waters of southern Alberta and its relation to manure sources. *Canadian Journal of Microbiology*, Vol. 49, pp. 326-335, ISSN 0008-4166.

Jokinen, C. C.; Schreier, H., Mauro, W., Taboada, E., Isaac-Renton, J. L., Topp, E., Edge, T., Thomas, J. E., & Gannon, V. P. J. (2010). The occurrence and sources of *Campylobacter* spp., *Salmonella enterica* and *Escherichia coli* O157:H7 in the Salmon River, British Columbia, Canada. *Journal of Water and Health*, Vol. 8, pp. 374-386, ISSN 1477-8920.

Jones, Y. E.; McLaren, I. M. & Wray, C. (2000). Laboratory aspects of *Salmonella*. In : Salmonella *in Domestic Animals*, Wray, C. & Wray A. (Eds), pp. 393-405, CAB International Publishing, ISBN 0851992617, Oxon, UK.

Kapperud, G. & Rosef, O. (1983). Avian wildlife reservoir of *Campylobacter fetus* subsp. *jejuni*, *Yersinia* spp., and *Salmonella* spp. in Norway. *Applied and Environmental Microbiology*, Vol. 45, pp. 375-380, ISSN 0099-2240.

Khakhria, R.; Woodward, D., Johnson, W. M. & Poppe, C. (1997). *Salmonella* isolates from humans, animals and other sources in Canada, 1983-92. *Epidemiology and Infection*, Vol. 119, pp. 15-23, ISSN 0950-2688.

Kinde, H.; Castellan, D. M., Kerr, D., Campbell, J., Breitmeyer, R. & Ardans, A. (2005). Longitudianl monitoring of two commercial layer flocks and their environments for *Salmonella enterica* serovar Enteritidis and other salmonellae. *Avian Diseases*, Vol. 49, pp. 189-194, ISSN 0005-2086.

Kirk, J. H.; Holmberg, C. A. & Jeffrey, J. S. (2002). Prevalence of *Salmonella* spp in selected birds captured on California dairies. *Journal of American Veterinary Medical Association*, Vol. 220, pp. 359-362, ISSN 0003-1488.

Kobayashi, H.; Kanazaki, M., Shimizu, Y., Nakajima, H., Khatun, M. M., Hata, E. & Kubo, M. (2007). *Salmonella* isolates from cloacal swabs and footpads of wild birds in the immediate environment of Tokyo bay. *Journal of Veterinary Medical Science*, Vol. 69, pp. 309-311, ISSN 0916-7250.

Leclerc, H.; Schwartzbrod, L. & Dei-Cas, E. (2004). Microbial agents associated with waterborne diseases. In: *Microbial Waterborne Pathogens*, Cloete, T. E., Rose, J., Nel, L. H. & Ford, T. (Eds), pp. 1-54, IWA Publishing, ISBN 1-84339-055-8, London, UK.

Lemarchand, K. & Lebaron, P. (2003). Occurrence of *Salmonella* spp. and *Cryptosporidium* spp. in a French coastal watershed: relationship with fecal indicators. *FEMS Microbiology Letters*, Vol. 218, pp. 203-209, ISSN 1574-6968.

Lightfoot, D. (2004). *Salmonella* and other enteric pathogens. In: *Waterborne Zoonoses: Identification, Causes and Control*, Cotruvo, J. A., Dufour, A., Rees, G., Bartram, J., Carr, R., Cliver, D. O., Craun, G. F., Fayer, R. & Gannon, V. P. J. (Eds), pp. 228-241, IWA Publishing, ISBN 9241562730, London, UK.

Lim, C. H. & Flint, K. P. (1989). The effects of nutrients on the survival of *Escherichia coli* in lake water. *Journal of Applied Bacteriology*, Vol. 66, pp. 559-569, ISSN 0021-8847.

Ling, J. M.; Koo, I. C., Kam, K. M. & Cheng, A. F. (1998). Antimicrobial susceptibilities and molecular epidemiology of *Salmonella enterica* serotype Enteritidis strains isolated in Hong Kong from 1986 to 1996. *Journal of Clinical Microbiology*, Vol. 36, pp. 1693-1699, ISSN 0095-1137.

Lin-Hui, S. & Cheng-Hsun, C. (2007). *Salmonella*: clinical importance and evolution of nomenclature. *Chang Gung Medical Journal*, Vol. 30, pp. 210-219, ISSN 2072-0939.

Linton, A. H. & Hinton, M. H. (1988). Enterobacteriaceae associated with animals in health and diseases. *Journal of Applied Bacteriology Symposium Supplement*, Vol. 65, pp. 71S-85S. ISSN 1365-2672.

Literák, I.; Vanko, R., Dolejská, M., Čížek, A. & Karpíšková, R. (2007). Antibiotic resistant *Escherichia coli* and *Salmonella* in Russian rooks (*Corvus frugilegus*) wintering in the Czech Republic. *Letters in Applied Microbiology*, Vol. 45, pp. 616-621, ISSN 0266-8254.

Liu, W. -B.; Chen, J., Huang, Y. -Y., Liu, B. & Shi, X. -M. (2010). Serotype, genotype and antimicrobial susceptipility profiles of *Salmonella* from chicken farms in Shanghai. *Journal of Food Protection*, Vol. 73, pp. 562-567, ISSN 0362-028X.

Mafu, N. C.; Pironcheva, G. & Okoh, A. I. (2009). Genetic diversity and in vitro antibiotic susceptibility profile of *Salmonella* species isolated from domestic water and wastewater sources in the eastern Cape province of South Africa. *African Journal of Biotechnology*, Vol. 8, pp. 1263-1269, ISSN 1684-5315.

Martinez-Urtaza, J. & Liebana, E. (2005). Investigation of clonal distribution and persistence of *Salmonella* Senftenberg in the marine environment and identification of potential sources of contamination. *FEMS Microbiology Ecology*, Vol. 52, pp. 255-263, ISSN 0168-6469.

Martinez-Urtaza, J.; Saco, M., de Novoa, J., Perez-Pineiro, P., Peiteado, J., Lozano-Leon, A. & Garcia-Martin, O. (2004a). Influence of environmental factors and human activity on the presence of *Salmonella* serovars in a marine environment. *Applied and Environmental Microbiology*, Vol. 70, pp. 2089-2097, ISSN 0099-2240.

Martinez-Urtaza, J.; Liebana, E., Garcia-Migura, L., Perez-Pinerio, P. & Saco, M. (2004b). Characterization of *Salmonella* serovar Typhimurium from marine environments in coastal waters of Galicia (Spain). *Applied and Environmental Microbiology*, Vol. 70, pp. 4030-4034, ISSN 0099-2240.

McKay, A. M. (1992). Viable but non-culturable forms of potentially pathogenic bacteria in water. *Letters in Applied Microbiology*, Vol. 14, pp. 129-135, ISSN 0266-8254.

McMahon, M. A. S.; Xu, J., Moore, J. E., Blair, I. S. & McDowell, D. A. (2007). Environmental stress and antibiotic resistance in food-related pathogens. *Applied and Environmental Microbiology*, Vol. 73, pp. 211-217, ISSN 0099-2240.

Melloul, A. A. & Hassani, L. (1999). *Salmonella* infection in children from the wastewater-spreading zone of Marrakesh city (Morocco). *Journal of Applied Microbiology*, Vol. 87, pp. 536-539, ISSN 1364-5072.

Melloul, A. A.; Hassani, L. & Rafouk, L. (2001). *Salmonella* contamination of vegetables irrigated with untrated wastewater. *World Journal of Microbiology and Biotechnology*, Vol. 17, pp. 207-209, ISSN 1573-0972.

Melloul, A.; Amahmid, O., Hassani, L. & Bouhoum, K. (2002). Health effect of human wastes use in agriculture in El Azzouzia (the wastewater spreading area of Marrakesh city, Morocco). *International Journal of Environmental Health Research*, Vol. 12, pp. 17-23, ISSN 0960-3123.

Mohanty, S.; Renuka, K., Sood, S., Das, B. K. & Kapil, A. (2006). Antibiogram pattern and seasonality of *Salmonella* serotypes in North Indian tertiary care hospital. *Epidemiology and Infection*, Vol. 134, pp. 961-966, ISSN 0950-2688.

Mølbak, K. (2004). Spread of resistant bacteria and resistance genes from animals to humans - The public health consequences. *Journal of Veterinary Medicine B*, Vol. 51, pp. 364-369, ISSN 0931-1793.

Mølbak, K. (2005). Human health consequence of antimicrobial drug-resistant *Salmonella* and other foodborne pathogens. *Clinical Infectious Diseases*, Vol. 41, pp. 1613-1620, ISSN 1058-4838.

Moore, B. C.; Martinez, E., Gay, J. M. & Rice, D. H. (2003). Survival of *Salmonella enterica* in freshwater and sediments and transmission by the aquatic midge *Chironomus tentans* (Chironomidae: Diptera). *Applied and Environmental Microbiology*, Vol. 69, pp. 4556-4560, ISSN 0099-2240.

Morgan, J. A. W.; Cranwell, P. A. & Pickup, R. W. (1991). Survival of *Aeromonas salmonicida* in lake water. *Applied and Environmental Microbiology*, Vol. 57, pp. 1777-1782, ISSN 0099-2240.

Morinigo, M. A.; Córnax, R., Castro, D., Jimenez-Notaro, M., Romero, P. & Borrego, J. J. (1990). Antibiotic resistance of *Salmonella* strains isolated from natural polluted waters. *Journal of Applied Bacteriology*, Vol. 68, pp. 297-302, ISSN 0021-8847.

Morinigo, M. A.; Córnax, R., Munoz, M. A., Romero, P. & Borrego, J. J. (1990). Relationships between *Salmonella* spp and indicator microorganisms in polluted natural waters. *Water Research*, Vol. 24, pp. 117-120, ISSN 0043-1354.

Morinigo, M. A.; Martinez-Manzanares, E., Munoz, M. A., Balebona, M. C. & Borrego, J. J. (1993). Reliability of several microorganisms to indicate the presence of *Salmonella* in natural waters. *Water Science and Technology*, Vol. 27, pp. 471-474, ISSN 0273-1223.

Murakami, K.; Horikawa, K., Ito, I. & Otsuki, K. (2001). Environmental survey of *Salmonella* and comparison of genotypic character with human isolates in Western Japan. *Epidemiology and Infection*, Vol. 126, pp. 159-171, ISSN 0950-2688.

Murray, C. J. (2000). Environmental aspects of *Salmonella*. In: Salmonella *in Domestic Animals*, Wray, C. & Wray A. (Eds), pp. 265-283, CAB International Publishing, ISBN 0851992617, Oxon, UK.

Naumova, E. N.; Jagai, J. S., Matyas, B., De Maria, A., McNeill, I. B. & Griffiths, J. K. (2007). Seasonality in six enterially transmitted diseases and ambient temperature. *Epidemiology and Infection*, Vol. 135, pp. 281-292, ISSN 0950-2688.

Nyeleti, C.; Cogan, T. A. & Humphrey, T. J. (2004). Effect of sunlight on the survival of *Salmonella* on surfaces. *Journal of Applied Microbiology*, Vol. 97, pp. 617-620, ISSN 1364-5072.

Oboegbulem, S. I. & Okoronkwo, I. (1990). Salmonellae in the African great cane rat (*Thryonomys swinderianus*). *Journal of Wildlife Diseases*, Vol. 26, pp. 119-121, ISSN 0090-3558.

Olańczuk-Neyman, K.; Geneja, M., Quant, B., Dembińska, M., Kruczalak, K., Kulbat, E., Kulik-Kuziemska, Mikolajski, S. & Gielert, M. (2003). Microbiological and biological aspects of the wastewater treatment plant 'Wschód'. *Polish Journal of Environmental Studies*, Vol. 12, pp. 747-757, ISSN 1230-1485.

Oliver, J. D. (2000). The public health significance of viable but nonculturable bacteria. In : *Nonculturable Microorganisms in the Environment*, Colwell, R. R. & Grimes, D. J. (Eds), pp. 277-300, ASM Press, ISBN 1-55581-196-5, Washington D. C., USA.

Oliver, J. D. (2005). The viable but noncluturable state in bacteria. *Journal of Microbiology*, Vol. 43, pp. 93-100, ISSN 1225-8873.

Oliver, J. D. (2010). Recent findings on the viable but nonculturable state in pathogenic bacteria. *FEMS Microbiology Reviews*, Vol. 34, pp. 415-425, ISSN 0168-6445.

Oliver, J. D.; Dagher, M. & Linden, K. (2005). Induction of *Escherichia coli* and *Salmonella typhimurium* into the viable but nonculturable state following chlorination of wastewater. *Journal of Water and Health*, Vol. 3, pp. 249-257, ISSN 1477-8920.

Olsen, S. J.; Bishop, R., Brenner, F. W., Roels, T. H., Bean, N., Tauxe, R. V. & Slutsker, L. (2001). The changing epidemiology of *Salmonella*: trends in serotypes isolated from humans in the United States, 1987-1997. *The Journal of Infectious Diseases*, Vol. 183, pp. 753-761, ISSN 0022-1899.

Padungtod, P. & Kaneene, J. B. (2006). *Salmonella* in food animals and humans in northern Thailand. *International Journal of Food Microbiology*, Vol. 108, pp. 346-354, ISSN 0168-1605.

Palmgren, H.; Sellin, M., Bergström, S. & Olsen, B. (1997). Enteropathogenic bacteria in migrating birds arriving in Sweden. *Scandinavian Journal of Infectious Diseases*, Vol. 29, pp. 565-568, ISSN 0036-5548.

Palmgren, H.; Broman, T., Waldenström, J., Lindberg, P., Aspán, Björn, O. (2004). *Salmonella* Amager, *Campylobacter jejuni*, and urease-positive thermophilic *Campylobacter* found in free-flying peregrine falcons (*Falco peregrinus*) in Sweden. *Journal of Wildlife Diseases*, Vol. 40, pp. 583-587, ISSN 0090-3558.

Palmgren, H.; Aspán, A., Broman, T., Bengtsson, K., Blomquist, L., Bergström, S., Sellin, M., Wollin, R. & Olsen, B. (2006). *Salmonella* in black-headed gulls (*Larus ridibundus*); prevalence, genotypes and influence on *Salmonella* epidemiology. *Epidemiology and Infection*, Vol. 134, pp. 635-644, ISSN 0950-2688.

Pedersen, K.; Clark, K., Andelt, W. F. & Salman, M. D. (2006). Prevalence of shiga toxin-producing *Escherichia coli* and *Salmonella enterica* in rock pigeons captured in Fort Collins, Colorado. *Journal of Wildlife Diseases*, Vol. 42, pp. 46-55, ISSN 0090-3558.

Percival, S. L..; Chalmers, R. M., Embrey, M., Hunter, P. R., Sellwood, J. & Wyn-Jones, P. (2004). *Microbiology of Waterborne Diseases*, Elsevier Academic Press, ISBN 0-12-551570-7, San Diego, California, USA.

Pfleger, S.; Benyr, G., Sommer, R. & Hassl, A. (2003). Pattern of *Salmonella* excretion in amphibians and reptiles in a vivarium. *International Journal of Hygiene and Environmental Health*, Vol. 206, pp. 53-59, ISSN 1438-4639.

Pianetti, A.; Baffone, W., Burscolini, F., Barbieri, E., Biffi, M. R., Salvaggio, L. & Albano, A. (1998). Presence of several pathogenic bacteria in the Metauro and Foglia rivers (Pesaro-Urbino, Italy). *Water Research*, Vol. 32, pp. 1515-1521, ISSN 0043-1354.

Plummer, R. A. S.; Blissett, S. J. & Dodd, C. E. R. (1995). *Salmonella* contamination of retail chicken products sold in the UK. *Journal of Food Protection*, Vol. 58, pp. 843-846, ISSN 0362-028X.

Pokorný, J. (1988). Survival and virulence of salmonellae in water. *Journal of Hygiene, Epidemiology, Microbiology and Immunology*, Vol. 32, pp. 361-366, ISSN 0022-1732.

Polo, F.; Figueras, M. J., Inza, I., Sala, J., Fleisher, J. M. & Guarro, J. (1998). Relationship between presence of *Salmonella* and indicators of faecal pollution in aquatic habitats. *FEMS Microbiology Letters*, Vol. 160, pp. 253-256, ISSN 0378-1097.

Polo, F.; Figueras, M. J., Inza, I., Sala, J., Fleisher, J. M. & Guarro, J. (1999). Prevalence of *Salmonella* serotypes in environmental waters and their relationships with indicator organisms. *Antonie van Leeuwenhoek*, Vol. 75, pp. 285-292, ISSN 0003-6072.

Poppe, C. (2000). *Salmonella* infections in the domestic fowl. In: Salmonella *in Domestic Animals*, Wray, C. & Wray A. (Eds), pp. 107-132, CAB International Publishing, ISBN 0851992617, Oxon, UK.

Pui, C. F.; Wong, W. C., Chai, L. C., Tunung, R., Jeyaletchumi, P., Noor Hidayah, M. S., Ubong, A., Farinazleen, M. G., Cheah, Y. K. & Son, R. (2011). *Salmonella*: A foodborne pathogen. *International Food Research Journal*, Vol. 18, PP. 465-473, ISSN 1985-4668.

Reche, M. P.; Jiménez, P. A., Alvarez, F., De Los Ríos, J. E. G., Rojas, A. M. & De Pedro, P. (2004). Incidence of salmonellae in captive and wild free-living raptorial birds. *Journal of Veterinary Medicine B*, Vol. 50, pp. 42-44, ISSN 1439-0450.

Refsum, T.; Handeland, K., Baggesen, D. L., Holstad, G. & Kapperud, G. (2002). Salmonellae in avian wildlife in Norway from 1969 to 2000. *Applied and Environmental Microbiology*, Vol. 68, pp. 5595-5599, ISSN 0099-2240.

Roszak, D. B.; Grimes, D. J. & Colwell, R. R. (1984). Viable butnonrecoverable stage of *Salmonella enteritidis* in aquatic systems. *Canadian Journal of Microbiology*, Vol. 30, pp. 334-338, ISSN 0008-4166.

Rusin, P.; Enriquez, C. E., Johnson, D. & Gerba, C. P. (2000). Environmentally transmitted diseases. In: *Environmental Microbiology*, Maier, R. M., Pepper, I. L. & Gerba, C. P. (Eds), pp. 447-489, Academic Press, ISBN 0-12-497570-4, London, UK.

Sato, Y.; Mori, T., Koyama, T. & Nagas, H. (2000). *Salmonella* Virchow infection in an infant transmitted by household dogs. *Journal of Veterinary Medical Science*, Vol. 62, pp. 767-769, ISSN 0916-7250.

Sahlström, L.; Aspan, A., Bagge, E., Danielsson-Tham, M. -L. & Albihn, A. (2004). Bacterial pathogens in sludge from Swedish sewage treatment plants. *Water Research*, Vol. 38, pp. 1989-1994, ISSN 0043-1354.

Sahlström, L.; de Jong, B. & Aspen, A. (2006). *Salmonella* isolated in sewage sludge traced back to human cases of salmonellosis. *Letters in Applied Microbiology*, Vol. 43, pp. 46-52, ISSN 0266-8254.

Schlundt, J.; Toyofuku, H. Jansen, J. & Herbst, S. A. (2004). Emerging food-borne zoonoses. *Revue Scientifique et Technique Office International des Epizooties*, Vol. 23, pp. 513-533, ISSN 0253-1933.

Schröter, M.; Roggentin, P., Hofmann, J., Speicher, A., Laufs, R. & Mack, D. (2004). Pet snakes as a reservoir for *Salmonella enterica* subsp. Diarizonae (serogroup IIIb): a prospective study. *Applied and Environmental Microbiology*, Vol. 70, pp. 613-615, ISSN 0099-2240.

Scott, E. & Bloomfield, S. F. (1990). The survival and transfere of microbial contamination via cloths, hands and utensils. *Journal of Applied Bacteriology*, Vol. 68, pp. 271-278, ISSN 0021-8847.

Seepersadsingh, N. & Adesiyun, A. A. (2003). Prevalence and antimicrobial resistance of *Salmonella* spp. in pet mammals, reptiles, fish aquarium water, and birds in Trinidad. *Journal of Veterinary Medicine B*, Vol. 50, pp. 488-493, ISSN 0931-1793.

Setti, I; Rodriguez-Castro, A., Pata, M. P., Cadarso-Suarez, C., Yacoubi, B., Bensamel, L., Moukrim, A. & Martinez-Urtaza, J. (2009). Characteristics and dynamics of *Salmonella* contamination along the coast of Agadir, Morocco. *Applied and Environmental Microbiology*, Vol. 75, pp. 7700-7709, ISSN 0099-2240.

Sharma, A. & Rajput, S. (1996) *Salmonella* as an index of pollution of fresh-water environments. *Environmental Monitoring and Assessment*, Vol. 41, pp. 67-76, ISSN 1573-2959.

Shellenbarger, G. G.; Athearn, N. D., Takekawa, J. Y. & Boehm, A. B. (2008). Fecal indicator bacteria and *Salmonella* in ponds managed as bird habitat, San Francisco Bay, California, USA. *Water Research*, Vol. 42, pp. 2921-2930, ISSN 0043-1354.

Simental, L. & Martinez-Urtaza, J. (2008). Climate patterns governing the presence and permanence of salmonellae in coastal areas of Bahia de Todos Santos, Mexico. *Applied and Environmental Microbiology*, Vol. 74, pp. 5918-5924, ISSN 0099-2240.

Simpson, V. R. (2002). Wild animals as reservoir of infectious diseases in the UK. *The Veterinary Journal*, Vol. 163, pp. 128-146, ISSN 1090-0233.

Sinton, L.; Hall, C. & Braithwaite, R. (2007). Sunlight inactivation of *Campylobacter jejuni* and *Salmonella enterica*, compared with *Escherichia coli*, in seawater and river water. *Journal of Water and Health*, Vol. 5, pp. 357-365, ISSN 1477-9820.

Skova, M. N.; Spencer, A. G., Hald, B., Petersen, L., Nauerby, B., Carstensen, B. & Madsen, M. (2004). The role of litter beetles as potential reservoir for *Salmonella enterica* and thermophilic *Campylobacter* spp. between broiler flocks. *Avian Diseases*, Vol. 48, pp. 9-18, ISSN 0005-2086.

Smith, R. J.; Newton, A. T., Harwood, C. R. & Barer, M. R. (2002). Ative but nonculturable cells of *Salmonella eterica* serovar Typhimurium do not infect or colonize mice. *Microbiology*, Vol. 148, pp. 2717-2726, ISSN 1350-0872.

Stenstrom, T. A. (1989). Bacterial hydrophobicity, an overall parameter for the measurement of adhesion potential to soil particles. *Applied and Environmental Microbiology*, Vol. 55, pp. 142-147, ISSN 0099-2240.

Suk-Kyung, L.; Byun, J. –R., Nam, H. – M., Lee, H. –S. & Jung, S. – C. (2011). Phenotypic and genotypic characterization of *Salmonella* spp. isolated from pigs and their farm environment in Korea. *Journal of Microbiology and Biotechnology*, Vol. 21, pp. 50-54, ISSN 1017-7825.

Tanaka, C.; Miyazawa, T., Watari, M. & Ishiguro, N. (2005). Bacteriological survey of feces from feral pigeons in Japan. *Journal of Veterinary Medical Science*, Vol. 67, pp. 951-953, ISSN 1347-7439.

Threlfall, E. J. (2002). Antimicrobial drug resistance in *Salmonella*: problems and perspective in food- and water-borne infections. *FEMS Microbiology Reviews*, Vol. 26, pp. 141-148, ISSN 0168-6445.

Timbury, M. C.; McCartney, A. C., Thakker, B. & Ward, K. K. (2002). *Notes on Medical Microbiology*, Churchill Livingstone, ISBN 0-443-07164-0, London, UK.

Tizard, I. (2004). Salmonellosis in wild birds. *Seminars in Avian and Exotic Pet Medicine*, Vol. 13, pp. 50-66, ISSN 1055-937X.

Tsai, H. -J. & Hsiang, P. -H. (2005). The prevalence and antimicrobial susceptibilities of *Salmonella* and *Campylobacter* in ducks in Taiwan. *Journal of Veterinary Medical Science*, Vol. 67, pp. 7-12, ISSN 1347-7439.

Tsiodras, S.; Kelesidis, T., Kelesidis, I., Bauchinger, U. & Falagas, M. E. (2008) Human infections associated with wild birds. *Journal of Infection*, Vol. 56, pp. 83-98, ISSN 0163-4453.

Uyanik, M. H.; Yazgi, H. & Ayyildiz, A. (2008). Survival of *Salmonella typhi* and *Shigella flexneri* in different water samples and at different temperatures. *Turkish Journal of Medical Science*, Vol. 38, pp. 307-310, ISSN 1300-0144.

Van Donsel, D. J. & Geldreich, E. E. (1971). Relationships of salmonellae to fecal coliforms in bottom sediments. *Water Research*, Vol. 5, pp. 1079-1087, ISSN 0043-1354.

Van Immerseel, F.; Pasmans, F., De Buck, J., Rychlik, I., Hradecka, H., Collard, J. -M, Wildemauwe, C., Heyndrickx, M., Ducatelle, R. & Haesebrouck, F. (2004). Cats as a risk for transmission of antimicrobial drug-resistant *Salmonella*. *Emerging Infectious Diseases*, Vol. 10, pp. 2169-2174, ISSN 1080-6059.

Venglovsky, J.; Martinez, J. & Placha, I. (2006). Hygienic and ecological risks connected with utilization of animal manures and biosolids in agriculture. *Livestock Science*, Vol. 102, pp. 197-203, ISSN 1871-1413.

Vlahović, K.; Matica, B., Bata, I., Pavlak, M., Pavičić, Ž., Popović, M., Nejedli, S. & Dovč, A. (2004). *Campylobacter*, *Salmonella* and *Chlamydia* in free-living birds of Croatia. *European Journal of Wildlife Research*, Vol. 50, pp. 127-132, ISSN 1612-4642.

Warwick, C.; Lambiris, A. J. L., Westwood, D. & Steedman, C. (2001). Reptile-related salmonellosis. *Journal of the Royal Society of Medicine*, Vol. 94, pp. 124-126, ISSN 0141-0768.

Weichart, D.; Oliver, J. D. & Kjelleberg, S. (1992). Low temperature induce non-culturability and killing of *Vibrio vulnificus*. *FEMS Microbiology Letters*, Vol. 100, pp. 205-210, ISSN 0378-1097.

Weinstein, J. W.; Seltzer, E. G. & Nelson, R. S. (1995). Reptile-associated salmonellosis-selected states. *Morbidity and Mortalitiy Weekley Report*, Vol. 44, pp. 347-350, ISSN 0149-2195.

Winfield, M. & Groisman, E. A. (2003). Role of nonhost environment in the lifestyles of *Salmonella* and *Escherichia coli*. *Applied and Environmental Microbiology*, Vol. 69, pp. 3687-3694, ISSN 0099-2240.

Woodward, D. L.; Khakhria, R. & Johnson, W. M. (1997). Human salmonellosis associated with exotic pets. *Journal of Clinical Microbiology*, Vol. 35, pp. 2786-2790, ISSN 0095-1137.

Wray, C. & Davies, R. H. (2000). *Salmonella* infections in cattle. In: Salmonella *in Domestic Animals*, Wray, C. & Wray A. (Eds), pp. 169-190, CAB International Publishing, ISBN 0851992617, Oxon, UK.

Wray, C. & Linklater, K. A. (2000). *Salmonella* infections in sheep. In: Salmonella *in Domestic Animals*, Wray, C. & Wray A. (Eds), pp. 209-218, CAB International Publishing, ISBN 0851992617, Oxon, UK.

Yokoyama, E.; Maruyama, S., Kabeya, H., Hara, S., Sata, S., Kuroki, T. & Yamamoto, T. (2007). Prevalence and genetic properities *Salmonella enterica* serovar Typhimurium definitive phage type 104 isolated from *Rattus norvegicus* and *Rattus rattus* house rats in Yokohama city, Japan. *Applied and Environmental Microbiology*, Vol. 73, pp. 2624-2630, ISSN 0099-2240.

Xu, H. -S.; Roberts, N., Singleton, F. L., Attwell, R. W., Grimes, D. J. & Colwell, R. R. (1982). Survival and viability of nonculturable *Escherichia coli* and *Vibrio cholerae* in the estuarine and marine environment. *Microbial Ecology*, Vol. 8, pp. 313-323, ISSN 0095-3628.

Zhao, S.; Datta, A. R., Ayers, S., Friedman, S., Walker, R. D. & White, D. G. (2003). Antimicrobial-resistant *Salmonella* serovars isolated from imported foods. *International Journal of Food Microbiology*, Vol. 84, pp. 87-92, ISSN 0168-1605.

3

Prevalence, Detection and Antimicrobial Resistance Pattern of *Salmonella* in Sudan

Adil A. El Hussein[1,*], Halima S. Mohy-Eldin[1],
Mayha M. Nor Elmadiena[2] and Marmar A. El Siddig[1]
[1]*Botany Dept., Faculty of Science, University of Khartoum*
[2]*University of Medical Sciences and Technology*
Sudan

1. Introduction

Infectious microbial diseases constitute a major cause of death in many parts of the world, particularly in developing countries. *Salmonella* has been identified as an important food and water-borne pathogen that can infect human and animals resulting in significant morbidity and mortality (Akkina et al., 1999). *Salmonella* is a facultative anaerobe, Gram-negative rod-shaped, 2 - 3 x 0.4 - 0.6 µm in size and motile by peritrichous flagella except for *S.* Gallinarum and *S.* Pullorum which are immotile. Members of the genus have a % G+C content of 50-53. They are urease and Voges-Proskauer negative and citrate utilizing (Montville and Matthews, 2008).

Salmonellae are typically non-lactose, non-sucrose fermenting but are able to ferment glucose, maltose and mannitol with the production of acid only as in the case of *S.* Typhi and acid with H_2S in the case of *S.* Paratyphi and for most other *Salmonella* serovars (Cruickshank, 1975). Optimum temperature for growth is in the range of 35 - 37°C but some can grow at temperatures as high as 54°C and as low as 2°C (Gray & Fedorka-Cray, 2002). *Salmonella* grow in a pH range of 4 - 9 with the optimum being 6.5 - 7.5. They require high water activity for growth (> 0.94) but can survive at a_w of < 0.2 such as in dried foods. Inhibition of growth occurs at temperatures < 7°C, pH < 3.8 or a_w < 0.94 (Hanes, 2003).

Based on differences in 16S rRNA sequence data, the genus *Salmonella* is divided into two species: *S. enterica* and *S. bongori*. *S. enterica* is further divided into six subspecies: subspecies *enterica, salamae, arizonae, diarizonae, houtenae* and subspecies *indica* (Popoff & Minor, 2001). Kauffmann-White scheme classifies members of *Salmonella* species according to three major antigenic determinants composed of somatic (O-antigens), flagellar (H-) and virulence (K-) antigens. Agglutination by antibodies specific for the various O-antigens, groups the salmonellae into six serogroups: A, B, C_1, C_2, D and E. Rarely cross reactivity between O-antigens of *Salmonella* and other genera of Enterobacteriaceae do occur. Therefore further classification of serotypes is based on the highly specific H-antigens (Scherer & miller, 2001). H-antigens can be expressed in one of two phases: phase 1 H-antigens are serovar specific while phase 2 antigens are not. However K-antigens are produced by serovars that are

* Corresponding Author

characterized by extracellular polysaccharide capsules (Hu & Kopecko, 2003; Yousef & Carlstrom, 2003). Currently, Kauffmann-White scheme recognizes 2610 *Salmonella* serovars, the majority (2587) belongs to *S. enterica* while the remaining (23 serovars) are assigned to *S. bongori* (Guibourdenche et al., 2010).

The incidence of typhoid salmonellosis is stable, with comparatively few cases in developing countries. Cases of typhoid salmonellosis are estimated to be in the range of 16-17 million resulting in about 600,000 deaths annually (Pang et al., 1995). However, cases of non-typhoid salmonellosis are increasing worldwide. The World Health Organization (WHO) estimates 1.3 billion cases with 3 million deaths annually. Data on salmonellosis cannot be ascertained in most developing countries because many patients with acute gastroenteritis do not visit a health care provider or do not submit a specimen for laboratory testing (Portillo, 2000; Hanes, 2003; Hu & Kopecko, 2003). An unpublished data of Sudan Ministry of Health indicated that the incidence of salmonellosis has markedly increased. In 2004 these were 43,144 cases and 68 deaths in different hospitals. However, a more accurate figure of salmonellosis is difficult to determine because only large outbreaks are investigated whereas sporadic cases are under-reported.

Since *Salmonella* is closely related to both human and animal health, more rapid and sensitive methods for the identification of this bacterium are required (Schrank et al., 2001). In the regions where enteric fever is common, clinical diagnosis of typhoid fever is inadequate, as the symptoms it causes are non-specific and overlap with those of other febrile illness. Serological tests, predominantly the Widal test, are available but have very low sensitivity and specificity, and no practical value in endemic areas despite their continued use (Levine et al., 1978). Isolation of the causative organism remains the most effective diagnostic method in suspected typhoid fever (Zhou & Pollard, 2010). Standard culture methods for detecting *Salmonella* spp. include non-selective pre-enrichment followed by selective enrichment and plating on selective and differential media (Whyte et al., 2002). These methods take approximately 4-7 days (Harvey & Price, 1979; Perales & Audicana, 1989), so they are considered laborious and time consuming.

In a clinical setting, suspected Enterobacteriaceae are often subjected to biochemical testing to investigate the ability of an isolate to grow upon certain substrates, produce various metabolic products or alter the pH. In the 1970s, efforts were being made to collect together multiple biochemical tests to allow rapid and relatively high throughput identification of clinical bacterial isolates (Lindberg et al., 1974). Numerous test kits of varying accuracy became available for the identification of the Enterobacteriaceae. The API 20E system (BioMérieux, France) was found to be the most reliable, having a 99% correlation with standard biochemical tests and a 94% identification rate (Nord et al., 1974). Over 60 bacterial species can currently be identified with the API20E, with identification extending to the serovar level for Typhi and Paratyphi A among others. However, results of such tests are open to interpretation and require experience and a high level of technical skill to generate reproducible results (Jamshidi et al., 2007). Therefore, several alternative faster methods for the detection of *Salmonella* have been suggested.

Molecular methods have been applied in the identification of *Salmonella* and were found to be very useful in differentiating between species. These methods include pulsed field gel electrophoresis (PFGE) (Mohand et al., 1999; Nair et al., 1994), IS200 fingerprinting (Ezquerra et al., 1993), PCR ribotyping (Lagatolla et al., 1996), ribosomal DNA intergenic spacer amplification and heteroduplex analysis (Jensen and Hubner, 1996), amplification fragment length polymorphism (Aarts et al., 1998; Nair et al., 2000), automated nuclease PCR assay (Hoorfar et al., 2000) and random amplification of polymorphic DNA (RAPD) (Shangkuan and Lin, 1998). Since all molecular techniques are based on variability of microbial chromosomes or plasmids, then DNA sequencing would appear to be the best approach for differentiating subtypes (Liebana et al., 2001)

Many oligonucleotide primer sets have been described for the detection of *Salmonella* using the PCR technique. These primers include those associated with the invasion genes *inv*A and *inv*E (Stone et al., 1994), histidine transport operon *hit*J (Cohen et al., 1993), *SPI*1 invasion gene *hil*A (Guo et al., 2000), virulence plasmid gene *spv* (Gulig et al., 1993), virulence gene *sip*C (Sharma and Carlson, 2000), enterotoxin gene *stn* (Makino et al., 1999), *omp*C (Amavisit et al., 2001), *spa*Q (Kurowski et al., 2002), *ori*C (Widjojoatmodjo et al., 1992), *fim*A (Swenson et al., 1991), 16S rRNA (Lin and Tsen, 1996), *iro*B (Bäumler et al., 1998) and a repetitive DNA fragment (Jitrapakdee et al., 1995). Recent studies described a serotype-specific PCR method for differentiating *Salmonella* Pullorum from other serotypes using the *rfb*S gene (Desai et al., 2005). Most researchers agree that in the future more serotype-specific PCR assays will be developed.

Resistance of infectious microorganisms to commonly prescribed antibiotics has emerged and spread in both developed and developing countries (Zhao et al., 2003; Ahmed et al., 2000; Grob et al., 1998). This imposes serious constraints on the options available for the treatment of many infections (Kunin et al., 1990). In the case of salmonellae, resistance to tetracyclines or chloramphenicol was first reported in 1961 (Ramsey and Edwards, 1961). Since then, reports on salmonellae resistance to one or more antibiotics have increased substantially and resistance has emerged even to newer more potent antimicrobial agents (Montville and Matthews, 2008; Piddock, 2002). In addition, multidrug resistance in *Salmonella* has become a public health concern (Crump and Mintz, 2010; Asai et al., 2010; Singh et al., 2010).

In the Sudan, as in most other developing countries, resistance and multiple resistance to antimicrobial agents among members of Enterobacteriaceae including some *Salmonella* serovars was found to increase during the last decades (Yagoub et al., 2005; Ahmed et al., 2000; Hassan, 1985, Shears et al., 1988; Musa and Shears, 1998). The sensitivity of *Salmonella* Typhi, *S.* Paratyphi A and *S.* Paratyphi B to ten antibiotics was examined in Sudan (Ahmed et al., 2000). The examined strains were sensitive to all drugs tested except for one *S.* Typhi strain which was resistant to cotrimaxazole; tetracycline and sulfonamide and one *S.* Paratyphi A which was resistant to tetracycline. The sensitivity of *Salmonella* Paratyphi A and *S.* Paratyphi B which were isolated from Sudanese white cheese was tested against 9 antibiotics (Yagoub et al., 2006). ciprofloxacin, chloramphenicol and ofloxacin were the most effective drugs against the tested isolates. The resistance was more frequent to ampicillin, tetracycline, penicillin, gentamicin and co-trimoxazole.

Due to the indiscriminate and injudicious use of antibiotics in human and veterinary medicine as well as for the promotion of growth in food animals, *Salmonella* strains resistant to first line antibiotics will continue to develop at an increasing rate. Therefore updated knowledge of *Salmonella* serotypes resistance patterns is important for the proper selection and use of antimicrobial drugs and for the development of appropriate prescribing policies.

1.2 History of *Salmonella* research in Sudan

In Sudan, the prevalence of *Salmonella* serovars is not well documented, as salmonellae are not routinely isolated and identified. Only a few studies have been reported by few workers.

Horgan (1947) made the first report on *Salmonella* infections in cattle. He investigated a food poisoning outbreak at Wad Madani town and isolated *Salmonella* serovar Dublin from faeces of two persons who fell sick after eating meat. Again the serovar Dublin was isolated from infected calves and from one of the apparently healthy animals (Soliman and Khan, 1959). A survey to ascertain the incidence rate of *Salmonella* infection in animals was made in Khartoum (Khan, 1970). During the survey, 230 *Salmonella* cultures were recovered from different sources belonging to 63 serotypes.

Subsequent *Salmonella* surveys which have been conducted at Khartoum and Malakal added 15 serovars to the list of Sudan. The serovars reported were: *S.* Amager, *S.* Derby, *S.* Kandle, *S.* Reading, *S.* Salford, *S.* Adelaide, *S.* Amersfoort, *S.* Bertin, *S.* Chester, *S.* Mushmar-haemek, *S.* Muenche, *S.* Muensters, *S.* Newport, *S.* Pomona and *S.* Poona (Khan, 1970). In his attempt to assess the quality of fresh meats in Sudan, Sariy Eldin (1971) reported the occurrence of *Salmonella* Wein, *S.* Dublin, *S.* Havana, *S.* Typhimurium, *S.* Senegal and *S.* Braenderup. *S.* Dublin was also isolated from sheep liver (Salih and Ibrahim, 1972). Fifty-eight *Salmonella* strains were isolated from slaughtered chicken in Khartoum North and Omdurman (Yagoub and Mohamed, 1987). The most common serotypes reported were: *S.* Mons, *S.* Amek and *S.* Uganda. The incidence of *S.* Dublin in the mesenteric lymph nodes and faeces of sick calves in Kuku dairy cooperative farm, Omdurman and El Obeid slaughter houses was also reported (Saliem, 1987).

Forty-five *Salmonella* isolates (not serotyped) were isolated from carcasses, liver, spleen, intestinal contents of chickens from a poultry farm in El Obeid (unpublished data). The isolation of *Salmonella enterica* subspecies *enterica* serotype San-Diego from three goats (3.84%) at Omdurman Central Abattoir was reported (El Tom et al., 1999). Recently, *Salmonella* Umbadah plus 19 new serovars were reported from different sources at Khartoum (Hag Elsafi et al., 2009; El Hussein et al., 2010).

2. Materials and methods

2.1 Isolation and identification of *Salmonella*

Salmonellae were isolated and identified according to the techniques recommended by the International Organization for Standardization described by Molla et al. (2004).

For confirmation, presumptive salmonellae were subjected to biochemical tests (Macfaddin, 1980), further identified with API 20E identification kits (Bio Merieux, Marcy, France) and a slide agglutination test was employed thereafter, using a commercially available *Salmonella* polyvalent O (Denkafeiken, Japan) and H antisera (Mast Diagnostic, UK). Presumptive *Salmonella* isolates were shipped to the Public Health Agency, Office International des´ Epizooties (OI´E) Reference Laboratory for salmonellosis, Guelph, Ontario, Canada or to the Egypt Management Central Laboratory for serotyping and phage typing.

2.2 Serotyping and phage typing

For serotyping, the somatic (O) antigens of the *Salmonella* isolates were determined with the slide-agglutination test as described by Ewing (1986), whereas the flagellar (H) antigens were identified by a microtechnique (Shipp and Rowe, 1980) that uses microtitre plates (Poppe et al., 2001). The antigenic formulae of *Salmonella* serovars as listed by Popoff (2001) were used to name the serovars.

The standard phage typing technique described by Anderson and Williams (1956) was used. Strains that did not conform to any recognized phage type were considered atypical (AT). *Salmonella* Enteritidis strains were phage typed according to Ward et al. (1987) with typing phages obtained from the International Centre for Enteric Phage Typing (ICEPT), Central Public Health Laboratory, Colindale, United Kingdom via the National Laboratory for Enteric Pathogens (NLEP), Health Canada, Winnipeg, Manitoba. The phagetyping-scheme and phages for *S.* Typhimurium, developed by Callow (1959) and further extended by Anderson (1964) and Anderson et al. (1977), were obtained from the ICEPT via the NLEP.

2.3 Antimicrobial susceptibility testing

The antimicrobial resistance of the isolates was tested against ten antimicrobial agents by the agar diffusion method with Mueller Hinton agar and antibiotic disks (Hi Media), following the guidelines of the National Committee for Clinical Laboratory Standards (NCCLS, 2000). *E. coli* ATCC 25922 was used for quality control. The categories susceptible or resistant were assigned on the basis of the critical points recommended by the NCCLS (2007).

The antibiotics tested were those commonly used in poultry, animals or in human, they are in mcg/disc: tetracycline (Te) 10; gentamicin (Cn), 10; nalidixic acid (Na) 25; streptomycin (St), 25; co-trimoxazole (Cot), 25; chloramphenicol (C), 30; ciprofloxacin (Cip), 5; ampicillin (Amp), 25; norfluxacin, (Nor), 10 and apramycin (Apr), 15.

2.4 Plasmid profiling analysis

For each isolate a single colony was grown overnight in 1ml LB media at 37°C. The bacterial cells were harvested by centrifugation for 30s in a micro-centrifuge (Sanyo), the supernatant was discarded and the pellet was subjected to Plasmid DNA extraction according to alkaline - detergent method (Dillon et al., 1985). The plasmids extracted were stored at -20°C till used for further analysis. Later, the extracted plasmid for each isolate was analyzed electrophoretically on a 0.8% agarose gel. The gel was then exposed to ultraviolet transillumination and photographed in a gel documentation system (Model GAS Uvitec. Product). One Kb DNA ladder (Invitrogen, Germany) was also used to determine the plasmids sizes.

2.5 Specificity of PCR primer sets

Ten specific primer sets (Invitrogen, Germany) each targeting a different gene were evaluated for their specificity and sensitivity to detect locally isolated *Salmonella* serovars. DNA from each *Salmonella* serovar and non-*Salmonella* strain was extracted according to the boiling - centrifugation method (Soumet et al., 1994). A single colony of a pure nutrient agar culture was grown overnight at 37°C in 1ml Luria - Bertani broth. Bacterial cells were precipitated by centrifugation at 13,000 rpm for 5min in a micro-centrifuge (MSE, MSBo1o.cx2.5, Sanyo, UK). The supernatant was discarded and the pellet was re-suspended in 500µl deionized distilled water. The suspension was boiled for 10min in a water bath then immediately cooled on ice. Extracted DNA was then stored refrigerated at 4oC until used as a template for PCR amplification.

The extracted chromosomal DNA was amplified by an established PCR technique (Sambrook et al., 1989). PCR amplification reactions were carried out in 25 µl total volume of PCR mixture containing 5 µl of template DNA, 12.5µl of the PCR master mix (Promega) (50 unit/ml Taq DNA polymerase in an appropriate reaction buffer {pH 8.5}, 400 µM each dNTPs and 3mM MgCl2) and 0.1 µM of each of primer pair. DNA was amplified according to reaction conditions published for each primer pair in a thermal cycler (Techne/ Flexigene - biotech).

Appearance of the target band specified for each primer set on the 1.2% agarose gel under specified gel electrophoresis conditions is considered as a positive amplification product.

2.6 Sensitivity of PCR primers

To determine the sensitivity of each PCR primer set, a single colony of a pure culture of *Salmonella* Typhi was grown overnight at 37ºC in 10ml Luria - Bertani broth. After incubation for 24 hours ten-fold dilutions (10 to 10-9) of the broth culture were made. The viable cell count in each dilution was determined using plate count media. For each mixture 100µl was cultured immediately in a plate count media (Somasegaran and Hoben, 1985; Vincent, 1970). The cultures were incubated overnight at 37ºC. The numbers of formed colonies were then counted (each colony is considered to be formed by a single cell). The DNA from each dilution was extracted as previously described and was used as a PCR template for each primer set.

3. Results

3.1 Prevalence

Out of 1921 collected and examined samples; 833 (43.4%) belonged to poultry, 680 (35.4%) to food items, 224 (11.7%) to human faeces, 107 (5.6%) to chlorinated drinking water and 77 (4%) to food animal faeces (Table 1). In Total, 213 (11.09%) *Salmonella* strains belonging to 54 different serovars were isolated. Of these, 210 were members of *S. enterica* subspecies *enterica*,

Source	Total Samples Examined	Total +ve samples	% from Source	% from +ve samples	% from total examined
Food	680	32	4.7	15.0	1.7
Poultry	833	70	8.4	32.8	3.6
Water	107	10	9.3	4.7	0.5
Animal faeces	77	8	10.4	3.8	0.4
Human Faeces from handlers	224	93	41.5	43.7	4.8
Total	1921	213	-	100	11.09

Table 1. Number and percentage of *Salmonella* isolated from food, poultry, water, animal faeces and human

Serogroup	No. of Serovars	Serovars	Phagetype	Source					Total	%
				Food	Poultry	Water	Animal Faeces	Human Faeces		
S. *enterica*	52									
O:4(B)	15	Limete		0	0	0	0	2	2	0.94
		Stanleyville		5	12	0	1	0	18	8.45
		Sarajane		0	0	0	0	1	1	0.47
		Massenya		0	0	0	0	2	2	0.94
		Tudu		0	0	0	0	1	1	0.47
		Ituri		0	0	0	0	2	2	0.94
		Lagos		0	0	0	0	3	3	1.41
		Java		0	0	0	0	2	2	0.94
		Typhimurium	2	2	1	3	0	1	7	3.29
		Schwarzengrund		0	0	0	0	2	2	0.94
		Agona		0	0	0	1	5	6	2.82
		Stanley		0	0	0	0	2	2	0.94
		I:4,12:eh:-		0	0	0	1	0	1	0.47
		Paratyphi B		0	0	0	0	6	6	2.82
		Dragona		0	0	0	1	0	1	0.47
Total				**7**	**13**	**3**	**4**	**29**	**56**	**26.29**
O:7(C_1)	12	Menden		0	0	0	0	3	3	1.41
		Isangi		0	0	0	0	2	2	0.94
		Inganda		0	0	0	0	2	2	0.94
		Edinburg		0	0	0	0	4	4	1.88
		Montevideo		0	0	0	0	3	3	1.41
		Kisii		0	0	0	0	2	2	0.94
		Virchow		1	9	0	0	0	10	4.69
		Mbandaka		0	1	0	0	0	1	0.47
		Rissen		0	2	0	0	0	2	0.94
		Livingstone		5	0	2	0	1	8	3.76
		Infantis		0	0	0	0	2	2	0.94
		I:6,7:-:enz		1	0	0	0	0	1	0.47
Total				**7**	**12**	**2**	**0**	**19**	**40**	**18.78**

Serogroup	No. of Serovars	Serovars	Phagetype	Source					Total	%
				Food	Poultry	Water	Animal Faeces	Human Faeces		
S. *enterica*	52									
$O:3,10(E_1)$	7	Kalina		0	0	0	0	5	5	2.35
		Lexington		0	0	0	0	2	2	0.94
		Okerara		0	0	0	0	3	3	1.41
		Amoundernes		0	0	0	0	1	1	0.47
		Muenster		0	3	0	0	0	3	1.41
		Uganda		0	0	0	2	0	2	0.94
		Meleagridis		0	0	0	0	1	1	0.47
Total				**0**	**3**	**0**	**2**	**12**	**17**	**7.98**
$O:8(C_2)$	5	Albany		0	0	0	0	3	3	1.41
		Blockley		4	6	0	0	0	10	4.69
		Kentucky		0	17	0	0	2	19	8.92
		Hadar		0	6	0	0	0	6	2.82
		Molade		2	2	5	0	0	9	4.23
Total				**6**	**31**	**5**	**0**	**5**	**47**	**22.07**
O:40(R)	3	II (formarly Ottershaw)		0	0	0	0	2	2	0.94
		Saugus		0	0	0	0	3	3	1.41
		Johannesburg		0	0	0	0	3	3	1.41
Total				**0**	**0**	**0**	**0**	**8**	**8**	**3.76**
$O:1,3,19(E_4)$	2	Senftenburg		4	0	0	0	3	7	3.29
		Umbadah		0	0	0	2	0	2	0.94
Total				**4**	**0**	**0**	**2**	**3**	**9**	**4.23**
O:13(G)	2	Havana		0	2	0	0	0	2	0.94
		Poona		0	3	0	0	0	3	1.41
Total				**0**	**5**	**0**	**0**	**0**	**5**	**2.35**
O:35(O)	2	Alachua		1	6	0	0	0	7	3.29
		Adelaide		4	0	0	0	0	4	1.88
Total				**5**	**6**	**0**	**0**	**0**	**11**	**5.16**

Serogroup	No. of Serovars	Serovars	Phagetype	Source					Total	%
				Food	Poultry	Water	Animal Faeces	Human Faeces		
S. enterica	**52**									
O:9(D$_1$)	2	Enteritidis	21a, Atypical	2	0	0	0	4	6	2.82
		Typhi		0	0	0	0	9	9	4.23
Total				**2**	**0**	**0**	**0**	**13**	**15**	**7.04**
Other	2	I:rough-O:z29:-		0	0	0	0	1	1	0.47
		I:Rough-O:I,z13:1,5		1	0	0	0	0	1	0.47
Total				**1**	**0**	**0**	**0**	**1**	**2**	**0.94**
subsp. *salamae*	1	S. salamae		0	0	0	0	2	2	0.94
subsp. *arizonae*	1	S. arizonae		0	0	0	0	1	1	0.47
Total				**0**	**0**	**0**	**0**	**3**	**3**	**1.41**
Overall Total				32	70	10	8	93	213	100.00

Table 2. Prevalence of *Salmonella* serovars in different sources

two were *S. enterica* subspecies *salamae* and one belonged to subspecies *arizonae*. Serovars of *S. enterica* subsp. *enterica* reported here belonged to 10 serogroups as shown in Table 2. Serogroups B (56 isolates), C_1 (40 isolates), E_1 (17 isolates), C_2 (47 isolates) and R (8 isolates) were each represented by 15, 12, 7, 5 and 3 different serovars, respectively. The remaining serogroups (E_4, G, O, D_1 and other) were represented by two serovars each. The predominant serovars were: Kentucky (8.9%), Stanleyville (8.4%), Blockley and Virchow (each 4.7%), Molade and Typhi (each 4.2%), Livingstone (3.8%), Typhimurium, Senftenberg and Alachua (each 3.3%) and serovars Hadar, Agona, Paratyphi B and Enteritidis (2.8% each). The remaining 38 serovars were represented each by less than six isolates. S. Typhimurium isolates were phagetype 2 while five of S. Enteritidis isolates were 21a phenotype and one was an Atypical phenotype.

Table 2 shows that the serovar Typhimurium was isolated from four of five sources examined whereas Stanleyville, Livingstone and Molade were isolated from three of the Sources. The remaining serovars were isolated each from two or only one source. The most common serovar of the poultry isolates (n=70) was *S*. Kentucky (24.3%) followed by Stanleyville (17.1%), Virchow (12.9%) and Blockley, Hadar and Alachua (8.6% each). *S*. Typhi (9 isolates) was the most common (9.7%) serovar among human faeces isolates (n=93) followed by Paratyphi B (6.5%), Agona and Kalina (5.4 % each). Among the food isolates (n=32) *S*. Stanleyville and Livingstone were the most common (15.6%) with 5 isolates each. The most common serovars among water isolates (n=10) and animal faeces isolates (n=8) were *S*. Molade (50%) and Uganda (25%), respectively. To the best of our knowledge, 21 of the serovars reported here were isolated for the first time in Sudan and were all from human source only. These included: *S*. Stanley, Okerara, Sarajane, Limete, Massenya, Edinburg, Isangi, Inganda, Java, Alabany, Kalina, Tudu, Ottershaw, Saugus, Amoundrenes, Lexington, Kisii, Ituri, Lagos, salamae and arizonae.

3.2 Antimicrobial resistance and plasmid analysis

Results in Table 3 show that the highest frequency of resistance observed was to streptomycin (41.3%) followed by tetracycline (31.9%), gentamycin (28.2%), ampicillin (25.4%), nalidixic acid (22.1%), co-trimoxazole (17.4%), ciprofloxacin (8.9%), chloramphenicol (8%), norfloxacin (7.5%) and apramycin (5.6%). All isolates of the serovars Tudu, Montevideo, Meleagridis, Johannesburg, Umbadah, Poona, Kisii and one Rough isolate which were found infrequently (n ranging from 1-3) were susceptible to all of the antibiotics tested. Out of the 37 isolates which showed resistance against co-trimoxazole, 27 (73%) belonged to the serovars Sanleyville (11/18 isolates), Virchow (10/10 isolates) and Typhi (6/9 isolates). Similarly, out of the 68 tetracycline-resistant isolates, 40 (58.8%) belonged to the serovars Stanleyville, Virchow, Blockley and Kentucky, each contributing by 10 isolates. Isolates of S. Blockley (n=10) were all resistant to tetracycline but were fully sensitive to co-trimoxazole, chloramphenicol, ciprofloxacin, ampicillin, norfloxacin and apramycin. All *S*. Kentucky isolates (n=19) were resistant to nalidixic acid but fully sensitive to chloramphenicol. Of the 22 isolates belonging to *S*. Typhi (9), Paratyphi B (6) and Typhimurium (7), 14 were resistant to ampicillin, 6 to gentamycin, 4 to chloramphenicol and 3 to each of ciprofloxacin and nalidixic acid but none to norfloxacin.

Serovar	Antibiotics									
	Te	Cn	Na	St	Cot	C	Cip	Amp	Nor	Apr
Limete (n=2)	1	2	1	2	0	0	1	0	1	1
Stanleyville (n=19)	10	0	1	1	11	0	0	7	0	0
Sarajane (n=1)	1	0	0	0	0	1	0	0	1	0
Massenya (n=2)	2	0	0	0	0	2	2	0	0	0
Tudu (n=1)	0	0	0	0	0	0	0	0	0	0
Ituri (n=2)	0	2	0	2	0	0	0	0	0	0
Lagos (n=3)	0	0	0	3	0	0	0	0	0	0
Java (n=2)	0	2	1	2	0	0	1	0	0	0
Typhimurium (n=7)	0	1	0	1	0	0	0	3	0	2
Schwarzengrund (n=2)	0	0	0	1	0	0	0	0	0	0
Agona (n=6)	0	2	0	0	0	0	0	2	2	2
Stanley (n=2)	2	2	0	2	0	0	0	0	0	0
I:4,12:eh:- (n=1)	1	0	0	0	0	0	0	0	0	0
Paratyphi (n=6)	1	3	1	6	3	1	1	5	0	0
Dragona new variant (n=1)	1	0	0	1	0	0	0	0	0	0
Menden (n=3)	0	0	1	1	0	1	1	2	1	0
Isangi (n=2)	2	1	1	1	0	2	1	2	0	0
Inganda (n=2)	1	2	0	2	0	1	0	2	1	0
Edinburg (n=4)	2	4	0	4	0	4	1	4	1	0
Montevideo (n=3)	0	0	0	0	0	0	0	0	0	0
Kisii (n=2)	0	0	0	0	0	0	0	0	0	0
Virchow (n=10)	10	0	10	0	10	0	0	0	0	0
Mbandaka (n=1)	0	1	1	0	0	0	0	0	0	0
Rissen (n=2)	0	1	1	2	1	0	0	0	0	0
Livingstone (n=8)	0	5	7	2	0	0	0	2	0	0
Infantis (n=2)	2	0	0	0	0	0	0	2	0	0
I:6,7:-:enz (n=1)	1	0	0	0	1	0	0	0	0	0
Kalina (n=5)	0	5	0	5	0	0	0	0	0	2
Lexington (n=2)	0	0	0	1	0	0	0	0	0	0
Okerara (n=3)	0	0	0	3	0	0	0	0	0	0
Amoundernes (n=1)	0	1	0	1	0	0	0	0	0	0
Muenster (n=3)	0	0	0	1	0	0	0	0	0	0
Uganda (n=2)	1	0	0	0	0	0	0	0	0	0

Serovar	Antibiotics									
	Te	Cn	Na	St	Cot	C	Cip	Amp	Nor	Apr
Meleagridis (n=1)	0	0	0	0	0	0	0	0	0	0
Albany (n=3)	0	3	0	2	0	1	2	1	2	1
Blockley (n=10)	10	1	1	1	0	0	0	0	0	0
Kentucky (n=19)	10	12	19	12	1	0	6	6	6	1
Hadar (n=6)	0	0	0	6	0	0	0	3	0	0
Molade (n=9)	3	0	0	3	3	0	0	2	0	0
II (formarly Ottershaw) (n=2)	0	0	0	2	0	0	0	0	0	0
Saugus (n=3)	0	0	0	3	0	0	0	0	0	0
Johannesburg (n=3)	0	0	0	0	0	0	0	0	0	0
Senftenberg (n=7)	0	1	0	0	0	0	0	0	0	1
Umbadah (n=2)	0	0	0	0	0	0	0	0	0	0
Havana (n=2)	2	0	0	0	1	0	0	0	0	0
Poona (n=3)	0	0	0	0	0	0	0	0	0	0
Alachua (n=7)	0	0	0	1	0	0	0	2	0	0
Adelaide (n=4)	0	1	0	1	0	0	0	0	0	1
Enteritidis (n=5)	0	3	0	3	0	1	1	2	1	1
Typhi (n=9)	5	2	2	7	6	3	2	6	0	0
I:rough-O:z29:- (n=1)	0	0	0	0	0	0	0	0	0	0
I:Rough-O:I,z13:1,5 (n=1)	0	0	0	0	0	0	0	1	0	0
S. salamae (n=2)	0	2	0	2	0	0	0	0	0	0
S. arizonae (n=1)	0	1	0	1	0	0	0	0	0	0
Total of resistant isolates	68	60	79	54	37	18	15	54	16	12

Table 3. Number of isolates in different serovars resistant to different antibiotics

There were 164 *Salmonella* isolates belonging to 46 serovars exhibited 55 different resistance patterns. A percentage of 23.5 (50/213) of the isolates displayed a single type of resistance, 17.8% (38/213) showed resistance to two classes of antibiotics (data not shown) and 35.7% (76/213) were multidrug-resistant (resistant to more than two antimicrobials). Resistance patterns, MAR indices and plasmid profiles are presented in Table 4. As shown in this Table, the 76 multidrug-resistant isolates (MDR) exhibited 37 different MDR profiles. Of these profiles, 17, 10, 6 and 4 resulted from resistance to 3, 4, 5 and 6 antimicrobials. All of S. Virchow isolates (n=10) showed a resistance pattern of TeNaCot. One isolate of each of S. Enteritidis and S. Inganda and two isolates of S. Paratyphi B shared the pattern CnStAmp. One isolate of each of S. Inganda, S. Isangi, S. Limete and two isolates of S. Edinburg showed four different hexa-resistance patterns. Seven isolates of S. Kentucky, three of S. Typhi and one isolate of each of S. ParatyphiB and S. Albany had six penta-resistance patterns. Four isolates of *S*. Kentucky shared the same profile of TeCnNaStAmp while the three isolates of *S*. Typhi shared the pattern TeStCotCAmp.

Twenty-one isolates belonging to ten serovars showed resistance to four antibiotics and exhibited ten resistance patterns. Of these, three patterns (TeCnNaSt, NaCipNorAmp and NaCipNorApr) were shown by eight isolates of *S*. Kentucky. One of the patterns, TeCnNaSt, was displayed by five of the 19 *S*. Kentucky isolates while the three isolates of *S*. Molade and two of *S*. Typhi shared the pattern TeStCotAmp. The other six patterns were shown by eight isolates belonging to the serovars Edinburg (2), Paratyphi B (1), Rissen (1), Java (1), Livingstone (1), Enteritidis (1) and Albany (1).

Of the 76 isolates showing MDR, 42 (55.3%) originated from human sources, 26 (34.2%) from poultry, 3 (3.9%) from each of water and food and 2 (2.6%) from animal sources. Of the 26 poultry isolates showing MDR, 13 belonged to *S*. Kentucky and 9 to *S*. Virchow whereas 17 of the 42 MDR human isolates belonged to *S*. Typhi (7), *S*. Paratyphi (6) and *S*. Edinburg (4). Average of multiple antibiotic resistance indices (MAR indices) indicated that *Salmonella* isolated from water had the highest average MAR index (0.4) followed by human (0.39), poultry (0.37), animal (0.35) and food (0.3).

Pattern	Serovars	Source	MAR index	Plasmid Profile (Kb)
Cn,Nor,Apr	Agona	Human	0.3	ND
Cn,Nor,Apr	Agona	Human	0.3	ND
Cn,Amp,Apr	Albany	Human	0.3	ND
Te,Na,St	Blockley	Poultry	0.3	ND
Cn,St,Cip	Enteritidis	Human	0.3	12.5
Cn,St,Amp	Enteritidis	Human	0.3	12.2
Cn,St,Amp	Inganda	Human	0.3	ND
Te,C,Amp	Isangi	Human	0.3	10.6
Cn,St,Apr	Kalina	Human	0.3	ND
Cn,St,Apr	Kalina	Human	0.3	ND
Cn,St,Apr	Limete	Human	0.3	10.6
Na,St,Amp	Livingstone	Food	0.3	10.6
Te,C,Cip	Massenya	Human	0.3	12.2
Te,C,Cip	Massenya	Human	0.3	10.6, 12.2
St,C,Amp	Menden	Human	0.3	ND
St,Ct,Amp	Paratyphi B	Human	0.3	8.3
St,Ct,Amp	Paratyphi B	Human	0.3	10.6, 12.2
Cn,St,Amp	Paratyphi B	Human	0.3	7.9, 10.6
Cn,St,Amp	Paratyphi B	Human	0.3	10.6

Pattern	Serovars	Source	MAR index	Plasmid Profile (Kb)
Te,C,Nor	Saragane	Human	0.3	12.2
Te,Cn,St	Stanley	Human	0.3	ND
Te,Cn,St	Stanley	Human	0.3	7.9
Te,Na,Cot	Stanleyville	Poultry	0.3	8.3, 12.5
Te,Cot,Amp	Stanleyville	Animal	0.3	1.2, 12.2, 12.5
Te,Cot,Amp	Stanleyville	Food	0.3	1.2, 12.2, 12.5
Te,Cot,Amp	Stanleyville	Poultry	0.3	1.2, 12.5
Cn,Na,Amp	Typhi	Human	0.3	3.5, 8.3
Na,St,Cip	Typhi	Human	0.3	8.3, 12.2, 12.5
Te,Na,Cot	Virchow	Poultry	0.3	ND
Te,Na,Cot	Virchow	Poultry	0.3	ND
Te,Na,Cot	Virchow	Poultry	0.3	ND
Te,Na,Cot	Virchow	Poultry	0.3	ND
Te,Na,Cot	Virchow	Poultry	0.3	ND
Te,Na,Cot	Virchow	Poultry	0.3	ND
Te,Na,Cot	Virchow	Poultry	0.3	ND
Te,Na,Cot	Virchow	Poultry	0.3	ND
Te,Na,Cot	Virchow	Poultry	0.3	ND
Te,Na,Cot	Virchow	Food	0.3	ND
Cn,St,Cip,Nor	Albany	Human	0.4	12.5
Cn,Na,C,Amp	Edinburg	Human	0.4	12.2, 10.6
Cn,Na,C,Amp	Edinburg	Human	0.4	ND
Cn,Na,C,Amp	Enteritidis	Human	0.4	ND
Cn,Na,St,Cip	Java	Human	0.4	12.5
Te,Cn,Na,St	Kentucky	Poultry	0.4	ND
Te,Cn,Na,St	Kentucky	Poultry	0.4	ND
Te,Cn,Na,St	Kentucky	Poultry	0.4	2.9, 3.5
Te,Cn,Na,St	Kentucky	Poultry	0.4	2.9, 5.5
Te,Cn,Na,St	Kentucky	Poultry	0.4	5.5
Na,Cip,Nor,Amp	Kentucky	Poultry	0.4	15.6, 12.5, 12.2
Na,Cip,Nor,Amp	Kentucky	Poultry	0.4	15.6, 12.2
Na,Cip,Nor,Apr	Kentucky	Poultry	0.4	12.2

Pattern	Serovars	Source	MAR index	Plasmid Profile (Kb)
Cn,Na,St,Amp	Livingstone	Animal	0.4	8.3, 12.2
Te,St,Ct,Amp	Molade	Water	0.4	1.2, 2.9, 8.3
Te,St,Ct,Amp	Molade	Water	0.4	1.2, 8.3
Te,St,Ct,Amp	Molade	Water	0.4	1.2, 8.3
Te,St,Ct,C	Paratyphi B	Human	0.4	12.5
Cn,Na,St,Ct	Rissen	Poultry	0.4	12.2
Te,St,Ct,Amp	Tuphi	Human	0.4	12.2, 12.5
Te,St,Ct,Amp	Tuphi	Human	0.4	3.5, 12.2
Cn,St,C,Cip,Nor	Albany	Human	0.5	8.3, 12.2
Cn,Na,St,Cip,Nor	Kentucky	Human	0.5	12.2
Cn,Na,St,Cip,Nor	Kentucky	Human	0.5	5.5, 12.2
Te,Cn,Na,St,Ct	Kentucky	Poultry	0.5	ND
Te,Cn,Na,St,Amp	Kentucky	Poultry	0.5	7.9
Te,Cn,Na,St,Amp	Kentucky	Poultry	0.5	ND
Te,Cn,Na,St,Amp	Kentucky	Poultry	0.5	10.6
Te,Cn,Na,St,Amp	Kentucky	Poultry	0.5	7.9
Cn,Na,St,Cip,Amp	Paratyphi B	Human	0.5	12.2, 12.5
Te,St,Ct,C,Amp	Typhi	Human	0.5	8.3, 12.5
Te,St,Ct,C,Amp	Typhi	Human	0.5	3.5, 8.3, 12.5
Te,St,Ct,C,Amp	Typhi	Human	0.5	8.3, 12.5
Te,Cn,Ct,C,Cip,Amp	Edinburg	Human	0.6	15.6, 10.6
Te,Cn,Ct,C,Cip,Amp	Edinburg	Human	0.6	15.6, 12.5
Te,Cn,St,Ct,C,Amp	Inganda	Human	0.6	12.5
Te,Cn,Na,C,Cip,Amp	Isangi	Human	0.6	12.2, 15.6
Te,Cn,Na,St,Cip,Nor	Limete	Human	0.6	12.2, 12.5

Table 4. Multiple antibiotic resistance profile and MAR indices of individual *Salmonella* isolates

Results of plasmid profile for MDR *Salmonella* isolates is shown in Table 4. Plasmid DNA was detected in 67.1% of the multiple resistant isolates demonstrating nine plasmids which constituted four plasmid profiles among the 37 resistance patterns. The number of plasmids per isolate ranged from 1 - 3 and their sizes ranged from 1.2 - 15.6 Kb. The majority of isolates (31.6%) had two plasmids but 27.6% had a single plasmid while 7.9% of the isolates had three plasmids. MDR *Salmonella* isolates that not harboring plasmids showed ten different resistance patterns which includes all of the antibiotics examined except for ciprofloxacin. Plasmids were not detected in all *S.* Virchow isolates (n=10) which share the resistance profile TeNaCot, a profile which re-appeared only in one isolate of *S*. Stanleyville. The largest plasmid (15.6 Kb) was detected in two isolates of *S*. Edinburg, two isolates of *S*. Kentucky and one isolate of *S*. Isangi. They were all resistant to ampicillin and ciprofloxacin and showed three different resistance patterns. The smallest plasmid (1.2 Kb) detected in three isolates of each of *S*. Molade and *S*. Stainleyville. These isolates were resistant to tetracycline, co-trimoxazole and ampicillin. It is also clear that, all of the ciprofloxacin resistant isolates were found to contain at least one of the largest plasmids (12.2, 12.5 and 15.6 Kb). The 12.2 Kb plasmid was present, either alone or in combination with plasmids of other sizes, in 15 (40.5%) of the different resistance patterns.

3.3 Detection by PCR

DNA extracted from 213 *Salmonella* strains and 12 closely related non-*Salmonella* strains were used to evaluate the specificity and sensitivity of ten primer sets to detect *Salmonella* sp. using the polymerase chain reaction technique (Table 5). The primer pairs targeting *inv*A, *hil*A, *iro*B, *ori*C, *fim*A, *hit*J and *stn* genes successfully amplified the DNA extracted from all *Salmonella* isolates generating the specific amplicon for each primer, and no amplification products were detected with DNA from non-*Salmonella* strains. These primers were, therefore, recommended as reliable means for simple and rapid PCR - based detection of the locally isolated *Salmonella* serovars.

Primer	*Salmonella* isolates (n=213)		Non-*Salmonella** isolates (n=12)		Sensitivity limit as for *S*. Typhi (CFU/ml)
	No. of +ve	No. of -ve	No. of +ve	No. of -ve	
invA	213	0	0	12	6.07x10
hilA	213	0	0	12	6.07x10^2
ompC	203	10	0	12	6.07x10^2
iroB	213	0	0	12	6.07x10^2
oriC	213	0	0	12	6.07x10^2
fimA	213	0	0	12	6.07x10^2
16S rDNA	213	0	4	8	6.07x10^2
Rep.feg	201	12	5	7	6.07x10^2
Hist	213	0	0	12	6.07x10^2
Stn	213	0	0	12	6.07x10^2

Table 5. Interpretation and follow-up action for PCR-based detection results. * *E. coli, Klebsiella* sp., *Klebsiella pneumonia, Bacillus subtils, Serratia* sp., *Proteus* sp., *Shigella dysenteriae, Shigella flexneri, Citrobacter freundii, Pseudomonas aeroginosa, Staphylococcus* sp. (1), *Staphylococcus* sp. (2).

The ompC primer set produced the expected amplicon with the DNA extracted from most of the *Salmonella* isolates, but failed to do so with DNA of *S*. Molade and *S*. Meleagridis. Negative results were also obtained with all non-*Salmonella* strains. The primer set 16S rDNA generated target size amplicons with all *Salmonella* isolates. However, similar amplicons were produced from the DNA of some non-*Salmonella* strains including *Proteus sp., Shigella dysenteriae, Citrobacter freundii* and *Pseudomonas aeruginosa*. The repetitive fragment of DNA primer set failed to amplify the DNA of 2 isolates of each of *S*.

Adelaide, *S.* Senftenberg and *S.* Virchow, and one isolate of *S.* Blockley, *S.* Hadar, *S.* Molade, Poona, *S.* Schwazengrund and *S.* Stanlyville. Moreover, the repetitive fragment of DNA amplified a specific fragment from the DNA of *E. coli, Klebsiella pneumoniae, Bacillus subtilis, Proteus sp.* and *Shigella flexneri.*

4. Discussion

Salmonella was isolated from different sources with an overall prevalence of 11.09%, which is comparable to the isolation frequency (9.2 and 11.2%) reported by El Hussein et al. (2010) in Khartoum State, Sudan and by Mohammad et al. (2006) in Zahedan, Iran respectively. The prevalence percentage reported demonstrates the widespread occurrence and distribution of *Salmonella* in Sudan. This prevalence was clearly higher than the range of 3.34 - 4.0%, reported in the limited studies conducted previously (Soliman and Khan, 1959; Khan, 1962, 1970; Yagoub and Mohamed, 1987; El Tom et al., 1999; Yagoub et al., 2006 and Hag Elsafi et al., 2009). Several studies in other developing countries have reported a higher overall prevalence of *Salmonella* (human, food, and animal) such as 68.2% in Ethiopia, 51.2% in Argentina , 25.9% in Korea, and 72% in Thailand (Cardinale et al., 2003). It is important to recognize that the prevalence and distribution of *Salmonella* serovars varies from region to region (Dominguez et al., 2002; Uyttendaele et al., 1998) and isolation rates depend upon the country where the study was carried out, the sampling plan and the detection limit of the methodology (Roberts, 1982; Uyttendaele et al., 1998). Consequently, it is difficult to make comparisons between *Salmonella* surveillance conducted in different countries. However, the serovars isolated from the various sample types in our survey in Sudan were comparable to the results reported by various investigators in other countries. For example, Baudart et al. (2000) reported the prevalence of *S.* Agona, *S.* Enteritidis, *S.* Infantis, *S.* Mbandaka, *S.* Muenster, *S.* Rissen, *S.* Typhimurium, *S.* Montevideo and *S.* Virchow in different aquatic environments. The same serovars plus *S.* Senftenberg were isolated by Saha et al. (2001) from faecal samples taken from hospitalized diarrhoeal children in India. Similar to this study, Liebana et al. (2001, 2002)and Tamada et al. (2001) reported the isolation of *S.* Mbandaka, *S.* Montevideo and *S.* Livingstone from animal sources. The findings of Delicato et al. (2004) and of Fernandez et al. (2003) were also comparable to our results. They reported the isolation of *S.* Enteritidis, *S.* Infantis and *S.* Typhimurium from human faeces. *S.* Typhimurium and *S.* Enteritidis, in particular, are regarded worldwide as significant pathogenic serovars, with certain phagetypes being associated with serious illness in humans, chickens and animals (Dominguez et al., 2002; Jorgensen et al., 2002; Roy et al., 2002 & Mohammad et al., 2006). The predominant phagetype of *S.* Typhimurium was PT2, while those for *S.* Enteritidis were PT21a and Atypical. In Western Europe, phagetype 4 was generally reported as a dominant phage for S. Enteritidis (Humphrey et al., 1991), while in the United States, PT8 was generally dominant (Hickman-Brenner et al., 1991).

The most predominant serovar in this study was *S.* Kentucky constituting 8.9% of the recovered isolates. The ranking of this serovar among other serovars increased substantially during the past decade in most European countries (Gill et al., 2002; 2004; Gill and Threlfall, 2007; Bonalli et al., 2011). However, this serovar was considered an unsuccessful pathogen because it was rarely associated with human illness (Collard et al., 2007). *S.* Kentucky and *S.* Stanleyville were mostly isolated from poultry samples in comparison with other serotypes (24.3 and 17.1%, respectively). In chickens, it is well established that *S.* Enteritidis is the most predominant *Salmonella* serovar, followed by *S.* Typhimurium (Mohammad et al., 2006; Suresh et al., 2011). However, no S. Enteritidis and only one isolate of *S.* Typhimurium was isolated from poultry in this study.

Many animal species harbour *Salmonella* and can act as potential reservoirs for human infections. For example, *S.* Menden, *S.* Enteritidis, *S.* Montevideo and *S.* Senftenberg, which were recovered from humans in this study, were previously isolated from different animals in Sudan (Khan, 1970). *Salmonella* may enter the food chain through carcass contamination with animal faeces at slaughter and during processing, or through food or food handlers. However, human infection may also occur through contaminated water, pets, and exotic animals. Measures taken to control these routes of transmission are an effective way of preventing salmonellosis. The collection of prevalence data of *Salmonella* serovars is an important component of a successful epidemiological surveillance for public health management in any country.

Since all human isolates were recovered from stool samples of food handlers, it is likely that food can act as potential reservoirs for salmonellosis epidemics. More strict measures should be implemented in the food industry to curtail the spread of salmonellosis in Sudan. For example, monitoring of restaurant workers should be performed at more frequent intervals rather than the current mandatory annual check-up for renewal of work permits. This should be accompanied by organized training programs involving suppliers of food items and corporate administrators as well as front line restaurant employees. More involvement by public health authorities in surveillance programs is needed to ensure that public safety regulations are properly implemented.

This initial survey has provided useful information about the status of salmonellosis in Khartoum, Sudan. We have demonstrated that *Salmonella* was isolated mostly from humans followed by chickens suggesting that chicken and chicken-food products could be a potential source of salmonellosis in the food chain. The *S.* Kentucky serovar, which has a lesser potential for infection, was common to human, chicken and food items. Furthermore, *S.* Kentucky isolates are known for their resistance to ciprofloxacin, the antibiotic of choice for the treatment of typhoid in Sudan (Bonalli et al., 2011). Thus this phenotype may spread to other serovars which might have greater potential for infection.

The increased level of drug resistance in *Salmonella* has become a public health concern (Pui et al., 2011). As antibiotic usage varies among countries, different resistant phenotypes and genotypes can be expected. Thus monitoring of antimicrobial resistance patterns from different sources and regions is an important issue.

In this study, the rate of resistance to ampicillin (25.4%) and chloramphenicol (8.0%) was comparable to those detected for the same antibiotics in the year 2000. At that time, Ahmed et al. (2000) reported 25.0% and 13.0% resistance to ampicillin and chloramphenicol, respectively. However, the percentage of *Salmonella* isolates resistant to nalidixic acid and ciprofloxacin in Sudan has increased from zero percent (Ahmed et al., 2000) to 22.0 and 8.9%, respectively. The wide resistance to Nalidixic acid is a matter of concern, since nalidixic acid resistance has been associated with a decrease in susceptibility to fluoroquinolones, including ciprofloxacin, which are used to treat salmonellosis in humans (Gorman and Adley, 2004). The human isolates were more resistant to ciprofloxacin (16.1%) than the poultry isolates of which only 5.7% showed resistance to the antibiotic. Our results are consistent with what has been reported by Tassios et al. (1997), but disagree with the findings of Al-Bahry et al. (2007) who found that isolates of human origin were less resistant than those of chicken. In this study, resistance was 41.3% to streptomycin and 31.9% to tetracycline which is inconsistent with a report of complete susceptibility, to both antibiotics, by Singh et al. (2010) in India. Our results are in line with other investigators who observed high rates of resistance to streptomycin and tetracycline by *Salmonella* isolates (Zhao et al., 2005; Stevens et al., 2006; Dogru et al., 2009; Iseri and Erol, 2010). De Oliveira et al. (2010) attributed the prevalence of resistance to streptomycin and tetracycline to their frequent administration in veterinary medicine.

A lower percentage of resistance was observed for norfloxacin (7.5%), chloramphenicol (8.0%) and ciprofloxacin (8.9%). Lower resistance rates to these drugs were also reported by other workers (Gulsen et al., 2004; Zhao et al., 2006; Lestari et al., 2009). Therefore, these drugs may continue to be the drugs of choice for treatment of human salmonellosis in Sudan. apramycin, to which only 5.6% of *Salmonella* isolates were resistant, can replace the currently used antibiotics (mostly streptomycin and tetracycline) in the treatment of poultry.

Reduced susceptibility to fluoroquinolones and chloramphenicol has also been reported particularly for *S.* Kentucky isolates in many countries of the region such as Ethiopia (Molla et al., 2006), Morocco (Bouchrif et al., 2009) and Tunisia (Turki et al., 2011). Weill and Le Hello (2008) indicated that the acquisition and spread of distinct antibiotic resistance, especially resistance to ciprofloxacin, the drug of choice in Sudan, is associated with the emergence of S. Kentucky.

Turki et al. (2011) reported a correlation between resistance to nalidixic acid and ciprofloxacin. This was not the case in our study; instead, nalidixic acid resistance closely correlates with tetracycline resistance. Strong evidence of cross resistance between chloramphenicol and ampicillin was also observed. Of 17 chloramphenicol resistant isolates, 12 (70.6%) were also resistant to ampicillin. Values of 100%, 85% and 21% cross resistance between these two antibiotics was reported by different investigators (Goldstein et al., 1983; Rowe et al., 1992; Gupta et al., 1990).

This study demonstrated that 35.7% of the *Salmonella* isolates tested (n=213) were multidrug resistant. This level was comparable to that reported by Bouchrif et al. (2009) in Morocco (44%) and Van et al. (2007) in Vietnam (34%) but much lower than the level reported by Thong and Modarressi (2011) in Kuala Lumpur (67%). Among all *Salmonella* isolates from different sources, 37 antibiotic resistance patterns were detected, indicating wide spread multidrug resistance. This result is comparable with the findings of Singh et al. (2010) who identified 24 different resistance patterns among their *Salmonella* isolates. The authors attributed the observed high number in multidrug resistance patterns to the frequent use of antibiotics in the environments from which the isolates originated. It should be emphasized that most of the MDR isolates (n=76) in this study originated from human (42) and poultry sources (26). Nowroozi et al. (2004) demonstrated that indiscriminate use of antibiotics in poultry production has increased the emergence and maintenance of MDR bacteria in the environment. Similarly, Ahmed et al. (2000) attributed the high level of multiple resistance salmonellae among human isolates to the inordinate and irrational use of antimicrobial agents in the Sudan. The authors mentioned a number of factors that have led to the prevalence of antibiotic resistance. The most important among which are the deliberate self-administration of antibiotics by patients themselves, the wide use of antibiotics due to the high prevalence of infectious diseases, lack of laboratory support in rural areas and selective prescribing due to cost constrains.

Plasmid DNA was demonstrated in 67.1% of the multiple resistant isolates. Our results indicated the association of large integrons (12.2 - 15.6 Kb) with the resistance to ampicillin and/or ciprofloxacin. Certain plasmid sizes may be responsible for resistance to particular antibiotics (White et al., 2001). Resistance to ampicillin in *Salmonella* was mediated by a β-lactamase gene carried on a plasmid (Thong & Modarressi, 2011). Since some of the isolates were resistant to one or more antibiotics and yet did not harbour any plasmid, the antibiotic resistance might be chromosomally mediated or mediated by other mobile elements such as transposons (Yah & Eghafona, 2008). The finding of both plasmid and non-plasmid mediated antibiotic resistance is consistent with other studies (Rodrigue et al., 1992; Ansary et al., 2006). This implies that there is no consistent relationship between the detected plasmid profile and antibiotic resistance patterns. Similar conclusions were previously drawn by Shears et al. (1988) in Sudan and Mamun et al. (1993) in Bangladesh.

In summary, this study confirmed that food, water, poultry and food handlers might act as reservoirs for antimicrobial resistant *Salmonella*. To diminish contamination rates by *Salmonella*, risk reduction strategies such as training of food handlers regarding food safety, institutional periodic focused medical checkups for food handlers, more restrictions on the irrational use of antibiotics, and establishment of standardized monitoring systems for on-going drug resistance surveillance are required. Although the current study addressed a local problem in Sudan where it appears that there is a high incident of antibiotic resistant salmonellae, many other developing countries are faced with a similar situation (Al-Bahry et al., 2007; Turki et al., 2011; Thong and Modarressi, 2011). In addition, dissemination of information on antibiotic resistance is important for development of prescribing polices and for general medical practitioners in a remote area who may not have access to microbiology laboratory back-up and, hence, must depend on prevailing knowledge of antibiotic-resistant *Salmonella*.

Results of the primers pairs targeting *inv*A, *hil*A, *iro*B, *ori*C, *fim*A, *hit*J and *stn* genes indicated their reliability, sensitivity and accuracy for the detection of *Salmonella enterica*. These findings affirm results of the previous studies (Moganedi et al., 2007; Murphy et al., 2007; Narvaneni and Jamil, 2005; Moore and Feist, 2006). It has been shown that *inv*A and *hil*A genes are associated with pathogenicity of *Salmonella* spp. The former gene was reported to be essential for the invasion of epithelial cells by *Salmonella* (Moganedi et al., 2007); consequently, all *Salmonella* isolates studied are capable of invading the epithelial cells of the host (Bajaj et al., 1995). The *hil*A gene proved to be highly conserved among our *Salmonella* serovars. Being unspecific, the repetitive fragment of DNA, 16S rDNA and opmC primers were considered as unsuitable for PCR detection of locally isolated *Salmonella* serovars. The positive results obtained by the primer set 16S rDNA with some non-*Salmonella* strains could be explained by the fact that this primer set is constructed from 16SFl and 16SIII derived from the two regions of 16S rRNA gene. *16S*F1 is the reverse and complementary strand of *16S*I, which has been found to hybridize with *Salmonella* as well as with *Citrobacter* sp., while the *16S*III sequence was able to hybridize with *Klebsiella* and *Serratia* spp., in addition to *Salmonella* (Lin and Tsen, 1996). Similarly, the repetitive DNA fragment PCR assay was found to be unspecific for *Salmonella* as it failed to amplify the DNA of a number of *Salmonella* isolates and positive results were obtained for most of the non- *Salmonella* strains. Comparably, Ziemer and Steadham (2003) reported the ability of this primer set to amplify the DNA of bacteria commonly associated with intestinal samples.

5. Acknowledgements

The authors gratefully acknowledge the support of the Office International des Epizooties (OIÉ) Reference Laboratory for Salmonellosis, Laboratory for Foodborne Zoonoses, Public Health Agency of Canada and the help of Egypt Management Central Laboratory, Cairo, Egypt.

6. References

Aarts, H. J. M., Vanlith, L. A. J. T. & Keljer, J. (1998). High - resolution genotyping of *Salmonella* strains by AFLP fingerprinting. *Letters in Applied Microbiology*. Vol. 26, pp. (131 - 135). ISSN 0266-8254.

Ahmed, A. A., Osman, H., Mansour, A. M., Musa, H. A., Ahmed, H. A., Karrar, Z. & Hassan, H. S. (2000). Antimicrobial agent resistance in bacterial isolates from patients with diarrhea and urinary tract infection in the Sudan. *American Journal of Tropical Medicine and Hygiene*. Vol. 63, No. 5-6, pp. 259-263. ISSN 0002-9637.

Akkina, J. E., Hogue, A. T., Angulo, F. J., Johnson, R., Petersen, K. E., Saini, P. K., P. J. Fedorka-Cray, P. K. & Schlosser, W. D. (1999). Epidemiologic aspects, control, and importance of multiple-drug resistant *Salmonella* Typhimurium DT104 in the United States. *Journal of American Veterinary Medicine Association*, Vol. 214, pp. 790–798. ISSN 0003-1488. PMID: 10101410.

Al-Bahry, S. N., Elshafie, A. E., Al-Busaidy, S., Al-Hinai, J. & Al-Shidi, I. (2007). Antibiotic-resistant *Salmonella* spp. from human and non-human sources in Oman. *Eastern Mediterranean Health Journal*. Vol. 12, No. 1, pp. (49-55). ISSN 1687-1634.

Amavisit, P., Browning, G. F., Lightfoot, D., Church, S., Anderson, G. A., Whithear, K. G. & Markham, P. F. (2001). Rapid PCR detection of *Salmonella* in horse faecal samples. Veterinary Microbiology. Vol. 79, No. 1, pp. (63-74). ISSN 0378-1135.

Anderson, E. S. & Williams, R.E.O. (1956). Bacteriophage typing of enteric pathogens and staphylococci and its use in epidemiology. *Journal of Clinical Pathology*. Vol. 9, pp. 94-127. ISSN 0021-9746.

Anderson, E.S. (1964). The phage typing of salmonellae other than *S*. Typhi. In: *The World Problem of Salmonellosis*. van Oye, E. (ed.), pp. 89-110. The Hague: Dr W. Junk. ISBN 9061930669.

Anderson, E.S., Ward, L.R., De Saxe, M.J. & De Sa, J.D.H. (1977). Bacteriophage-typing designations of *Salmonella* Typhimurium. *Journal of Hygiene, Cambridge*. Vol. 78, pp. (297-300). ISSN 0022-1724

Ansary, A., Haneef, R., Torrres, J. & Yadav, M. (2006). Plasmid and antibiotic resistance in Aeromonas hydrophila isolated in Malaysia from healthy and diseased fish. *Journal of Fish Diseases*. Vol. 15, pp. (191-196). ISSN 0140-7775.

Asai, T., Namimatsu, T., Osumi, T., Kojima, A., Harada, K., Aoki, H., Toshiya, S. & Takahashi, T. (2010). Molecular typing and antimicrobial resistance of *Salmonella enterica* subspecies *enterica* serovar Choleraesuis isolates from diseased pigs in Japan. Comparative Immunology. Comparative Immunology, Microbiology and Infectious Disease. Vol. 33, No. 2, pp. (109-119). ISSN 0147-9571.

Bajaj, V., Hwang, C. & Lee, C. A. (1995). *hilA* is a novel *ompR/toxR* family member that activates expression of *Salmonella typhimurium* invasion genes. *Journal of Medical Microbiology*. Vol. 18, pp. (715-727). ISSN 0022-2615.

Baudart, J., Lemarchand, K., Brisabois, A. & Lebaron, P. (2000). Diversity of *Salmonella* strains isolated from the aquatic environment as determined by serotyping and amplification of the ribosomal DNA spacer regions. *Applied and Environmental Microbiology*. Vol. 66, No. 4, pp. (1544–1552). ISSN 0099-2240.

Baumler, A.J., Tsolis, R.M., Ficht, T.A. & Adams, L.G. (1998). Evolution of host adaptation in *Salmonella enterica*. *Infection and Immunity*. Vol. 66, No. 10, pp. (4579-4587). ISSN 1098-5522.

Bonalli, M., Stephen, R., Kappeli, U., Cernela, N., Adank, L. & Hachler, H. (2011). *Salmonella enterica* serotype Kentucky associated with human infections in Switzerland: Genotype and resistance trends 2004-2009. *Food Research International*. ISSN: 0963-9969.

Bouchrif, B., Paglietti, B., Murgia, M., Piana, A., Cohen, N., Ennaji, M., Rubino, S. & Timinouni, M. (2009). Prevalence and antibiotic-resistance of *Salmonella* isolated from food in Morocco. *Journal of Infection in Developing Countries*. Vol. 28, No. 3, pp. (35-40). ISSN 1972-2680.

Callow, B. R. (1959). A new phage-typing scheme for *Salmonella* typhimurium. *Journal of Hygiene*. Vol. 57, pp. (346-359). ISSN 0022-1724.

Cardinale, E., Perrier Gros-Claude, J. D., Tall, F., Cissé, M., Guèye, E. F. & Salvat, G. (2003). Prevalence of *Salmonella* and *Campylobacter* in retail chicken carcasses in Senegal. *Revue d Elevage et de Medecine Veterinaire des Pays Tropicaux (Paris)*. Vol. 56, pp. (13-16). ISSN 0035-1865.

Cohen, N.D., Neibergs, H.L., McGruder, E.D., Whitford, H.W., Behle, R.W., Ray, P.M. & Hargis, B.M. (1993). Genus-specific detection of salmonellae using the polymerase chain reaction (PCR). *Journal of Veterinary Diagnostic Investigation*. Vol. 5, No. 3, pp. (368-371). ISSN 1040-6387.

Collard, J.M., Place, S., Denis, O., Rodriguez-Villalobos, H., Vrints, M., Weill, F.X., Baucheron, S., Cloeckaert, A., Struelens, M. & Bertrand, S. (2007). Travel-acquired salmonellosis due to *Salmonella* Kentucky resistant to ciprofloxacin, ceftriaxone and co-trimoxazole and associated with treatment failure. *Journal of Antimicrobial Chemotherapy*. Vol60, No. 1, pp (190-192). ISSN 0305-7453.

Cruickshank, R. (1975). Medical Microbiology (12th ed. Vol. 2), 587 p., Churchill -Livingstone, ISBN 0443010994 . Edinburgh, London and New York.

Crump, J. A. & Mintz, E. D. (2010). Global trends in typhoid and paratyphoid fever. *Emerging Infections*. Vol. 50, pp. (241-246). ISSN 1058-4838.

De Oliveira, F. A., Pasqualotto, A. P., da Silva, W. P. & Tondo, E. C. (2010). Characterization of *Salmonella* enteritidis isolated from human samples. *Food research International*, In press, Corrected Proof. doi:10.1016/j.foodres.2010.09.040. ISSN: 0963-9969.

Delicato, E. R., Mikcha, J. M. G., Fernandes, S. A. & Peloyo, J. S. (2004). Resistance profile to antimicrobials of *Salmonella* spp. isolated from human infections. *Brazilian Archives of Biology and Technology*, Vol. 47, No. 2, pp. (193-197). ISSN 1516-8913.

Desai, A.R.; Shah, D.H.; Shringi, Smriti; Lee, M.J.; Li, Y.H.; Cho, M.R.; Park, J.H.; Eo, S.K.; Lee, J.H. and Chae, J.S. (2005). An allele-specific PCR assay for the rapid and serotype-specific detection of *Salmonella pullorum*. *Avian Diseases*. Vol. 49, No. 4, pp. (558-561). ISSN 0005-2086.

Dillon, J. R., Nasim, A. & Nestmann, E. R. (1985). Recombinant DNA Methodology. John Wiley & Sons, Inc., pp. (1- 39). ISSN 0471898511.

Dogru, A. K., Ayaz, N. D. & Gencay, Y. E. (2009). Serotype identification and antimicrobial resistance profiles of *Salmonella* spp. isolated from chicken carcasses. *Tropical Animal Health and Production*. Vol. 42, No. 5, pp. 893-897. ISSN 0049-4747.

Dominguez, C., Gómez, I. & Zumalacarregui, J. (2002). Prevalence of *Salmonella* and *Campylobacter* in retail chicken meat in Spain. *International Journal of Food Microbiology*. Vol. 72, pp. (165-168). ISSN 0168-1605.

El Hussein, A. A., Nor Elmadiena, M. M., Elsaid, S. M., Siddig, M. A. M., Muckle, C. A., Cole, L., Wilkie, E. & Mistry, K. (2010). Prevalence of *Salmonella enterica* subspecies *enterica* Serovars in Khartoum State, Sudan. *Research Journal of Microbiology*. Vol. 5, No. 10, pp. (966-973). ISSN 1816-4935.

El Tom G.M., Abdel Rahman, S.M., Elamin, E.D.M. & Yassin, T.E. (1999). Isolation of the *Salmonella* Serotype San-Diego from Lymph Nodes of Slaughtered Goats. *The Sudan Journal of Veterinary Research*. Vol. 16, pp (61-65). ISSN 1028-9437.

Ewing, W. H. (1986). Serologic identification of *Salmonella*. In: *Edwards and Ewing's Identification of Enterobacteriaceae*, 4th (edn.) Ewing W. H. (Eds), Elsevier Science Publishing Co., Inc. pp. (201-238), ISBN 0-444-00981-7 New York.

Ezquerra, E., Burnens, A., Jones, C. and Stanley, J. (1993). Genotyping and phylogenetic analysis of *Salmonella* Paratyphi B and S. Java with IS200. *Journal of General Microbiology*. Vol. 139, pp. (2409–2414). ISSN 0022-1287.

Fernandez, J., Fica, A., Ebensperger, G., Calfullan, H., Prat, S., Fernandez, A., Alexandre, M. & Heitmann, I. (2003). Analysis of molecular epidemiology of Chilean *Salmonella enterica* serotype Enteritidis isolates by pulsed-field gel electrophoresis and bacteriophage typing. *Journal of Clinical Microbiology*. Vol. 41, pp. (1617-1622). ISSN 0095-1137.

Gill, N., & Threlfall, J. (2007). Enter-net quarterly *Salmonella* report-06/4. European Centre for Disease Prevention and Control. Retrieved from: http://www.ecdc.europa.eu/en/publications/Publications/0702_SUR_Enter-net_Salmonella_Report_00_4.pdf

Gill, N., Reilly, B., & Smith, H. (2002). Enter-net quarterly *Salmonella* report-00/4. European Centre for Disease Prevention and Control. Retrieved from: http://www.ecdc.europa.eu/en/publications/Publications/0205_SUR_Enter-net_Salmonella_Report_00_4.pdf

Gill, N., Reilly, B., & Smith, H. (2004). Enter-net quarterly *Salmonella* report-03/4. European Centre for Disease Prevention and Control. Retrieved from: http:// www.ecdc.europa.eu/en/activities/surveillance/pages/Enter-net_aspx

Goldstein, F., Chumpitaz, J., Guevara, J., Papadapoolou, B., Acar, J., Vieu, J. (1983). Plasmid-mediated resistance to multiple antibiotics in *Salmonella* Typhi. *Journal of Infectious Diseases*. Vol. 153, pp. (261-266). ISSN 0022-1899.

Gorman, R. & Adley, C. (2004). Characterization of *Salmonella enterica* serotype Typhimurium isolates from human, food and animal sources in the Republic of Ireland. *Journal of Clinical Microbiology*. Vol. 42, pp. 2314-2316. ISSN 0095-1137

Gray, J. T. & Fedorka-Gray, P. J. (2002). *Salmonella*. In: *Foodborne Diseases* (2nd edn.), Cliver, D. O. & H. P. Riemann (Eds.), pp. 55–68. Academic Press, ISBN 0121765598.

Grob, U., Tschape, H., Bednarek, I. & Frosch, M. (1998). Antibiotic resistance in *Salmonella enteric* serotype Typhimurium. *European Journal of Clinical Microbiology & Infectious Diseases*. Vol. 17, pp. (385-387). ISSN 0934-9723.

Guibourdenche, M., Roggentin, P., Mikoleit, M., Fields, P.I., Bockemuhl, J., Grimont, P.A.D. & Weill, F-X. (2010). Supplement 2003 - 2007 (No. 47) of the White-Kauffmann-Le Minor scheme. *Research in Microbiology*. Vol. 161, pp. 26-29. ISSN 0923-2508.

Gulig, P.A., Danbara, H., Guiney, D.G., Lax, A.J., Norel, F. & Rhen, M. (1993). Molecular analysis of spv virulence genes of the *Salmonella* virulence plasmids. *Molecular Micriobiology*. Vol. 7, No. 6, pp. (825-830). ISSN 1365-2958.

Gulsen, G., Eloin, G. N. & Arli, K. T. (2004). Antibiotic resistance of Salmonella Enteritidis of human and chicken origin. *Turkish Journal of Veterinary and Animal Science*. Vol. 28, pp. (911-914). ISSN 1300-0128.

Guo, X., Chen, J., Beuchat, L. R. & Brackett, R. E. (2000). PCR Detection of *Salmonella enterica* Serotype Montevideo in and on Raw Tomatoes Using Primers Derived from *hil*A. *Applied and Environmental Microbiology*. Vol. 66, pp. (5248-5252). ISSN 0099-2240.

Gupta, B., Bhujwala, R. & Shriniwas, R. (1990). Multiresistant Salmonella typhi in India (letter). *Lancet*. Vol. 336, No. 8709, pp. (252). ISSN 0140-6736.

Hag Elsafi H. E., Nor Elmadiena, M. M., El Hussein, A. A., Siddig, M. A. M., Muckle, C. A., Cole, L., Wilkie, E. & Mistry, K. (2009). *Salmonella* Umbadah: A new *Salmonella* serovar isolated from cattle in Sudan. *Tropical Animal Health and Production*. Vol. 41, pp. (1605-1606). ISSN 0049-4747.

Hanes, D. (2003). Nontyphoid *Salmonella*. In: *International handbook of foodborne pathogens*, Henegariu, O., Heerema, N. A., Dloughy, S. R., Vance, G. H and Vogt, P. H. (Eds.)., pp. 137-149. Marcel Dekker, Inc., ISBN 0-8247-0685-4, New York.

Harvey, R.W. & Price, T. H. (1979). Principles of *Salmonella* isolation. *Journal of Applied Bacteriology*. Vol. 46, pp. (27-56). ISSN 0021-8847.

Hassan, S.H. (1985). Sensitivity of *Salmonella* and *Shigella* species to antibiotics and chemotherapeutic agents in Sudan. *Journal of Tropical Medicine and Hygiene*. Vol. 88, pp. (243-248). ISSN 0022-5304.

Hickman-Brenner, F.W., Stubbs, A.D. & Farmer, J.J. (1991). Phage typing of Salmonella enteritidis in the United States. *Journal of Clinical Microbiology*. Vol. 29, pp. (2817-2823). ISSN 0095-1137.

Hoorfar, J., Ahrens, P. & Radstrom, P. (2000). Automated 5_ nuclease PCR assay for identification of *Salmonella enterica*. *Journal of Clinical Microbiology*. Vol. 38, pp. (3429–3435). ISSN 0095-1137.

Horgan, N. E. (1947). Annual Report. Sudan Medical Service, Vol. 1, pp. 51.

Hu, L. & Kopecko, D. J. (2003). Typhoid *Salmonella*. In: *International handbook of foodborne pathogens*, Millotis, M. D. and Bier, J. W. (Eds.). p. 151-165, Marcel Dekker, Inc., ISBN 0-8247-0685-4, New York.

Humphrey, T.J., Whitehead, A., Gawler, A.H., Henley, A., Rowe, B. (1991). Numbers of *Salmonella* enteritidis in the contents of naturally contaminated hens' eggs. *Epidemiology and Infection*. Vol. 106, No. 3, pp. (489–496). ISSN 1469-4409.

Iseri, O. & Erol, I. (2010). Incidence and antibiotic resistance of *Salmonella* spp. in ground turkey meat. *British Poultry Science*. Vol. 51, No. 1, pp. (60-66). ISSN 0007-1668.

Jamshidi, A., Zahraei-Salehi, T. & Afshari-Nic, S. (2007). Detection of *Salmonella spp* contamination of carcasses slaughtered in poultry abattoir in Mashhad, Iran. *Archives of Razi Institute*. Vol. 62, No. 4, pp. (229-233). ISSN 3439-0365.

Jensen, M. A. & Hubner, R. J. (1996). Use of homoduplex ribosomal DNA spacer amplification products and heteroduplex cross - hybridization products in the identification of

Salmonella serovars. *Applied and Environmental Microbiology*, Vol. 62, pp. (2741 - 2746). ISSN 0099-2240.

Jitrapakdee, S., Tassanakajon, A., Boonsaeng, V., Piankijagum, S. & Panyim, S. (1995). A simple, rapid and sensitive detection of *salmonella* in food by polymerase chain reaction. Molecular and Cellular Probes, Vol. 9, No. 6, pp. (375-382). ISSN 0890-8508.

Jorgensen, F., Bailey, R., Williams, S., Henderson, P., Wareing, D. R., Bolton, F. J., Frost, J. A., Ward, L. & Humphrey, T. J. (2002). Prevalence and numbers of *Salmonella* and *Campylobacter* spp. on raw, whole chickens in relation to sampling methods. *International Journal of Food Microbiology*. Vol. 76, pp. (151-164). ISSN 0168-1605

Khan, A.Q. (1962). Salmonellosis in the Sudan. *Sudan Journal of Veterinary Science and Animal Husbandry*. Vol. 3, pp. (84-89). ISSN: 0562-5084.

Khan, A.Q. (1970). *Salmonella* infections in dogs and cats in the Sudan. *British Veterinary Journal*. Vol. 126, pp. 607-611. ISSN 0007-1935

Kunin, C. M., Johansen, S., Worning, A. M., Daschner, F. D. (1990). Report of a symposium on use and abuse of antibiotics worldwide. *Review of Infectious Disease*. Vol. 12, pp. 12-19. ISSN 0162-0886.

Kurowski, P.B., Traub-Dargatz, J.L., Morley, P.S., Gentry-Weeks, C.R. (2002). Detection of *Salmonella* spp in fecal specimens by use of real-time polymerase chain reaction assay. *American Journal of Veterinary Research*. Vol. 63, No. 9, pp. (1265-1268). ISSN 0002-9645.

Lagatolla, C., Dolzani, L., Tonin, E., Lavenia, A., Dimichele M., Tommansin, T. & Monti-Bragadin, C. (1996). PCR - ribotyping and characterizing *Salmonella* isolates of different serotypes. *Journal of Clinical Microbiology*, Vol. 34, pp. (2440 - 2443). ISSN 0095-1137.

Lestari, S. I., Han, F., Wang, F. & Ge, B. (2009). Prevalence and antimicrobial resistance of *Salmonella* serovars in conventional and organic chickens from Louisiana retail stores. *Journal of Food Protection*. Vol. 72, pp. (1165-1172). ISSN 0362-028X.

Levine, M.M., Grados, O., Gilman, R.H., Woodward, W.E., Solis-Plaza, R., Waldman, W. (1978). Diagnostic value of the Widal test in areas endemic for typhoid fever. *American Journal of Tropical Medicine and Hygiene*, Vol. 27, No.4, pp. (795-800), ISSN 0002-9637.

Liebana, E., Garcia-Migura, L. Clouting, C., Clifton-Hadley, F. Lindsay, E. Threlfall, E. J., McDowell, S. W.J. & Davies, R. H. (2002). Multiple genetic typing of *Salmonella enterica* serotype Typhimurium isolates of different phage types (DT104, U302, DT204b, and DT49) from animals and humans in England, Wales, and Northern Ireland. *Journal of Clinical Microbiology*. Vol. 40, pp. (4450-4456). ISSN 0095-1137.

Liebana, E., Guns, D., Woodward, M.J. *et al.* (2001). Molecular typing of *Salmonella* serotypes prevalent in animals in England: Assessment of Methodology. *Journal of Clinical Microbiology*. Vol. 39, pp. (3609-3616). ISSN 0095-1137.

Lin, C. K. & Tsen, H. Y. (1996). Use of two 16S DNA targeted oligonucleotides as PCR primers for the specific detection of Salmonella in foods. *Journal of Applied Bacteriology*. Vol. 80, No. 6, pp. (659-666). ISSN 0021-8847.

Lindberg, A.A., Nord, C.E., Hellgren, M. & Sjöberg, L. (1974). Identification of gram-negative aerobic fermentors in a clinical bacteriological laboratory. *Medical Microbiology and Immunology*. Vol. 159, pp. (201-210). ISSN 0300-8584.

MacFaddin, J. F. (1980). Biochemical test for identification of medical bacteria, 3rd (Edn). Lippincott Williams & Wilkins, 912 p. ISBN 0683053183.

Makino, S., Kurazono, H., Chongsanguam, M., Hayashi, H., Cheun, H., Suzuki, S. & Shirahata, T. (1999). Establishment of the PCR system specific to *Salmonella* spp. and its application for the inspection of food and fecal samples. *Journal of Veterinary Medical Sciences*. Vol. 61, No. 11, pp. (1245-1247). ISSN 0916-7250.

Mamun, K.Z., Shears, P. & Hart, C. A. (1993). The prevalence and Genetics of resistance to commonly used antimicrobial agents in faecal Enterobacteriaceae from children in Bangladesh. *Epidemiology and Infection*. Vol. 110, pp. (447-458). ISSN 1469-4409.

Moganedi K. L. M., Goyvaerts E. M. A., Venter S. N. and Sibara M. M. (2007). Optimisation of PCR-*inv*A primers for the detection of *Salmonella* in drinking and surface waters following a pre-cultivation step. *Water SA*. Vol. 33, No. 2, pp. (195-202). ISSN 0378-4738.

Mohammad, B., Mohagheghi, F. A. H. & Roqiah, G. (2006). An investigation on contamination of poultries by *Salmonella* species in Zahedan (South-East Iran) during 2004. *Research Journal Microbiology*. Vol. 1, No. 5, pp. (463-466). ISSN 1816-4935.

Mohand, R. V., Brahimi, N.m Moustaoui, N., Mdaghri, N. E., Amarouch, H., Grimont, F., Bingen, E. and Benbachir, M. 1999. Characterization of extended spectrum β-lactamase producing *Salmonella* Typhymirium by phenotypic and genotypic typing methods. *Journal Clinical Microbiology*. Vol. 37, pp. (3769 – 3773). ISSN 0095-1137.

Molla, B., Berhanu, A., Muckle, A., Cole, L., Wilkie, E., Kleer, J. & Hildebrandt, G. (2006). Multidrug resistance and distribution of Salmonella serovars in slaughtered pigs. *Journal of veterinary medicine. B, Infectious diseases and veterinary public health*. Vol. 53, pp. (28-33). ISSN 0931-1793.

Molla, B., Mohammed, A. & Salah, W. (2004). *Salmonella* prevalence and distribution of serotypes in apparently healthy slaughtered camels (*Camelus dromedarius*) in Eastern Ethiopia. *Tropical Animal Health Production*. Vol. 36, No. 5, pp. (451–458). ISSN 0049-4747.

Montville, T. J. & Matthews, K. R. (2008). Food microbiology: An introduction (2nd ed.). 428 p., United States of America: ASM Press, Washington, DC. ISBN 9781-1-55581-396-3.

Moore, M. M. and M. D. Feist. (2006). Real-time PCR method for *Salmonella* spp. targeting the *stn* gene. Journal of Applied Microbiology . Vol. 102, No. 2, pp. (516 – 530). ISSN 1365-2672.

Murphy, N. M., Mclauchlin J., Ohai C., Grant K. A. (2007). Construction and valuation of a microbiological positive process internal control for PCR-based examination of food samples for *Listeria monocytogenes* and *Salmonella enterica*. International Journal of Food Microbiology. Vol. 120, No. 1-2, pp. (110-119). ISSN 0168-1605.

Musa, H. A. & Shears, P. (1998). Antibiotic resistant Escherichia coli in a Sudanese hospital. *Journal of Hospital Infection*. Vol. 38, No. 2, pp. (148-150). ISSN 0195-6701.

Nair, S., Poh, C. L., Lim, Y. S., Tay, L. & Goh, K. T. (1994). Genome fingerprinting of *Salmonella* Typhi by pulsed – field gel electrophoresis for subtyping common phage types. *Epidemiology and Infection*. Vol. 113, pp. (391 – 402). ISSN 1469-4409.

Nair, S., Schreiber, E., Thong, K-L., Pang, T. & Altwegg, M. (2000). Genotypic characterization of *Salmonella typhi* by amplified fragment length polymorphism fingerprinting provides increased discrimination as compared to pulsed-field gel electrophoresis and ribotyping. Journal of Microbiological Methods. Vol. 41, No. 1, pp. (35-43). ISSN 0167-7012.

Naravaneni, R. & Jamil, K. (2005). Rapid detection of food-borne pathogens by using molecular techniques. *Journal of Medical Microbiology,* Vol. 54, pp. (51 -54). ISSN 0022-2615.

Nord, C.E, Lindberg, A.A. & DahlbÄck, A. (1974). Evaluation of five test-kits—API, AuxoTab, Enterotube, PathoTec and R/B—for identification ofEnterobacteriaceae. *Medical Microbiology and Immunology.* Vol. 159, pp. (211-220). ISSN 0300-8584.

Nowroozi, J., Mirzaii, M. & Norauzi, M. (2004). Study of Lactobacillus as probiotic bacteria. *Iranian Journal of Public Health.* Vol. 33, No. 1, pp. (1-7). ISSN 0304-4556.

Pang, T., Bhutta, Z. A., Finally, B. B. & Altwegg, M. (1995). Typhoid fever and other salmonellosis: a continuing challenge. *Trends in Microbiology,* Vol. 3, pp. (35–43), ISSN 0966-842X.

Perales I. & Audicana, A. (1989). Semisolid media for isolation of Salmonella spp. from coastal waters. *Applied and Environmental Microbiology,* Vo. 55, No. 11, pp. (3032-3033). ISSN 0099-2240.

Piddock, L. J. V. (2002). Fluoroquinolone resistance in *Salmonella* serovars isolated from human and food animals. *FEMS Micobiology Reviews.* Vol. 26. pp. (3-16). ISSN 0168-6445.

Popoff, M. Y. & Le Minor, L. (2001). Antigenic formulas of the *Salmonella* serovars, 8th revision. WHO Collaborating Center for Reference and Research on *Salmonella,* Pasteur Institute, Paris, France. Retrieved from: < www.prise-pcp.org/.../cd/.../antigenic-formulas-salmonella-serovars.pdf>

Poppe, C., Ayroud, M., Ollis, G., Chirino-Trejo, M., Smart, N., Quessy, S. & Michell, P. (2001). Trends in antimicrobial resistance of *Salmonella* isolated from animals, foods of animal origin and the environment of animal production in Canada, 1994–1997. *Microbial Drug Resistance.* Vol. 7, No. 2, pp (197-212). DOI:10.1089/ 10766290152045084.

Portillo, F. G. (2000). Molecular and cellular biology of *Salmonella* pathogenesis. In: *Microbial foodborne Diseases: Mechanisms of Pathogenesis and Toxin Synthesis,* Gary, J.W. & Bhatnagar, D. (Eds.). pp. 3-34, Technomic Publishing Company, Inc., USA. ISBN 1566767873.

Pui, C. F., Wong, W. C., Chai, L. C., Tunung, R., Jeyaletchumi, P., Noor Hidayah, M. S., Ubong, A., Farinazleen, M. G., Cheah, Y. K. & Son, R. (2011). Review Article *Salmonella*: A foodborne pathogen. *International Food Research Journal.* Vol. 18, pp. (465-473). ISSN 19854668.

Ramsey, C. H. & Edwards, P. R. (1961). Resistance of Salmonellae Isolated in 1959 and 1960 to Tetracyclines and Chloramphenicol. *Applied and Environmental Microbiology.* Vol. 9, No. 5, pp. (389-391). ISSN 0099-2240.

Roberts, D. (1982). Bacteria of public health significance. In: *Meat Microbiology,* Brown, M.H. (Eds.), Applied Science Publishers, pp. (319- 386), ISBN 0853341389, London.

Rodrigue, D.C., Cameron, D.N., Puhr, N.D., Brenner, F., Louis, M. Wachsmuth, I.K. et al. (1992). Comparison of plasmid profiles, phage types, and antimicrobial resistance patterns of *Salmonella* Enteritidis isolates in the United States. *Journal of Clinical Microbiology.* Vol. 30, pp. (854-857). ISSN 0095-1137.

Rowe, B., Ward, L. & Threlfall, E. (1992). Ciprofloxacin and typhoid fever (letter). *Lancet.* Vol. 339, No. 8795, pp. (740). ISSN 0140-6736.

Roy, P., Dhillon, A. S., Lauerman, L. H., Schaberg, D. M., Bandli, D., Johnson, S. (2002). Results of *Salmonella* isolation from poultry products, poultry, poultry environment, and other characteristics. *Avian Diseases.* Vol. 46, pp. (17-24). ISSN 0005-2086.

Saha, P. D., Mitra, U. & Bhattachary, S. K. (2001). Isolation of *Salmonella enterica* serotypes from children with diarrhoea in Calcutta. *Journal of Health Population and Nutrition*. Vol. 19, No. 4, pp. (301-305). ISSN 1606-0997. PMID: 11855352.

Saliem, M. (1987). Bovine Salmonellosis in the Sudan. M.Sc. Thesis, University of Khartoum. Retrieved from:
< http://etd.uofk.edu/uofketdalllist.php?t=uofketdall&RecPerPage=ALL>

Salih, M. S.M. & Ibrahim, A. E. (1972). Bacteriological studies on raw edible sheep and cattle offal. *Sudan Medical Journal*. Vol. 10, pp. (183-193). Retrieved from:
< http://sudanmedicaljournal.net/index1.html#>

Sambrook, J., Fritsh, E.F. & Maniatis, T. (1989). Molecular Cloning: A laboratory manual, 2nd edn., vol. 1, pp. (21-32), Cold Spring Harber: Cold Spring Harber Laboratory Press. ISBN 0-87969-309-6.

Sariy Eldin, M. (1971). Studies on bacteriological quality of fresh meat. Ph.D. Thesis, University of Khartoum. Retrieved from:
<http:// etd.uofk.edu/uofketdalllist.php?t=uofketdall&RecPerPage=ALL >

Scherer, C. A. & Miller, S. I. (2001). Molecular pathogenesis of salmonellae. In: *Principles of Bacterial Pathogenesis*, Groisman. E. A. (Eds.), pp. 265-316. ISBN 0123042208, United States of America: Academic Press.

Schrank, I. S., Mores, M. A. Z., Costa, J. L. A., Frazzon, A. P. G., Soncini, R., Schrank, A., Vainstein, M. H. & Silva, S. C. (2001). Influence of enrichment media and application of a PCR based method to detect *Salmonella* in poultry industry products and clinical samples. *Veterinary Microbiology*, Vol. 82, pp. (45-53). ISSN 0378-1135.

Shangkuan, Y. H., & Lin, H. C. (1998). Application of random amplified polymorphic DNA analysis to differentiate strains of *Salmonella* Typhi and other *Salmonella* species. *Journal of Applied Microbiology*, Vol. 85, pp. (693 – 702). ISSN 1365-2672.

Sharma, V.K. & Carlson, S.A. (2000). Simultaneous detection of *Salmonella* strains and Escherichia coli O157:H7 with fluorogenic PCR and single-enrichment-broth culture. *Applied and Environmental Microbiology*. Vol. 66, No. 1, pp. (5472-5476). ISSN 0099-2240.

Shears, P., Suliman, G. & Hart, C. A. (1988). Occurrence of multiple resistance and R. Plasmids in Enterobacteriaceae isolated from children in the Sudan. *Epidemiology and Infection*. Vol. 100, pp. (73-81). ISSN 1469-4409.

Shipp, C. R. & Rowe, B. (1980). A mechanized microtechnique for *Salmonella* serotyping. *Journal of Clinical Pathology*. Vol. 33, pp. (595-597). ISSN 0021-9746.

Singh, S., Yadav, A. S., Singh, S. M. & Bharti, P. (2010). Prevalence of *Salmonella* in chicken eggs collected from poultry farms and marketing channels and their antimicrobial resistance. *Food Research International*. Vol. 43, No. 8. Pp. (2027-2030). ISSN 0963-9969.

Soliman, K. N. & Khan, A. Q. (1959). A note on *Salmonella* infection of livestock in Upper Nile Province, Sudan. *Bulletin of Epizootic Diseases of Africa*. Vol. 7, pp. (371-377). ISSN 0049-4747.

Somasegaran P. & Hoben H. J. (1985). Handbook for Rhizobia: Methods in Legume - Rhizobium Technology. Springer-Verlag, 450 p., ISBN 3540941347.

Soumet, C., Ermel, G., Fach, P. & Colin, P. (1994). Evaluation of different DNA extraction procedures for the detection of *Salmonella* from chicken products by polymerase chain reaction. *Letters in Applied Microbiology*, Vol. 19, pp. (294-298). ISSN ISSN 0266-8254.

Stevens, A., Kabore, Y., Perrier-Gros-Claude, J.D., Millemann, Y., Brisabois, A., Catteau, M., Cavin, J. and Dufour, B. (2006). Prevalence and antibiotic-resistance of *Salmonella* isolated from beef sampled from the slaughterhouse and from retailers in Dakar (Senegal). *International Journal of Food Microbiology*. Vol. 110, pp (178-86). DOI:10.1016/j.ijfoodmicro.2006.04.018.

Stone, G. G., Oberst, R. D., Hays, M. P., McVey, S. & Chengappa, M. M. (1994). Detection of *Salmonella* serovars from clinical samples by enrichment broth cultivation-PCR procedure. *Journal of Clinical Microbiology*. Vol. 32, pp. (1742–1749). ISSN 0095-1137.

Suresh, T., Hatha, A. A., Harsha, H. T. & Lakshmanaperumalsamy, P. (2011). Prevalence and distribution of *Salmonella* serotypes in marketed broiler chickens and processing environment in coimbatore city of southern India. *Food Research International*. Vol. 44, pp. (823-825). ISSN: 0963-9969.

Swenson, D. L., Clegg, S. & Old, D. C. (1991). The frequency of the *fim* genes among *Salmonella* serovars. *Microbial Pathogenesis*. Vol. 10, pp. (487–490). ISSN 0882-4010.

Tamada, Y., Nakaoka, Y., Nishimori, K., Doi, A., Kumaki, T., Uemura, N., Tanaka, K., Makino, S. I., Sameshima, T., Akiba, M., Nakazawa, M. & Uchida, I. (2001). Molecular typing and epidemiological study of *Salmonella enterica* serotyping Typhimurium isolates from cattle by fluorescent amplified –fragment length polymorphism fingerprinting and pulsed-filed gel electrophoresis. *Journal of Clinical Microbiology*. Vol. 39, pp. (1057-1066). ISSN 0095-1137.

Tassios, P. T., Markogiannakis, A., Vatopoulos, A.C., Katsanikou, E., Velonakis, E. N., Kourea-Kremastinou, J. & Legakis, N. J. (1997). Molecular epidemiology of antibiotic resistance of *Salmonella enteritidis* during a 7-year period in Greece. *Journal of Clinical Microbiology*. Vol. 35, pp. (1316–1321). ISSN 0095-1137.

Thong, K.L. & Modarressi, S. (2011). Antimicrobial resistant genes associated with *Salmonella* from retail neats and street foods. *Food Research International*. In press. DOI: 10.1016/j.foodres.2011.05.013. ISSN: 0963-9969.

Turki, Y., Mehri, I., Cherif, H., Najjari, A. & Aissa, R. B. (2011). Epidemiology and antibiotic resistance of *Salmonella enterica* serovar Kentucky isolates from Tunisia: The new emergent multi-drug resistance serotype. *Food Research International*. In press. DOI: 10/1016/j.foodres.2011.03044. ISSN: 0963-9969.

Uyttendaele, M. R., Debevere, J. M., Lips, R. M. & Neyts, K. D. (1998). Prevalence of *Salmonella* in poultry carcass and their products in Belgium. *International Journal of Food Microbiology*. Vol. 40, pp. 1-8. ISSN 0168-1605.

Van, T. T. H., Moutafis, G., Istivan, T., Tran, L. T. & Coloe, P. J. (2007). Detection of *Salmonella* spp. in retail raw food samples from Vietnam and characterization of their antibiotic resistance. *Applied and Environment Microbiology*. Vol. 73, No. 21, pp. (6885-6890). ISSN 0099-2240

Vincent J. M. (1970). A Manual for the Practical Study of Root-Nodule Bacteria. Blackwell, 176 p., ISBN 0632064102, Oxford.

Ward, L. R., De Sa, J. D. & Rowe, B. (1987). A phage-typing scheme for *Salmonella* Enteritidis. *Epidemiology and Infection*. Vol. 99, No. 2, pp. (291 - 294). ISSN 1469-4409.

Weill, F.-X. & Le Hello, S. (2008). F.-X. Weill and S. Le Hello, Rapport d'activité annuel 2008. Centre National de Référence des *Salmonella*. Retrieved from: http://www.pasteur.fr/ip/portal/action/WebdriveActionEvent/oid/01s-00003k-03o (2008) accessed 11-30-2010

White, D. G., Zhao, S., Sudler, R., Ayers, S., Friedman, S., Chen, S., et al. (2001). The isolation of antibiotic-resistant *Salmonella* from retail ground meat. *The New England Journal of Medicine*. Vol. 345, pp. (1147-1154). ISSN 0028-4793.

Whyte, P., Mc Gill, K., Collins, J.D., & Gormley, E. (2002). The prevalence and PCR detection of *Salmonella* contamination in raw poultry. *Veterinary Microbiology*, Vol. 89, pp. (53-60). ISSN 1476-0711.

Widjojoatmodjo, M. N., Fluit, A. C., Torensma, R., Verdonk, G. P. H. T. & Verhoef, J. (1992). The magnetic immuno polymerase chain reaction assay for direct detection of salmonellae in fecal samples. *Journal of Clinical Microbiology*. Vol. 30, pp. 3195– 3199. ISSN 0095-1137.

Yagoub, I. A. & Mohammed, T. E. (1987). Isolation and identification of *Salmonella* from chickens in Khartoum Province of Sudan. *British Veterinary Journal*. Vol. 143, No. 6, pp. (537-540). ISSN 0007-1935

Yagoub, S.O., Awadalla, N. E. & El Zubeir, I. E. M. (2005). Incidence of some potential pathogens in raw milk in Khartoum North (Sudan) and their susceptibility to antimicrobial agents. *Journal of Animal and Veterinary Advances*. Vol. 4, No. 3, pp. 341-344. ISSN 1680-5593.

Yagoub, S.O., Oshi, N. A. M. & El Zubeir, I. E. M. (2006). Isolation and susceptibility to antimicrobial agent of *Salmonella* Paratyphi from Cheese in Khartoum (Sudan). *Research Journal of Microbiology*. Vol. 1, No. 2, pp. (110-114). ISSN 1816-4927.

Yah, C.S. & Eghafona, N. O. (2008). Plasmids: A Vehicle for rapid transfer of antibiotic resistance markers of *Salmonella* species in animals. International *Journal of Integrative Biology*. Vol. 2, No. 1, pp. (55-61). ISSN 0973-8363.

Yousef, A. E. & Carlstrom, C. (2003). *Salmonella*. In: *Food microbiology: A laboratory manual*, Yousef, A. E. and Carstrom, C. (Eds.). p. 167-205, John Wiley & Sons, Inc., ISBN 0471391050, New Jersey.

Zhao, S., Datta, A. R., Ayers, S., Friedman, S., Walker, R. D. & White, D. G. (2003). Antimicrobial-resistant *Salmonella* serovars isolated from imported foods. *International Journal of Food Microbiology*. Vol. 84, No. 1, pp. (87-92). ISSN 0168-1605.

Zhao, S., Fedorka-Cray, P. J., Friedman, S., Mcdermott, P. F., Walker, R. D., Qaiyumi, S., et al (2005). Characterization of *Salmonella* Typhimurium of animal origin obtained from the national antimicrobial resistance monitoring system. *Foodborne Pathogens and Disease*. Vol. 2, pp. 169-181. ISSN 1535-3141.

Zhao, S., McDermott, P. F., Friedman, S., Abbott, J., Ayers, S., Glenn, A., et al. (2006). Antimicrobial resistance and genetic relatedness among Salmonella from retail foods of animal origin: NARMS retail meat surveillance. *Foodborne Pathogens and Disease*. Vol. 3, No. 1, pp. 106-117. ISSN 1535-3141.

Zhou, L. & Pollard, A. J. (2010). A fast and highly sensitive blood culture PCR method for clinical detection of *Salmonella enteric* serovar Typhi. *Annals of Clinical Microbiology and Antimicrobials*, Vol. 9:14. DOI: 10.1186/1476-0711-9-14, retrieved from <http://www.ann-clinmicrob.com/content/9/1/14>

Ziemer, C. J., & Steadham, S. R. (2003). Evaluation of the Specificity of *Salmonella* PCR primers using various Intestinal bacteria species. *Letters in Applied Microbiology*. pp. (263 - 269). ISSN 0266-8254.

4

Salmonella Associated with Snakes (Suborder Serpentes)

Henrique Marçal Bastos
Clínica Veterinária Vila Sabrina, São Paulo, SP
Brazil

1. Introduction

In modern society, snakes (suborder Serpentes) are valued for their use in scientific research. Although being perceived with fear and repugnance by many people, snakes play an essential role in nature and influence many aspects of human life and culture. For centuries, snakes have developed significant scientific, ecologic, economic, cultural, and religious importance (Table 1).

Scientific	Laboratory animals for biomedical research
	Research on venoms for the development of new therapeutic drugs
	Venom collection for antiserum production
Ecologic	Control of rodents and other vertebrates
	Prey items for several carnivore species (mammals, birds and reptiles)
	Important components of the food web
	Ambassadors for environmental education programs and zoological parks
Economic	Exotic pets
	Skin and meat production
Cultural	Popular symbolism, including as the symbol of the medical sciences
	Mythological symbolism
	Subjects in public demonstrations and entertainment
Religious	As a symbol and representation of gods and other religious elements
	Use in various modern religious cults

Table 1. Importance of snakes

Direct contact is necessary between humans and snakes for many of the activities described above; however during such handling, one is susceptible to contamination by any microbe or pathogen that may be on the animal surface or in its secretions. Such contamination may occur not only by direct contact, but also indirectly through objects, food and inanimate surfaces that had previously been in contact with reptiles.

Among the several microorganisms inhabiting the body of snakes, Gram-negative bacteria are considered one of the most significant groups. Although they may be part of the saprophytic microbiota, oftentimes they can behave as pathogens and lead to well-defined diseases or act as opportunistic invaders of their animal or human hosts. There are many

Gram-negative bacteria of medical significance, and *Salmonella* is a particularly important genus due to its implication for public health.

2. Etiology

The current classification of *Salmonella* is complex. The genus is divided into two major species: *S. enterica* and *S. bongori* (subspecies V). *S. enterica* is further divided into six distinct subspecies based on biochemical differences: *enterica* (subspecies I), *salamae* (subspecies II), *arizonae* (subspecies IIIa), *diarizonae* (subspecies IIIb), *houtenae* (subspecies IV), and *indica* (subspecies VI). *Salmonella* strains may be further classified by serology into over 2500 serotypes (serovars) using the Kauffman and White classification scheme. This scheme defines the serogroup according to the expression of somatic lipopolysaccharide O antigens (LPS), and the serotype based on the expression of flagellar H antigens (Barrow et al., 2010; Grimont & Weill, 2007; Mitchell & Shane, 2001). Besides serving for classification purposes, the variations in LPS structure provide each serotype a different degree of virulence (Paré et al., 2006). Serotypes may be referred to by a name or an antigenic formula. In this chapter, strains will be referred to by the genus followed by the serotype or the number of the subgroup: *Salmonella enterica enterica* serotype Typhimurium will be referred to as "*S.* Typhimurium", *Salmonella enterica diarizonae* 60:r:z_{15} as "*S.* 60:r:z_{15}", *Salmonella enterica diarizonae* (IIIb) as "*S.* IIIb", and so forth.

Distinct patterns of infection (pathovars) may also be used to classify serotypes. There are three pathovars: the first includes a few serotypes that produce severe systemic disease in healthy animals; the second pathovar comprises serotypes that affect young animals and pregnant or egg-laying females; the third pathovar includes serotypes that cause infection in immunocompromised animals (Barrow et al. 2010).

The classification of strains based on their host range (host-specific, host-restricted, ubiquitous) is controversial (Barrow et al., 2010). Clinical signs involving the digestive tract are the predominant manifestations of the infections by the generalist serotypes. These infections are characterized by high morbidity but low mortality. In contrast, infections caused by serotypes adapted to specific animal species or a restrict group of hosts will tend to present low morbidity and high mortality (Hoelzer et al., 2011).

In reptiles, *Salmonella* inhabits the distal small intestine and the colon (Carvalho, 2006); however its presence seldom produces primary disease, as the bacteria seem to be part of the indigenous gut flora of these animals (Mitchell, 2004).

The first reports of *Salmonella* isolation from reptiles date back to cases involving lizards in 1939. In 1944, the bacterium was first isolated from a Bull Snake (*Pituophis catenifer*) and in 1946 from a turtle. However it was not until 1953, when a human was shown to have probably acquired salmonellosis from a chelonian, that these isolations were considered relevant (Mathewson, 1979). Hinshaw & McNeil (1944, 1945, 1946, 1947) were two researchers that greatly contributed on the first *Salmonella* isolations from reptiles.

There is a very broad diversity of serotypes amongst reptiles (Pedersen et al., 2009). From all known serotypes, approximately 40% are predominantly associated with these animals (Hoelzer et al., 2011). Even though there are no reptile-specific serotypes, subspecies III is known to be the most common in snakes (Warwick et al., 2001). Other studies have also demonstrated that *Salmonella enterica diarizonae* (IIIb) corresponds to 92.8% of the serotypes isolated from *Bothrops jararaca* (Bastos et al., 2008) and to 100% of the isolates from *Bitis nasicornis* and *Bothriechis schlegelii* (Schröter et al., 2004), and that the subspecies *S.* IIIa and *S.* IIIb are also generally predominant in various other snake species (Sá & Solari, 2001).

In the past it was generally believed that subspecies III was a part of the reptile normal gastrointestinal microbiota (Orós et al., 1996). While serotypes of all *Salmonella* subspecies have been isolated from snakes (Bemis et al., 2007), *S.* IIIa seems to be the most pathogenic for these animals as it is most frequently isolated in cases with clinical disease (Lamberski et al., 2002; Ramsay et al., 2002). It must be taken into account, however, that due to recent changes in the nomenclature and structure of antigenic formulas used to classify *Salmonella* strains it is often difficult to determine to what extent the previous reports involved the subspecies IIIa and IIIb (Bemis et al., 2007). In Brazil, the subgroup III (formerly classified as genus *Arizona*) was first isolated in snakes in 1973, by Moreno and colleagues.

The retrieval of *Salmonella* strains from a reptile does not *per se* elucidate its role as a disease or potential zoonosis, as clinically healthy snakes may host highly virulent serotypes (Johnson-Delaney, 2006). Furthermore, the development of disease depends on a variety of factors such as animal species, individual susceptibility, stress, and inoculated dose (Carvalho, 2006).

3. Epidemiology

3.1 Prevalence

One of the first estimates of *Salmonella* prevalence among snakes was performed by Chiodini & Sundberg in 1981, who described rates of infection ranging from 16 to 92%. Another study conducted by Chiodini (1982), found that 55 out of 56 snakes (98%) were naturally infected with *Salmonella*. Several other studies determined the prevalence of these bacteria in snakes throughout the world: 92.5% and 69.2% in Australia (Iveson et al., 1969; Scheelings et al., 2011), 24% in Austria (Pfleger et al., 2003), 64.7% in Brazil (Bastos et al., 2008), 71.6% in Germany and Austria (Geue & Löschner, 2002), 69.7% in Taiwan (Chen et al., 2010), and 15% in Trinidad (Gopee et al., 2000). Prevalence is generally high in snakes; however it is important to consider these numbers may vary broadly depending on the evaluation methods (Johnson-Delaney, 2006).

The most prevalent *Salmonella* strains in snake fecal samples may vary over time (Schröter et al., 2004), however such fluctuations have yet to be understood (Schröter et al., 2006), but it has been suggested that failures of the isolation methods and intermittent elimination of the bacteria in the feces may be involved (Chiodini & Sundberg, 1981).

3.2 Sources of infection

Fecal shedding is well documented in snakes (Ramsay et al., 2002) however other potential sources of infection must be considered (Warwick et al., 2001). The bacteria may be present in the oral cavity and there is a remote possibility of transmission through bites (see Treatment). The bacteria can also be eliminated via the cloaca in the eggs, feces, urine, and possibly other secretions.

Ramsay et al. (2002) reported that in a colony of rattlesnakes, some of which presented *Salmonella*-associated osteomyelitis, contaminated wood shaving substrate might have been a source of infection when snakes were transferred among cages. The transmission of *Salmonella* through inanimate objects has been well described in a *Salmonella* outbreak in Komodo Dragons (*Varanus komodoensis*) held captive at a zoo (Friedman et al., 1998). Furthermore, considering the natural tongue-flicking behavior of snakes, the ingestion of substrate during prey consumption is probably not necessary to cause infection, as the briefest contact of the tongue with a contaminated surface could be sufficient to acquire *Salmonella*. Although the bacterium is frequently present in the environment, large outbreaks in humans are rarely caused solely due to environmental contamination (Friedman et al., 1998).

Some reptiles may inoculate *Salmonella* through bites and claw scratches. It is also possible that humans could be infected through ear or eye contact with feces, urine or water from the snakes' cages (Warwick et al., 2001). A snake may become infected when maintained in poor hygiene conditions, in cages or exhibits with accumulation of excrements (Fornazari & Teixeira, 2009).

3.3 Methods of transmission

Transmission occurs primarily through the fecal-oral route, but may also occur through the ingestion of contaminated food or water. Bacteria present in inanimate surfaces or in the animals may also be transmitted indirectly (Carvalho, 2006).

Snake prey, whether wild animals captured by free-ranging snakes or laboratory animals used to feed captive snakes, may present distinct species-specific characteristics that influence the acquisition of *Salmonella*. This bacterium has been frequently retrieved from wild rodents (Hoelzer et al., 2011) and other vertebrates upon which free-ranging snakes feed, however its prevalence tends to be generally lower in wild than in captive reptiles (Gray, 2011).

Although most snakes feed on vertebrates, some have specialized on invertebrate-based diets. Mollusks and crustaceans may also be consumed by snakes and it is believed that they may be a source of *Salmonella* to humans and other animals. Information is yet insufficient to confirm whether they could be potential sources of infection for snakes, but it has been suggested that they could maintain these bacteria in natural environments (Minette, 1984).

The indirect transmission from reptiles may occur because *Salmonella* can retain its virulence for several days or months in the environment. This has been shown to be particularly important for small children, as they may often become infected without ever touching the pet reptile (Bays, 2005; Hoelzer et al., 2011).

Mermin et al. (2004) reported that *Salmonella* can been isolated from the aquarium water of chelonians several weeks following contamination, and the bacteria can be recovered from the reptiles' feces even several months after defecation. It is likely that strains from semi-aquatic snakes may persist for several weeks in the water of their cages.

Salmonella has been used for several decades in an unusual manner: as a rodenticide. Even nowadays these products are still produced in some countries, despite the risk they are known to pose to human health (Painter et al., 2004). Such rodenticides are prepared using *Salmonella* Typhimurium and *S.* Enteritidis (Hoelzer et al., 2011). In addition to the unnecessary risk of transmission to humans, the strains used in these products may infect food, livestock and wildlife.

Another form of *Salmonella* infection is vertical transmission. Investigating chelonians, Kaufmann and colleagues (1972) reported that the first studies on this subject indicated trans-ovarian infection may occur, but with unknown frequency and likely with less relevance than post-laying contamination of the eggs. Those authors did not succeed in isolating *Salmonella* from the ovarian tissues of the turtles as they had done before (Kaufmann & Morrison, 1966) and suggested their previous findings could be due to rapid bacterial penetration through the egg shell after oviposition, resulting in infected newborn animals. In the 1960s, it was already known that *Salmonella* quickly penetrated turtle eggs, contaminating them as they passed through the cloaca or were laid in contaminated soil (Chiodini & Sundberg, 1981). In the following decades, the isolation of *Salmonella* from turtle ovarian tissues and egg contents as had been performed by Kaufmann and Morrison (1966) was not reproduced (Kaufmann et al., 1972) nor investigated in other reptiles (Chiodini & Sundberg, 1981).

Snake fetuses are not sterile, and the shedding of *Salmonella* by hatchlings does not necessarily occur even when the fetuses are already infected by that microorganism (Chiodini, 1982). *Salmonella* is only shed in the feces when the digestive tract of the fetus is infected, not in systemic or coelomic infections. Moreover, because *Salmonella* may be isolated in one fecal culture and not in another, it is possible that fetuses positive to *S. arizonae* may be delivered by a female that had negative fecal cultures during pregnancy (Chiodini, 1982).

In a study carried out in Germany, Schröter et al. (2006) observed 65% *Salmonella* prevalence in newborn snakes, suggesting that colonization may have occurred during pregnancy or upon birth. There seems to be no correlation between a specific serotype and its success in being transmitted to the host's progeny.

Discussions on the vertical transmission of a pathogen are generally focused on the female, whether it is an oviparous or viviparous species. The male is not often considered, either because it is not recognized as playing a significant role in vertical transmission or simply because it is forgotten. In certain snake species sperm transfer during copulation may be very prolonged, the cloacae remaining in intimate contact during this period, which may be sufficient for the exchange of bacteria between male and female. Moreover, it has been shown that some female snakes can store viable sperm from copulation for up to 6 years, a phenomenon called *amphigonia retardata* (Mader, 2006). There is research that can help us evaluating the possibility of sexual transmission of *Salmonella* from male to female, and the potential hazard for posterior vertical transmission to the progeny (Hidalgo-Vila, 2007, as cited in Pedersen et al., 2009). For instance, Chiodini (1982) did not succeed in isolating *Salmonella* from snake testes, whilst Ramsay et al. (2002) successfully isolated *S. arizonae* from the testes of a *Crotalus willardi*, and noted that active spermatogenesis occurred despite the presence of granulomatous infiltrates.

Behavioral characteristics may interfere with the acquisition and elimination of *Salmonella* by a snake. The high prevalence of *Salmonella* in terrestrial (ground-dwelling) snakes when compared to arboreal snakes may be explained by behavioral differences and by the higher risk for the terrestrial species to come in contact with contaminated excrements in the soil or substrate (Schröter et al., 2004). Semiaquatic snakes, which spend most of their time inside water, present a greater probability to acquire *Salmonella* by hydric transmission. This becomes particularly relevant for snakes in captivity, where the concentration of bacteria may become high depending on the maintenance routine and the characteristics of their tank or artificial lake. There is a case report of fatal bacterial sepsis in Water Snakes (*Helicops modestus*) in which the lack of flowing water was considered a contributing factor for the contamination of the cages with *Proteus vulgaris* (Coutinho et al., 2001).

Although they often prefer to place their feces on a corner of the cage, snakes may defecate and urinate in various locations, including in watering bowls, particularly after ecdysis. Urine may be contaminated by fecal debris upon expelling through the cloaca. Some freshwater chelonians can drain water into the cloaca and release it at the nesting site to soften the soil and facilitate oviposition (Warwick et al., 2001), a behavior that may lead to the contamination of the nest and eggs.

4. Diagnostic techniques

The diagnostic method most frequently used to isolate *Salmonella* is microbiological culture (Mitchell, 2006). Isolation protocols and information on culture media are easily found in the vast scientific literature on this topic. The isolation of this bacterium generally involves: direct culture, enrichment, inoculation on culture plates, screening for suspect colonies and confirmation through biochemical and serological tests (Waltman, 2000). Most techniques and protocols used for the isolation of *Salmonella* from other sources are also used for its isolation from reptiles.

Although microbiological culture may fail to detect some asymptomatic carriers (Bradley & Angulo, 2008), it may assist investigations concerning the transmission of *Salmonella* from reptiles to humans (Gray, 2011), while biomolecular assays such as pulsed-field gel electrophoresis (PFGE) provide additional confirmatory clues.

Tetrathionate, Rappaport-Vassiliadis and selenite broths are the selective-enrichment media used to isolate *Salmonella*. To isolate this bacterium from reptiles, Mitchell (2006) recommends selenite broth. After incubation, a small aliquot of the primary enrichment broth is transferred to a selective medium. Although the direct culturing of a sample is usually unsuccessful, Bastos et al. (2008) were able to isolate multiple *Salmonella* and other enterobacteria from intestinal mucosa swabs of *Bothrops jararaca*.

Most of the broad variety of selective media used to isolate *Salmonella* from other animals has already been tested for reptiles, and the XLT4 agar has been shown to provide the best results (Bastos et al., 2008; Mitchell, 2006). In spite of the morphologic similarity of *Salmonella* colonies with those of other Enterobacteriaceae in MacConkey agar, Bastos et al. (2008) isolated 7 colonies on this agar (poorly selective media) when compared to the 13 colonies obtained from the same samples using the XLT4 agar (highly selective media); MacConkey agar is seldom used to specifically isolate *Salmonella*.

Selective screening media are used to confirm or rule out suspect colonies. The most commonly used are lysine iron agar (LIA), urea and triple sugar iron agar (TSI), besides a variety of commercial biochemical test kits (Mitchell, 2006).

After confirmation of the *Salmonella* genus, colonies can be submitted for serotyping. Subsequently, the isolates may be further identified using molecular methods such as ribotyping and PFGE (Ghilardi et al., 2006; Nair et al., 2002). Non-culture diagnostic methods can also be used for the detection of *Salmonella*, such as enzyme-linked immunosorbent assays (ELISA) and polymerase chain reactions (PCR). Both techniques can detect low numbers of bacteria in a sample (Mitchell, 2006); however are seldom applied for reptiles.

Rough phase strains are frequently isolated (Bastos et al., 2008; Geue & Löschner, 2002; Pedersen et al., 2009; Pfleger et al., 2003; Ramsay et al., 2002). These isolates agglutinate spontaneously during the agglutination serotyping tests (Difco, 2011), producing negative results that render these strains non-typable. Non-typable strains are also frequent in *Salmonella* isolated from reptiles (Bastos et al., 2008; Chen et al., 2010; Pedersen et al., 2009; Sá & Solari, 2001). Salb et al. (2002) were able to identify 42% of the isolates retrieved from Green Iguanas (*Iguana iguana*). Isolates from other vertebrates may also be similarly difficult to characterize.

Knowledge on the dynamics of this bacterium may be obtained through antigenic characterization and molecular methods (Nair et al., 2002; Sá & Solari, 2001). However, studies on the virulence of *Salmonella* in snakes still lack appropriate infection models (Bernis et al., 2007).

5. Clinical signs

In reptiles, *Salmonella* gastroenteritis leads to diarrhea (Funk, 1996), particularly in acute form. Other clinical signs include coelomitis, pneumonia, and septicemia. Hypovolemic shock and death may also occur. The feces may become green-grayish and contain mucus or blood. Small hemorrhagic spots may appear on the mucous membranes and ventral scales in animals with sepsis. Reptiles in this condition may also exhibit muscle weakness (Messonnier, 1996).

Inappetance and regurgitation with blood and mucus were observed in a Rosy Boa (*Lichanura trivirgata*) with gastrointestinal lesions (Orós et al., 1996). Extra-intestinal salmonellosis may also occur. *S. arizonae* has been associated with extensive bone lesions on the vertebrae and ribs of snakes, leading to limited mobility and prostration. Severely affected animals lose their righting reflexes and fail to capture prey (Ramsay et al., 2002). *Salmonella*-associated pneumonias in *Boa constrictor* may also lead to dyspnea (Onderka & Finlayson, 1985).

6. Pathological findings

Several reports dating back to the 1940s demonstrated that snakes may harbor *Salmonella*, often without any clinical manifestations (asymptomatic carriers) or with clinical signs and lesions typically related to the disease. Although this does not occur frequently, the first descriptions reported hepatic lesions and intestinal inflammation (Page, 1966). Inflammation and necrosis are often present in many organs. However, *Salmonella* can occur in virtually any visceral tissue of clinically healthy snakes (Chiodini, 1982) and its implication in the death of snakes and other reptiles is uncommon. In snakes, salmonellosis may manifest as necrotizing subacute severe enteritis, normally involving the distal half of the intestines (Onderka & Finlayson, 1985). The intestinal tract of two *Crotallus willardi* that died from enteritis presented heterophilic necrotizing and granulomatous lesions (Ramsay et al., 2002). A Rosy Boa (*Lichanura trivirgata*) with gastrointestinal clinical signs presented diffuse thickening of the gastric wall with necrotic and fibrinonecrotic lesions (Orós et al., 1996).

Besides the digestive tract, the urinary tract and the liver were found to be frequently infected in a survey conducted by Chiodini (1982). In snakes, *Salmonella* septicemia produced hepatitis associated to granulomas (Onderka & Finlayson, 1985).

Salmonella was speculated to be involved in a case of septic endocarditis of a Burmese Python (*Python molurus bivittatus*) (Murray, 1996), and was proven to have caused granulomatous myocarditis in a Madagascar Dumerili's Boa (*Acrantophis dumerili*) (Schilliger et al., 2003).

Lesions associated with *S. arizonae* are frequently observed in the gastrointestinal tract, spleen, liver, oviduct and ureter. Lesions in the respiratory tract are less common. Orós et al. (1996) observed tracheal necrosis and inflammation caused by *S. arizonae* in a double-headed Honduran Milksnake (*Lampropeltis hondurensis*) which had been found dead without previous clinical signals. Onderka & Finlayson (1985) reported fibrinous alveolar exudation and interstitial inflammatory infiltration in the lungs of a *Boa constrictor* deceased from a pneumonia caused by *Salmonella*.

In snakes with osteomyelitis, the bone lesions presented heterophilic-granulomatous inflammation, osteonecrosis and sequestra, periosteal bone proliferations in the form of exostoses accompanied by heterophilic-granulomatous inflammation, and trabecular and cortical osteopenia; oophoritis and salpingitis also occured (Ramsay et al., 2002).

7. Treatment

7.1 Antibiotics

It is not possible to eliminate *Salmonella* from the digestive tract of reptiles. Experience has shown it is impossible to raise *Salmonella*-free reptiles (Association of Reptilian and Amphibian Veterinarians [ARAV], 2009), suggesting a participation of environmental contamination in the infection, and indicating that the animals may maintain latent infections (Mermin et al., 2004).

The administration of antimicrobial agents is not recommended for enteric salmonellosis in reptiles, as some studies have demonstrated that the course of the disease is not affected by the antimicrobial therapy. On the other hand, treatment of systemic salmonellosis should include intensive care and appropriate antimicrobial therapy (Hirsh, 2004).

Whenever possible, antibiotic choice should be based on antimicrobial sensitivity testing. When this is not possible, information from the literature may be useful: *Salmonella* strains isolated from snakes are generally sensitive to aminoglycosides, quinolones and trimethoprim-sulfamethoxazole, and are often resistant to ampicillin, cefoperazone, chloramphenicol, neomycin, streptomycin and tetracycline (Bastos et al., 2008; Chen et al., 2010; Gopee et al., 2000). Multi-resistant strains are uncommon.

Bastos et al. (2008) demonstrated that *Salmonella* isolates from Jararacas were sensible to most antimicrobials tested. *Salmonella* strains carried by free-ranging snakes are also generally sensitive to antibiotics. Indiscriminate use of antibiotics can select resistant strains, however Jijón et al. (2007) pointed out that the emergence of drug-resistant bacteria is not mandatorily associated to prior antimicrobial therapy.

Several bacterial genera, including *Salmonella*, may be isolated from the mouth of snakes that are clinically healthy or with stomatitis (Mehler & Bennett, 2006). However, prophylactic antibiotic administration is not recommended for victims of ophidism if the snake species involved has venom lacking strong cytotoxic effects, such as is the case for South American Rattlesnakes (*Crotalus durissus*) (Nishioka et al., 2000). Although the incidence of abscesses on the bite wound area is approximately 12% for accidents involving South American *Bothrops* spp. (Ribeiro & Jorge, 1990, 1997), the specific involvement of *Salmonella* is clearly not a problem (Andrade et al., 1989; Jorge et al., 1990). This also applies to large constrictor snakes and small colubrids. Among several hundred snake-bite accidents involving numerous Brazilian species, in only one case (0.4%) there was the formation of a small, easily treatable abscess (Bastos, pers. obs.). Interestingly, snake venom contains biologically active peptides with antimicrobial activity (Lima et al., 2005; Wang et al., 2008).

It is likely that the bacterial diversity found in the snake oral microbiota reflects the variation in the fecal microbiota of the live prey they ingested, particularly as the prey often defecates while it is being killed and consumed (Goldstein et al., 1979). These researchers mentioned that live rodents were used to feed the studied captive snakes, however oftentimes the studies on differences in the microbiota of wild and captive snakes do not specify which food items were offered to the animals. Another important consideration is that food and stress may alter the snake oral microbiota depending on the lifetime spent in captivity.

7.2 Probiotics and prebiotics

The capacity of the microbial flora to prevent the multiplication of a given microorganism is called competitive exclusion (Schneitz & Mead, 2000). Probiotics act in this manner: they are live microorganisms that provide beneficial effects to their host's health that go beyond their inherent nutritional value. Studies demonstrate that only a few organisms truly act as probiotics (Myers, 2007).

Studies from the 1980s and the early 1990s demonstrated that the successful colonization of the cecum of turkeys by bacteria such as *Lactobacillus reuteri* and *Bacillus subtilis* may provide protection against the establishment of *Salmonella* in the microbiota; these findings were accompanied by general improvements in viability, body mass, and feed conversion efficiency. Research on hens, however, have generally failed to reproduce those results and did not provide protection against the colonization by *Salmonella* (Hafez & Jodas, 2000). Recent studies have indicated some organisms that might be more successful in preventing *Salmonella* colonization in the ceca of hens, and Pascual and colleagues (1999) demonstrated that *Lactobacillus salivarius* strain CTC2197 may be an effective competitor against the establishment of *S.* Enteritidis in the intestinal epithelium of hens.

The administration of probiotics on the feed of Green Iguanas (*Iguana iguana*) is anecdotally said to eliminate *Salmonella* from their gastrointestinal tract. However, such effect was not demonstrated in Carpet Pythons (*Morelia spilota*), as the probiotics did not prevent the shedding of the bacterium in the feces (Holz & Middleton, 2002). Although at the moment no tests on the use of probiotics in snakes have produced successful results, efforts to characterize their intestinal microflora have been conducted aiming to identify microorganisms that may be used for the competitive exclusion of *Salmonella* (Gray, 2011).

Prebiotics are another group of substances intended to modify the intestinal environment, favoring the growth of beneficial microorganisms while preventing the proliferation of pathogens. Lactulose is a prebiotic with beneficial effects on the health of domestic animals, and has also been used to prevent the growth of *Salmonella* in their digestive tract (Holz & Middleton, 2005). This compound is used as a nutritional substrate, to promote the growth of desirable bacteria. Pathogenic bacteria, on the other hand, are unable to use this energetic substrate and their growth is suppressed by the acidification of the intestinal environment (Jankowski, 2009). Unfortunately, however, lactulose failed to prevent the elimination of *Salmonella* in the feces on studies conducted with Carpet Pythons (*Morelia spilota*) and Scrub Pythons (*Morelia amethystina*) (Holz & Middleton, 2005).

8. Prevention and control

A number of measures may be taken to interrupt the proliferation of *Salmonella* in the environment, eliminate it whenever possible and prevent it from reaching specific areas: rigorous hygiene and disinfection of facilities and equipment, isolation of sick animals and asymptomatic carriers, measures of animal welfare, and the complete removal of organic matter to facilitate disinfectant action. Sodium hypochlorite (bleach) is an effective and low-cost disinfectant that may be used for the sanitation of exhibits and cages. It should also be kept in mind that asymptomatic carriers are important sources of infection (Carvalho, 2006), as infected animals are normally isolated and monitored, thus reducing transmission (Fornazari & Teixeira, 2009).

The general public is often unaware of the risks associated to salmonellosis, failing to take basic hygiene practices while handling reptiles. Simple hygiene procedures alone can considerably decrease the probability of transmission (Hoelzer et al., 2011). Friedman et al. (1998) demonstrated that washing hands after attending a reptile exhibit or before the next meal is sufficient to prevent reptile-associated salmonellosis. This hygiene routine oftentimes is not properly followed by children under the age of five, and as a result this age group is more prone to become contaminated (Centers for Disease Control and Prevention [CDC], 2010).

The release of animals to their natural habitats, as performed by wildlife rehabilitation centers, should be thoughtful to avoid spreading *Salmonella* to free-ranging populations (Jijón et al., 2007).

Table 2 presents a list of instructions cooperatively elaborated by the Association of Reptilian and Amphibian Veterinarians (ARAV) and the Center for Disease Control and Prevention (CDC) to reduce human exposure and disease development risks involving reptiles. Table 3 provides a client educational handout developed by the ARAV.

Veterinarians who treat reptiles should educate their clients who own reptiles about *Salmonella* and provide information on the recommended precautions for reducing the risk of transmission of *Salmonella* from reptiles to humans. This is especially important in households with infants and children under 5 years of age or with immunocompromised persons. The CDC recommends that households with children less than 5 years of age not own reptiles.

All veterinarians, staff and clients who handle reptiles should follow recommended precautions for reducing the risk of transmitting *Salmonella* from reptiles to humans. These precautions are also included in the ARAV client education handout and are based on good personal hygiene and not allowing reptiles to soil the owners' domicile.

All reptiles should be presumed to be carrying *Salmonella* in their intestinal tract and to be continuously or intermittently shedding it in their feces. Bacterial culture of fecal specimens from reptiles to determine *Salmonella* infection status is discouraged. If veterinarians are called upon to assist health officials in determining the cause of salmonellosis in a person, bacterial culture of combined fecal and cloacal specimens from reptiles with which that person has had direct or indirect contact are recommended. Serotyping of *Salmonella* isolates is usually needed to help discern the source of the *Salmonella* in human infections.

It is not recommended to treat healthy reptiles with antimicrobial agents with the intention of eliminating *Salmonella* from the intestinal tract. Clients who request treatment of healthy reptiles for *Salmonella* should be discouraged from such treatment and cautioned about the possibility of causing the emergence of antimicrobial-resistant *Salmonella* strains that might pose a greater health risk to humans (Bradley & Angulo, 2008).

Table 2. *Salmonella* and reptiles: veterinary guidelines

Always wash your hands with hot, soapy water after handling reptiles, reptile cages and equipment, and the feces of reptiles.
Do not allow reptiles to have access to the kitchen, dining room, or any other area in which food is prepared or eaten. Also, do not allow reptiles to have access to bathroom sinks and tubs or to any area where infants are bathed. Consider keeping your reptiles caged or limiting the parts of the house where reptiles are allowed to roam free. Always wash your hands after coming into contact with any area where reptiles are allowed to roam free.
Do not eat, drink, or smoke while handling reptiles, reptile cages, or reptile equipment. Do not kiss reptiles or share food or drink with them.
Do not use the kitchen sink, kitchen counters, bathroom sinks or bathtubs to bathe reptiles or to wash reptile cages, dishes or aquariums. Reptile owners may wish to purchase a plastic basin or tub in which to bathe or swim their reptiles. Waste water and fecal material should be disposed of in the toilet instead of the bathtub or household sink.
The CDC recommends that children less than five years of age avoid contact with reptiles and those households with children less than five years of age not own reptiles. The ARAV encourages reptile owners with young children to discuss steps to minimize risks associated with owning reptiles with their reptiles' veterinarian and their physician. Children should be supervised when they are handling reptiles to ensure that they do not place their hands or objects that a reptile has contacted in their mouths. Reptiles should not be kept in childcare centers.
Immunocompromised persons should avoid contact with reptiles.
Follow instructions from your reptile's veterinarian concerning proper diet and environment for your reptile. Healthy reptiles living in proper environments are less likely to shed *Salmonella* bacteria (ARAV, 2008).

Table 3. *Salmonella* bacteria and reptiles: client educational handout

9. Zoonotic aspects

9.1 Snake-associated human salmonellosis

Animal transmitted-salmonellosis is thought to be underreported, and the registered cases are probably biased towards uncommon or unusual characteristics. For instance, less than

1% of the reported cases of human salmonellosis are caused by reptile-associated strains (Hoelzer et al., 2011). Moreover, many patients recover rapidly without having received any treatment, further increasing underreporting (Gray, 2011).

Human salmonellosis is most frequently associated with food ingestion, however direct or indirect contact with animals in public or private environments may also be sources of infection (Hoelzer et al., 2011). Reptile-associated human infections only occur if the reptile or a feces-contaminated object is placed in the mouth. Physical contact with a reptile alone is thus not sufficient to produce infection in humans (ARAV, 2008).

Immunological, biological and behavioral characteristics are probably the reason why human salmonellosis is most frequent in children, especially the youngest (Hoelzer et al., 2011), although the disease may also occur in other age groups, including healthy adults (Warwick et al., 2001).

Many reports associate human *Salmonella* infections with isolates from snakes. Four cases were selected for discussion here; these cases will be presented in chronological order and were chosen because they are representative, interesting and illustrate the diversity of manners in which these exposures may occur. It is important to note that the development of molecular assays and their incorporation to the set of diagnostic techniques results in chronologically-increasing precision in comparing isolates retrieved from humans and reptiles in each case.

In July 1977, for the first time, *S. eingedi* was isolated from a snake in Israel and from a child that had diarrhea shortly after that. That serotype was also isolated from another child with diarrhea in the same Israeli community (Cahan, 1980).

In 1997, Paton & Mirfattahi presented the case of a 5-month-old boy with bacterial meningitis. *S. uzaramo* was isolated from the cerebrospinal fluid, blood and stool samples of the patient. The same serotype was isolated from the feces of an Indian Python (*Python molurus*) and two Ball Pythons (*P. regius*); *S. arizonae* and an unidentified isolate were also cultured from the Ball Pythons.

Jafari et al. (2002) reported *S.* Enteritidis infections resulting from a platelet donation. The apparently healthy donor had acquired an asymptomatic *S. enterica* bacteremia from his Boa Constrictor. Two patients receiving the platelet donation developed sepsis, and one of them died. The reptilian origin of the infection was confirmed through the determination of the serotype by PFGE.

A large *S.* Typhimurium outbreak occurred in the United States in 2005 and 2006. Several people had direct or indirect contact with snakes that had been fed with commercially-raised mice. The rodents had been captive raised, euthanized, vacuum-packed, frozen and sold through the internet. Cultures from three of those mice yielded pure isolates of *S.* Typhimurium that were indistinguishable by PFGE from the isolates obtained from the human cases, snakes, and environmental samples (Fuller et al., 2008).

9.2 Snake products as food items, folk remedies, and human salmonellosis

Despite the legal prohibitions and the risks of foodborne bacterial infections, many communities worldwide consume sea turtle meat and eggs. The raw or undercooked meat, often prepared in unsanitary conditions, may result in human salmonellosis (Aguirre et al., 2006). In an outbreak of salmonellosis that occurred in Australia in 1988 it was found that 62% of the victims had ingested green turtle meat. Several people were hospitalized, and *S. chester* was isolated from undercooked sea turtle meat samples and from fecal samples of the patients (O'Grady & Krause, 1999).

Similarly to the consumption of chelonians, snakes are also used for meat production (Magnino et al., 2009). Although in the USA and in some Asian countries there are specific breeding facilities for this purpose, snakes may also often be collected from the wild. The consumption of snake meat poses a risk to the development of salmonellosis due to the high prevalence of this microorganism in these animals, and also probably because oftentimes the adequate hygiene measures are not properly carried out.

Snake powder and dried meat, especially those prepared from rattlesnakes, are often used in folk medicine. However, several reports have associated the consumption of these products to the development of salmonellosis in humans (Babu et al., 1990), as well as infections by other Enterobacteriacea. Most of these cases occur in Mexican-American patients. Consumers often ingest such products while presenting underlying chronic and immunosuppressive conditions such as cancer, diabetes, arthritis, systemic lupus erythematosus, or acquired immunodeficiency syndrome (AIDS) (Sharma et al., 1993; Waterman et al., 1990). These conditions further complicate the cases, as *Salmonella* infections will tend to produce much more severe clinical manifestations and complications. For example, patients with AIDS may present recurrent bacteremia (Babu et al., 1990) and patients with gastric cancer may develop peritonitis (Sharma et al., 1993). Not only many *Salmonella* serotypes can be isolated from such rattlesnake capsules (Cone et al., 1990) but it also seems likely that all types of folk medicine preparations generally involve poor conditions of hygiene during their preparation, which may be yet another factor for the contamination of these products.

10. Conclusion

Numerous authors argue that *Salmonella* is a normal component of the reptilian intestinal microbiota and that 90% or more of reptiles harbor *Salmonella,* however some European researchers do not share that opinion (Hassl & Benyr, 2003), and there is evidence in other continents that some serotypes may be considerably pathogenic for the snakes (Bemis et al., 2007; Ramsay et al., 2002).

Basic hygiene practices may be sufficient to prevent most cases of human salmonellosis (Mitchell, 2004), even when it is known that snakes are very likely to be infected by *Salmonella* in both domestic and natural environments (Mermin et al., 2004).

It is vital to acknowledge *Salmonella* as an inhabitant of the digestive tract of reptiles, as this basic understanding is a solid basis to interpret the disease it may cause, to improve the life quality of these animals in captivity, and to take appropriate prevention and control measures.

11. References

Aguirre, A.A. et al. (2006). Hazards associated with the consumption of sea turtle meat and eggs: a review for health care workers and the general public. *EcoHealth,* Vol. 3, No. 3, pp. 141-153

Andrade, J.G. et al. (1989). Estudo bacteriológico de abscessos causados por picada de serpentes do gênero *Bothrops*. *Revista do Instituto de Medicina Tropical de São Paulo*, Vol. 31, No. 6, pp. 363-367

ARAV Special Publications. (2008). *Salmonella* bacteria and reptiles: client educational handout revised, In: *Association of Reptilian and Amphibian Veterinarians*, 23.04.2011, Available from: <http://www.arav.org/ECOMARAV//timssnet/pdf/SalmonellaBacteriaandReptiles_client_final_11apr08.pdf>

Babu, K. et al. (1990). Isolation of salmonellae from dried rattlesnake preparations. *Journal of Clinical Microbiology*, Vol. 28, No. 2, pp. 361-362

Barrow, P.A.; Jones, M.A. & Thomson, N. (2010). *Salmonella*, In: *Pathogenesis of bacterial infections in animals*, 4. ed., Gyles, C.L.; Prescott, J.F.; Songer, G. & Thoen, C.O., pp. 231-265, Blackwell Publishing, Ames

Bastos, H.M.; Lopes, L.F.L.; Gattamorta, M.A. & Matushima, E.R. (2008). Prevalence of enterobacteria in *Bothrops jararaca* in São Paulo State: microbiological survey and antimicrobial resistance standards. *Acta Scientiarum. Biological Sciences*, Vol. 30, No. 3, pp. 321-326

Bays, T.A.B. (2005). Equipping the reptile practice. *Veterinary Clinics of North America Exotic Animal Practice*, Vol. 8, No. 3, pp. 437-461

Bemis, D.A., et al. (2007). Clonal relatedness of *Salmonella* isolates associated with invasive infections in captive and wild-caught rattlesnakes. *Veterinary Microbiology*, Vol. 120, No. 3-4, pp. 300-307

Bradley, T. & Angulo, F.J. (2008). *Salmonella* and reptiles: veterinary guidelines revised, In: *Association of Reptilian and Amphibian Veterinarians*, 23.04.2011, Available from: <http://www.arav.org/ECOMARAV//timssnet/pdf/SalmonellaandReptiles_vetguideline_FINAL_11apr08.pdf>

Cahan, D. et al. (1980). New *Salmonella* serovar, *Salmonella eingedi* [6_1,6_2,7:f,g,t:1,(2),7]. *Journal of Clinical Microbiology*, Vol. 11, No. 3, pp. 292

Carvalho, V.M. (2006). Colibacilose e salmonelose, In: *Tratado de animais selvagens: medicina veterinária*, Cubas, Z.S.; Silva J.C.R. & Catão-Dias, J.L., pp. 742-750, Roca, São Paulo

Centers for Disease Control and Prevention (CDC). (2010). Multistate outbreak of human *Salmonella* Typhimurium infections associated with aquatic frogs - United States, 2009. *Morbidity and Mortality Weekly Report (MMWR)*, Vol. 58, No. 51-52, pp. 1433-1436

Chen, C.Y. et al. (2010). Prevalence and antimicrobial susceptibility of salmonellae isolates from reptiles in Taiwan. *Journal of Veterinary Diagnostic Investigation*, Vol. 22, No. 1, pp. 44-50

Chiodini, R.J. (1982). Transovarian passage, visceral distribution, and pathogenicity of *Salmonella* in snakes. *Infection and Immunity*, Vol. 36, No. 2, pp. 710-713

Chiodini, R.J. & Sundberg, J.P. (1981). Salmonellosis in reptiles: a review. *American Journal of Epidemiology*, Vol. 113, No. 5, pp. 494-499

Cone, Lionel A.; Boughton, W.H.; Cone, Lawrence A. & Lehv, L.H. (1990). Rattlesnake capsule-induced *Salmonella arizonae* bacteremia. *The Western Journal of Medicine*, Vol. 153, No. 3, pp. 315-316

Coutinho, S.D.A. et al. (2001). Bacterial septicemia in water snakes (*Helicops modestus*) in Brazil. *Arquivo Brasileiro de Medicina Veterinária e Zootecnia*, Vol. 53, No. 4, pp. 1-2

Difco. *Difco Salmonella O Antisera, Difco Salmonella H Antisera, Difco Salmonella Antiserum Vi.* Product label, 23.04.2011, pp. 18

Fornazari, F. & Teixeira, C.R. (2009). Salmonelose em répteis: aspectos epidemiológicos, clínicos e zoonóticos. *Veterinária e Zootecnia,* Vol. 16, No. 1, pp. 19-25

Friedman, C.R. et al. (1998). An outbreak of salmonellosis among children attending a reptile exhibit at a zoo. *The Journal of Pediatrics,* Vol. 132, No. 5, pp. 802–807

Fuller, C.C. et al. (2008). A multi-state *Salmonella* Typhimurium outbreak associated with frozen vacuum-packed rodents used to feed snakes. *Zoonoses and Public Health,* Vol. 55, No. 8-10, pp. 481-487

Funk, R.S. (1996). Diarrhea, In: *Reptile medicine and surgery,* Mader, D.R., pp. 364-365, W.B. Saunders, Philadelphia

Geue, L. & Löschner, U. (2002). *Salmonella enterica* in reptiles of German and Austrian origin. *Veterinary Microbiology,* Vol. 84, No. 1-2, pp. 79-91

Ghilardi, A.C.R.; Tavechio, A.T. & Fernandes, S.A. (2006). Antimicrobial susceptibility, phage types, and pulsetypes of *Salmonella* Typhimurium, in São Paulo, Brazil. *Memórias do Instituto Oswaldo Cruz,* Vol. 101, No. 3, pp. 281-286

Goldstein, E.J.C. et al. (1979). Bacteriology of rattlesnake venom and implications for therapy. *The Journal of Infectious Diseases,* Vol. 140, No. 5, pp. 818-821

Gopee, N.V.; Adesiyun, A.A. & Caesar, K. (2000). Retrospective and longitudinal study of salmonellosis in captive wildlife in Trinidad. *Journal of Wildlife Diseases,* Vol. 36, No. 2, pp. 284-293

Gray, T.Z. (2011). Update: reptiles and *Salmonella. Journal of Exotic Pet Medicine,* Vol. 20, No. 1, pp. 14-17

Grimont, P.A.D. & Weill, F.X. (2007). Antigenic formulas of the *Salmonella* serovars, 9. ed., revision, *WHO Collaborating Center for Reference and Research on Salmonella,* Institut Pasteur, Paris

Hafez, H.M. & Jodas, S. (2000). *Salmonella* infections in turkeys, In: Salmonella *in domestic animals,* Wray, C. & Wray, A., pp. 133-135, CABI Publishing, Oxon

Hassl, A. & Benyr, G. (2003). Hygienic evaluation of terraria inhabited by amphibians and reptiles: cryptosporidia, free-living amebas, salmonella. *Wien Klin Wochenschr,* Vol. 115, Suppl. 3, pp. 68-71

Hidalgo-Vila, J. et al. (2008). *Salmonella* in free-living exotic and native turtles and in pet exotic turtles from SW Spain. *Research in Veterinary Science,* Vol. 85, No. 3, pp. 449-452

Hinshaw, W.R. & McNeil, E. (1944). Gopher snakes as carriers of salmonellosis and paracolon infections. *The Cornell Veterinarian,* Vol. 34, pp. 248-254

Hinshaw, W.R. & McNeil, E. (1945). *Salmonella* types isolated from snakes. American Journal of Veterinary Research, Vol. 6, pp. 264-266

Hinshaw, W.R. & McNeil, E. (1946). Paracolon type 10 from captive rattlesnakes. *Journal of Bacteriology,* Vol. 51, No. 3, pp. 397-398

Hinshaw, W.R. & McNeil, E. (1947). Lizards as carriers of *Salmonella* and paracolon bacteria. *Journal of Bacteriology,* Vol. 53, No. 6, pp. 715-718

Hirsh, D.C. (2004). Enterobacteriacea: *Salmonella,* In: *Veterinary microbiology,* 2. ed., Hirsh, D.C.; MacLachlan, N.J. & Walker, R.L., pp. 69-74, Blackwell Publishing, Ames

Hoelzer, K.; Switt, A.I.M. & Wiedmann, M. (2011). Animal contact as a source of human non-typhoidal salmonellosis. *Veterinary Research,* Vol. 42, No. 34, pp. 1-27

Holz, P.H. & Middleton, D.R. (2002). The effect of probiotic feeding on *Salmonella* excretion in carpet pythons, *Morelia spilota. Journal of Herpetological Medicine and Surgery,* Vol. 12, No. 3, pp. 5-7

Holz, P.H. & Middleton, D.R. (2005). The effect of feeding a prebiotic on *Salmonella* excretion in carpet pythons, *Morelia spilota,* and scrub pythons, *Morelia amethystine. Journal of Herpetological Medicine and Surgery,* Vol. 15, No. 1, pp. 4-6

Iveson, J.B.; Mackay-Scollay, E.M. & Bamford, V. (1969). *Salmonella* and *Arizona* in reptiles and man in Western Australia. *The Journal of Hygiene (London),* Vol. 67, No. 1, pp. 135-145

Jafari, M. et al. (2002). *Salmonella* sepsis caused by a platelet transfusion from a donor with a pet snake. *The New England Journal of Medicine,* Vol. 347, No. 14, pp. 1075-1078

Jankowski, G. (2009). Lactulose. *Journal of Exotic Pet Medicine,* Vol. 18, No. 2, pp. 156-159

Jijón, S.; Wetzel, A. & LeJeune, J. (2007). *Salmonella enterica* isolated from wildlife at two Ohio rehabilitation centers. *Journal of Zoo and Wildlife Medicine,* Vol. 38, No. 3, pp. 409-413

Johnson-Delaney, C.A. (2006). Reptile zoonoses and threats to public health, In: *Reptile medicine and surgery,* 2. ed., Mader, D.R., pp. 1017-1030, Saunders Elsevier, St. Louis

Jorge, M.T. et al. (1990). Flora bacteriana da cavidade oral, presas e veneno de *Bothrops jararaca*: possível fonte de infecção no local da picada. *Revista do Instituto de Medicina Tropical de São Paulo,* Vol. 32, No. 1, pp. 6-10

Kaufmann, A.F. & Morrison, Z.L. (1966). An epidemiologic study of salmonellosis in turtles. *American Journal of Epidemiology,* Vol. 84, No. 2, pp. 364-370

Kaufmann, A.F. et al. (1972). Turtle-associated salmonellosis: III. The effects of environmental salmonellae in commercial turtle breeding ponds. *American Journal of Epidemiology,* Vol. 95, No. 6, pp. 521-528

Lamberski, N. et al. (2002). Recovery of a pathogenic *Salmonella arizona* from four snakes at the Riverbanks Zoo. *Journal of Herpetological Medicine and Surgery,* Vol. 12, No. 4, pp. 17-22

Lima, D.C. et al. (2005). Snake venom: any clue for antibiotics and CAM? *Evidence-Based Complementary and Alternative Medicine,* Vol. 2, No. 1, pp. 39-47

Mader, D.M. (2006). Perinatology, In: *Reptile medicine and surgery,* 2. ed., Mader, D.R., pp. 365-375, Saunders Elsevier, St. Louis

Magnino, S. et al. (2009). Biological risks associated with consumption of reptile products. *International Journal of Food Microbiology,* Vol. 134, No. 3, pp. 163-175

Mathewson, J.J. (1979). Enterobacteriaceae isolated from iguanid lizards of west-central Texas. *Applied and Environmental Microbiology,* Vol. 38, No. 3, pp. 402-405

Mehler, S.J. & Bennett, R.A. (2006). Upper alimentary tract disease, In: *Reptile medicine and surgery,* 2. ed., Mader, D.R., pp. 924-930, Saunders Elsevier, St. Louis

Mermin, J. et al. (2004). Reptiles, amphibians, and human *Salmonella* infection: a population-based, case-control study. *Clinical Infectious Diseases,* Vol. 38, Suppl. 3, pp. 253-261

Messonnier, S.P. (1996). *Common reptile diseases and treatment,* Blackwell Science, Cambridge

Minette, H.P. (1984). Epidemiologic aspects of salmonellosis in reptiles, amphibians, mollusks and crustaceans - a review. *International Journal of Zoonoses,* Vol. 11, No. 1, pp. 95-104

Mitchell, M.A. (2004). Snake care and husbandry. *Veterinary Clinics of North America Exotic Animal Practice,* Vol. 7, No. 2, pp. 421-446

Mitchell, M.A. (2006). *Salmonella*: diagnostic methods for reptiles, In: *Reptile medicine and surgery*, 2. ed., Mader, D.R., pp. 900-905, Saunders Elsevier, St. Louis

Mitchell, M.A. & Shane, S.M. (2001). *Salmonella* in reptiles. *Seminars in Avian and Exotic Pet Medicine*, Vol. 10, No. 1, pp. 25-35

Moreno, G. et al. (1973). Enterobactérias isoladas de anfíbios e répteis. *Revista do Instituto de Medicina Tropical de São Paulo*, Vol. 15, No. 3, pp. 122-126

Murray, M.J. (1996). Cardiology and circulation, In: *Reptile medicine and surgery*, Mader, D.R., pp. 95-104, W.B. Saunders, Philadelphia

Myers, D. (2007). Probiotics. *Journal of Exotic Pet Medicine*, Vol. 16, No. 3, pp. 195-197

Nair, S.; Lin, T.K.; Pang, T. & Altwegg, M. (2002). Characterization of *Salmonella* serovars by PCR-single-strand conformation polymorphism analysis. *Journal of Clinical Microbiology*, Vol. 40, No. 7, pp. 2346–2351

Nishioka, S.A.; Jorge, M.T.; Silveira, P.V.P. & Ribeiro, L.A. (2000). South American rattlesnake bite and soft-tissue infection: report of a case. *Revista da Sociedade Brasileira de Medicina Tropical*, Vol. 33, No. 4, pp. 401-402

O'Grady, K.A. & Krause, V. (1999). An outbreak of salmonellosis linked to a marine turtle. *Southeast Asian Journal of Tropical Medicine and Public Health*, Vol. 30, No. 2, pp. 324-327

Onderka, D.K. & Finlayson, M.C. (1985). Salmonellae and salmonellosis in captive reptiles. *Canadian Journal of Comparative Medicine*, Vol. 49, No. 3, pp. 268-270

Orós, J. et al. (1996). Respiratory and digestive lesions caused by *Salmonella arizonae* in two snakes. *Journal of Comparative Pathology*, Vol. 115, No. 2, pp. 185-189

Page, L.A. (1966). Diseases and infections of snakes: a review. *Bulletin of the Wildlife Disease Association*, Vol. 2, No. 4, pp. 111-126

Painter, J.A. et al. (2004). *Salmonella*-based rodenticides and public health. *Emerging Infectious Diseases*, Vol. 10, No. 6, pp. 985-987

Paré, J.A.; Sigler, L.; Rosenthal, K.L. & Mader, D.R. (2006). Microbiology: fungal and bacterial diseases of reptiles, In: *Reptile medicine and surgery*, 2. ed., Mader, D.R., pp. 217-238, Saunders Elsevier, St. Louis

Pascual, M. et al. (1999). *Lactobacillus salivarius* CTC2197 prevents *Salmonella enteritidis* colonization in chickens. *Applied and Environmental Microbiology*, Vol. 65, No. 11, pp. 4981-4986

Paton, J.H. & Mirfattahi, M.B. (1997). *Salmonella* meningitis acquired from pet snakes. *Archives of Disease in Childhood*, Vol. 77, No. 1, pp. 91

Pedersen, K.; Lassen-Nielsen, A.M.; Nordentoft, S. & Hammer, A.S. (2009). Serovars of *Salmonella* from captive reptiles. *Zoonoses and Public Health*, Vol. 56, No. 5, pp. 238-242

Pfleger, S.; Benyr, G.; Sommer, R.; Hassl, A. (2003). Pattern of *Salmonella* excretion in amphibians and reptiles in a vivarium. *International Journal of Hygiene and Environmental Health*, Vol. 206, No. 1, pp. 53-59

Ramsay, E.C. et al. (2002). Osteomyelitis associated with *Salmonella enterica* ss *arizonae* in a colony of ridgenose rattlesnakes (*Crotalus willardi*). *Journal of Zoo and Wildlife Medicine*, Vol. 33, No. 4, pp. 301-310

Ribeiro, L.A. & Jorge, M.T. (1990). Epidemiologia e quadro clínico dos acidentes por serpentes *Bothrops jararaca* adultas e filhotes. *Revista do Instituto de Medicina Tropical de São Paulo*, Vol. 32, No. 6, pp. 436-442

Ribeiro, L.A. & Jorge, M.T. (1997). Acidente por serpentes do gênero *Bothrops*: série de 3.139 casos. *Revista da Sociedade Brasileira de Medicina Tropical*, Vol. 30, No. 6, pp. 475-480

Sá, I.V.A. & Solari, C.A. (2001). *Salmonella* in Brazilian and imported pet reptiles. *Brazilian Journal of Microbiology*, Vol. 32, No. 4, pp. 293-297

Salb, A.; Mitchell, M.A.; Riggs, S. & Diaz-Figueroa, O. (2002). Characterization of the aerobic and anaerobic intestinal flora of the green iguana (*Iguana iguana*), *Proceedings of ARAV Conference*, Reno, NV

Scheelings, T.F.; Lightfoot, D. & Holz, P. (2011). Prevalence of *Salmonella* in Australian reptiles. *Journal of Wildlife Diseases*, Vol. 47, No. 1, pp. 1-11

Schilliger, L.; Vanderstylen, D.; Piétrain, J. & Chetboul, V. (2003). Granulomatous myocarditis and coelomic effusion due to *Salmonella enterica arizonae* in a Madagascar Dumerili's boa (*Acrantophis dumerili*, Jan. 1860). *Journal of Veterinary Cardiology*, Vol. 5, No. 1, pp. 43-45

Schneitz, C. & Mead, G. (2000). Competitive exclusion, In: Salmonella *in domestic animals*, Wray, C. & Wray, A., pp. 301-322, CABI Publishing, Oxon

Schröter, M. et al. (2004). Pet snakes as a reservoir for *Salmonella enterica* subsp. *diarizonae* (serogroup IIIb): a prospective study. *Applied and Environmental Microbiology*, Vol. 70, No. 1, pp. 613-615

Schröter, M.; Speicher, A.; Hofmann, J. & Roggentin, P. (2006). Analysis of the transmission of *Salmonella* spp. through generations of pet snakes. *Environmental Microbiology*, Vol. 8, No. 3, pp. 556–559

Sharma, J.; Von Hoff, D.D. & Weiss, G.R. (1993). *Salmonella arizonae* peritonitis secondary to ingestion of rattlesnake capsules for gastric cancer. *Journal of Clinical Oncology*, Vol. 11, No. 11, pp. 2288-2289

Waltman, W.D. (2000). Methods for the cultural isolation of *Salmonella*, In: Salmonella *in domestic animals*, Wray, C. & Wray, A., pp. 355-372, CABI Publishing, Oxon

Wang, Y. et al. (2008). Snake cathelicidin from *Bungarus fasciatus* is a potent peptide antibiotics. *PLoS ONE*, Vol. 3, No. 9, pp. 1-9

Warwick, C.; Lambiris, A.J.L.; Westwood, D. & Steedman, C. (2001). Reptile-related salmonellosis. *Journal of the Royal Society of Medicine*, Vol. 94, No. 3, pp. 124-126

Waterman, S.H. Juarez, G.; Carr, S.J. & Kilman, L. (1990). *Salmonella arizona* infections in Latinos associated with rattlesnake folk medicine. *American Journal of Public Health*, Vol. 80, No. 3, pp. 286-289

5

Salmonella Control Measures at Farm in Swine Production

Héctor Argüello, Pedro Rubio and Ana Carvajal
Animal Health Department
University of León
Spain

1. Introduction

Salmonella is one of the most important food-borne pathogens. Each year a high number of cases as well as outbreaks of *Salmonella* in humans are reported (EFSA, 2011). Despite the fact that *Salmonella* can cause disease in pigs mainly associated to infections by *Salmonella enterica* subsp. *enterica* serovar Cholerasuis, the importance of swine salmonellosis is related to human infections caused by pork products. During the nineties and the first years of the present century it was estimated that 10% of the human salmonellosis cases were attributed to pork products (Hald *et al.*, 2004), classically categorized as the third most common source of human infections after poultry and turkey meat. Nevertheless with the implementation of control programs in avian production with the subsequent prevalence reduction, the role of pork products have been enhanced and nowadays it is the second most common source of human salmonellosis after laying hens (Pires *et al.*, 2011). Regarding swine salmonellosis, control programs are not compulsory at the moment but the EU Regulation 2160/2003 has established the need for developing proper and effective measures to detect and control *Salmonella* at all relevant stages of pork production chain and particularly at the primary production level in order to reduce the prevalence and the risk that *Salmonella* poses to public health (EU Regulation 2160/2003). From our point of view, *Salmonella* control should start at the end of the pork production chain (slaughterhouses and finishing farms) and go back to the first steps of the production system (breeding herds and feed suppliers). The compulsory or voluntary *Salmonella* control programmes that have already been established in several European countries base their *Salmonella* evaluation on serological and carcass microbiological contamination results principally (Alban et al., 2002; Nielsen et al., 2001). At the farm level, these control programmes include the implementation of specific measures to reduce the *Salmonella* prevalence in those herds identified as highly contaminated according to their serological results.

The present chapter aims to give a view of the most relevant control measures that can be used to reduce *Salmonella* prevalence in swine farms including a deep review of scientific research as well as our personal experience with control strategies at swine finishing farms. They will be presented into three different categories: 1) measures related to feeding practices, 2) vaccination and 3) generic measures of hygiene and biosecurity.

2. *Salmonella* control in the pork production chain

Focused in food safety, the control of *Salmonella* must be carried out taking into account the philosophy *"from farm to fork"* which implies the participation of all sectors involved throughout the food chain. Due to the complexity of its epidemiology and ecology, *Salmonella* control is a great challenge. As it has been proposed by Davies *et al.* (2004) the food supply should be seen as a linear series of sectors engaged in production, harvest, distribution and consumption and the goal of control programmes is to define the optimal combination of interventions at each sector that delivers the maximum risk reduction at minimal cost. It has been demonstrated that the risk of *Salmonella* contamination increases across the pork production chain and reaches its maximum in the slaughterhouse (Duggan *et al.*, 2010; Argüello *et al.*, 2011a; Visscher *et al.*, 2011). Therefore, the slaughter process seems to be the main target to implement control measures and its importance has been pointed by many studies (Hurd *et al.*, 2002, Argüello *et al.*, 2011a). According to this, several countries, led by Denmark with more than twenty years of experience with a national swine *Salmonella* control program are pointing nowadays their reduction strategies towards slaughterhouse interventions (Alban *et al.*, 2005; Goldbach *et al.*, 2006). Nevertheless there are some aspects that make us to include pig finishing farms, together with the slaughterhouses, as the primary control points in the pork production chain. On the one hand sometimes it is difficult to implement slaughterhouse strategies due to policy restrictions at this level. On the other hand, it has been clearly demonstrated that infected pigs are the main source of *Salmonella* at the slaughterhouse (Argüello *et al.*, 2011a; Visscher *et al.*, 2011), thus in order to reduce the risk of *Salmonella* transmission in the food chain including feasible cost and success, finishing farms should be taken into consideration.

Although sows have been implicated as the primary source of infection to finishers (Lettelier *et al.*, 1999; Kranker *et al.*, 2003), other studies have demonstrated that this transmission can be controlled or interrupted by proper handling practices (Dahl *et al.*, 1997). Several surveys have also supported that vertical transmission is not the main source of *Salmonella* in finishers (Berends *et al.*, 1996; Stege *et al.*, 2000; Funk *et al.*, 2001; Argüello *et al.*, 2010a). According to this, finishing farms should be the main target of *Salmonella* control programmes at the primary level.

3. Feeding practices for *Salmonella* control in swine farms

The role of feed in the control of *Salmonella* in swine farms includes two different views. On the one hand, feed can be a source of *Salmonella* contamination while on the other hand there are several feeding practices that are useful tools to be used in the control of *Salmonella.* Several studies have demonstrated the relative low importance of feed as a primary source of infection to pigs (Harris *et al.*, 1997). *Salmonella* is rarely detected after feed processing at the feed mills due to the thermal treatment coupled with good manufacturing practices, and moreover *Salmonella* serotypes sporadically isolated from feed are not related to those usually identified at the farm level (Harris *et al.*, 1997; Davies *et al.*, 2004; Torres *et al.*, 2011). However, most researchers agree that feed can be easily contaminated at the farm level.

Feeding practices include many strategies for the control of *Salmonella.* Most of them are based on the same principle: the modification of the intestinal environment and the promotion of the normal microbial flora within the gastrointestinal tract, creating a healthier environment. Even when the feeding practices that are exposed in this chapter are very different, the main mechanisms elicited to reduce or prevent *Salmonella* contamination are shared. Briefly, these feeding control strategies reduce directly or indirectly the pH within the intestinal tract and create an environment which is adverse to *Salmonella* and favours the growth of other bacteria. In a second step, this beneficial gut microflora contributes to maintain a hostile environment to *Salmonella* by lowering the pH and/or producing several anti-*Salmonella* compounds and metabolites.

3.1 Feed composition and feed physical structure

It is well documented that feed presentation, pelletized or not, coupled with the milling type, coarse or fine, has an influence on the gut microflora and therefore determines the success in the establishment and multiplication of *Salmonella* in the intestinal tract of swine. Although, pelleting and thermal-treatment processes can reduce the *Salmonella* contamination in compound feed, it has been demonstrated that non-pelleted feed has a clear protective effect against *Salmonella* compared to the use of pelleted feed (Jørgensen *et al.*, 1999; Kjeldsen & Dahl, 1999; Kranker *et al.*, 2001; Leontides *et al.*, 2003; Lo Fo Wong *et al.*, 2004; Rajik *et al.*, 2007; García-Feliz *et al.*, 2009). In a similar way, coarsely ground meal has been demonstrated to have a protective effect compared to fine grounded meal (Jørgensen *et al.*, 1999; Kjeldsen & Dahl, 1999; Jørgensen *et al.*, 2001; Mikkelsen *et al.*, 2004). It is important to remark that more than defining pelleted or fined ground meal as risk factors that promote the presence of *Salmonella* at farm level, we should define non-pelleted feed or coarsely meal as efficient protective elements against *Salmonella* in swine farms.

As we have already indicated, the anti-*Salmonella* activity seems to be related to the changes in the intestinal microflora that are associated with these types of feed. The effect of feed grinding and feed processing on physicochemical properties and microbial populations in the gastrointestinal tract of pigs were evaluated by Mikkesen *et al.* (2004). Those pigs fed a coarse non-pelleted feed showed a significant increase in the number of total anaerobic bacteria within the stomach as well as higher concentrations of various organic acids and lower pH compared to those pigs fed other diets suggesting a higher microbial fermentation in the stomach, fact that was also asserted by a slower gastric passage rate. These environmental conditions in the stomach would reduce the population of *Salmonella* populations by 1000-fold (Mikkesen *et al.*, 2004). Other effects were also observed, to a leser extent, in other parts of the gastrointestinal tract with a lower number of coliform bacteria in the distal small intestine, in the colon and in the caecum and higher concentrations of butyric acid (Mikkesen *et al.*, 2004). Apart from these findings, it is well known that the digestibility of non-pelleted and coarse feed is lower than that of fine pelleted feed. Consequently, higher amounts of carbohydrates reach the last part of the small intestine and the large intestine providing a source of energy for anaerobic bacteria settled there.

3.2 Dry or liquid feed

It is well documented that liquid feed has a protective effect against *Salmonella* as compared to dry feed (Van der Wolf *et al.*, 2001a; Højberg *et al.*, 2003). Basically, this feeding strategy can be accomplished by using non-fermented liquid feed or fermented feed. In the first case, water or food industry derivates such as serum from dairy industry are added to the mixed feed immediately before its administration while when using fermentation, the feed and the water are mixed and stored at a certain temperature for a period of time, prior to its use. Traditionally, liquid feeding systems are much extended in areas where liquid co-products from the human food industry are abundant and cheap. Industries involved in potato, vegetable, milk and fish processing, starch and sugar manufacture, baking, brewing and bio-ethanol production generate co-products that can be valuable and cost-saving inclusions in liquid diets.

The beneficial effects of liquid diets in the gastrointestinal tract are related to the stimulation of epithelial cells growth, the reduction of the intestinal pH and the increase in the lactic acid microbial flora. Its anti-*Salmonella* activity is based on the effect of the fermented feed against *Salmonella* itself since fermented liquid feed contains high concentrations of acids including lactic acid and short chain fatty acids and decreases the pH level in the gastrointestinal tract which in turn influence the ecology of the gastrointestinal microflora. In a study carried out in Canada, Farzan *et al.* (2006) compared *Salmonella* infection between 20 liquid-feeding farms and 61 dry-feeding farms. The use of liquid feed was associated to a lower number of *Salmonella* positive farms by both serological and bacteriological analysis. Moreover, a reduced usage of antimicrobials and consequently an improved pig health status was reported in those farms using liquid feed. Winsen *et al.* (2001) carried out a clinical trial comparing two groups of pigs, one fed with a dry-diet and the other with a *Lactobacillus plantarum* supplemented fermented liquid diet. A reduction in the total counts of *Enterobacteriaceae* within the gastrointestinal tract was reported in those animals receiving the supplemented fermented liquid food and was associated with an increase in the concentration of undissociated lactic acid and short chain fatty acids in the stomach content. According to these results, many risk factor studies have also described the protective effect of the liquid feed in *Salmonella* infection in swine farms (Beloeil *et al.*, 2004; Lo Fo Wong *et al.*, 2004; Poljak *et al.*, 2008; Farzan *et al.*, 2010; Hotes *et al.*, 2010).

It is important to remark that in contrast to other feeding practices, the use of liquid feed and particularly of fermented liquid feed has been associated with an improvement in the growth performance. However, this feed system is not feasible economically in all herds due to the investment needed for storage capacity, mixers, pumps, pipelines and computers (Van der Wolf *et al.*, 2001a).

3.3 Probiotics

Feeding antibiotics is one of the most effective strategies of prophylactically controlling gastrointestinal infections but this practice is in decline because of the concern with antibiotic resistance in human medicine (Fairbrother *et al.*, 2005). Even more, the European Union banned the use of antibiotics as growth promoters in food animals in 1999, on the basis of the "*precautionary principle*". One of the most promising and attractive alternatives to in-feed antibiotics is the use of probiotics and according to this, several researchers have also proposed their utility in the control of *Salmonella* infections in swine farms.

Probiotic treatment is based on the oral administration of viable bacteria, generally non-pathogenic anaerobic bacteria, with the objective to establish the first indigenous flora in newborn piglets or remove the pathogenic flora already established in growers or finishers. The two main actions of probiotics include the nutritional effect and the sanitary effect (Anadon *et al.*, 2006). The nutritional effect is attributed to a reduction of the metabolic reactions that produce toxic substances, a stimulation of the indigenous enzymes and a production of vitamins. The sanitary effect of probiotics is linked to several actions including the creation of a restrictive environment by reducing the pH at the intestinal tract, the competition for gut surface adhesion, the production of anti-bacterial substances such as bacteriocins, the competition for the nutrients, the improvement of the epithelial gut cells health and the stimulation of the immune system acting as bio-regulators of the gut microflora and reinforcing the host natural defences.

At the moment most of the probiotics that are in use consist in a well-defined mix of microorganisms. The main bacterial genera used in these probiotics include *Clostridium, Enterococcus, Bacteroides, Streptococcus, Pediococcus, Bifidobacterium* or *Lactobacillus* as well as yeast such as *Saccharomyces (S. cerevesiae)* or *Kluyveromyces*. According to the guidelines from the EFSA, the identification of all the bacteria included in the mixture and the determination of the absence of antimicrobial resistance genes or plasmids and toxic metabolites are recommended for all probiotic products in the market (Anadon *et al.*, 2006).

Despite the fact that anti-*Salmonella* activity of several lactic acid bacteria has been already demonstrated using *in vitro* procedures (Hume *et al.*, 2001; Harvey *et al.*, 2002; Casey *et al.*, 2004), the literature regarding the efficacy of probiotics in clinical trials is scarce, above all in pig surveys. According to the idea that the efficiency of probiotics is strongly related to the host animal where they have been developed (Ozawa *et al.*, 1983), we will focus the discussion on trials performed in pigs even when there is not too much data available. Genovese *et al.* (2000 and 2003) evaluated the effect of an undefined mixture of lactic acid bacteria of porcine origin previously developed by Harvey *et al.* (2002) on caecal colonization and faecal shedding of *S.* Cholerasuis in neonatal and weaned pigs. Their results showed a significant decrease in colonization as well as a reduced shedding after experimental infection with *S.* Cholerasuis in treated animals as compared with the control group. In a similar way, Fedorka-Cray *et al.* (1999) demonstrated the usefulness of a mixed and undefined culture from caecal mucosa of a 6-week-old healthy pig for the control of *Salmonella* infection. A 2- to 5-log reduction of *Salmonella* in the caecal content or ileocolic junction was observed in the pigs that received this probiotic mixture when compared with the controls. Moreover, 28% of the gut tissues from the treated pigs were positive versus 79% from the control pigs. More recently, the effect of a defined mixture of lactic acid bacteria of porcine origin containing *Lactobacillus murinus, L. pentosus, L. salivarus* and *Pediococcus pentosaceus* developed by Casey *et al.* (2004) was evaluated in weaned pigs (Casey *et al.*, 2007). The study design included three groups of five pigs: two treated groups that were administered the probiotic directly or fermented prior to its use and a control group in which milk was used as a placebo. All the animals from the treated groups were administered $4x10^9$ colony forming units (CFU) of the probiotic bacteria during 6 days. On day 7, all the pigs were challenged with 10^9 CFUs of *S.* Typhimurium and were monitored for 23 days. Probiotic treated animals showed reduced incidence, severity and duration of diarrhoea as well as a lower concentration of *Salmonella* in faeces. In contrast Zsabo *et al.* (2009) did not find differences in clinical symptoms after a probiotic treatment based on *Enterococcus faecium* and subsequent challenge with *S.* Typhimurium DT104. Moreover the invasiveness was greater in the treated group than in the control one, showing that not all the potential probiotic bacteria offer protection against *Salmonella.*

Our research group has evaluated hundreds of lactic acid bacteria recovered from faeces, intestinal content or intestinal mucosa of healthy pigs and selected according to their potential probiotic properties including their anti-*Salmonella* effect. Among those with high anti-bacterial activity against *Salmonella* we found isolates from the *Streptococcus* and *Lactobacillus* genera, including *L. reuteri, S. gallolyticus* subsp. *gallolyticus, L. delbrueckii, S. alactolyticus, L. animalis, L. salivarius, L ruminis* and *L. murinus* (Collazos *et al.*, 2008a). In general, *L. reuteri* and *L. animalis* isolates are particularly resistant to the gastrointestinal environment of swine. Although *L. delbrueckii* isolates exhibited a strong anti-*Salmonella* activity, they were particularly sensitive to gastric conditions. When a defined probiotic mixture of five lactobacilli containing *L. reuteri, L. delbrueckii, L. animalis, L. murinus* and *L. ruminis* was administered to 5-weeks old piglets for 7 days before the challenge with *S.* Typhimurium (10^9 CFU) a significant reduction in the pathogen shedding and its dissemination to different organs and tissues as well as an alleviation of the clinical signs of the infection as compared with the pigs from the control group was demonstrated (Collazos *et al.*, 2008b). Similar results were previously reported by Casey *et al.* (2007).

In spite of all these promising results from experimental trials, there is very little experience regarding the effect of such probiotic treatments in *Salmonella* infected swine farms. Moreover, at least two relevant questions regarding the probiotic use in the real practice still arise: (1) how can or should be administered the probiotic and (2) at which growth stage should it be used in order to reduce *Salmonella* contamination at the time of the slaughtering. Regarding the first question, two main possibilities should be considered. On the one hand, direct administration of the probiotic bacteria should be very effective and consequently high ratios of viable bacteria would reach the gastrointestinal tract. However it is almost impossible to use this administration in field conditions at farm level, particularly if the product is going to be used in growers or finishers. On the other hand, probiotic bacteria could be mixed with feed or drinking water allowing a very easy administration that could be extended for large periods of time. According to this, De Angelis *et al.* (2006) proposed that one of the main prerequisites for the selection of probiotic bacteria in swine is that these bacteria should be able to survive and maintain their health-promoting properties during feed manufacturing and storage. Our research group have evaluated the survival of five lactic acid bacteria of porcine origin incorporated into pelleted feed and stored for 24 days at farm conditions. Although one of the evaluated isolates was not included because its performance in the previous steps of fermentation and lyophilisation, was not satisfactory, stable numbers of the other four bacteria were recovered from pelleted feed stored in the farm until the end of the experiment allowing us to conclude that pelleted feed can apparently be used as a vehicle to administer probiotics in swine. Regarding the second question elicited, the moment of administration of the probiotic in a *Salmonella* control strategy in a swine farm, to our knowledge there is no field study in a *Salmonella* infected farm that can be used to give a well-grounded answer. In general, probiotics can be used to establish the flora in a newborn piglet, strengthen colonization resistance to pathogenic bacteria, or to compete with potential pathogenic bacteria already established in the gastrointestinal tract. Hence, the administration of probiotics is recommended during critical periods such as weaning (3 or 4 age-weeks) or at the beginning of the fattening period, when intestinal disorders are common. Focusing on the control of *Salmonella* infection in swine farms, both periods seem to be also suitable to establish a health intestinal status which would increase the resistance to *Salmonella* colonization. However, special attention should be paid in order to avoid infections by *Salmonella* during the fattening period. Other option would be the administration of the probiotic during this fattening period or even at the end of the fattening period to reduce the risk of *Salmonella* transmission in the food chain.

3.4 Acids

A well studied strategy for the control of *Salmonella* infection on swine farms is the addition of acidic compounds to feed or drinking water. The main idea is not new and acids have been evaluated to replace growth promoters and to improve the hygiene and quality of the gut microflora since the 1980's (Giesting & Easter, 1985). It has been demonstrated that the un-dissociated form of various acids can freely cross the bacterial cell membrane and enter the bacterial cell, causing cell death (Van Immersel *et al.*, 2006). Moreover, acids decrease the pH at the gastrointestinal tract and they could serve as carbon source, taking part in several bacterial metabolic routes.

The anti-*Salmonella* effect of many acids have been tested and evaluated in several experimental and field studies. The fact that short chain volatile fatty acids are produced by anaerobic bacteria of the gut microflora has focused many studies on their effectiveness against *Salmonella*. Propionic acid has shown satisfactory results against *Salmonella* in poultry (Hume *et al.*, 1993). To our knowledge, there is no reported clinical trial based on the use of butyric acid, nevertheless its activity against *Salmonella* has been documented *in vitro*. The increase of butyric acid concentration in the gut has been associated with a decrease in *Enterobacteriaceae* and *Salmonella* populations (Van Immerseel *et al.*, 2006) and an inhibition of the pathogenicity island I of *Salmonella*, involved in the gut cells invasion, after exposure to butyric acid has been reported (Gantois *et al.*, 2005). Acetic acid is probably the most evaluated short chain volatile fatty acid in clinical trials. However, several studies have concluded that this acid does not show a relevant anti-*Salmonella* activity (Dahl *et al.*, 1996; Van Immerseel *et al.*, 2006) and further, it increases the development of resistance against acids by the mechanisms defined as acid tolerance response (Known *et al.*, 1998). The anti-*Salmonella* effect of lactic and propionic acids have also been evaluated in several studies with promising results (Tsiloyiannis *et al.*, 2001; Wingstrand *et al.*, 1996; Creus *et al.*, 2007). Apart from these five acids described here, many other studies have been carried out using other products such as citric acid, fumaric acid, malic acid and many other acid products that can be found in the market. At the same time, some of these acids have been coated in an attempt to avoid an early absorption in the small intestine. The most relevant results of clinical trials evaluating the use of acids in the control of *Salmonella* infection in swine farms are summarized in Table 1 (Dahl *et al.*, 1996; Wolf *et al.*, 2001b; Tsiloyiannis *et al.*, 2001; Anderson *et al.*, 2004; Creus *et al.*, 2007; Boyen *et al.*, 2008; De Busser *et al.*, 2008; Argüello *et al.*, 2010b).

Our research group carried out an interventional study in a pig fattening unit infected *by Salmonella* to assess the effectiveness of an acid treatment administered in drinking water for the control of salmonellosis (Argüello *et al.*, 2011b). Animals from the experimental group were administered a commercial acid, composed of lactic acid (56%), formic acid (23%), propionic acid (13%) and acetic acid (5%), that was added to drinking water during the last 40 days of the fattening period at a concentration of 0.035%. This treatment was able to reduce the number of *Salmonella* shedders as well as the number of *Salmonella* seropositive animals at the end of the fattening period.

Study	Trial type	Production Stage	Acid selected	Vehicle	Concentration used	Treatment duration	Results and discussion
Anderson, 2004	Clinical trial	Weaning and fattening	Sodium chlorate	Water	30-80 mg/kg bw	36 h.	24 h. of administration in weaned pigs are enough to reduce the qualitatively recovery of *Salmonella* from gut and rectum. Proportions of *Salmonella* positive pigs were not significant reduced in finishers
Arguello, 2011	Field trial	Fattening	Mixture of Lactic (56 %), formic (23 %) propionic (13 %) and acetic acid (5 %).	Water	0.035 %[1]	60 days	Reduction at farm in bacteriological (faces) and serological results at the end of the fattening period. Reduced positive lymph nodes and cecal samples at the slaughterhouse (no reach significance).
Boyen, 2008	Clinical trial	6-week old piglets	1-. Coated butyric 2-. Coated caprilyc 3- Uncoated butyric 4-. Uncoated caprilyc	Feed	1-. Butyric 0.02% 2-. Caprylic 0.03% 3-. Butyric 0.01% 4-. Caprylic 0.017%	12 days	Treatment with coated butyric acid decreased the intestinal *Salmonella* load and shedding. (the concentration of butyric acid used in the uncoated treatment was half the coated).
Creus, 2007	Field trial	Finishers	Formic-propionic (50:50)	Feed	a) 1.2 % b) 0.8 %	a) 14 weeks b) 8 weeks	a) Reduction of percentage of *Salmonella* carriage in lymph nodes. b) Clear serological reduction and partial reduction of carriers in lymph nodes or cecal content.
Dahl, 1996	Field trial	Finishers	Formic, propionic, ammoniumformiate ammoniumpropionate	Feed	0.4%	14 days	No differences in shedding or serological prevalence. The treatment was not effective in previously infected pigs.
De Busser, 2008	Field trial	Finishers	-	Water	-	14 days	No beneficial effect in samples collected (carcass, lymph nodes or rectum)
Tsiloyiannis, 2001	Field trial	Weaners	Separately diets of: - Propionic acid (1 %) / Malic acid (1.2 %) / Formic acid (1.2 %) / Lactic acid (1.6 %) / Citric acid (1.5 %) / Fumaric acid (1.5 %)	Feed	Cited in acids colums	14 days	Thse study was carried out in a famr with clinical post-weaning diarrhoea syndrome caused by ECET. All the treatments reduced the numbers of ECET and showed ain improved growing specially the lactic acid group.
Wolf, 2000	Field trial	Finishers	Acid mixture: Lactic (8 %), formic (23 %), ammonium formiat (28 %), acetic (4 %), propionic (3 %) sorbic (1 %).	Water	0.2 %	12 weeks	The overall prevalence in control group was three times the treated groups, but just in a situation with clinical problems would justify the use of acids to the authors.

Table 1. Summary of experimental and field trials carried out using acid treatments to control *Salmonella.*

In summary and taking into account all the information provided by the different studies, it seems that the success in the control of *Salmonella* infection by using acids is related to several factors. The concentration given must be related to the pH value (Boyen *et al.,*

2008) and the duration of the treatment should be higher than a few weeks. No differences have been demonstrated between their administration in the feed or water. While the incorporation of the acids in the drinking water allows an easy regulation of the concentration and duration of the treatment, it has been associated with damages in the supply water circuits (Van der Wolf *et al.*, 2001b). Moreover, it has been proposed that the success of these acid treatments administered at the end of the fattening period is related to the establishment of the *Salmonella* infection before the acid addition (Dahl *et al*, 1996; Creus *et al.*, 2007).

3.5 Other feed strategies

Other products such as prebiotics, mainly fructo-oligosacharides that cannot be digested by the animal but serve as carbon source for intestinal bacteria, or herbal extracts with significant anti-*Salmonella* activities have been proposed as potential options in the control of *Salmonella* infection in swine farms. However, further studies evaluating their usefulness in *Salmonella* infected swine units are required.

4. Vaccination

Immune response stimulation by vaccines has been a useful mechanism to battle against pathogens. In this subheading of the chapter, vaccinology to control *Salmonella* in pigs will be reviewed including the different types of vaccines tested against *Salmonella* in swine, discussing their efficacy, advantages and disadvantages. In order to develop a useful vaccine against *Salmonella,* the mechanisms involved in the defence of the host as well as those by which the bacteria is able to establish the infection in the host have to be taken into consideration. Hence, a brief revision of the *Salmonella* transmission, pathogenesis and host immune response will be included to improve the reader comprehension about vaccination theories.

4.1 *Salmonella* transmission, pathogenesis and immune response

The fecal-oral route is the typical mode of transmission of *Salmonella.* Once it is ingested, *Salmonella* is able to resist the acid environment in the stomach and the bactericidal effect of compounds such as bile salts in the first part of the small intestine (Fedorka-Cray *et al.*, 1994). In the ileum, the peristalsis together with the indigenous microflora are the main difficulties that *Salmonella* has to overcome to reach its main target, the gut associated lymphoid tissue forming the Peyer's patches in the ileum wall and more exactly the microfold or 'M' cells of this tissue. The virulence genes encoded in the *Salmonella* pathogenicity island I allow the bacteria to trigger macropinocytosis (a form of endocytosis of large particles such as bacteria) in these M cells and also in enterocytes and goblet cells (Frances *et al.*, 1993; Ginocchio *et al.*, 1994). After intestinal wall colonization *Salmonella* is presented to macrophages where it is able to survive by inhibiting the endosome-lysosome fusion through virulence genes encoded in the *Salmonella* pathogenicity island II (Hensel, 2004; Gal-Mor & Finlay, 2006). This allows the bacteria to reach the reticulloendothelial system as previous stage prior to systemic infection. Most of the swine infections caused by *Salmonella* serotypes different from the host-specific serotype *S.* Cholerasuis are restricted to the follicle associated epithelium that surrounds the intestine. That is why we will focus this description of the immune response elicited by the host in this first stage of the infection to the gut and lymphoid tissue associated thereof.

Immediately after entering in the gastrointestinal tract, a complex and concerted immune response involving epithelial cells and both innate and adaptive immune response is mounted against pathogenic *Salmonella.* Although the microfold or M cells aforementioned are the main target to cross the intestinal wall, it has been described that *Salmonella* is also able to disrupt tight junctions between epithelial cells allowing paracellular transit into gastrointestinal tract tissue (Boile *et al.,* 2006). The approach that *Salmonella* uses to cross the epithelial cell barrier is a critical step in the immune responses generated. Those invasive bacteria that cross through the M cells activate particularly the secretion of IgA in the lamina propia; in contrast those non-invasive *Salmonella* that use mainly the paracellular transport do not induce the secretion of IgA.

Once the epithelial barrier is breached, the innate immune cells stimulate the pattern recognition receptors. Macrophages localized in the interfollicular region, neutrophils and monocytes (which will be differentiated in dendritic cells or macrophages) accumulated in the gut associated lymphoid tissue induce the classic T helper 1 immune response and provide the first cellular defence against invasion. Interleukins such as IL-12, IL-1 or those more recently found participating in the immune response to *Salmonella* such as IL-23, IL-22 (Schulz *et al.,* 2008; Godinez *et al.,* 2009) and IL-17 (Raffatelu *et al.,* 2008) as well as TNFα and IFNγ take part in the organism defence.

In later stages of the infection, *Salmonella* clearance is mediated by the specific immune response. Humoral response can be detected one week after the infection of the pigs (Gray *et al.,* 1996a; 1996b), firstly represented by IgM and followed by IgG and IgA (Hasan *et al.,* 1991). The levels of IgM and IgA decrease gradually while IgG persist during extended periods of time, being detected at the time of slaughtering in finisher pigs. Cell immune response is principally represented by $CD4^+$ T lymphocytes (Hess *et al.,* 1996). The exact mechanism by which $CD4^+$ T-cells are able to control bacterial growth is unknown and seems not to be related to the production of TNFα and IFNγ. The antibody production against various *Salmonella* antigens also plays a role in the *Salmonella* clearance from systemic sites. This antibody production is stimulated by T-cells and the $CD8^+$ cytotoxic lymphocytes (Mastroeni *et al.,* 2009) and is directed against antigens such as the lipopolysaccharides, the capsular Vi polysaccharide or flagelins.

Salmonella is a potential intra-cellular pathogen. Its ability to survive and replicate in the macrophages and the reticulloendothelial system let it to avoid, at least partially, the immune response (Hormaeche *et al.,* 1993). Nevertheless it has been described that control and clearance of *Salmonella* rely in the cell immune response mediated by $CD4^+$ and $CD8^+$. (Mastroeni *et al.,* 1997). The specific humoral immune response, except for the IgA presented in the intestinal mucosa, is at least partially avoided by the fact that *Salmonella* is "protected" by the cells which infects and also the innate response (mediated by neutrophils and macrophages) even being the first barrier and also participating in antigens presentation, does not offer protection against *Salmonella.* So to summarize it seems that vaccines should stimulate the cell immune response to protect pigs against *Salmonella* infection.

4.2 Vaccination in pigs against *Salmonella*

The stimulation of the immune system by vaccines against *Salmonella* in swine aims to prevent gut colonization and faecal shedding as well as the development of a carrier state; in a word, bring to end the infection cycle at the farm level (Haesebrouck *et al.,* 2004). The disappearance of clinical symptoms is not the goal of this vaccination since most of the infections by *Salmonella* are not associated with clinical disease in pigs.

Several vaccines have been tested against *Salmonella* including live vaccines, attenuated or genetically modified, inactivated vaccines and also subunit vaccines. Live vaccines have the ability to arouse the best immune response; they stimulate the production of IgA in the intestinal mucosa since they can be used by oral administration and on the other hand they are theoretically able to produce a strong cell-mediated immune response (Lindberg & Robbertson, 1983). Besides, antibody titres seem to be lower than those induced by inactivated vaccines (Springer *et al.*, 2001; Husa *et al.*, 2008) and this fact is relevant if the vaccine is going to be used in the course of control programmes based on serological detection and quantification of the infection. Live vaccines against *Salmonella* included (i) attenuated vaccines obtained by the dwindling of at least one of the virulence mechanisms of the bacteria without localizing or characterizing the molecular basis of attenuation; and (ii) genetically modified vaccines which in contrast to attenuated vaccines are those in which identified genes for the bacterial metabolism such as *aroA* (Lumsden *et al.*, 1991), global regulator genes or virulence genes such as *spv* genes located in *Salmonella* virulence plasmid (Kramer *et al.,* 1992) have suffered induced mutations to attenuate the bacteria.

Many studies have tested live vaccines in both challenge and clinical trials. We will focus our attention on those studies that have reported bacteriological results and therefore have measured the impact of vaccination in the *Salmonella* shedding and *Salmonella* infection in the gut or the associated lymphoid tissue. Several live vaccines including those based on modifications of their genome such as *aroA* mutants, *Δcya-Δcrp, gyrA-cpxA-rpoB* or *adenine-histidine* auxotrophy organisms (Lumsden *et al.*, 1991; Lumsden *et al.*, 1992; Springer *et al.,* 2001; Denagamage *et al.,* 2007; Selke *et al.,* 2007; Husa *et al.,* 2008) have demonstrated a reduction in the faecal shedding and isolation of *Salmonella* from the gut and lymphoid tissues. When piglets were vaccinated with these vaccines and challenged with the bacteria, a diminution in the infection pressure based on a reduction of the *Salmonella* faecal shedding and isolation from the gut and the lymphoid tissue associated was demonstrated. Nevertheless in most of these challenge experiments, the monitoring of the piglets was only carried out during the subsequent days or weeks after the experimental infection and therefore there are doubts regarding the duration of this protection. The experience from field trials has provided scarce but very interesting data; an *adenine-histidine* auxotrophy *S.* Typhimurium vaccine was tested for a period of six months in a farrow-to-finish farm. The prevalence of *Salmonella* infection in the unit decreased from 65% to 23% in 6 weeks. Unfortunately, this study does not include a control group and comparison was made using historical data. More recently, Farzan & Frienship (2009) have evaluated a commercial *S.* Cholerasuis live vaccine in a clinical field trial. The prevalence of *Salmonella* shedding animals decreased as immunized pigs aged but the results were not conclusive since this fact was also reported to a lesser degree in the control pigs. The point that the pigs were probably infected before their vaccination together with the coexistence of three different serotypes of *Salmonella* involved in the infection at the farm could explain at least part of the low efficacy of vaccination against *Salmonella* found in this study. Finally another study using a *S.* Cholerasuis live vaccine (Maes *et al.*, 2001) showed a reduction in the positive ileocaecal lymph nodes (ILN) in the vaccinated group, 0.6%, compared to the control 7.2% while 24% and 9% of the vaccinated and control animals were positive in serology at 24 weeks (cut-off > 10).

Although theoretically live vaccines offer the best protection, they have also several disadvantages; firstly they are not as secure as inactivated vaccines since reversion to virulence can theoretically occur. Besides, transport and storage conditions are more demanding and finally if they are going to be administered orally several factors such as handling, withdrawal of antimicrobial treatments during administration or negative effects such pyrexia or reduced daily gain have to be taken into consideration (Husa *et al.*, 2008). For these reasons, there is still interest in *Salmonella* inactivated vaccines, which are easier to administer, more secure and also cheaper than attenuated life vaccines. In general, inactivated vaccines are useful against extracellular or toxin producer bacteria because humoral immune response can easily and effectively protects the host. It could be expected that no protective or a very limited effect would be seen with intracellular bacteria since the cell-mediated response is not stimulated directly. However, it is important to take into account that at least part of the infection cycle of *Salmonella* takes place in the extracellular space being vulnerable to the action of specific antibodies.

Inactivated vaccines are easy to produce and there are a number of clinical field and experimental trials to evaluate their effectiveness against *Salmonella* in different stages of the swine production including breeding herds, nursery pigs and finishers. A homologous inactivated *S.* Typhimurium vaccine was applied to sows in a research performed by Roesler *et al.* (2006). The results of this vaccination were measured in the offspring and revealed a decreased in the prevalence of *Salmonella* shedders as well as in the prevalence of seropositive piglets. According to these results, vaccination with an inactivated vaccine could be a proper tool to control *Salmonella* transmission from the sows to their progeny, easy to apply and cheap. On the contrary, Farzan & Friendship (2009) failed to demonstrate a clear protection in piglets after vaccination with an autogenous *S.* Typhimurium bacterin probably because the vaccine failed to elicit cross-protection against other serovars and piglets were suffering a multiple-serovar infection. The effectiveness of vaccination of finishers at the beginning of the fattening period with a whole-cell inactivated *S.* Typhimurium bacterin was tested in a field trial carried out by our research group (Argüello *et al.*, 2010c). Vaccinated pigs showed lower faecal shedding throughout the fattening period as well as lower serological response at the slaughter time. Moreover *Salmonella* prevalence in caecal content and mesenteric lymph nodes were also lower in vaccinated pigs as compared with control animals. However, the undesirable effect of vaccination was the strong humoral immune response which would interfere with a serological surveillance on the farm since more than a forty percent of the vaccinated pigs were seropositive (OD cut-off >40%) at the end of the fattening period.

In spite of their limitations, inactivated vaccines as well as subunit vaccines can increase in usefulness by taking advantage of the improvements in DIVA vaccines (Differenciating Infected from Vaccinated Animals) which have already been tested (Selke *et al.*, 2006; Leyman *et al.*, 2011) and also in adjuvants which should be able to increase the immunostimulation boost of these vaccines (Leclerc, 2003). The application of such technology in conjunction with the ongoing developments in identifying new virulence determinants such as purified recombinant proteins, synthetic peptides or plasmid DNA could induce protective immunity by the selective activation of immune effectors mechanisms. The next generation of *Salmonella* vaccines could be based on these premises, to overcome the problems discussed above and improve the protections elicited by vaccines against *Salmonella.*

Despite the fact that the vaccine field has been the target of many surveys since decades, there are still many gaps. Most of the investigations regarding *Salmonella* immunity have been done in a murine model without taking account that *S.* Typhimurium is the host-specific pathogen for this specie. Moreover, most of the challenge trials carried out in piglets do not perform an extended monitoring of the animals until the market-weigh. Further research should be done to increase the knowledge in the immune response against *Salmonella* in production animal species and to non-host specific serotypes as well as in vaccine field trials in both finishers and sows (transmission of the immunity to the piglet).

5. Hygiene, handling practices and biosecurity

At farm level there are many factors that can modify the epidemiology of the infection determining the success of *Salmonella* colonization. Throughout this chapter we have mentioned that *Salmonella* needs to overcome the hostile environment of the gastrointestinal tract of the host as well as the immune response mechanisms elicited in order to establish an infection. In the pig, *Salmonella* can survive in the gut associated lymphoid tissue with reactivation of infection and shedding in favourable conditions, a fact which implies that infected animals are always a risk of infecting other animals throughout their lives. Moreover, *Salmonella* is perfectly adapted to the external environment and is able to survive outside the host for extended periods of time. These two premises, the carriage of *Salmonella* by apparently healthy animals and the ability of these bacteria to survive in the environment, determine the importance of hygiene and biosecurity practices in the control of the infection. None of the control measures aforementioned will be successful if they are not accompanied by adequate hygiene and biosecurity practices on the farm.

Hygiene standards are based on cleaning and disinfection procedures. All-in/all-out systems, where each room or building is completely emptied and sanitized between groups of pigs, are used frequently in finishing units in swine production and it is during the period of time comprised between two consecutive batches when the effort must be paid in order to prevent the infection of the incoming pigs. *Salmonella* can survive in the environment for long periods of time, for instance 14 days on smooth metallic surfaces, one year in wet soil or even up to two and four years in dry excrements and dust respectively (Murray, 2000). Its ability to persist in the environment enhances its transmission capacity. Apart from the direct transmission from pig to pig, the environment is the most important source of *Salmonella* infection in finishing units, being more relevant than contaminated sows at breeding herds (Berends *et al.,* 1996). As was demonstrated by Dahl *et al.* (1997) pigs coming from infected breeding herds, allocated in an environment perfectly cleaned and free of *Salmonella,* can arrive at the slaughterhouse without any positivity in bacteriological or serological samples. Hence, special attention should be paid to avoid the presence of *Salmonella* in the environment.

An effective cleaning protocol should cover the following premises: (i) clean the facilities with pressured water to remove the organic matter with special attention to holes and corners where it can be accumulated, (ii) apply detergents together with the pressured water to enhance the organic matter removal and finally (iii) apply a disinfectant after the proper cleaning protocol. Regarding useful disinfectants, it can be said that *Salmonella* is susceptible to most of the disinfectants used, such chlorine, iodine derivates, phenols, peroxides or quaternary ammonium compounds. However it is surprising that being susceptible to most disinfectants it can be found after cleaning and disinfection protocols routinely applied at farm level (Argüello *et al.*, 2011b).

We have evaluated the effectiveness of routinely cleaning and disinfection procedures against *Salmonella* in swine farms (Argüello *et al.*, 2011). A total number of thirty-six pig finishing farms performing a strict all-in/all-out management (AI/AO) were studied by collecting twelve samples within each farm including samples from pen floors (5 samples), pen walls (5 samples), corridors (1 sample) and dust (1 sample). All the farms were studied after cleaning and disinfection procedures, just before the entrance of a new batch of animals. Despite the fact that cleaning procedures were classified as satisfactory by clinicians and a phenol derivate disinfectant was used, *Salmonella* was still detected in one of each five investigated farms (22.2%). *Salmonella* was recovered mainly from floor samples (6 out of 8 positive farms were positive in floor samples) followed by pen walls (three farms). It is remarkable that in two of the positive farms the contamination was only detected in corridors. In contrast, *Salmonella* was not isolated from dust samples in any of the farms. In a similar farm environmental study performed in Germany, Gotter *et al.* (2011) reported *Salmonella* positive results in 22% of the pens floors, 28% of the pen walls and 32% of the central hallway. Gebrelles *et al.* (1999) also found that 80% of the pens were contaminated after cleaning and disinfection procedures in swine farms. Moreover, *Salmonella* serotypes isolated were related to new infections in the incoming pigs. Regarding these results, it is important to note that it has been described that holes in floors and walls make difficult the penetration of disinfectant solutions along with the biofilm formation by *Salmonella* can make the action of the disinfectants difficult (Marin *et al.*, 2009). Surprisingly, it has been reported that farms using cleaning protocols without disinfectants had lower *Salmonella* levels than those using disinfectants (Van der Wolf *et al.*, 2001a). This fact indicates that disinfection protocols are sometimes not carried out properly and points towards the importance of performing adequate cleaning protocols if we want to achieve an effective disinfection. Moreover, particular attention should be paid not only to pens but also to corridors in order to prevent infections between batches and also to the instruments employed at farm level since they can constitute a source of *Salmonella* contamination. Gotter *et al.* (2011) found that elements such as driving boards, pig toys or boots, presented the higher contamination values, showing that the farm equipment can be a source of contamination that sometimes is underestimated. These results together with the risk factors studies in which not beneficial effects were found in AI/AO systems (Nollet *et al.*, 2004; Rajic *et al,*. 2007; García-Feliz *et al.*, 2010) show that cleaning protocols carried out routinely at farm sometimes do not reach their goal and so special attention should be paid in the cleaning and disinfection carried out between batches removing the organic matter present, cleaning not only the surfaces visible to the naked eye but also equipments, corners, and other surfaces in which dust and contamination can be stored.

Regarding management and handling by farmers the main premises that should be taken into consideration are as follows; large facilities are usually supplied by several breeding origins and then *Salmonella*-free pigs can be mixed with infected pigs at the fattening unit. Thus, in order to avoid the risk of contamination by potentially infected pigs, the origin status of the piglets should be confirmed, above all in low *Salmonella* contaminated farms included in control programmes. Moreover, it is believed that mixing animals with different ages increases the risk of *Salmonella* transmission, so pig handling is also important in avoiding or minimizing *Salmonella* infections at the farm. Adequate handling and caring of the animals is also necessary to diminish the stress, which is related to an increase in pig susceptibility to *Salmonella* infection as well as to an increase in faecal shedding by carriers (Verbrugghe *et al.*, 2011).

Biosecurity is essential at farm level to avoid the entrance of infectious diseases and most of the swine farms fulfil the basic biosecurity measures. General biosecurity measures such as double external fence, footbaths, changing rooms with showers and farm clothes to staff and visitors, external access to feed and dead animal trucks are essential in farms and several risk factor studies have associated them to a lower *Salmonella* prevalence (Amass *et al.*, 2000; Lo Fo Wong *et al.*, 2004).

Apart from infected animals, which constitute the main source of *Salmonella* infection, the indirect transmission of disease by feed or wild animals present at the farm can be also relevant. The importance of feed as *Salmonella* vehicle has been already discussed in the feeding strategies subheading. As it was pointed out if feed transport or storage in the farm are not carried out under strict isolation conditions, feed can be easily contaminated by *Salmonella*. Water supply can also be a significant vehicle to indirect *Salmonella* transmission. The ability of *Salmonella* to survive in water supply depends on the nature of the water and factors such as the presence of protozoa, the concentration of organic matter, toxins, heavy metals, and several physicochemical properties. Fish & Petiborne (1995) estimated that *Salmonella* can survive at least 56 days in water. Farmers should pay attention to water quality and also to guarantee a supply of potable water on their farms. At the same time, wild birds or rodents can also contaminate the feed if they can access to the places where it is stored. Feed and water are effective vehicles to *Salmonella* transmission because they are supplied to all the animals and bring *Salmonella* directly to the gastrointestinal tract. So appropriate production and feed handling as well as water treatment has to be done in order to avoid contamination by *Salmonella* from these two sources.

Probably one of the main factors implied in the spreading of *Salmonella* is its ability to colonize a wide range of animal species including warm or cold blooded animals; this fact implies that most of the animals, birds or insects present in an environment with *Salmonella* will be infected or will carry *Salmonella*. This fact implies that all domestic and wild animals that get in touch with the farm can constitute a source of *Salmonella* for pigs. *Salmonella* has been isolated from rodents in several studies (Healing, 1991) and their faecal pellets can contain up to 10^5 CFU of *Salmonella* (Henzler & Opitz, 1992). Although wild birds have been recognised as carriers of *Salmonella*, evidence suggests that infected birds are rarely identified. It seems that birds are infected by their feeding environment with a short term carriage (Murray, 2000). *Salmonella* has been also isolated from insects including cockroaches, flies, and beetles (Benett, 1993; Davies & Wray 1995; Olsen & Hammack, 2000).

Other wild animals are more related with the maintenance and perpetuation of the infection in the farm more than with the introduction of *Salmonella* thereof; finding positive mice or rats or cats for instance in the farm proves that *Salmonella* is distributed in the environment and the elimination of these animals is crucial if other efforts are taken at the same time to reduce the *Salmonella* prevalence.

Hygiene, handling practices or biosecurity are not sometimes taken into account to battle against a pathogen but in facultative environmental pathogens such *Salmonella,* they can play a crucial role in its maintenance and perpetuation and must be included in the practices to reduce the prevalence at farm level if practitioners want to have success reducing *Salmonella.*

6. Conclusions

The main objective of this chapter was to identify the main potential control strategies applicable in swine production to reduce *Salmonella* prevalence. Fortunately there is enough background to discern which measures seem to be most efficient in general, but we must stress that *Salmonella* epidemiology is not completely understood and that there are many factors that can influence its presence at farm level. The achievement of success in a reduction programme will depend in which measures, of those described here, may be feasible applied taking into account the serotype involved in the infection, its prevalence, type of farm etc, and also factors such economical resources.

7. References

Alban, L.; Stege H., Dahl J., (2002). The new classification system for slaughter-pig herds in the Danish *Salmonella* surveillance-and-control program. *Preventive Veterinary Medicine,* No. 14 pp 133-146.

Alban, L. & Stärk, K.D. (2005). Where should the effort be put to reduce the *Salmonella* prevalence in the slaughtered swine carcass effectively? Preventive Veterinary Medicine., No. 68 pp 63-79.

Amass, S.F.; Vyverberg, B.D., Ragland, D., Dowell, C.A., Anederson, C.D., Stover, J.H., & Beaudry, D.J. (2000). Evaluating the efficacy of boot baths in biosecurity protocols. *Swine Health and Production,* Vol. 4 No. 8 pp. 169-173.

Anadón, A.; Martínez-Larrañaga, M.R. & Aranzazu Martínez, M. (2006). Probiotics for animal nutrition in the European Union. Regulation and safety assessment. *Regulatory, Toxicology and Pharmacology.,* No. 45 pp. 91-95.

Anderson, R.C.; Hume, M.E., Genovese, K.J., Callaway, T.R., Jung, Y.S., Edrington, T.S., Poole, T.L., Harvey, R.B., Bischoff, K.M. & Nisbet, D.J. (2004). Effect of drinking-water administration of experimental chlorate ion preparations on Salmonella enterica serovar Typhimurium colonization in weaned and finished pigs. *Veterinary. Research Communications.,* No. 28 pp. 179-189.

Argüello, H.; Carvajal, A., Alvarez, S., Osorio, J., Hidalgo, A., & Rubio, P., (2010a). Salmonellosis in fattening period: relative importance of sows in two points multiple-site production. *Proceedings of 2nd ESPHM,* Hannover, Germany, 26-28 May 2010.

Argüello, H.; Carvajal, A., Osorio, J., Martin, D. & Rubio, P. (2010b). Evaluation of a commercial acid mixture administered in drinking water as a control measure in swine salmonellosis. Proccedings of International Symposium Salmonella and Salmonellosis, pp: 455-466. Saint Malo, France 28-30 June, 2010.

Argüello, H.; Carvajal, A., Osorio, J., Martin, D. & Rubio, P. (2010c). Efficacy of vaccination with an inactivated vaccine to reduce *Salmonella* prevalence in a pig fattening unit. Proccedings of International Symposium Salmonella and Salmonellosis, pp: 465-466. Saint Malo, France 28-30 June, 2010

Argüello, H.; Carvajal, A., Collazos, J.A., García-Feliz, C., Rubio, P., (2011a). Prevalence and serovars of *Salmonella enterica* on pig carcasses, slaughtered pigs and the environment of four Spanish slaughterhouses. *Journal Food Research.* (in press).

Argüello, H.; Rubio, P., Jaramillo, A., Barrios, V., García, M., & Carvajal, A., (2011b). Evaluation of cleaning and disinfection procedures against *Samonella enterica* at swine farms, transport and lairage facilities. *Procidings of International Safepork congress, pp: 254-256.* Maastrich, Netherlands, 18-20 June 2011.

Beloeil, P.A.; Fravalo, P., Fablet, C., Jolly, J.P., Eveno, E., Hascoet, Y., Chauvin, C., Salvat, G. & Madec, F. (2004). Risk factors for *Salmonella enterica* subsp. *enterica* shedding by market-age pigs in French farrow-to-finish herds. *Preventive Veterinary Medicine,* No. 63 pp. 103-120.

Bennett, G. (1993). Cockroaches as carriers of bacteria. *Lancet,* No. 341 pp. 732.

Berends, B.R.; Urlings, H.A., Snijders, J.M., & Van Knapen, F. (1996). Identification and quantification of risk factors in animal management and transport regarding *Salmonella spp.* in pigs. *International Journal Food Microbiology.* No. 30 pp. 37-53.

Boyle, E.C.; Bishop, J.L., Grassl, G.A., & Finlay, B.B., (2006). *Salmonella*: from pathogenesis to therapeutics. *Journal of Bacteriology. Vol. 5 No. 189 pp. 1489-1495.*

Boyen, F.; Haesebrouck, F., Vanparys, A., Volf, J., Mahu, M., Van Immerseel, F., Rychlik, I., Dewulf, J., Ducatelle, R. & Pasmans, F. (2008). Coated fatty acids alter virulence properties of *Salmonella* Typhimurium and decrease intestinal colonization of pigs. *Veterinary Microbiology,* No. 132 pp. 319-327.

Casey, P.G.; Gardiner, G.E., Casey, G., Bradshaw, B., Lawlor, P.G., Lynch, P.B., Leonard, F.C., Stanton, C., Ross, R.P., Fitzgerald, G.F. & Hill, C. (2007). A five-strain probiotic combination reduces pathogen shedding and alleviates disease signs in pigs challenged with *Salmonella enterica* Serovar Typhimurium. *Applied Environmental Microbiology.* No. 73 pp. 1858-1863.

Casey, P.G.; Casey, G.D., Gardiner, G.E., Tangney, M., Stanton, C., Ross, R.P., Hill, C. & Fitzgerald, G.F. (2004). Isolation and characterization of anti-*Salmonella* lactic acid bacteria from the porcine gastrointestinal tract. *Letters of Applied Microbiology,* No. 39 pp. 431-438.

Collazos, J.A.; Samaniego, L.M., García, C., de Castro, L., Carvajal, A. & Rubio, P. (2008a). Selection and characterization of anti-salmonella lactic acid bacteria of porcine origin. *Proccedings of 20th International Pig Veterinary Society Congress,* pp. 317, Durban, South Africa, 20.25 June, 2008.

Collazos, J.A.; Samaniego, L.M., García, C., de Castro, L., Carvajal, A. & Rubio, P. (2008b). Effect of a probiotic mixture of porcine origin on experimental salmonellosis in swine. *Proccedings of 20th International Pig Veterinary Society Congress*, pp. 317, Durban, South Africa, 20.25 June, 2008.

Creus, E.; Pérez, J.F., Peralta, B., Baucells, F. & Mateu, E. (2007). Effect of acidified feed on the prevalence of *Salmonella* in market-age pigs. Zoonoses and Public Health, No. 54 pp. 314-319.

Dahl, J.; Wingstrand, A., Baggesen, D.L., Nielsen, B. & Thomsen, L.K. (1996). The effect of a comercial, organic acid preparation on seroprevalence and shedding of *Samonella* in finishing herds. *Proccedings of 14th International Pig Veterinary Society Congress*, pp. Bologna, Italy, 1996.

Dahl, J.; Wingstrand, A., Nielsen, B. & Baggesen, D.L. (1997). Eradication of *Salmonella* Typhimurium infection by the strategic movement of pigs. *The Veterinary Record*, No. 140 pp. 679-681.

Davies, P.R.; Scott Hurd, H., Funk, J.A., Fedorka-Cray, P.J. & Jones, F.T. (2004). The role of contaminated feed in the epidemiology and control of *Salmonella enterica* in pork production. Foodborne Pathogens and Disease. No. 1. pp. 202-215.

Davies, R.H. & Wray C. (1997). Distribution of *Salmonella* on 23 pig farms in the U.K. *Proceedings of the 2nd International Symposium on the Epidemiology and Control of Salmonella in Pork*. p.137-141. Copenhagen, Denmark, 1997.

De Angelis, M.; Siragusa, S., Berloco, M., Caputo, L., Settanni, L., Alfonsi, G., Amerio, M., Grandi, A., Ragni, A. & Gobbetti, M. (2006). Selection of potential probiotic lactobacilli from pig feces to be used as additives in pelleted feeding. *Research in Microbiology*, No. 157 pp. 792-801.

De Busser, E.V.; Dewulf, J., Nollet, N., Houf, K., Schwarzer, K., De Sadeleer, L., De Zutter, L. & Maes, D. (2008). Effect of organic acids in drinking water during the last 2 weeks prior to slaughter on *Salmonella* shedding by slaughter pigs and contamination of carcasses. Zoonoses and Public Health, No. 56 pp. 129-136.

Duggan, S.J.; Mannion, C., Prendergast, D.M., Leonard, N., Fanning, S., Gonzales-Barron, U., Egan, J., Butler, F. & Duffy, G. (2010). Tracking the Salmonella status of pigs and pork from lairage through the slaughter process in the Republic of Ireland. *Journal of Food Protection*, No. 73 pp. 2148-2160.

EFSA, 2008. Analysis of the baseline survey on the prevalence of *Salmonella* in slaughtered pigs in the European Union. Part A *Salmonella* prevalence estimates. *EFSA Journal*, No. 135: 1-111.

EFSA, 2009. Analysis of the baseline survey on the prevalence of *Salmonella* in holding with breeding pigs in the European Union, (2008). Part A *Salmonella* prevalence estimates. *EFSA Journal*, No. 7 pp. 1377.

EFSA, 2011. The European Union summary report on trends and sources of zoonosis, zoonotic agents and food-borne outbreaks in (2009). *EFSA Journal*, No. 9 pp. 2090.

Fairbrother, J.M.; Nadeau, E. & Gyles, C.L. (2005). Escherichia coli in postweaning diarrhea in pigs: an update on bacterial types, pathogenesis, and prevention strategies. *Animal Health Reseseach Review*, No 6. pp. 17-39.

Farzan, A.; Friendship, R.M., Dewey, C.E., Warriner, K., Poppe, C. & Klotins, K. (2006). Prevalence of *Salmonella* spp. on Canadian pig farms using liquid or dry-feeding. *Preventive Veterinary Medicine*, No. 73 pp. 241-254.

Farzan, A.; Friendship, R.M., Dewey, C.E., Poppe, C. & Funk, J. (2010). Evaluation of the risk factors for shedding Salmonella with or without antimicrobial resistance in swine using multinomial regression method. *Zoonoses Public Health,* No. 57 pp. 85-93

Fedorka-Cray, P.J.; Whipp S.C., Isaacson R.E., Nord N., & Lager K. (1994). Transmission of *Salmonella* typhimurium to swine. Veterinary Microbiology, Vol. 4 No. 41 pp. 333-344.

Fedorka-Cray, P.J.; Bailey, J.S., Stern, N.J., Cox, N.A., Ladely, S.R. & Musgrove, M. (1999). Mucosal competitive exclusion to reduce *Salmonella* in swine. Journal of Food Protection, No. 62 pp. 1376-1380.

Fish J.T.; & Pettibone G.W. (1995). Influence of freshwater sediment on the survival of Escherichia coli and Salmonella sp. as measured by three methods of enumeration. Letters of Applied Microbiology, Vol., 5 No 20 pp 277-281.

Funk, J.A.; Davies, P.R. & Nichols, M.A. (2001). Longitudinal study of *Salmonella enterica* in growing pigs reared in multiple-site swine production systems. Veterinary Microbiology, No. 83 pp. 45-60.

Gal-Mor, O., & Finlay, B.B. (2006). Pathogenicity islands: a molecular toolbox for bacterial virulence. Cell Microbiology. Vol. 8 No.11 pp. 1707-1719.

Gantois, I.; Ducatelle, R., Pasmans, F., Haesebrouck, F., Hautefort, I., Thompson, A., Hinton, J.C. & Van Immerseel, F. (2005). Butyrate specifically down-regulates Salmonella pathogenicity island 1 gene expression. *Applied Environmental Microbiology,* No 72 pp. 946-949.

García-Feliz, C.; Carvajal, A., Collazos, J.A. & Rubio, P. (2009). Herd-level risk factors for faecal shedding of *Salmonella enterica* in Spanish fattening pigs. *Preventive Veterinary. Medicine,* No. 91 pp. 130-136.

Gebreyes, W.A.; Turner M.B., Funk J.A., Altier C., & Davies P.R. (1999). *Salmonella* prevalence, serotypes, and patterns of antimicrobial resistance in cohorts of nursery and finishing pigs. *Proceedings of the 3rd International Symposium on the Epidemiology and Control of Salmonella in Pork,* p.250-251. Washington, D.C. USA.

Genovese, K.J.; Anderson, R.C., Harvey, R.B. & Nisbet, D.J. (2000). Competitive exclusion treatment reduces the mortality and fecal shedding associated with enterotoxigenic *Escherichia coli* infection in nursery-raised neonatal pigs. Canadian. Journal of Veterinary Research, No. 64 pp. 204-207.

Genovese, K.J.; Anderson, R.C., Harvey, R.B., Callaway, T.R., Poole, T.L., Edrington, T.S., Fedorka-Cray, P.J. & Nisbet, D.J. (2003). Competitive exclusion of *Salmonella* from the gut of neonatal and weaned pigs. Journal of Food Protection, No. 66 pp. 1353-1359.

Giesting, D.W. & Easter, R.A. (1985). Response of starter pigs to supplementation of corn-soybean meal diets with organic acids. Journal of Animal Science, No. 60 pp. 1288-1294.

Ginocchio, C.C.; Olmsted, S.B., Wells, C.L., & Galán, J.E. (1994). Contact with epithelial cells induces the formation of surface appendages on Salmonella typhimurium. Cell. Vol. 4 No. 76 pp. 717-724.

Goldbach, S.G., & Alban, L. (2006). A cost-benefit analysis of *Salmonella*-control strategies in Danish pork production. Preventive Veterinary Medicine. No 77pp. 1-14.

Godinez I.; Raffatellu M., Chu H., Paixão T.A., Haneda T., Santos R.L., Bevins C.L., Tsolis R.M., Bäumler A.J. (2009). Interleukin-23 orchestrates mucosal responses to Salmonella enterica serotype Typhimurium in the intestine. Infection and Immunity. Vol. 1 No. 77 pp. 387-398.

Gotter, V.; Blaha, T., & Klein, G. (2011). A case-control study on the occurrence of *Salmonella* spp. in the environment of pigs. Epidemiology and Infection. No. 16 pp. 1-7.

Gray, J.T.; Fedorka-Cray, P.J., Stabel, T.J., Kramer, T.T. (1996a). Natural transmission of *Salmonella* choleraesuis in swine. Applied Environmental Microbiology. Vol. 1 No. 62 pp. 141-146.

Gray, J.T.; Stabel, T.J., Fedorka-Cray, P.J. (1996b). Effect of dose on the immune response and persistence of Salmonella choleraesuis infection in swine. Amercan Journal Veterinary Research. Vol. 3 No. 57. pp 313-319.

Hald, T., & Wegener, H.C. (1999). Quantitative assesement of the sources of human salmonellosis attributable to pork. *Proceedinings of 3th International Symposium on the Epidemiology and Control of Salmonella in Pork*, pp. 200-205. Washington, D.C., USA.

Hald, T.; Vose D., Wegener H.C., Koupeev, T. (2004). A Bayesian approach to quantify the contribution of animal-food sources to human salmonellosis. *Risk Analysis* No. 24. pp 255-269.

Harris, I.T.; Fedorka-Cray, P.J., Gray, J.T., Thomas, L.A. & Ferris, K. (1997). Prevalence of *Salmonella* organisms in swine feed. Journal of the American. Veterinary Medical Association. No. 210 pp 382-385.

Harvey, R.B.; Droleskey, R.E., Hume, M.E., Anderson, R.C., Genovese, K.J., Andrews, K. & Nisbet, D.J. (2002). In vitro inhibition of *Salmonella enterica* serovars Choleraesuis and Typhimurium, *Escherichia coli* F-18, and *Escherichia coli* O157:H7 by a porcine continuous-flow competitive exclusion culture. *Current Microbiology.* No 45 pp 226–229.

Healing, T.D. (1991). *Salmonella* in rodents: a risk to man? *CDR (London, England Review.* Vol. 10 No.1 pp 114-116.

Hensel, M. (2004). Evolution of pathogenicity islands of *Salmonella enterica*. International Journal of Medicine Microbiology. Vol. 2-3 No. 294 pp. 95-102.

Henzler, D.J.; Opitz, M.H. (1992). The role of mice in the epizootiology of *Salmonella* Enteritidis infection in chicken layer farms. *Avian Diseases*, No 36 pp. 625-631.

Hess, J.; Ladel C., Miko, D., & Kaufmann, S.H. (1996). *Salmonella* typhimurium aroA-infection in gene-targeted immunodeficient mice: major role of CD4+ TCR-alpha beta cells and IFN-gamma in bacterial clearance independent of intracellular location. Journal of Immunology. Vol 9 No. 156 pp. 3321-3326.

Højberg, O.; Canibe, N., Knudsen, B. & Jensen, B.B. (2003). Potential rates of fermentation in digesta from the gastrointestinal tract of pigs: effect of feeding fermented liquid feed. *Applied Environmental Microbiology. No.* 69 pp. 408-418.

Hormaeche, C.E.; Villareal, N., Dougan, G., and Chatfield, S.N. (1993). Immunity mechanisms in experimental Salmonellosis. In: Cabello, F., Hormaeche ,C.E., MAstroeni , P., and Bonina, P.,(eds). *Biology of Salmonella*. Plenum press, New York, pp. 223-235.

Hotes, S.; Kemper, N., Traulsen, I., Rave, G. & Krieter, J. (2010). Risk factors for Salmonella infection in fattening pigs - an evaluation of blood and meat juice samples. *Zoonoses and Public Health,* No. 57 pp. 30-38.

Hume.; M.E., Corrier, D.E., Ambrus, S., Hinton, A. & DeLoach, J.R. (1993). Effectiveness of dietary propionic acid in controlling Salmonella typhimurium colonization in broiler chicks. *Avian Dissease.* No 37 pp. 1051-1056.

Hume, M.E.; Nisbet, D.J., Buckley, S.A., Ziprin, R.L., Anderson, R.C. & Stanker, L.H. (2001). Inhibition of in vitro *Salmonella* Typhimurium colonization in porcine cecal bacteria continuous-flow competitive exclusion cultures. *Journal of Food Protection* No 64 pp. 17–22.

Hurd, H.S.; McKean, J.D., Griffith, R.W., Wesley, I.V. & Rostagno, M.H. (2002). Salmonella enterica infections in market swine with and without transport and holding. *Applied Environmental Microbiology.* No 68 pp. 2376-2381.

Jørgensen, L.; Dahl, J. & Wingtrand, A. (1999). The effect of feeding pellets, meal and heat treatment on the *Salmonella*-prevalence of finishing pigs, *Procceedings 3th International. Symposium on Epidemiology and Control of Salmonella in Pork* pp. 308-312 Washington D.C., USA, 1999.

Jørgensen, L.; Kjærsgaard, H.D., Wachamann, H., Jensen, B. & Knudsen, B. (2001). Effect of pelleting and use of lactic acid in feed on *Salmonella* prevalence and productivity in weaners. P*rocceedings 4th International Symposium on the Epidemiology and Control of Salmonella in Pork.* Pp109-111 Leipzig, 2001.

Kjeldsen, N.J. & Dahl, J. (1999). The effect of feeding non-heat treated, non-pelleted feed compared to feeding pelleted, heat-treated feed on the *Salmonella*-prevalence of finishing pig. *Procceedings 3th International. Symposium on Epidemiology and Control of Salmonella in Pork* pp. 313-316 Washington D.C., USA, 1999.

Kranker, S.; Alban, L., Boes, J. & Dahl, J. (2003). Longitudinal study of *Salmonella enterica* serotype Typhimurium infection in three Danish farrow-to-finish swine herds. Journal of Clinical. *Microbiology.* No 41 pp. 2282-2288.

Kranker, S.; Dahl, J. & Wingstry, A. (2001). Bacteriological and serological examination and risk factor analysis of *Salmonella* occurrence in sow herds, including risk factors for high *Salmonella* seroprevalence in receiver finishing herds. *Berliner und Münchener Tierärztliche Wochenschrif.* No 114 pp. 350-352.

Kwon, Y.M. & Ricke, S.C. (1998). Induction of acid resistance of *Salmonella* typhimurium by exposure to short-chain fatty acids. Applied Environmental Microbiology. 64: 3458-3463.

Leyman, B.; Boyen F., Parys, A., Verbrugghe, E., Haesebrouck, F., Pasmans, F. (2011). Application of the DIVA principle to *Salmonella* Typhimurium vaccines in pigs avoids interference with serosurveillance programmes. *Procedings in International Safepork congress,* pp: 254-256 Maastrich, The Netherlands, 18-20 June, 2011.

Leontides, L.S.; Grafanakis, E. & Genigeorgis, C. (2003). Factors associated with the serological prevalence of *Salmonella enterica* in Greek finishing swine herds. *Epidemiology and Infection.* No. 131 pp. 599-606.

Letellier, A.; Messier, S., Pare, J., Menard, J. & Quessy, S., 1999. Distribution of *Salmonella* in swine herds in Quebec. *Veterinary Microbiology.* No. 67 pp. 299-306.

Lo Fo Wong, D.M.A.; Dahl, J., Stege, H., van der Wolf, P.J, Leontides, L., von Altrock, A. & Thorberg, B.M. (2004). Herd-level risk factors for subclinical *Salmonella* infection in European finishing-pig herds. *Preventive Veterinary Medicine*. No 62 pp. 253-266.

Maes, D.; Gibson K., Trigo, E., Saszak, A., Grass, J., Carlson, A., & Blaha, T. (2001). Evaluation of cross-protection afforded by a *Salmonella* Choleraesuis vaccine against *Salmonella* infections in pigs under field conditions. Berliner und Münchener Tierärztliche Wochenschrif. Vol 9-10. No 114. pp. 339-41.

Marin, C.; Hernandiz, A., & Lainez, M. (2009). Biofilm development capacity of *Salmonella* strains isolated in poultry risk factors and their resistance against disinfectants. Poultry Science. Vol 2. No 88. pp 424-431.

Mastroeni, P.; Grant, A., Restif, O., & Maskell, D. (2009). A dynamic view of the spread and intracellular distribution of *Salmonella* enterica. Natural Reviews, Microbiology. Vol. 1 No 7. pp. 73-80.

Mikkelsen, L.L.; Naughton, P.J., Hedemann, M.S. & Jensen, B.B. (2004). Effects of physical properties of feed on microbial ecology and survival of *Salmonella enterica* serovar Typhimurium in the pig gastrointestinal tract. Applied Environmental Microbiology No. 70 pp. 3485-3492.

Murray, C.J. (2000). Environmental aspects of *Salmonella.* In: WRAY, C; WRAY, . *Salmonella in Domestic Animals.* CABI Publishing, Wallingford pp. 265-283.

Nielsen, B.; Alban, L., Stege, H., Sørensen, L.L., Møgelmose, V., Bagger, J., Dahl, J., & Baggesen, D.L. (2001). A new *Salmonella* surveillance and control programme in Danish pig herds and slaughterhouses. *Berliner und Münchener Tierärztliche Wochenschrif,* No. 114 pp. 323-326.

Nollet, N., Maes, D., De Zutter, L., Duchateau, L., Houf, K., Huysmans, K., Imberechts, H., Geers, R., de Kruif ,A., & Van Hoof, J. (2004). Risk factors for the herd-level bacteriologic prevalence of *Salmonella* in Belgian slaughter pigs. Preventive Veterinary Medicine. Vol 1,2 No 65 (1-2) pp. 63-75.

Olsen, A.R., & Hammack, T.S. (2000). Isolation of *Salmonella* spp. from the housefly, Musca domestica L., and the Dump fly, Hydrotaea aenescens (Wiedemann) (Diptera: Muscidae), at caged-layer houses. *Journal of Food Protection,* No.63 pp. 958-960.

Ozawa, K.; Yabuuchi, K., Yamanaka, K., Yamashita, Y., Nomura, S. & Oku, I. (1983). Effect of *Streptococcus faecalis* BIO-4R on intestinal flora of weaning piglets and calves. *Applied Environmental. Microbiology.* No. 45 pp. 1513-1518.

Pires, S.M.; Knegt, L., and Hald, T (2011). Estimation of the relative contribution of different food and animal sources to human Salmonella infections in the European Union. *EFSA-Q-*2010-00685.

Poljak, Z.; Dewey, C.E., Friendship, R.M., Martin, S.W. & Christensen, J., (2008). Multilevel analysis of risk factors for Salmonella shedding in Ontario finishing pigs. *Epidemiology and Infection.* No. 136 pp. 1388-1400.

Raffatellu, M.; Santos, R.L., Verhoeven, D.E., George, M.D., Wilson, R.P., Winter, S.E., Godinez, I., Sankaran, S., Paixao,T.A., Gordon, M.A., Kolls, J.K., Dandekar, S., & Bäumler, A.J., (2008). Simian immunodeficiency virus-induced mucosal interleukin-17 deficiency promotes Salmonella dissemination from the gut. *Nature Medicine.* Vol. 4 No. 14 pp. 421-428.

Rajic, A.; O'Connor, B.P., Deckert, A.E., Keenliside, J., McFall, M.E., Re-Smith, R.J., Dewey, C.E. & McEwen, S.A. (2007). Farm-level risk factors for the presence of *Salmonella* in 89 Alberta swine-finishing barns. *Canadian Journal of Veterinary Research.* No 71 pp. 264-270.

Stege, H.; Christensen, J., Nielsen, J.P., Baggesen, D.L., Enoe, C. & Willeberg, P. (2000). Prevalence of subclinical *Salmonella enterica* infection in Danish finishing pig herds. *Preventive Veterinary Medicine* No. 44 pp. 175-188.

Schulz, S.M.; Köhler, G., Schütze, N., Knauer, J., Straubinger, R.K., Chackerian, A.A., Witte, E., Wolk, K., Sabat, R., Iwakura, Y., Holscher, C., Müller, U., Kastelein, R.A., & Alber, G. (2008). Protective immunity to systemic infection with attenuated *Salmonella enterica* serovar enteritidis in the absence of IL-12 is associated with IL-23-dependent IL-22, but not IL-17. *Journal of Immunology.* Vol. 11 No. 181 pp. 7891-7901.

Szabó, I.; Wieler. L.H., Tedin, K., Scharek-Tedin, L., Taras, D., Hensel, A., Appel, B., Nöckler K. (2009). Influence of a probiotic strain of Enterococcus faecium on *Salmonella* enterica serovar Typhimurium DT104 infection in a porcine animal infection model. Applied Environmental Microbiology. Vo. 9 No. 75 pp: 2621-2628.

Torres, G.J.; Piquer, F.J.; Algarra, L., de Frutos, C. & Sobrino, O.J., (2011). The prevalence of *Salmonella enterica* in Spanish feed mills and potent*ial feed-related risk factors for contamination. Preventive Veterinary Medicine.* No 98 pp. 81-87.

Tsiloyiannis, V.K.; Kyriakis, S.C., Vlemmas, J. & Sarris, K., (2001). The effect of organic acids on the control of porcine post-weaning diarrhoea. *Research in Veterinary Science.* No 70 pp. 287-293.

Van der Wolf, P.J.; Wolbers, W.B., Elbers, A.R.W., van der Heijden, H.M.J.F., Koppen, J.M.C.C., Hunneman, W.A., van Schie, F.W. & Tielen, M.J.M., (2001a). Herd level husbandry factors associated with the serological *Salmonella* prevalence in finishing pig herds in The Netherlands. *Veterinary Microbiology* No 78 pp. 205-219.

Van der Wolf, P.J.; van Schie, F.W., Elbers, A.R., van der Heijden, H.M., Hunneman, W. A., Tielen, M.J. (2001b). Administration of acidified drinking water to finishing pigs in order to prevent *Salmonella* infections. *The Veterinary Quarterly* No. 23 pp. 121-125

Van Immerseel, F.; Russell, J.B., Flythe, M.D., Gantois, I., Timbermont, L., Pasmans, F., Haesebrouck, F. & Ducatelle, R. (2006). The use of organic acids to combat *Salmonella* in poultry: a mechanistic explanation of the efficacy. Avian Pathology. No 35 pp. 182-188.

Verbrugghe, E.; Haesebrouck, F., Boyen, F.L., Leyman, B., Van Deun, K., A. Thompson, A., Shearer, N., Van Parys, A., & Pasmans, F. (2011). Stress induced *Salmonella* Typhimurium re-excretion by pigs is associated with cortisol induced increased intracellular proliferation in porcine macrophages. *Proceedings of International Safepork congress, pp: 49-52.* Maastrich, Netherlands, 18-20 June 2011.

Visscher, C.F., Klein, G., Verspohl, J., Beyerbach, M., Stratmann-Selke, J. & Kamphues, J., 2011. Serodiversity and serological as well as cultural distribution of Salmonella on farms and in abattoirs in Lower Saxony, Germany. *International. Journal of Food Microbiology.* No. 146 pp. 44-51.

Wingstrand, A.; Jorgensen, L., Christensen, G., Thomsen, L.K., Dahl., J. & Jensen, B. (1996). Reduction of subclinical *Salmonella* infection by feeding coarse ground feed and adding formic acid to water. *Proceedings of 14th International Pig Veterinary Society Congress*. pp. 180 Bologna, Italy. 1996.

Van Winsen, R.L.; Lipman, L.J., Biesterveld, S., Urlings, B.A., Snijders, J.A., & van Knapen, F. (2001). Mechanism of *Salmonella* reduction in fermented pig feed. *Journal of the Science of Food and Agriculture*, No. 81 pp. 342-346.

6

Adaptation of *Salmonella* to Antimicrobials in Food-Processing Environments

Florence Dubois-Brissonnet
AgroParisTech, UMR MicAliS, Massy
INRA, UMR 1319, MicAliS, Jouy-en-Josas
France

1. Introduction

Salmonella remains an important concern in food processing environments as it causes salmonellosis, a major public health problem throughout the world (Anonymous, 2004; Mead et al., 1999). This review deals with the ability of *Salmonella* to survive and adapt to the antimicrobial stresses encountered in food processing environments. It illustrates how bacteria can develop greater tolerance to these stresses and cross-protection with other environmental stresses, thus increasing their persistence throughout the food chain. Two types of antimicrobial agents are primarily encountered in food-processing environments, food preservatives and disinfectants.

Food preservatives are directly included in food products. Their use is the most common method to guarantee microbial food safety until the end of shelf-life. Among these substances, traditional chemical preservatives should be distinguished from naturally-occurring antimicrobial compounds. The former group includes officially approved compounds such as organic acids (lactic, acetic, sorbic, benzoic acids) and their salts, nitrites and nitrates, or sulfites (Roller, 2003). The latter group includes compounds which come from a natural source: whether they are produced by a microorganism, e.g. several weak acids or bacteriocins, or whether they are extracted from a plant or animal product, e.g. essential oil compounds, lactoperoxidase or lactoferrin (Roller, 2003). In most cases, these natural antimicrobials are used in foods for their acidifying or flavoring properties, but they also play an important role in maintaining microbiological food safety. Indeed, it has been long recognized that numerous natural compounds have antimicrobial properties (Naidu, 2000; Roller, 2003), among them, weak organic acids (Doores, 2005) and essential oil compounds (Burt, 2004). The inhibition of Gram-negative bacteria by bacteriocins produced by lactic acid bacteria is limited because of the impermeability of the outer membrane (Abee et al., 1995), even though treatment with EDTA (which permeabilizes the membrane) can render these bacteria sensitive to nisin but not to pediocin (Schved et al., 1994). Nevertheless, microcin L, a bacteriocin produced by *E. coli,* is highly efficient against *S.* Typhimurium (Morin et al., 2011).

Disinfectants are chemical agents used on inanimate surfaces to inactivate all recognized pathogenic microorganisms (Centers for Disease Control and Prevention, USA). They are applied regularly in food processing environments in order to control surface biocontamination, and must be officially approved (Anonymous, 1998). Numerous disinfectants with different mechanism of action are widely employed by the food industry, such as peroxygens, quaternary ammonium compounds, halogen-realizing agents or aldehydes (McDonnell & Russell, 1999). But regulations are currently being revised (Reach, biocide directive) and some of these molecules would no longer be permitted in the future years (Anonymous, 2006; Anonymous, 2009).

Antimicrobial properties of a compound can be characterized with respect to its bacteriostatic and/or bactericidal activities. The bacteriostatic activity of an antimicrobial is determined by its minimum inhibitory concentration (MIC); i.e. the minimum concentration that can completely inhibit growth of the target pathogen. The bactericidal activity can be evaluated using a survival curve (a single concentration is applied and survivors are enumerated over time) or by establishing the Minimum Bactericidal Concentration (MBC: a range of concentrations are applied for a specific period of time and survivors are then numbered). Food antimicrobials are intended to eradicate or inhibit the growth of pathogenic microorganisms, whereas disinfectants are only designed to kill the microbial population rapidly.

Although bacterial resistance can be characterized regularly using one of these techniques, it is important to know that, like in numerous pathogens, the resistance of *Salmonella* to antimicrobials can evolve as a function of its living conditions. If bacteria are subjected to stressful conditions, they can increase their survivability under conditions that would normally be lethal. Induced tolerance was first demonstrated in *Salmonella* after a heat pre-shock at 48°C which induced an increase in the further thermotolerance of the strain (Mackey & Derrick, 1986). Preservative factors can impose non-lethal stresses upon bacteria in foods, potentially eliciting stress tolerance. Moreover, consumers today are looking for additive-free, fresh and more natural foodstuffs. In this context, combinations of treatments may be a way to enable their use at low doses while maintaining microbial food safety. The term "hurdle technology" is widely employed to describe these combinations of technologies with preservative effects (Leistner, 1995) and, because these treatments are often applied at the same time, the term multifactorial preservation has been proposed as being more appropriate (Roller, 2003). However, because these cumulative processes are all applied at sub-inhibitory concentrations, they may promulgate an adaptive stress response and enable the survival of a greater fraction of the bacterial population.

Moreover, in food processing or farming environments, *Salmonella* biofilms can settle on surfaces, despite disinfection procedures (Vestby et al., 2009). A biofilm is a bacterial community that adheres to a surface and is embedded in a matrix of microbial extracellular polymeric substances (Costerton et al., 1995; Hoiby et al., 2010). Protected by this matrix, *Salmonella* cells in the deeper layers of the biofilm thus become less accessible to the disinfectant because of diffusion limitations and can develop adaptive stress responses to sub-lethal concentrations of disinfectant.

The ability of the pathogen to respond to stressful conditions has been described as bacterial stress adaptation, stress adaptive response, habituation, induced tolerance, acclimatization or stress hardening (Yousef & Courtney, 2003). Numerous physiological responses are implicated in this increase in bacterial survival and tolerance in harsh environments (Wesche et al., 2009). Many physiological modifications occur concomitantly in the cell, including protein up- or down-regulation, modifications to the cell membrane composition and altered morphology. In addition, these physiological changes following stressful conditions can induce cross resistance to other stressful environmental conditions, modifications to colonization or virulence (Figure 1). In all cases, bacterial stress will exert a considerable impact on the persistence of *Salmonella* throughout the food chain because of the modifications they induce to cell physiology, reactivity and tolerance. This is therefore a major concern in the area of food microbiology because it may constitute an emergent microbiological hazard.

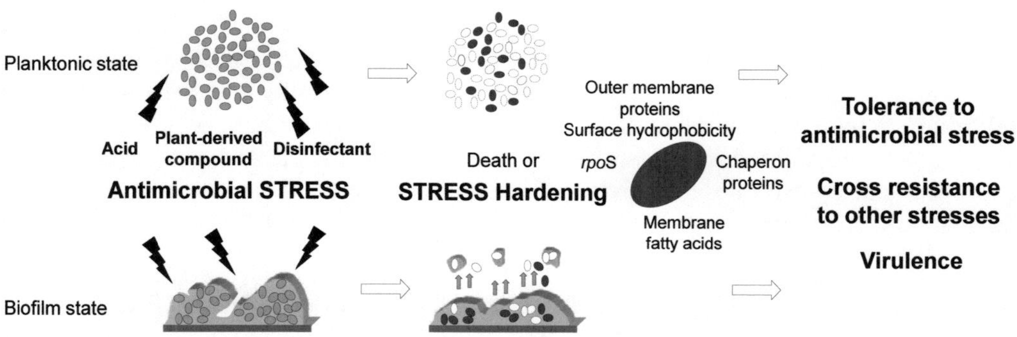

Fig. 1. Adaptation of *Salmonella* to antimicrobial stresses in food processing environments and consequences

Adaptation of *Salmonella* to both food antimicrobials and disinfectants will be discussed in the next three parts. Among the former group, we will focus on the two main groups of natural compounds which have demonstrated their efficiency against *Salmonella* and many other Gram-negative bacteria; i.e. weak acids and essential oil compounds.

2. Adaptation of *Salmonella* to weak organic acids

This section reviews the ability of *Salmonella* to grow and survive under acidic conditions. We will also discuss its capacity to develop acid adaptation and the consequences relative to its cross resistance to other stresses and virulence.

Salmonella may encounter a variety of acidic stress situations in both natural and industrial environments, as well as during pathogenesis. In foodstuffs, weak organic acids (e.g. acetic, lactic, citric acids, etc.) are either present naturally as constituents of the food, are produced by fermentation or are added during food formulation in order to protect against deterioration. For example, acetic acid is widely employed as a food acidulant to inhibit microbial growth and extend the shelf-life of food. Within the human digestive system, *Salmonella* must endure an extreme pH in the stomach and survive in the presence of weak acids in the intestinal environment before reaching the epithelial cells (Baik et al., 1996).

2.1 Growth or survival under acidic conditions

The optimum pH for *Salmonella* growth is generally said to be between 6.5 and 7.5, but the minimum pH value depends on many factors such as the strain and type of acid. For example, *Salmonella* Typhimurium can grow at 25-37°C at pH 4.5 when the pH is adjusted with citric acid, while it has to be over 5.4 with lactic acid and 6.4 with acetic acid (Alvarez-Ordonez et al., 2010a). These findings can be explained because the undissociated form is that which is primarily responsible for antimicrobial activity, as it is able to penetrate into the cell and reduce the cytoplasmic pH by intracellular dissociation. For a given acid, the lower the pH, the higher the proportion of the undissociated form (Dziezak, 1986). However, the activity of each acid will depend on its pKa; the higher the pKa, the higher is the proportion of undissociated form at a given pH. For example, at pH 5, 34.9% of acetic acid is undissociated, as opposed to 0.41% of citric acid at the same pH. Inhibitory efficiency, thus, decreases as follows: acetic acid (pKa 4.75) > lactic acid (pKa 3.08) > citric acid (pKa1 3.14; pKa2 4.77; pKa3 6.39) (Doores, 2005). Acid preservatives are therefore more efficient in acid or acidified foods. Lactic, acetic, and benzoic acids are authorized in foodstuffs at *quantum satis* concentrations ("the amount which is needed"). They are generally added to foodstuffs at a rate of 1% or higher. Above the pH mode of action, some acids exert specific toxicity; for example propionic, sorbic or benzoic acids, which should therefore be used at lower concentrations such as 0.05% to 0.2% (Mescle & Zucca, 1996).

The minimum growth pH of *Salmonella* is also temperature-dependent. The minimum growth pH is increased by about 1 pH unit at high (45°C) or low (10°C) temperatures, compared to the minimum pH at 25-37°C (Alvarez-Ordonez et al., 2010a).

Above the minimum pH level, growth kinetics can be characterized by modeling the growth rate versus the concentration of acid (Guillier et al., 2007). Inhibitory activity will depend on the type of acid, its concentration and the pH. Beyond the MIC determination, one parameter is particularly useful for characterizing acid inhibition: the Non-Inhibitory Concentration (NIC) which is the higher concentration at which no inhibition is observed. Different models can be utilized in this respect, including a square-root model based on the Lambert and Pearson model (Lambert & Pearson, 2000). The growth rate (μmax) as a function of acid concentration (c) is expressed as follows, where MIC, NIC and μmax(c=0) are the model parameters (Guillier et al., 2007):

$$\sqrt{\mu_{\max}(c)} = \sqrt{\mu_{\max}(c=0) \cdot g(c)} \text{ where } g(c) = \exp\left[-\left(\frac{c}{MIC \Big/ \exp\left(\frac{\ln(NIC/MIC)}{-e}\right)}\right)^{\left(\frac{-e}{\ln(NIC/MIC)}\right)}\right]$$

Depending on the acid, different growth rate inhibition profiles have been generated while acid concentration increases in the medium (Figure 2). There was no pH adjustment. For example, the inhibitory effect of lactic acid on *S.* Typhimurium starts above 36.6 mM, while citric acid is effective up to 9.9 mM. The MIC values for citric, lactic and acetic acids in these conditions are respectively 30 mM, 40 mM and 52 mM (Guillier et al., 2007). In addition to the MIC, determining the NIC is of great importance because for some compounds, the difference between NIC and MIC values is very small. Thus a small error made when adjusting the concentration in a food product can lead to a level that is the wrong side of the growth-no growth limit.

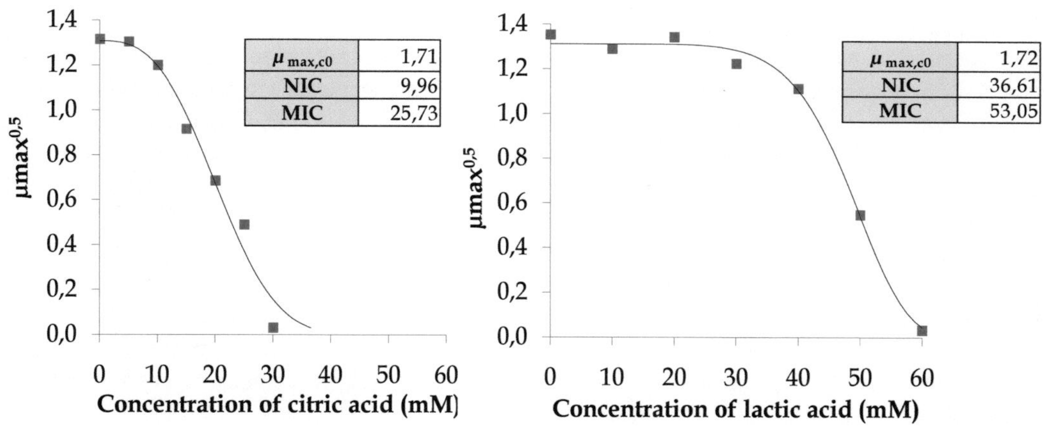

Fig. 2. *S.* Typhimurium growth rate inhibition versus concentration of citric acid or lactic acid (data from Guillier et al., 2007).

Below the minimum growth pH, *Salmonella* can nevertheless survive. The minimum survival pH has usually been stated to be at about 3.0 for *Salmonella*, unlike *E. coli* or *Shigella* that can survive at pH 2 or 2.5 in complex media (Lin et al., 1995). However, different strains of *Salmonella* have been shown to survive at pH 2.5 for prolonged periods of time (de Jonge et al., 2003). The emergence of these acid-resistant strains suggests a preconditioning in acidic conditions, most probably within the intestinal tract of ruminants fed with a carbohydrate-rich diet (de Jonge et al., 2003) as it will be described in the next paragraph.

Furthermore, acid compounds can also have a bactericidal activity against *Salmonella*. This can be evaluated in the same way as other inactivation treatments, using a survival curve or by determining *D*-values (number of minutes required to reduce the number of viable organisms by a factor of 10).

2.2 Onset of acid tolerance response (ATR)

Some early studies showed that the exposure of *Salmonella* to mild acidic conditions could protect it against extreme acid conditions (Huhtanen, 1975). When log-phase cells grown at pH 7.6 were shifted to mildly acidic conditions (pH 5.8) for one generation, they were able to develop 100- to 1,000-fold higher tolerance to extreme acid conditions (pH 3.3) than non-adapted cells shifted directly from pH 7.6 to 3.3 (Foster & Hall, 1990). The increased tolerance to a low pH following acid habituation was referred to as the Acid Tolerance Response (ATR) (Foster & Hall, 1990). Even if the majority of studies investigating acid resistance of *Salmonella* were first conducted with inorganic acids, it was later shown that organic acids also have the ability to induce resistance to many other stresses. Acid shock confers protection on *Salmonella* against the lethal effect of a low pH under different conditions (see some examples in Table 1) obtained with different types of acids (citric, lactic, malic, acetic acids, HCl, etc.), challenge media (laboratory media or foodstuffs), or growth conditions during adaptation. More than just the pH value, it has been shown that the type of acid can influence the amplitude of the ATR. For *S.* Typhimurium, higher ATR values are obtained in order using citric, acetic, lactic, malic acids (Alvarez-Ordonez et al., 2009). Moreover, food composition can influence the stress responses and subsequent tolerance properties of adapted cells. For example, acid-adapted *S.* Typhimurium was more resistant to extreme acidic conditions when meat extract was used as a challenge medium rather than BHI (Alvarez-Ordonez et al., 2009). Recently, growth temperature has also been shown to be an important factor affecting the *Salmonella* ATR. Acid tolerance was increased 2-fold in cells grown at 10°C while it increased more than 3.5-fold at a temperature higher than 25°C (Alvarez-Ordonez et al., 2010a). Moreover, higher ATR obtained with citric acid occurred only at 25-37°C but not at 10°C or 45°C (Alvarez-Ordonez et al., 2010a). More than preventing growth, maintaining a low temperature may therefore constitute a means of limiting induction of the *Salmonella* ATR. In addition, the ATR may emerge with some strains more than others. For example, *S.* Typhimurium demonstrated a higher degree of acid tolerance than *S.* Typhi (Arvizu-Medrano & Escartin, 2005).

The acid tolerance response is a major concern in terms of food safety as it could permit *Salmonella* survival in acidic environments such as fermented foods, following acid cleaning treatments of industrial surfaces or the gastrointestinal tract. For example, acid-adapted cells were able to survive for a period of two months in cheddar, Swiss and mozzarella cheeses stored at 5°C (Leyer & Johnson, 1992).

2.3 ATR mechanism

The ATR mechanism of *Salmonella* has been widely described (Bearson et al., 1997; Foster, 1991; Foster & Hall, 1990; Lee et al., 1994). *Salmonella* possesses both log-phase and stationary-phase ATR systems. The log-phase ATR appears to be a two-stage inducible system (Foster, 1991) with complex regulation systems detailed below. The higher level of acid tolerance provided in stationary-phase appears to differ from log-phase ATR. It has been attributed to a pH-dependant system called stationary-phase ATR, together with a generalized stress response (Lee et al., 1994).

The two-stage system of log-phase ATR consists of pre-acid and post-acid shocks. Pre-acid shock, activated at pH 6, involves an emergency pH homeostatic system, designed to maintain the intracellular pH higher than 5. It induces several amino acid decarboxylases, such as lysine decarboxylase, which decarboxylates intracellular lysine to cadaverine while consuming a proton. Cadaverine is then exchanged for another lysine from the medium *via* a CadB antiporter (Bearson et al., 1997). A higher relative expression of the lysine and arginine decarboxylase systems was demonstrated in acid-adapted *Salmonella* Typhimurium (Alvarez-Ordonez et al., 2010b). The existence of these homeostatic systems, that can use the extracellular amino acids present in foodstuffs such as meat extract, explains the higher acid tolerance observed in these media. However, prolonged exposure (6h) to mild acid stress causes a loss of homeostasis, resulting in more susceptibility to lethal stress (Greenacre et al., 2003).

Post-acid shock is induced when the pH falls below 4.5. Acid shock proteins (ASP) are required for the adaptive acid tolerance response. Their synthesis is dependent on several regulatory genes: the alternative sigma factor σ^S encoded by *rpoS*, the iron regulator Fur and the two-component signal transduction system PhoPQ (Baik et al., 1996; Bearson et al., 1997; Foster, 1991; Foster, 1999). The alternative sigma factor σ^S has been recognized as a key factor in increasing the stress resistance of *Salmonella* cells in stationary phase but it can also be induced by stresses that bacteria may encounter during processing, such as acid stress (Dodd & Aldsworth, 2002). It controls the expression of about 40 genes/operons involved in generating the physiological changes associated with survival processes, among them ASP synthesis. For example, *S.* Typhimurium produces forty-three ASPs at pH 4.5 (Foster, 1993). At pH values lower than 2.6, the addition of chloramphenicol (which inhibits protein synthesis) has been found to reduce subsequent acid resistance, although the cells were not as sensitive as control cultures grown at pH 7.0 (Humphrey et al., 1993). Some ASPs are chaperon proteins which may protect internal proteins from denaturation (Foster, 1991). The pre-acid shock stage offers the cell an enhanced ability to synthesize APSs following acidification of the medium. The long-term adaptation of *S.* Enteritidis to propionate acid induces the differential expression of over twenty proteins. Of the five over-expressed proteins, two were clearly found to be implicated in acid induced resistance: Dps, a DNA-binding protein from starved cells and CpxR, a transcriptional regulatory protein (Calhoun et al., 2010). These two proteins are normally associated with virulence and pathogenesis.

Moreover, acid adaptation in log-phase has been shown to induce increased production of specific outer membrane proteins and enhanced surface hydrophobicity without lipopolysaccharide alteration (Leyer & Johnson, 1993). These surface modifications may be of considerable concern because they may affect the ability of *Salmonella* to adhere to inert surfaces in food processing environments, and then to form biofilms. Alongside proteome modifications, some other physiological modifications appear following acid adaptation, such as modifications of fatty acid profiles. The proportions of membrane cyclopropane fatty acid (CFA) in *S.* Typhimurium were found to be higher at a pH lower than 6 when compared with those of cells grown at pH 7.5 (de Jonge et al., 2003). CFA levels were also found to be 1.5-fold higher in acid-adapted cells (grown in the presence of acids at pH values of 6.4, 5.4, or 4.5 in BHI) than in non-adapted cells (Alvarez-Ordonez et al., 2008). It could be speculated that acid-induced RpoS in the exponential phase might increase CFA synthase activity in *S.* Typhimurium (Kim et al., 2005). CFAs are produced by the addition of a methyl group from *S*-adenosyl methionine across a *cis*-double bond of unsaturated fatty acids (UFAs). They are generally known to be preferentially synthesized when cells enter the stationary phase in *Salmonella,* as in numerous other bacteria (Kim et al., 2005). The conversion of UFAs into CFAs induces a decrease in membrane fluidity. This may be a way for stressed cells to limit exchanges with the external medium and conserve energy. The membrane fluidity of *Salmonella* adapted to citric acid was measured by fluorescence anisotropy of a fluorescent probe (DPH) and the results showed that it was lower than that of control cells (Alonso-Hernando et al., 2010). The over-synthesis of CFA is considered to be a major factor in the acid resistance of Gram-negative bacteria (Brown et al., 1997; Chang & Cronan, 1999).

Another concern is that, following acid adaptation, some injured cells may shift into a viable but non-cultivable (VBNC) state, which is one of the current mechanisms that allows non-sporulating cells to survive. These cells cannot grow on the selective media used to detect pathogens in foods, typically xylose lysine desoxycholate agar for *Salmonella*. They can escape the microbiological controls, but can slowly repair themselves and then re-grow in foodstuffs while being able to maintain their metabolic activity and pathogenicity (Xu et al., 2008).

Acid adaptation appears to be a multiple adaptive response related to the synthesis of several regulatory systems and leading to major modifications of cytoplasmic proteins, together with modifications to membrane protein and fatty acid contents. It is essential to understand these physiological adaptations as they can induce bacterial resistance and hence the persistence of pathogens in the food chain.

2.4 Cross resistance in acid-adapted *Salmonella*

In foods or food processing environments, *Salmonella* can encounter multiple subsequent stressor treatments. Numerous studies have demonstrated that acid adaptation can ensure cross-resistance (or cross-protection) to stresses other than acid stress, such as heat, biocide damage or high osmolarity.

Heat tolerance was the first cross-protection which was demonstrated after *Salmonella* was exposed to acid. For example, a 10-fold difference in survivors was seen between acid-adapted or non-adapted populations after a 20 min challenge at 50°C (Leyer & Johnson, 1993). Heat tolerance was also shown after acid adaptation in orange or watermelon juices (Mazzotta, 2001; Sharma et al., 2005). Several acid shock proteins, including chaperon proteins, are similar to those induced by heat shock, such as GroEL or Dnak (Foster, 1993). This may be one explanation for the cross resistance observed.

Acid adaptation has also been described to enhance tolerance towards osmotic stress (Leyer & Johnson, 1993; Tosun & Gönül, 2003) but it was dependent upon the acid used for adaptation. Acetic acid adaptation provided cells with protection against both NaCl and KCl stresses, while lactic acid adaptation did not protect against osmotic stressors (Greenacre and Brocklehurst, 2006). In the same way, *S.* Enteritidis adapted to acid in marinades did not display any increased resistance to drying processes (Calicioglu et al., 2003).

Acid adaptation provoked dramatic sensitization (~10,000-fold) of *Salmonella* to halogen-based sanitizers including chlorine and iodine (Leyer & Johnson, 1997). This was explained because hypochlorous acid oxidized a higher percentage of cell surface sulfhydryl groups in acid-adapted cells than in non-adapted cells, and sulfhydryl oxidation was correlated to cell inactivation. In the same way, *Salmonella* adapted with lactic acid displays sensitivity to hydrogen peroxide which is concomitant with down-regulation of the OxyR regulon (Greenacre et al., 2006). These results could have an interesting application in maintaining microbial food safety. The weakening of *Salmonella* defenses by acid shock could constitute a potential strategy to enhance the action of halogen-based sanitizers. However, it has been shown that the long-term adaptation of *Salmonella* to propionate induces strong tolerance to the *in vitro* oxidative and nitrosative stresses that may be encountered in mammalian hosts (Calhoun & Kwon, 2010).

Salmonella serotype	Acid pretreatment conditions	Exposure to acid shock	ATR (versus non adapted cells)	Reference
S. Typhimurium	From mid-log phase cells, one cell doubling in Minimal E glucose pH 5.7 (HCl) (vs control at pH 7.0)	Challenge at pH 3.2 - 45 min	16% survival vs 0.25%	(Foster & Hall, 1990)
S. Enteritidis	From mid-exponential phase cells, Lemco broth for 3h at pH 3 (HCl) vs pH 7 (control)	Survival curves at pH 2.5 D-value is the number of minutes required to reduce the number of viable organisms by a factor of 10	D-value 1.9 min vs 0.4 min	(Humphrey et al., 1993)
S. Typhimurium	TSB 37°C 1h in aerobic conditions 100mM propionate vs NaCl (control)	TSB pH 3.0 1h	42% survival vs 0.2%	(Kwon & Ricke, 1998)
S. Typhimurium	2h at 20°C in TSBG in mid-exponential phase Acetic acid pH 5.5 vs TSBG pH 7 (control) Acetic acid pH 5.8 vs TSBG pH 7 Lactic acid pH 5.5 vs TSBG pH 7 Lactic acid pH 5.8 vs TSBG pH 7	Survival curves at pH 3.0 Kmax is the slope of the survival curve	Death rate Kmax 1 h^{-1} vs 28.5 h^{-1} Kmax 1.7 h^{-1} vs 28.5 h^{-1} Kmax 2.4 h^{-1} vs 28.5 h^{-1} Kmax 5.4 h^{-1} vs 28.5 h^{-1}	(Greenacre et al., 2003)
S. Typhimurium	90 min at 30°C in TSB without dextrose lactic acid pH 4.5 vs TSB pH 7.0 (control) lactic acid pH 5.0 vs TSB pH 7.0	Survival curves at pH 3.5 Kmax is the slope of the survival curve	Death rate Kmax 4.6 h^{-1} vs 9.4 h^{-1} Kmax 7.7 h^{-1} vs 9.4 h^{-1}	(Koutsoumanis & Sofos, 2004)
S. Typhimurium	4h at 25°C in PBS pH 5.5 (HCl)	Survival curves in commercial yoghurt at 5°C for 10 days	Reduction of the population 0.6 log vs. 1.34	(Shen et al., 2007)
S. Enteritidis	Adaptation at pH 5.0 for 2h vs control pH 7.3	Survival curves at pH 4.0 and 20°C obtained using the Weibull model $logN=logN_0-b.t^n$	b: 0.93 vs 2.96; n: 0.86 vs 0.42	(Xu et al., 2008)
S. Enteritidis	Adaptation at pH 5.0 for 2h vs control pH 7.3	Survival curves at pH 4.0 and 4°C obtained using the Weibull model $logN=logN_0-b.t^n$	b: 0.11 vs 0.75; n: 0.99 vs 0.74	(Xu et al., 2008)
S. Typhimurium	Growth until stationary phase in: BHI acetic pH 6.4 - 37°C vs non acidified BHI pH 7.4 BHI citric pH 6.4 - 37°C vs non acidified BHI pH 7.4 BHI HCl pH 6.4 - 37°C vs non acidified BHI pH 7.4 BHI citric pH 4.5 - 37°C vs non acidified BHI pH 7.4 BHI HCl pH 4.5 - 37°C vs non acidified BHI pH 7.4	Survival curve at pH 3 (HCl) The negative reciprocal of the survival curve was used for the D-value	D-value : 15.7 min vs 11.8 min D-value : 22.0 min vs 11.8 min D-value : 15.5 min vs 11.8 min D-value : 24.6 min vs 11.8 min D-value : 22.2 min vs 11.8 min	(Alvarez-Ordonez et al., 2010a)

Table 1. Examples of conditions for acid adaptation and tolerance in *Salmonella*

2.5 Virulence of acid-adapted *Salmonella*

The infectivity of *Salmonella* is based on its ability to overcome numerous lethal environments in order to reach the site of infection. These include the acid barrier of the stomach, the physical barrier of epithelial cells and various immune defenses. To survive in these acidic environments, *Salmonella* has developed elaborate systems to sense stresses and adaptive response to acid stresses. The connection between ATR and virulence is a matter of debate. On the one hand, an acid tolerant S. Enteritidis isolate was found to be more virulent in mice than an acid-sensitive isolate (Humphrey et al., 1996). ATR is known to be regulated by RpoS, which also influences the expression of specific virulence factors (Fang et al., 1992; Gahan & Hill, 1999). Mutations in the *rpoS* gene of virulent S. Typhimurium strains render them incapable of developing a full ATR and significantly reduce their virulence potential (Fang et al., 1992; Lee et al., 1995). On the other hand, one study demonstrated that low pH environments could select persistent phenotypes of *Salmonella* with increased acid tolerance, but these were less virulent (Karatzas et al., 2008a). Similarly, the long-term adaptation of *Salmonella* to propionate reduced the overall infectivity of the adapted cells by inhibiting the colonization ability of the organism (Calhoun & Kwon, 2010). Moreover, flagella motility, which is fundamental to the virulence process, was shown to be repressed at a low pH in order to allow the conservation of ATP for survival processes (Adams et al., 2001).

3. Adaptation of *Salmonella* to plant-derived antimicrobials

Among naturally occurring antimicrobials that can be used in foods, we will focus here on phyto-antimicrobials which have seen a considerable resurgence of interest during the past 10 years among both consumers and industry. Essential oils and their compounds are known to have antimicrobial properties against numerous bacteria and fungi, including *Salmonella* (Burt, 2004; Kim et al., 1995b). Most of these compounds are "generally recognized as safe" (GRAS) and have been registered by the European Commission for their use as flavoring compounds in food products.

3.1 Growth inhibition of *Salmonella* by plant-derived antimicrobials

The antibacterial activity of essential oils and their components is due to the permeabilization of the cytoplasmic membrane that leads to a loss of cellular constituents (Burt, 2004; Helander et al., 1998). Its characterization has been widely reported in laboratory media. As previously described, the mimimum inhibitory concentration (MIC) and non-inhibitory concentration (NIC) can be determined by modeling growth rate as a function of the antimicrobial concentration (Guillier et al., 2007). As for acid compounds, the growth rate curves versus concentrations have different profiles depending on the compound. For example, menthol is efficient above 0.91 mM for a MIC of 3.3 mM, while the inhibitory effect of carvacrol starts at 0.73 mM for a MIC at 0.90 mM (Guillier et al., 2007). Among 14 natural antimicrobials, phenolic compounds were shown to be the most efficient in inhibiting the growth of S. Typhimurium. The MICs of carvacrol, thymol, eugenol, geraniol, menthol, α-terpineol and *trans*-cinnamaldehyde in BHI at 37°C after 24h were respectively 0.9, 0.9, 3.0, 2.9, 3.3, 4.1 and 3.7 (Guillier et al., 2007). Similar MICs have been found in various media for thymol and carvacrol (Cosentino et al., 1999; Helander et al., 1998; Kim et al., 1995a; Olasupo et al., 2003).

Plant-derived compounds have also been shown to retain a degree of efficacy in foods, but they generally need to be used at higher concentrations to achieve the same level of inhibition. Carvacrol at 3% succeeded in eradicating *Salmonella* in fish cubes after 4 days at 4°C while citral and geraniol were less efficient (Kim et al., 1995b). Basil oil at 50 ppm reduced the number of bacteria in food from 5 to 2 log cfu/g after storage for 3 days (Rattanachaikunsopon & Phumkhachorn, 2010). The susceptibility of bacteria to the antimicrobial effect of essential oils appears to be dependent on the composition and pH of the food, and the storage temperature (Juven et al., 1994; Tassou et al., 1995). Proteins and lipids, among other food constituents, can interact with essential oils, thus limiting their activity. For example, neutralization of the antibacterial effect of thymol was demonstrated by the addition of bovine serum albumin, which probably binds thymol and thus prevents it from penetrating through the bacterial membrane (Juven et al., 1994). Moreover, the activity of thymol on *Salmonella* is greater under anaerobic conditions (Juven et al., 1994).

The concentrations used in food products are to a great extent governed by their effect on the organoleptic properties. The concentrations thus needed to inhibit bacteria often exceed the flavor threshold acceptable to consumers. In that context, multifactorial preservation is highly appropriate for these compounds. Characterization of the synergy between two compounds can be achieved using the isobologram method or by calculating the fractional inhibitory concentration (Najjar et al., 2007), but different experimental designs are necessary if the combinations involve numerous compounds. Some combinations have been shown to be highly effective against the growth of *Salmonella,* such as the use of two plant-derived compounds (cinnamaldehyde-thymol, cinnamaldehyde-carvacrol, thymol-carvacrol) (Zhou et al., 2007b), three compounds (thymol-carvacrol-citral) (Nazer et al., 2005), or plant-derived compounds associated with EDTA, acetic or citric acid (Zhou et al., 2007a).

Some of these compounds can be also used in the vapor phase. For example, allyl isothiocyanate (8.3 µL/liter of air), carvacrol (41.5 µL/liter) or cinnamaldehyde (41.5 µL/liter) were able to inactivate *Salmonella* (decrease of population > 5 log) on sliced tomatoes at 4°C in 10 days (Obaidat & Frank, 2009).

3.2 The tolerance response of *Salmonella* to plant-derived compounds

In the context of multifactor preservation, when bacteria are subjected to sub-inhibitory concentrations of antimicrobials, attention should be paid to the potential for bacterial adaptation and the induction of cross-resistance to other treatments. Little is known today about bacterial adaptation to plant-derived compounds, notably in the case of *Salmonella*. Nevertheless, the presence of thymol during the growth of *S.* Thompson induced the up- or down-regulation of many proteins (Di Pasqua et al., 2010). Different chaperon proteins were up-regulated or *de novo* synthesized, such as GroEL and Dnak which are key proteins in protecting cells against stress. Outer membrane proteins were also up-regulated in the presence of thymol (Di Pasqua et al., 2010). Moreover, the membrane fatty acid composition was markedly modified during growth in the presence of plant-derived terpenes such as carvacrol, thymol, citral or eugenol (Dubois-Brissonnet et al., 2011). The saturated fatty acids became more abundant in the cell membrane of *Salmonella* grown in the presence of these terpenes. Membrane saturation appears to be a primary response of bacteria in order to maintain both membrane integrity and functionality. Moreover, compared with control cells, the cyclization of unsaturated fatty acids (UFA) to cyclopropane fatty acids (CFA) was markedly reduced when cells entered the stationary phase. It was hypothesized that terpenes, that have log $P_{o/w}$ values of about 3, probably accumulate between the acyl chains of fatty acids, thus limiting the accessibility of *S*-adenosylmethionine to the UFA *cis*-double bond (Dubois-Brissonnet et al., 2011).

A few studies have demonstrated cross-resistance induced by plant-derived compounds. *Salmonella* exposed to sublethal concentrations of tea tree oil displayed reduced susceptibility to a range of antibiotics when compared to non-habituated cultures (McMahon et al., 2007). For example, with a MIC of mupirocin of 64 mg/L in control *S.* Enteritidis, 1024 mg/L was not efficient against adapted cells (McMahon et al., 2007). *S.* Typhimurium cells adapted to carvacrol, thymol, citral or eugenol have all displayed higher tolerance to the bactericidal activity of two disinfectants used in industrial and medical environments, peracetic acid and didecyl dimethyl ammonium bromide (Dubois-Brissonnet et al., 2011). Because these two antimicrobials have different modes of action, it was hypothesized that this induced tolerance could be a general response to the stress induced by slow growth rates and by the reduction in membrane permeability caused by membrane saturation and terpene intercalation (Dubois-Brissonnet et al., 2011).

4. *Salmonella* adaptation to disinfectants – The biofilm implication

Disinfectants are chemical agents used to decontaminate inanimate surfaces. Several groups of disinfectants are regularly used in food processing environments; e.g. halogen-realizing agents, aldehydes, peroxygens or quaternary ammonium compounds (McDonnell & Russell, 1999). The mode of action of these disinfectants has been described extensively in numerous reviews (McDonnell & Russell, 1999; Russell, 2003). Unlike antibiotics, they have a broad spectrum of antimicrobial activity and generally act on several targets in microbial cells, such as outer and cytoplasmic membranes, functional and structural proteins, DNA, RNA and other cytosolic constituents (Russell, 2003).

4.1 *Salmonella* tolerance response to disinfectants

As disinfectants are intended to inactivate rapidly the biocontamination of surfaces, bacterial resistance to a disinfectant is generally evaluated by determining the minimum bactericidal concentration. The MBCs of *Salmonella* to three widely used disinfectants (peracetic acid, benzalkonium chloride and ortho-phthalaldehyde) were evaluated comparative to those of seven other bacterial species (Bridier et al., 2011a). The MBCs, defined here as the concentrations enabling a 5-log reduction in the initial population within 5 minutes at 20°C, were 8.2, 42 and 175 mg/L for the three disinfectants, respectively. Compared with other species, *Salmonella* did not display a remarkable resistance to these three disinfectants. There were only slight intra-specie variations among the ten different *Salmonella* strains, whatever their serotype (Bridier et al., 2011a).

Nevertheless, *Salmonella* is frequently isolated from food-processing environments. For example, *Salmonella* was isolated in 5.3% of 3485 samples of pork and 13.8% of 3573 environmental samples from seven slaughterhouses in four European countries (Hald et al., 2003). In Canada, 37.5% of the 1295 samples collected from 65 abattoirs were positive for *Salmonella* (Bohaychuk et al., 2009). The link between a persistence of *Salmonella* in the food-processing environment and its adaptation to the disinfectants used in that environment has been discussed. On the one hand, some authors have demonstrated that there was no obvious association between the susceptibility of isolates to disinfectants, their tendencies to persist and the previous use of biocides (Gradel et al., 2005). A few serotypes isolated from Danish broiler houses tended to have higher MICs to some disinfectants, but not necessarily those they had encountered previously (Gradel et al., 2005). Similarly, some Norwegian isolates found to be persistent in fish feed factories were no more resistant to nine disinfectants used in these than isolates from other sources (Moretro et al., 2003). On the other hand, *Salmonella* is known to be able to adapt itself to some disinfectants and to demonstrate increased resistance to disinfection procedures. For example, the benzalkonium chloride (BKC) MIC of *S.* Virchow was shown to rise from 4 to 256 µg/mL after repeated exposure to sublethal concentrations (Braoudaki & Hilton, 2004). This strain was also able to adapt to chlorhexidine. Moreover, the benzalkonium adapted-strain displayed elevated tolerance to both BKC and chlorhexidine; however, the chlorhexidine-adapted strain did not display reciprocal cross-resistance to benzalkonium chloride, suggesting specific resistance mechanisms (Braoudaki & Hilton, 2004). Growth in the presence of increasing sub-inhibitory concentrations of tri-sodium phosphate or acidified sodium chlorite also caused a significant increase in their MICs for *Salmonella* (Alonso-Hernando et al., 2009). Furthermore, 7-day passages of *S.* Typhimurium in sub-inhibitory concentrations of an ammonium quaternary compound containing formaldehyde and glutaraldehyde (AQCFG) selected variants with reduced susceptibility to antibiotics (Karatzas et al., 2007).

Cross resistance to other environmental stresses was also demonstrated following disinfectant adaptation. Significant increase in thermotolerance and resistance to high pH occurred after 1h shock with 1.5% tri-sodium phosphate (TSP) (Sampathkumar et al., 2004). But sensitivity to acid and hydrogen peroxide concomitantly increased.

The impact of disinfectant adaptation on virulence is dependent on the type of biocide and conditions of stress. AQCFG-adapted variants displayed an altered expression of several virulence proteins and reduced invasiveness in an epithelial cell line (Karatzas et al., 2008b). Conversely, *S.* Typhimurium LT2 retained its adhesive and invasive abilities after treatment with 5 mg/L peracetic acid for 1h in sewage effluent (Jolivet-Gougeon et al., 2003).

Like for many other stresses, differential protein expression seems concomitant to increased tolerance. In AQCFG-variants, it has been demonstrated higher levels of the different proteins that protect against stressors such as oxidants or peroxides (Karatzas et al., 2008b). Following chlorine shock, *Salmonella* genes that were associated with stress response, biofilm formation or energy metabolism were also over-expressed (>1.5-fold) (Wang et al., 2010) and hydrogen peroxide treatment induced the synthesis of 30 proteins in *Salmonella,* including that of Dnak, a chaperon protein (Morgan et al., 1986). Moreover, the resistance of BKC-adapted *Salmonella* is related to the up-regulation of an active efflux system (Braoudaki & Hilton, 2005). Similarly, in pre-mentioned variants, bacterial adaptation to disinfectants coincides with the up-regulation of the AcrAB efflux pump, which is responsible for producing the multiple-antibiotic-resistance *mar* strains that are resistant to many agents (Karatzas et al., 2007).

In addition, membrane composition can sometimes be altered with disinfectant adaptation. *S.* Enteritidis grown in the presence of three sanitizers, including a chlorinated product, an alkaline cleaner and a phenolic solution, was shown to increase its short-chain polysaccharide fractions of the LPS (Venter et al., 2006). A reduction in cell hydrophobicity was induced following the adaptation of *S.* Enteritidis to BKC at sub-inhibitory concentrations, although no change to the LPS or outer membrane composition was noticed (Braoudaki & Hilton, 2005). When *Salmonella* cells were exposed to 1.5% TSP for 1 h, significant changes were seen to affect the membrane fatty acid composition: the saturated and cyclic to unsaturated fatty acid ratio increases which leads to a increase in membrane saturation (Sampathkumar et al., 2004). But modifications to membrane fluidity were not related with the induction of resistance following growth in increasing sub-inhibitory concentrations of tri-sodium phosphate (TSP) (Alonso-Hernando et al., 2010).

Because the mechanisms of *Salmonella* adaptation to disinfectants are not fully understood, it is wise to continue the widely accepted practice of rotating the use of disinfectants in the food industry to prevent the development of adaptation and increased resistance.

4.2 Implication of biofilms in the tolerance response of *Salmonella* to disinfectants

The persistence of *Salmonella* in food processing environments is often related to their survival on the surface of equipment. For example, an *S.* Enteritidis strain isolated from an egg conveyor belt was found to be a source of persistent infection in poultry (Stocki et al., 2007). Similarly, *Salmonella* was able to persist in food bowls that had contained raw meat contaminated by this pathogen (Weese & Rousseau, 2006). The survival of microorganisms in food-processing environments is frequently linked to the presence of three-dimensional biofilm structures on surfaces. *Salmonella* produces a biofilm matrix that is mainly composed of fimbriae (curli) and cellulose (Solomon et al., 2005). A study of 111 *Salmonella* strains isolated in Norwegian feed and fish meal factories demonstrated that persistent strains were those that could produce more biofilm than presumably non-persisting strains (Vestby et al., 2009). Images of *Salmonella* biofilms (Figure 3) were acquired using scanning electron microscopy at the MIMA2 microscopy platform (http://voxel.jouy.inra.fr/mima2).

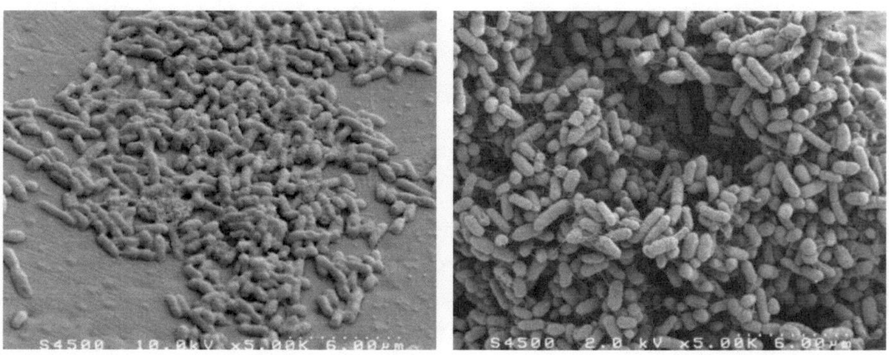

Fig. 3. Images of *Salmonella* biofilms obtained by scanning electron microscopy

Like many other biofilms, *Salmonella* biofilms display specific properties that include increased resistance to biocide treatment (Wong et al., 2010). Reductions in surface-attached

Salmonella using 256 ppm of sodium hypochlorite and BKC were respectively decreased 2.1 and 3-fold compared to the planktonic population (Riazi & Matthews, 2011). Sodium hypochlorite was shown to be more efficient than BKC and hydrogen peroxide against *Salmonella* biofilms formed in the Calgary Biofilm Device (Rodrigues et al., 2011). *S.* Typhimurium is more resistant to chlorine treatments when associated with *Pseudomonas fluorescens* in a mixed biofilm (Leriche & Carpentier, 1995).

Rather than a true resistance, biofilm insusceptibility is sometimes referred to as a tolerance because it is mainly induced by physiological adaptation to the biofilm mode of life (Russell, 1999). Biofilm resistance is multifactorial, resulting from the addition of different mechanisms such as diffusion and/or reaction problems affecting the sanitizers in the structure, the appearance of resistant biofilm-specific phenotypes (persister cells), of physiological and genetic heterogeneity, and adaptation to sanitizers (Bridier et al., 2011b). In deeper regions of the three-dimensional structures of biofilms, *Salmonella* may be protected against biocide activity because of the limited reaction-diffusion penetration of antimicrobial agents (Figure 4). Only sub-lethal concentrations of disinfectants can reach the bacteria which may thus develop adaptation mechanisms.

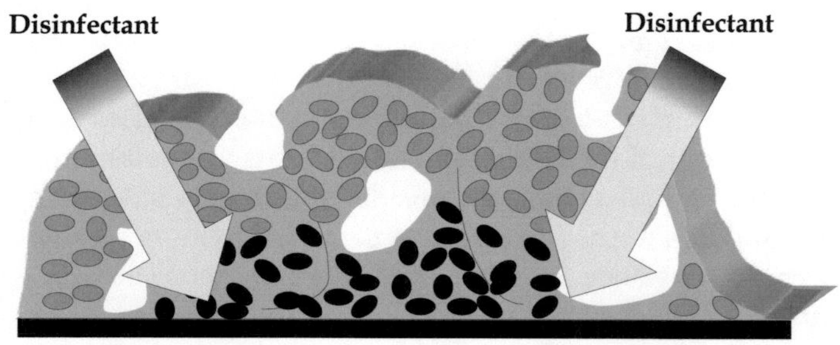

Fig. 4. Limited penetration of antimicrobial agents within the biofilm architecture due to diffusion-reaction problems (black cells can survive and adapt themselves to sub-lethal concentrations of disinfectants)

A few studies have described the adaptation of biofilm cells to disinfectants. One early study showed that when *S.* Typhimurium biofilm was disinfected daily, the proportion of viable but nonculturable cells increased in a 4-day biofilm (Leriche & Carpentier, 1995). Chlorine consumption of such biofilm was increased, suggesting that adaptation to chlorine stress induces a hyper-production of exopolymeric substances that can protect the viable cells. *Salmonella* biofilm cells were also reported to display a greater adaptation than their planktonic counterparts to BCK after continuous exposure to 1 µg/mL of this disinfectant (Mangalappalli-Illathu & Korber, 2006). Specific proteins involved in energy metabolism, protein biosynthesis, nutrient binding, cold shock and detoxification were up-regulated. Conversely, proteins involved in proteolysis, cell envelope formation, universal stress, heat shock response (Dnak) and broad regulatory functions (Hns) were down-regulated following adaptation (Mangalappalli-Illathu & Korber, 2006).

However, surface-attached *Salmonella* exposed sequentially to 100 ppm chlorhexidine digluconate remained susceptible to the action of the sanitizer. The bacteria were not able to adapt neither develop induced resistance (Riazi & Matthews, 2011). During this experiment, the disinfectant is applied at a much higher concentration than that used by Mangalappali-

Illathu et al., and it can more easily reach the surface-attached cells which are not embedded in an exopolymeric matrix. This therefore can explain why, in this case, the attached cells were not able to adapt and develop increased resistance.

Very little is known about cross-resistance and virulence abilities of biofilm cells adapted to disinfectant. A recent study has shown that following a disinfection treatment, surviving biofilm *Salmonella* cells demonstrated significantly up-regulated virulence genes (Rodrigues et al., 2011).

Therefore, in order to guarantee microbial food safety, cleaning procedures must be applied regularly in order to prevent biofilm formation, and the concentrations used should be high enough to eradicate surface-attached bacteria. Under these conditions, biofilm formation and adaptation to disinfectants should be limited.

5. Conclusion

Because antimicrobials are currently used to ensure microbiological food safety, the potential for the development of bacterial adaptation and induced tolerance to antimicrobial stresses must be taken into account. Although the mechanisms of acid adaptation are now well understood, knowledge on the adaptation of *Salmonella* to naturally occurring compounds and disinfectants needs to be improved. Research must be carried out to monitor the evolution of stress-tolerant pathogens in foods and to generate appropriate methods to detect and control them. Studies should focus on food matrix systems or food-processing plants because these should be considered as highly stressful environments. The ultimate purpose should be to predict and control the behavior of *Salmonella* in terms of its stress tolerance, cross resistance to other stresses, persistence in the environment and virulence in the host.

6. Acknowledgments

I thank Dr. R. Briandet (INRA) for helpful discussions and Dr. M. Naïtali (AgroParisTech) for critical reading of the manuscript.

7. References

Abee T, Krockel L, Hill C. (1995). Bacteriocins: modes of action and potentials in food preservation and control of food poisoning. *International Journal of Food Microbiology*, Vol.28, pp.169-185, 0168-1605

Adams P, Fowler R, Kinsella N, Howell G, Farris M, Coote P, O'Connor CD. (2001). Proteomic detection of PhoPQ- and acid-mediated repression of *Salmonella* motility. *Proteomics*, Vol.1, pp.597-607, 1615-9853

Alonso-Hernando A, Alonso-Calleja C, Capita R. (2010). Effects of exposure to poultry chemical decontaminants on the membrane fluidity of *Listeria monocytogenes* and *Salmonella enterica* strains. *International Journal of Food Microbiology*, Vol.137, pp.130-136, 0168-1605

Alonso-Hernando A, Capita R, Prieto M, Alonso-Calleja C. (2009). Adaptation and cross-adaptation of *Listeria monocytogenes* and *Salmonella enterica* to poultry decontaminants. *J Microbiol*, Vol.47, pp.142-146, 1225-8873

Alvarez-Ordonez A, Fernandez A, Bernardo A, Lopez M. (2009). Comparison of acids on the induction of an Acid Tolerance Response in *Salmonella typhimurium*, consequences for food safety. *Meat Sci*, Vol.81, pp.65-70, 0309-1740

Alvarez-Ordonez A, Fernandez A, Bernardo A, Lopez M. (2010a). Acid tolerance in *Salmonella* Typhimurium induced by culturing in the presence of organic acids at different growth temperatures. *Food Microbiol*, Vol.27, pp.44-49, 0740-0020

Alvarez-Ordonez A, Fernandez A, Bernardo A, Lopez M. (2010b). Arginine and lysine decarboxylases and the Acid Tolerance Response of *Salmonella* Typhimurium. *International Journal of Food Microbiology*, Vol.136, pp.278-282, 0168-1605

Alvarez-Ordonez A, Fernandez A, Lopez M, Arenas R,B ernardo A. (2008). Modifications in membrane fatty acid composition of *Salmonella* Typhimurium in response to growth conditions and their effect on heat resistance. *International Journal of Food Microbiology*, Vol.123, pp.212-219, 0168-1605

Anonymous. 1998. Directive 98/8/CE of the european parliament and of the council of 16 February 1998 concerning the placing of biocidal products on the market. In: Official Journal of the European Communities.

Anonymous. 2004. Morbidité et mortalité dues aux maladies infectieuses d'origine alimentaire en France. In: Rapport Institut de Veille Sanitaire -Agence Française de Sécurité Sanitaire des Aliments.

Anonymous. 2006. Regulation (EC) N° 1907/2006 of the european parliament and of the council of 18 december 2006 concerning the registration, evalution, authorisation and restriction of chemicals (REACH). In: Official Journal of the European Union.

Anonymous. 2009. Proposal for a regulation of the european parliament and of the council concerning the placing on the market and use of biocidal products. In: Commission of the European Communities.

Arvizu-Medrano SM, Escartin EF. (2005). Effect of acid shock with hydrochloric, citric, and lactic acids on the survival and growth of *Salmonella* Typhi and *Salmonella* Typhimurium in acidified media. *Journal of Food Protection*, Vol.68, pp.2047-2053, 0362-028X

Baik HS, Bearson S, Dunbar S, Foster JW. (1996). The acid tolerance response of *Salmonella typhimurium* provides protection against organic acids. *Microbiology*, Vol.142, pp.3195-3200,

Bearson S, Bearson B, Foster JW. (1997). Acid stress responses in enterobacteria. *FEMS Microbiol Lett*, Vol.147, pp.173-180,

Bohaychuk VM, Checkley SL, Gensler GE, Barrios PR. (2009). Microbiological baseline study of poultry slaughtered in provincially inspected abattoirs in Alberta, Canada. *Can Vet J-Rev Vet Can*, Vol.50, pp.173-178, 0008-5286

Braoudaki M, Hilton AC. (2005). Mechanisms of resistance in *Salmonella enterica* adapted to erythromycin, benzalkonium chloride and triclosan. *Int J Antimicrob Agents*, Vol.25, pp.31-37, 0924-8579

Braoudaki M, Hilton C. (2004). Adaptive resistance to biocides in *Salmonella enterica* and *Escherichia coli* 0157 and cross-resistance to antimicrobial agents. *Journal of Clinical Microbiology*, Vol.42, pp.73-78,

Bridier A, Briandet R, Thomas V, Dubois-Brissonnet F. (2011a). Comparative biocidal activity of peracetic acid, benzalkonium chloride and *ortho*- phthalaldehyde on 77 bacterial strains. *Journal of Hospital Infection*, Vol.78, pp.208-213,

Bridier A, Briandet R, Thomas V, Dubois-Brissonnet F. (2011b). Resistance of bacterial biofilms to disinfectants: a review. *Biofouling*, Vol.27, pp.1017-1032,

Brown JL, Ross T, McMeekin TA, Nichols PD. (1997). Acid habituation of *Escherichia coli* and the potential role of cyclopropane fatty acids in low pH tolerance. *International Journal of Food Microbiology*, Vol.37, pp.163-173,

Burt S. (2004). Essential oils: their antibacterial properties and potential applications in foods - a review. *International Journal of Food Microbiology*, Vol.94, pp.223-253,

Calhoun LN, Kwon YM. (2010). The effect of long-term propionate adaptation on the stress resistance of *Salmonella* Enteritidis. *J Appl Microbiol*, Vol.109, pp.1294-1300, 1364-5072

Calhoun LN, Liyanage R, Lay JO, Kwon YM. (2010). Proteomic analysis of *Salmonella enterica* serovar Enteritidis following propionate adaptation. *BMC Microbiol*, Vol.10, pp.11, 1471-2180

Calicioglu M, Sofos JN, Samelis J, Kendall PA, Smith GC. (2003). Effect of acid adaptation on inactivation of *Salmonella* during drying and storage of beef jerky treated with marinades. *International Journal of Food Microbiology*, Vol.89, pp.51-65, 0168-1605

Chang YY, Cronan JE. (1999). Membrane cyclopropane fatty acid content is a major factor in acid resistance of *Escherichia coli*. *Molecular Microbiology*, Vol.33, pp.249-259, 0950-382X

Cosentino S, Tuberoso CIG, Pisano B, Satta M, Mascia V, Arzedi E, Palmas F. (1999). In-vitro antimicrobial activity and chemical composition of Sardinian *Thymus* essential oils. *Letters in Applied Microbiology*, Vol.29, pp.130-135,

Costerton J, Lewandowski Z, Caldwell D, Korber D, Lappin-Scott H. (1995). Microbial biofilms. *Annu Rev Microbiol*, Vol.49, pp.711-745,

de Jonge R, Ritmeester WS, van Leusden FM. (2003). Adaptive responses of *Salmonella enterica* serovar Typhimurium DT104 and other *S.* Typhimurium strains and *Escherichia coli* O157 to low pH environments. *J Appl Microbiol*, Vol.94, pp.625-632, 1364-5072

Di Pasqua R, Mamone G, Ferranti P, Ercolini D, Mauriello G. (2010). Changes in the proteome of *Salmonella enterica* serovar Thompson as stress adaptation to sublethal concentrations of thymol. *Proteomics*, Vol.10, pp.1040-1049, 1615-9853

Dodd CER, Aldsworth TG. (2002). The importance of RpoS in the survival of bacteria through food processing. *International Journal of Food Microbiology*, Vol.74, pp.189-194, 0168-1605

Doores S. (2005). Organic acids, In: Antimicrobials in food, Boca Raton, CRC Taylor & Francis, p. 91-142,

Dubois-Brissonnet F, Naitali M, Maf AA, Briandet R. (2011). Induction of fatty acid composition modifications and tolerance to biocides in *Salmonella enterica* serovar Typhimurium by plant-derived terpenes. *Applied and Environmental Microbiology*, Vol.77, pp.906-910,

Dziezak JD. (1986). Antioxidants and antimicrobial agents. *Food technology*, Vol.40, pp.94-111,

Fang FC, Libby SJ, Buchmeier NA, Loewen PC, Switala J, Harwood J, Guiney DG. (1992). The Alternative sigma-factor Katf (Rpos) regulates *Salmonella* Virulence. *Proc Natl Acad Sci U S A*, Vol.89, pp.11978-11982, 0027-8424

Foster JW. (1991). *Salmonella* acid shock proteins are required for the adaptive acid tolerance response. *Journal of Bacteriology*, Vol.173, pp.6896-6902, 0021-9193

Foster JW. (1993). The acid tolerance response of *Salmonella* Typhimurium involves transient synthesis of key acid shock proteins. *Journal of Bacteriology*, Vol.175, pp.1981-1987, 0021-9193

Foster JW. (1999). When protons attack: microbial strategies of acid adaptation. *Curr Opin Microbiol*, Vol.2, pp.170-174, 1369-5274

Foster JW, Hall HK. (1990). Adaptive acidification tolerance response of *Salmonella typhimurium*. *Journal of Bacteriology*, Vol.172, pp.771-778,

Gahan CGM, Hill C. (1999). The relationship between acid stress responses and virulence in *Salmonella typhimurium* and *Listeria monocytogenes*. *International Journal of Food Microbiology*, Vol.50, pp.93-100,

Gradel KO, Randall L, Sayers AR, Davies RH. (2005). Possible associations between *Salmonella* persistence in poultry houses and resistance to commonly used disinfectants and a putative role of *mar*. *Veterinary Microbiology*, Vol.107, pp.127-138,

Greenacre EJ, Brocklehurst TF, Waspe CR, Wilson DR, Wilson PDG. (2003). *Salmonella enterica* serovar Typhimurium and *Listeria monocytogenes* acid tolerance response induced by organic acids at 20 degrees C: optimization and modeling. *Applied and Environmental Microbiology*, Vol.69, pp.3945-3951, 0099-2240

Greenacre EJ, Lucchini S, Hinton JCD, Brocklehurst TF. (2006). The lactic acid-induced acid tolerance response in *Salmonella enterica* serovar typhimurium induces sensitivity to hydrogen peroxide. *Applied and Environmental Microbiology*, Vol.72, pp.5623-5625, 0099-2240

Guillier L, Nazer A, Dubois-Brissonnet F. (2007). Growth response of *Salmonella* Typhimurium in presence of natural and synthetic antimicrobials: estimation of MICs from three different models. *Journal of Food Protection*, Vol.70, pp.2243-2250,

Hald T, Wingstrand A, Swanenburg M, von Altrock A, Thorberg BM. (2003). The occurrence and epidemiology of *Salmonella* in European pig slaughterhouses. *Epidemiol Infect*, Vol.131, pp.1187-1203, 0950-2688

Helander IM, Alakomi H-L, Latva-Kala K, Mattila-Sandholm T, Pol IE, Smid EJ, Morris LGM,Von Wright A. (1998). Characterization of the action of selected essential oil components on gram-negative bacteria. *J Agric Food Chem*, Vol.46, pp.3590-3595,

Hoiby N, Bjarnsholt T, Givskov M, Molin S, Ciofu O. (2010). Antibiotic resistance of bacterial biofilms. *Int J Antimicrob Agents*, Vol.35, pp.322-332, 0924-8579

Huhtanen CN. (1975). Use of pH gradient plates for increasing acid tolerance of *Salmonellae*. *Applied Microbiology*, Vol.29, pp.309-312, 0003-6919

Humphrey TJ, Richardson NP, Statton KM, Rowbury RJ. (1993). Acid habituation in *Salmonella enteritidis* PT4: impact of inhibition of protein synthesis. *Letters in Applied Microbiology*, Vol.16, pp.228-230,

Humphrey TJ, Williams A, McAlpine K, Lever MS, GuardPetter J, Cox JM. (1996). Isolates of *Salmonella enterica* Enteritidis PT4 with enhanced heat and acid tolerance are more virulent in mice and more invasive in chickens. *Epidemiol Infect*, Vol.117, pp.79-88, 0950-2688

Jolivet-Gougeon A, Sauvager F, Arturo-Schaan M, Bonnaure-Mallet M, Cormier M. (2003). Influence of peracetic acid on adhesion/invasion of *Salmonella enterica* serotype Typhimurium LT2. *Cell Biol Toxicol*, Vol.19, pp.83-93, 0742-2091

Juven BJ, Kanner J, Schved F, Weisslowicz H. (1994). Factors that interact with the antibacterial action of thyme essential oil and its active constituents. *J Appl Bacteriol*, Vol.76, pp.626-631, 0021-8847

Karatzas KAG, Hocking PM, Jorgensen F, Mattick K, Leach S, Humphrey TJ. (2008a). Effects of repeated cycles of acid challenge and growth on the phenotype and virulence of *Salmonella enterica*. *J Appl Microbiol*, Vol.105, pp.1640-1648, 1364-5072

Karatzas KAG, Randall LP, Webber M, Piddock LJV, Humphrey TJ, Woodward MJ, Coldham NG. (2008b). Phenotypic and proteomic characterization of multiply antibiotic-resistant variants of *Salmonella* enterica serovar Typhimurium selected following exposure to disinfectants. *Applied and Environmental Microbiology*, Vol.74, pp.1508-1516, 0099-2240

Karatzas KAG, Webber MA, Jorgensen F, Woodward MJ, Piddock LJV, Humphrey TJ. (2007). Prolonged treatment of *Salmonella enterica* serovar Typhimurium with commercial disinfectants selects for multiple antibiotic resistance, increased efflux and reduced invasiveness. *J Antimicrob Chemother*, Vol.60, pp.947-955, 0305-7453

Kim BH, Kim S, Kim HG, Lee J, Lee IS, Park YK. (2005). The formation of cyclopropane fatty acids in *Salmonella enterica* serovar Typhimurium. *Microbiology-(UK)*, Vol.151, pp.209-218, 1350-0872

Kim J, Marshall MR, Wei C-I. (1995a). Antibacterial activity of some essential oil components against five foodborne pathogens. *Journal of Agricultural and Food Chemistry*, Vol.43, pp.2839-2845,

Kim JM, Marshall MR, Cornell JA, Preston JF, Wei CI. (1995b). Antibacterial activity of carvacrol, citral, and geraniol against *Salmonella* Typhimurium in culture medium and on fish cubes. *Journal of Food Science*, Vol.60, pp.1364-1374,

Koutsoumanis KP, Sofos JN. (2004). Comparative acid stress response of *Listeria monocytogenes, Escherichia coli* O157: H7 and *Salmonella* Typhimurium after habituation at different pH conditions. *Letters in Applied Microbiology*, Vol.38, pp.321-326, 0266-8254

Kwon YM, Ricke SC. (1998). Induction of acid resistance of *Salmonella typhimurium* by exposure to short-chain fatty acids. *Applied and Environmental Microbiology*, Vol.64, pp.3458-3463,

Lambert RJW, Pearson J. (2000). Susceptibility testing : accurate and reproducible minimum inhibitory concentration (MIC) and non-inhibitory concentration (NIC) values. *J Appl Microbiol*, Vol.88, pp.784-790,

Lee IS, Lin JS, Hall HK, Bearson B, Foster JW. (1995). The stationary-phase sigma-factor sigma(S) (Rpos) is required for a sustained acid tolerance response in virulent *Salmonella* Typhimurium. *Molecular Microbiology*, Vol.17, pp.155-167, 0950-382X

Lee IS, Slonczewski JL, Foster JW. (1994). A low pH inducible, stationary-phase acid tolerance response in *Salmonella* Typhimurium. *Journal of Bacteriology*, Vol.176, pp.1422-1426, 0021-9193

Leistner L. (1995). Food preservation by hurdle technology. *Trends in Food Science and Technology*, Vol.6, pp.41-46,

Leriche V, Carpentier B. (1995). Viable but nonculturable *Salmonella typhimurium* in single- and binary-species biofilms in response to chlorine treatment. *Journal of Food Protection*, Vol.58, pp.1186-1191,

Leyer GJ, Johnson EA. (1992). Acid adaptation promotes survival of *Salmonella* spp in cheese. *Applied and Environmental Microbiology*, Vol.58, pp.2075-2080, 0099-2240

Leyer GJ, Johnson EA. (1993). Acid adaptation induces cross-protection against environmental stresses in *Salmonella typhimurium*. *Applied and Environmental Microbiology*, Vol.59, pp.1842-1847,

Leyer GJ, Johnson EA. (1997). Acid adaptation sensitizes *Salmonella typhimurium* to hypochlorous acid. *Applied and Environmental Microbiology*, Vol.63, pp.461-467,

Lin JS, Lee IS, Frey J, Slonczewski JL, Foster JW. (1995). Comparative analysis of extreme acid survival in *Salmonella* Typhimurium, *Shigella flexneri*, and *Escherichia coli*. *Journal of Bacteriology*, Vol.177, pp.4097-4104, 0021-9193

Mackey BM, Derrick CM. (1986). Elevation of the heat resistance of *Salmonella typhimurium* by sublethal heat shock. *J Appl Bacteriol*, Vol.61, pp.389-393,

Mangalappalli-Illathu AK, Korber DR. (2006). Adaptative resistance and differential protein expression of *Salmonella enterica* serovar Enteritidis biofilms exposed to benzalkonium chloride. *Antimicrobial Agents and Chemotherapy*, Vol.50, pp.3588-3596,

Mazzotta AS. (2001). Thermal inactivation of stationary-phase and acid-adapted *Escherichia coli* O157: H7, *Salmonella*, and *Listeria monocytogenes* in fruit juices. *Journal of Food Protection*, Vol.64, pp.315-320, 0362-028X

McDonnell G, Russell AD. (1999). Antiseptics and disinfectants : activity, action, and resistance. *Clinical Microbiology Reviews*, Vol.12, pp.147-179,

McMahon MAS, Blair IS, Moore JE, McDowell DA. (2007). Habituation to sub-lethal concentrations of tea tree oil (Melaleuca alternifolia) is associated with reduced susceptibility to antibiotics in human pathogens. *J Antimicrob Chemother*, Vol.59, pp.125-127, 0305-7453

Mead PS, Slutsker L, Dietz V, McCaig LF, Bresee JS, Shapiro C, Griffin PM, Tauxe RV. (1999). Food-related illness and death in the United States. *Emerging Infectious Diseases*, Vol.5, pp.609-625,

Mescle JF, Zucca J. (1996). Les facteurs du développement, In: Microbiologie alimentaire - Tome 1 Aspect microbiologique de la sécurité et de la qualité des aliments, Paris, Tec et Doc Lavoisier,

Moretro T, Midtgaard ES, Nesse LL, Langsrud S. (2003). Susceptibility of *Salmonella* isolated from fish feed factories to disinfectants and air-drying at surfaces. *Veterinary Microbiology*, Vol.94, pp.207-217, 0378-1135

Morgan RW, Christman MF, Jacobson FS, Storz G, Ames BN. (1986). Hydrogen peroxide inducible proteins in *Salmonella* Typhimurium overlap with heat shock and other stress proteins. *Proc Natl Acad Sci U S A*, Vol.83, pp.8059-8063, 0027-8424

Morin N, Lanneluc I, Connil N, Cottenceau M, Pons AM, Sable S. (2011). Mechanism of bactericidal activity of microcin L in *Escherichia coli* and *Salmonella enterica*. *Antimicrobial Agents and Chemotherapy*, Vol.55, pp.997-1007, 0066-4804

Naidu AS. (2000). Natural food antimicrobial systems, Boca Raton, CRC Press LLC,

Najjar MB, Kashtanov D, Chikindas ML. (2007). e-poly-l-lysine and nisin A act synergistically against Gram-positive food-borne pathogens *Bacillus cereus* and *Listeria monocytogenes*. *Letters in Applied Microbiology*, Vol.45, pp.13-18,

Nazer A, Kobilinsky A, Tholozan JL, Dubois-Brissonnet F. (2005). Combinations of food antimicrobials at low levels to inhibit the growth of *Salmonella* sv.Typhimurium: a synergistic effect ? *Food Microbiol*, Vol.22, pp.391-398,

Obaidat MM, Frank JF. (2009). Inactivation of *Salmonella* and *Escherichia coli* O157:H7 on sliced and whole tomatoes by allyl isothiocyanate, carvacrol, and cinnamaldehyde in vapor phase. *Journal of Food Protection*, Vol.72, pp.315-324, 0362-028X

Olasupo NA, Fitzgerald DJ, Gasson MJ, Narbad A. (2003). Activity of natural antimicrobial compounds against *Escherichia coli* and *Salmonella* enterica serovar Typhimurium. *Letters in Applied Microbiology*, Vol.37, pp.448-451,

Rattanachaikunsopon P, Phumkhachorn P. (2010). Antimicrobial activity of basil (*Ocimum basilicum)* oil against *Salmonella* Enteritidis in vitro and in Food. *Biosci Biotechnol Biochem*, Vol.74, pp.1200-1204, 0916-8451

Riazi S, Matthews KR. (2011). Failure of foodborne pathogens to develop resistance to sanitizers following repeated exposure to common sanitizers. *Int Biodeterior Biodegrad*, Vol.65, pp.374-378, 0964-8305

Rodrigues D, Cerca N, Teixeira P, Oliveira R, Ceri H, Azeredo J. (2011). *Listeria monocytogenes* and *Salmonella enterica* Enteritidis biofilms susceptibility to different disinfectants and stress response and virulence gene expression of surviving cells. *Microb Drug Resist*, Vol.17, pp.181-189, 1076-6294

Roller S. (2003). Natural antimicrobials for minimal processing of foods, Cambridge, Woodhead Publishing Limited,

Russell AD. (1999). Bacterial resistance to disinfectants: present knowledge and future problems. *Journal of Hospital Infection*, Vol.43, pp.S57-S68, 0195-6701

Russell AD. (2003). Similarities and differences in the responses of microorganisms to biocides. *J Antimicrob Chemother*, Vol.52, pp.750-763, 0305-7453

Sampathkumar B, Khachatourians GG, Korber DR. (2004). Treatment of *Salmonella enterica* serovar Enteritidis with a sublethal concentration of trisodium phosphate or alkaline pH induces thermotolerance. *Applied and Environmental Microbiology*, Vol.70, pp.4613-4620, 0099-2240

Schved F, Henis Y, Juven BJ. (1994). Response of spheroplasts and chelator permeabilized cells of Gram-negative bacteria to the action of the bacteriocins pediocin Sj-1 and nisin. *International Journal of Food Microbiology*, Vol.21, pp.305-314, 0168-1605

Sharma M, Adler BB, Harrison MD, Beuchat LR. (2005). Thermal tolerance of acid-adapted and unadapted *Salmonella, Escherichia coli* O157 : H7, and *Listeria monocytogenes* in cantaloupe juice and watermelon juice. *Letters in Applied Microbiology*, Vol.41, pp.448-453, 0266-8254

Shen HW, Yu RC, Chou CC. (2007). Acid adaptation affects the viability of *Salmonella* Typhimurium during the lactic fermentation of skim milk and product storage. *International Journal of Food Microbiology*, Vol.114, pp.380-385, 0168-1605

Solomon EB, Niemira BA, Sapers GM, Annous BA. (2005). Biofilrn formation, cellulose production, and curli biosynthesis by *Salmonella* originating from produce, animal, and clinical sources. *Journal of Food Protection*, Vol.68, pp.906-912, 0362-028X

Stocki SL, Annett CB, Sibley CD, McLaws M, Checkley SL, Singh N, Surette MG, White AP. (2007). Persistence of *Salmonella* on egg conveyor belts is dependent on the belt type but not on the rdar morphotype. *Poult Sci*, Vol.86, pp.2375-2383, 0032-5791

Tassou CC, Drosinos EH, Nychas GJE. (1995). Effects of essential oil from mint (*Mentha piperita*) on *Salmonella* Enteritidis and *Listeria monocytogenes* in model food systems at 4 degrees and 10 degrees C. *J Appl Bacteriol*, Vol.78, pp.593-600, 0021-8847

Tosun H, Gönül SA. (2003). Acid adaption protects *Salmonella* Typhimurium from environmental stresses. *Turkish Journal of Biology*, Vol.27, pp.31-36,

Venter P,Abraham M,Lues JFR,Ivanov I. (2006). Influence of commercial sanitizers on lipopolysaccharide production by *Salmonella* Enteritidis ATCC 13076. *Journal of Food Protection*, Vol.69, pp.2889-2895, 0362-028X

Vestby LK, Moretro T, Langsrud S, Heir E, Nesse LL. (2009). Biofilm forming abilities of *Salmonella* are correlated with persistence in fish meal- and feed factories. *BMC Vet Res*, Vol.5, pp.6, 1746-6148

Wang SY, Phillippy AM, Deng KP, Rui XQ, Li ZX, Tortorello ML, hang W. (2010). Transcriptomic responses of *Salmonella enterica* serovars Enteritidis and Typhimurium to chlorine-based oxidative stress. *Applied and Environmental Microbiology*, Vol.76, pp.5013-5024, 0099-2240

Weese JS, Rousseau J. (2006). Survival of *Salmonella* Copenhagen in food bowls following contamination with experimentally inoculated raw meat: effects of time, cleaning, and disinfection. *Can Vet J-Rev Vet Can*, Vol.47, pp.887-889, 0008-5286

Wesche AM, Gurtler JB, Marks BP, Ryser ET. (2009). Stress, sublethal injury, resuscitation, and virulence of bacterial foodborne pathogens. *Journal of Food Protection*, Vol.72, pp.1121-1138, 0362-028X

Wong HS, Townsend KM, Fenwick SG, Trengove RD, O'Handley RM. (2010). Comparative susceptibility of planktonic and 3-day-old *Salmonella* Typhimurium biofilms to disinfectants. *J Appl Microbiol*, Vol.108, pp.2222-2228, 1364-5072

Xu H, Lee HY, Ahn J. (2008). Cross-protective effect of acid-adapted *Salmonella enterica* on resistance to lethal acid and cold stress conditions. *Letters in Applied Microbiology*, Vol.47, pp.290-297, 0266-8254

Yousef AE, Courtney PD. (2003). Basics of stress adaptation and implications in new-generation foods, In: Microbial stress adaptation and food safety, Boca Raton (USA), CRC Press,

Zhou F, Baoping JI, Zhang H, Jiang H, Yang Z, Li J, Li J, Ren Y, Yan W. (2007a). Synergistic effect of thymol and carvacrol combined with chelators and organic acids against *Salmonella* Typhimurium. *Journal of Food Protection*, Vol.70, pp.1704-1709

Zhou F, Ji B, Zhang H, Jiang H, Yang Z, Li J, Li J, Yan W. (2007b). The antibacterial effect of cinnamaldehyde, thymol, carvacrol and their combinations against the foodborne pathogens *Salmonella* Typhimurium. *J Food Saf*, Vol.27, pp.124-133

7

Influence of Trisodium Phosphate on the Survival of *Salmonella* on Turkey Carcasses

Anita Mikołajczyk
University of Warmia and Mazury in Olsztyn
Poland

1. Introduction

Combating *Salmonella* in the environment is a difficult problem for those involved in livestock and food production. Table poultry are one of the main reservoirs of *Salmonella*. Contamination with *Salmonella* of up to 7% has been found in slaughter chickens immediately after stunning, while this figure has been observed to rise even to 48% in chickens prior to chilling (Mikolajczyk & Radkowski 2002a, 2002b). Despite numerous attempts to avoid secondary contamination by *Salmonella* on the slaughter line and during processing, there is an ongoing search for methods of rendering these bacteria harmless.

The number of chemical additives used in food processing is limited because of human health concerns, limits to solubility and governmental regulatory approval for direct application to foods. Further, consumers are demanding more "all natural", "organic", and "additive-free" foods, which limits the use of many chemical compounds.

In the search for methods of rendering *Salmonella* harmless, phosphates are worth considering. They are used by the poultry industry in many countries. Internationally, in-depth research on the safe use of additives and their effects, suitability, and harmlessness to health is being done by the UNO through the Joint FAO/WHO Expert Committee on Food Additives (JECFA). Advanced legislative work is also being done, independently of the JECFA, within the European Union. Within the EU, it is obligatory to use additives defined according to the EU numerical designation system, using the symbol E and an appropriate number. The same numbers are often used in many non-European countries, without the letter E.

In line with the numerical designation system of the European Union, sodium phosphates are distinguished by the symbol E 339, while trisodium phosphate is designated E 339 (E 339 iii) (Official Journal of the European Communities, 1995; Official Journal of the European Union, 2008).

On the basis of Union legislation, in Poland a Directive of the Ministry of Health (Directive of the Ministry of Health, 18 September 2005) allows the use of sodium phosphates (E 339) in foods for babies and small children. The maximum input of sodium phosphates used in production of food preparations intended for initial and further feeding of healthy babies is 1g/l in terms of P_2O_5.

The lists of the International Food Additive Numbering System (INS), drawn up by the Codex Committee on Food Additives and Contaminants (CCFAC) feature synonyms and groups of additives. Some additives are multifunctional. Despite the international character of these lists, not all the additives are permitted to be used in individual countries. Individual country lists are subject to constant modification through removal, in other words, the introduction of prohibition of certain additives, and the addition of new ones. Sometimes substances previously denied approval are added to approved lists, following further research validation, as safe for health.

The Food Safety and Inspection Service (FSIS) of the U.S. Department of Agriculture (USDA) publishes, in the Federal Register, regulations defining the process of approving the use of food product ingredients and sources of radiation in meat products, with the aim of enabling parallel control, carried out by the FSIS and the Food and Drug Administration (FDA), of applications to introduce new procedures and new additives and colourings to food items generally recognized as safe. The FDA publishes among its regulations a list (21 CFR - Code of Federal Regulations) of additives to food products and sources of radiation which are safe and appropriate for the production of meat and poultry products. The FDA regulations allow producers of ingredients and food products to determine, independently and using their own experts, whether a given substance is generally recognised as safe (GRAS - Generally Recognised as Safe). Substances with the statutory designation GRAS granted by internal experts are not included on the FDA list in CFR 21. The FDA sets out GRAS notifications for meat and poultry products in the GRAS Notification List, which it publishes on its own internet site. Substances permitted by the FDA regulations are approved for general use in food products (CFR 21, parts 172-180) or designated as substances generally safe for use in food products (CFR 21, parts 182 and 184).

Trisodium phosphate (TSP) is listed as approved in the CFR 21 and in the GRAS Notification, and may be used in meat and poultry production. "Trisodium phosphate is listed by the FDA as GRAS when used in accordance with good manufacturing practice." [Anon., 2005].

Trisodium phosphate is approved by the FDA as a food additive and is thus in the register entitled "Everything Added to Food in the United States" (EAFUS) [Anon., 2009].

2. The Influence of Solutions of Trisodium Phosphate (E 339 iii) Concentrations on *Salmonella* spp. in Microbiological Media and on Turkey Carcasses and Duration of Storage upon the Survival Rate of *Salmonella* in Turkey Carcasses

In the published literature, significant amounts of data relate to the widely accepted use of trisodium phosphate within the food industry and meat processing, justifying a study of the effects of trisodium phosphate on *Salmonella* during storage of carcasses. Hence the initiation of research aimed at determining the influence of trisodium phosphate on *Salmonella* present in microbiological media, on turkey carcasses and in samples from turkey carcasses kept for a period of 6 days, the maximum length of time before the meat reaches the consumer, may lead to an improved level of food hygiene and human health.

2.1 The Influence of Solutions of Trisodium Phosphate (E 339 iii) Concentrations on *Salmonella* spp. in Microbiological Media

2.1.1 Materials and methods

During stage one of the study, the influence of trisodium phosphate (E 339 iii) on *Salmonella* spp. was investigated in microbiological media. The following concentrations of analytically pure trisodium phosphate (E 339 iii) (Na_3Po_4) were added to nutritive agar were applied: 0.01%, 0.02%, 0.03%, 0.05%, 0.1%, 0.25%, 0.5%, 1%, 1.5%, 2.0%. *Salmonella* serovars studies included Enteritidis no. 33/66, *Salmonella* Anatum No. 30/93 and *Salmonella* Typhimurium No. 227/84, obtained from the Museum of bacterial strains of the National Veterinary Research Institute in Puławy in Poland.

The trisodium phosphate (E 339 iii) was sterilised using the Millipore filter (Millex 9P, 022µ, Bedford), and added at appropriate concentrations to the medium at the temperature of 50°C. The *Salmonella* strains were inoculated into 9 ml of nutritive agar incubated for 24 hours at 37°C. This bacterial suspension was then used as an inoculum for further studies. Next, a ten-fold dilution of the culture was made and each serovar at each dilution was inoculated by spread plating on the nutritive agar without the TSP (negative control) as well as and on the nutritive agar supplemented with different quantities of trisodium phosphate (E 339 iii). Surface inoculation was applied. Plates were incubated at 37°C for 24 to 48 hours. Trials were replicated ten times and populations were averaged.

2.1.1 The Research Results

Table 1 and figure 1 detail results of the influence of various quantities of solutions of trisodium phosphate (E 339 iii) on *Salmonella* spp. in microbiological media. The average number of bacteria in control samples not supplemented with trisodium phosphate (E 339 iii) was 2.3×10^8 for *S.* Enteritidis, 7.25×10^7 for *S.* Anatum, and 2.6×10^8 for *S.* Typhimurium. Trisodium phosphate in agar medium at 1% concentration inhibited growth of *Salmonella* strains entirely. In the case of 0.5% concentration, the number of *S.* Anatum compared to the controls decreased by 3 logarithmic cycles, while *S.* Enteritidis and *S.* Typhimurium decreased by 4 logarithmic cycles. It was established that the addition of a concentration of up to 0.25% of sodium orthophosphate to an agar substrate had no substantial influence on the quantitative growth of any of the *Salmonella* examined. With a concentration of 1% trisodium phosphate, no increase in *Salmonella* in the substrate could be established.

Type of *Salmonella* spp.	Number of colonies [CFU/ml]										
	Concentration of trisodium phosphate [%]										
	0.00	0.01	0.02	0.03	0.05	0.1	0.25	0.5	1	1.5	2
S. Anatum	7.25×10^7	1.8×10^7	6.0×10^6	8.0×10^6	8.7×10^6	1.2×10^7	8.9×10^6	2.0×10^4	0	0	0
S. Enteritidis	2.3×10^8	2.5×10^7	2.2×10^7	2.4×10^7	2.4×10^7	2.5×10^7	2.6×10^7	3.0×10^4	0	0	0
S. Typhimurium	2.6×10^8	2.6×10^7	1.9×10^7	2.6×10^7	2.8×10^7	2.3×10^7	1.9×10^7	2.5×10^4	0	0	0

Table 1. The growth of *Salmonella* spp. on agar substrate with an addition of trisodium phosphate (n=10)

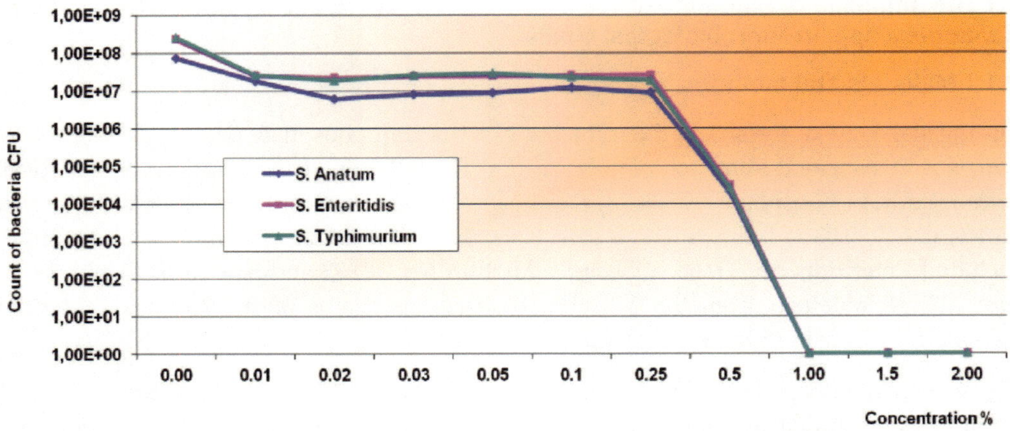

Fig. 1. The growth of *Salmonella* spp. on agar substrate with an addition of varying concentrations of trisodium phosphate

On the basis of the results displayed in table 1 and figure 1, it can be concluded that the addition of sodium orthophosphate had an influence on the survival of *Salmonella* in agar substrates. While the inhibiting influence of sodium orthophosphate in bacterial substrates was high, this compound may prove useful for destruction of *Salmonella* on poultry carcasses.

2.2 The Influence of Trisodium Phosphate (E 339 iii) on *Salmonella* Enteritidis on Turkey Carcasses

2.2.1 Materials and methods

This stage of the studies concerned analysis of the influence of trisodium phosphate (E 339 iii) on *Salmonella* Enteritidis present in elements of turkey carcasses.

Tests were conducted on 236 samples of turkey breast purchased from poultry processing plants. After delivery to the laboratory, the material was kept in a refrigerator at 4°C, and next used for preparation of 25 g samples for further analysis. No *Salmonella* spp. was detected when random samples (20% of all turkey breasts purchased) were examined for *Salmonella* spp.). *Salmonella* Enteritidis No. 33/66 was first inoculated in nutritive broth and incubated at 37°C for 24 hours. Turkey breast samples were then inoculated with 0.05 ml of the 24-hour broth culture of *S.* Enteritidis diluted to from 10^{-4} to 10^{-8} and initial inoculum of test samples was determined for each test series. The bacterial suspension was delicately spread with a special wide loop over the widest area possible. After inoculation with the bacteria, each sample was held for 20 minutes in a refrigerator at 4°C to fully dry the suspension. Next, each sample was transferred to a sterile beaker with 250 ml of a 1%, 2.5%, 5% or 10% trisodium phosphate (E 339 iii) solution for 15 minutes. Among the methods recommended for detection of *Salmonella* spp. on poultry carcasses, pluck and products the method given in ISO 6579, 1993; PN-ISO 6579, 1998 was applied.

Following 15 minutes of treatment in a trisodium phosphate (E 339 iii) solution, each sample was moved to a sterile beaker and covered with 225 ml of buffered peptone water (BPW, CM 509, Oxoid Basingstoke Hampshire, UK), and incubated at 37°C for 20 hours. Selective growth was achieved on SC medium (SC, 0 687-17-1, Difco Laboratories Detroit MI, USA),

Müller-Kauffman medium (MK, CM 343, Oxoid Basingstoke Hampshire, UK) and Rappaport-Vassiliadis medium (RV, CM 669, Oxoid Basingstoke Hampshire, UK) while the further culturing was done on brilliant green and phenol red agars (BGA, CM 329, Oxoid Basingstoke Hampshire, UK) on BSA medium (BSA, 00 73-01-1, Difco Laboratories Detroit MI, USA) and on XLD agar (XLD, CM 469 Oxoid Basingstoke Hampshire, UK). Colonies typical and suspected of belonging to *Salmonella* spp. were identified by serological and biochemical methods. Biochemical characteristics of *Salmonella* spp. were determined using API Test 20 E. Serological types were determined on the basis of the Kauffmann-White classification scheme as proposed by Popoff and Le Minor (1997) using the sera produced by the National *Salmonella* Centre.

Turkey breast samples inoculated with *Salmonella* spp. immersed in sterile water for 15 minutes were used as positive controls. Each variant of the experiment was done in ten repetitions.

2.2.2 Research results

Table 2 clearly demonstrates that inactivation of *Salmonella* on turkey carcasses is inversely proportional to the population of the original inoculum.

When 10 colony-forming units of *Salmonella* were inoculated onto the surface of a turkey carcass parts and treated for 15 minutes in 1%, 2.5%, 5% and 10% sodium orthophosphate, or either treated at 5% and 10% for 15 min., no *Salmonella* was detected. When 1% and 2.5% of sodium orthophosphate was used, there was a reduction in the number of samples in which *Salmonella* were found in relation to the control samples at both times as well as at a surface contamination of 10^3 colony-forming units and treatment for 15 minutes, , in a 5% or 10% solution. Where a surface contamination with 10^4 colony-forming units was applied to turkey meat immersed in the water solutions of the chemical substances in the study, their influence on detectability of *Salmonella* could not be confirmed (table 2).

Concentration [%]	Treatment time [minutes]	*Salmonella* Enteritidis nr 33/66 dilutions (inoculum)				
		4	5	6	7	8
		Number of positive results				
0	15	10	10	10	9	0
	45	10	10	10	9	0
1	15	10	10	9	0	0
	45	10	10	5	0	0
2.5	15	10	10	4	0	0
	45	10	10	2	0	0
5	15	10	9	0	0	0
	45	10	7	0	0	0
10	15	10	5	0	0	0
	45	0	0	0	0	0

Table 2. Number of samples from elements of turkey carcasses treated with trisodium phosphate, in which *Salmonella* Enteritidis was detected (n=10)

This study confirms the efficacy of the inhibiting influence of sodium orthophosphate on *Salmonella* on poultry carcasses. The unfavorable effect of this compound in relation to *Salmonella* was greater in bacterial substrates than on poultry carcasses.

2.3. The Influence of Trisodium Phosphate (E 339 iii) on survival of *Salmonella* Enteritidis on Turkey meat stored at a temperature of 4°C for 2, 4 & 6 Days

2.3.1 Materials and methods

Research was carried out on 192 samples of turkey breast purchased from poultry processing plants. Each sample was divided into two parts. One part was checked for the natural occurrence of *Salmonella*, while the other was inoculated with the relevant strain.

S. Enteritidis strain no. 33/66 was stored on agar strips in a refrigerator at a 4°C, then seeded into a nutrient broth and incubated at 37°C for 24 hours. After incubation, 10 ml of the broth were decanted into 4l of diluent consisting of: 1g peptone, 8.5% sodium chloride NaCl, and 1,000 ml distilled water, in which the turkey breast samples were immersed. After 5 minutes, the samples were extracted, drained for 2 minutes, placed on specially prepared sterile trays with drainage grids, and kept in a refrigerator at a temperature of 4°C for 20 minutes. The initial inoculum level of control samples was determined in each series of investigations. The samples were then transferred to sterile beakers containing 250ml of 1%, 2.5%, and 5% solutions of analytically pure (E 339 iii) trisodium phosphate (Na_3PO_4) for 15 minutes. The control material in this experiment consisted of breast samples inoculated with *Salmonella* and immersed in sterile water for 15 minutes. These were examined directly without decontamination, the number of bacteria being taken as the inoculum.

Swabs were taken from the exterior and interior surface of the turkey breasts using sterile tampons and templates. A stainless-steel template with a 25cm^2 aperture was applied to each surface examined. Two swabs were taken, one from the exterior, the other from the interior surface, the total surface area being 50 cm^2. The tampons with the swabs were placed in flasks with glass beads in 50ml of diluting fluid and shaken energetically for about 2 minutes. This achieved an initial dilution in which 1ml of fluid corresponded to 1cm^2 of surface examined. The fluid was then diluted tenfold and the level of *Salmonella* determined using the Most Probable Number method (ISO 7218, 1996). To achieve this, 1ml each of the initial suspension and its subsequent tenfold dilutions were decanted into 3 parallel test-tubes of buffered peptone water (BPW, CM 509, Oxoid, Basingstoke, Hampshire, UK). These were incubated at 37°C for 20 hours and then re-decanted onto a selenite cystine substrate (SC broth), a Müller-Kaufman substrate, and a Rappaport-Vassiliadis substrate. After 24 hour incubation at 41.5°C (RV) and 37°C (MK & SC), an inoculation was made into an agar substrate with brilliant green and phenol red (BGA, CM 329, Oxoid, Basingstoke, Hampshire, UK), a bismuth-sulphite substrate (BSA 00 71-01-1, Difco Laboratories, Detroit Mi., USA), and a substrate with xylose, lysine, and deoxycholane (XLD, CM 469, Oxoid, Basingstoke, Hampshire, UK). A reading of the most probable number of *Salmonella* was made using the Hoskins table.

The research was carried out in line with methods set out in PN-ISO 6579, 1998; PN-A-82055-3, 1994; ISO 6579, 1993; ISO 7218, 1996. Each turkey breast was quantitatively examined for *Salmonella* immediately and after 2, 4, and 6 days of refrigerated storage at 4°C. This process was repeated six fold for each experimental variant.

The numerical material collected in the experiment was processed statistically using Student's T - test and correlation analysis. Correlation analysis was carried out on numbers expressed as logarithms.

2.3.2 Results and discussion

Table 3 and figure 2 show the changing numbers of *Salmonella* during storage of turkey meat samples at 4°C. The average initial contamination of the turkey samples amounted to 2.3x 10^3 *Salmonella*. Following immersion in water, an average of 4.3x 10^2 *Salmonella* were recovered, which was used as the inoculum. The initial inoculum of *Salmonella* Enteritidis amounted to 10^2 colony-forming units per 1 cm^2 surface area of the turkey meat sample. Directly after application of the selected concentrations of trisodium phosphate (E 339 iii) solutions, it was possible to confirm their influence on the number of *Salmonella*, reflected by a substantial decrease in the number of colonies.

A concentration of 2.5% and 5% solution of (E 339 iii) trisodium phosphate caused a reduction of *Salmonella* on a poultry meat sample by 1 logarithmic cycle. It was also established that during storage in a refrigerator at a temperature of 4°C the number of *Salmonella* in the meat samples decreased. After 6 days, this reduction was greatest where a 5% solution of trisodium phosphate (E 339 iii) was used, amounting to 2 logarithmic cycles. A similar reduction of 2 log cycles was observed in the case of meat samples immersed in sterile water after 2 days of storage treated with a 5% solution. In the remaining variants of the experiment where a 5% solution of trisodium phosphate (E 339 iii) was used, *S.* Enteritidis was reduced by 1 logarithmic cycle. A 2.5% solution of trisodium phosphate (E 339 iii) , in the case of samples immersed in sterile water, reduced *Salmonella* on the meat samples by 1 logarithmic cycle both directly after contamination and after 2 and 6 days of storage. Nevertheless, after 4 days of storage, *S.* Enteritidis increased in numbers within the same logarithmic range. Where a 1% solution of trisodiumphosphate(E 339 iii) was used, *S.* Enteritidis increased in numbers within the same logarithmic range both directly after contamination and after 2 days of storage. During the remaining days of storage, the number of bacteria rose by 1 logarithmic cycle in the case of samples immersed in sterile water.

Substances examined	Concentration [%]	Days' storage				Dependence of number of bacteria on duration of storage	
		Directly after contamination	2	4	6	Correlation coefficient r	Level of significance p
		Number of bacteria					
Control	0	2.3×10^3	4.3×10^2	2.3×10^2	2.3×10^2	- 0.89	> 0.10
Water	0	4.3×10^2	2.4×10^2	9.3×10^1	4.3×10^1	- 0.99	0.01
Na_3PO_4	1	1.2×10^2	1.2×10^2	2.4×10^2	2.3×10^2	0.88	> 0.10
	2.5	9.3×10^1	4.1×10^1	9.3×10^1	2.3×10^0	- 0.76	> 0.10
	5	2.3×10^1	2.3×10^0	2.3×10^0	3.6×10^{-1}	- 0.94	0.05

Table 3. The influence of trisodium phosphate on survival of *Salmonella* Enteritidis on turkey carcass elements stored at 4°C for 2, 4 & 6 days (n=6)

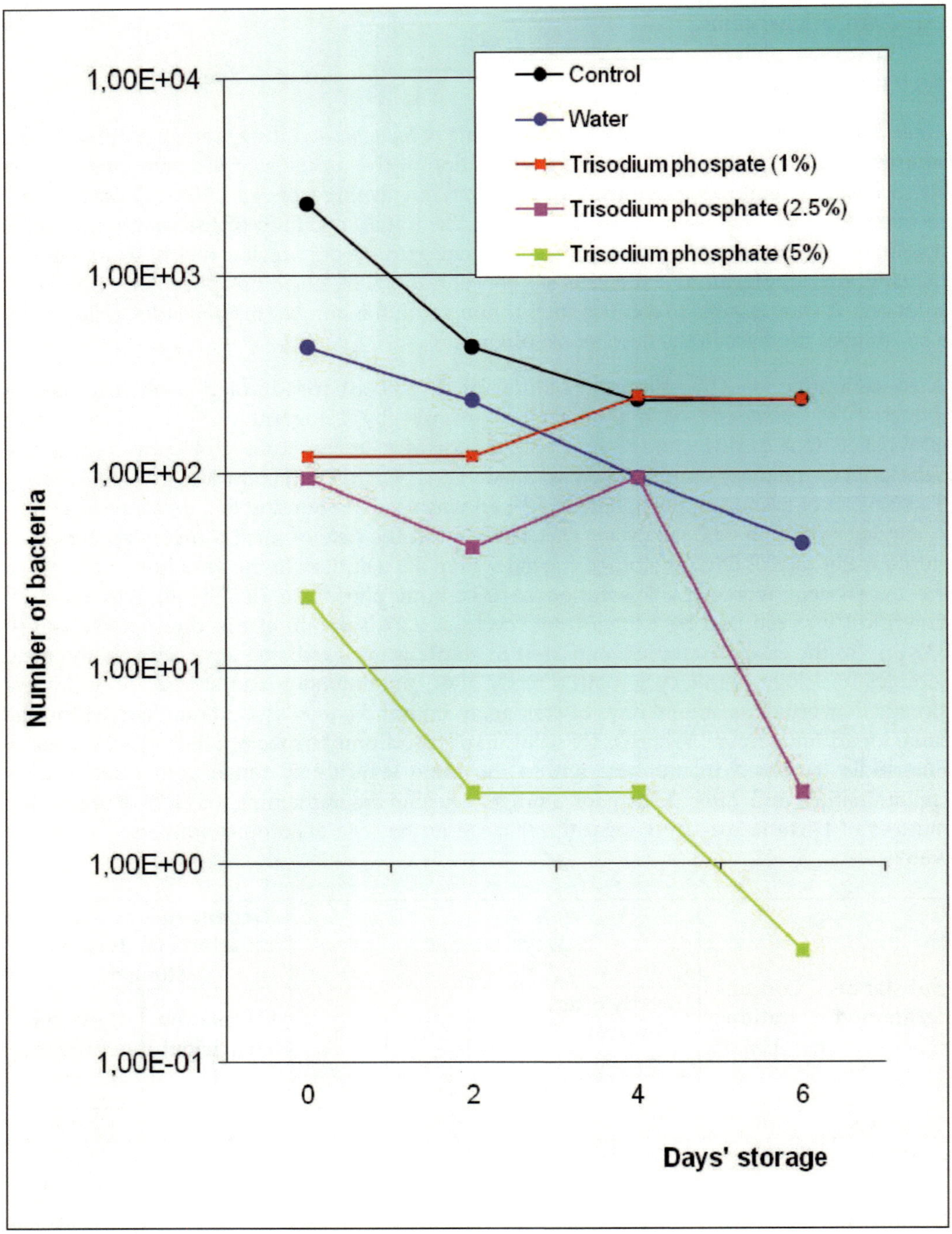

Fig. 2. The influence of sodium phosphate on survival of *Salmonella* Enteritidis bacteria on elements of turkey carcasses stored at 4°C for 2, 4, & 6 days

After slaughter, poultry carcasses with an internal muscle temperature of around 40°C must be subjected to chilling to reach a temperature of 4°C within approximately 2 hours or less, in order to extend the meat's keeping period and inhibit the growth of microorganisms. If poultry carcasses are contaminated with *Salmonella* during this production cycle, current technologies are not sufficient to render the pathogen harmless. Air temperatures in the range of 0°C to -1°C do not render *Salmonella* harmless and carcasses contaminated with them may be delivered for sale. The time before a carcass reaches the consumer after chilling is variable and depends on many factors. The producer, on the basis of research into storage, defines the date up to which fresh poultry is fit for consumption.

In the author's research, the influence of various concentrations of solutions of trisodium phosphate (E 339 iii) upon *Salmonella* was determined in conditions as near to natural as possible, in other words, using poultry meat originating directly from poultry processing plants, not subjected to any processes intended to eliminate accompanying microflora in the laboratory, and stored in conditions with a constant temperature of 4°C.

Hwang and Beuchat (1995), studying the effectiveness of reduction in the number of *Salmonella* on chicken skins under the infuence of trisodium phosphate (E 339 iii), confirmed a reduction in the number of these microorganisms only following immersion for 30 minutes at a temperature of 25°C in a 1% solution of NA_3PO_4 . Bender and Brodsky (1990) observed that neutralization of the bacteria under the influence of a 10% solution of potassium phosphate for 15 minutes was incomplete, probably because of the formation of a coating of fat on the poultry skin. According to Giese (1992) this observation should enable the removal of bacteria from the surface of carcasses.

The mechanism by which trisodium phosphate (E 339 iii) kills *Salmonella* is not fully known. As indicated by Giese (1992 &1993), the effectiveness of using this medium is linked not only with its strong antibacterial properties but also with the possibility of removing the thin lipid layer from the surface of poultry skin.

Benedict et al. (1991) confirmed that the high index of the bacterial suspension's adhesion to the skin is achieved thanks to immersion of the carcasses in it. The serotype of the *Salmonella* and the temperature of the bacterial suspension do not influence the adhesion of microorganisms on the skin (Conner & Bilgili, 1994). Cell structures such as fimbriae or cilia are essential in the mechanism of adhesion to the skin (Dickson, 1992; De Graft-Hanson & Heath, 1990). A very important role is played by the duration of contact between the bacterial suspension and the skin (Conner & Bilgili, 1994). Directly after applying the relevant bacterial culture to the skin, samples should be kept for an appropriate period with the aim of obtaining better adhesion of bacteria to the skin of the carcasses. According to Conner and Bilgili (1994), the optimal time needed for *Salmonella* to settle and attach themselves on the skin is 10 minutes if an inoculum of 10^4 is used. Where a lower inoculum is used, the time should be extended to 20 minutes with an inoculum of 10^3 and 30 minutes with one of 10^2.

Salmonella which are firmly attached to the skin ("firmly attached cells") are significantly more resistant to the effect of chemical media than those which have not succeeded in settling firmly but are loosely attached to the skin ("loosely attached cells") (Lillard, 1989a, 1989b; Tamblyn et al., 1997). Bailey et al. (1986) observed a 90-96% reduction in *S.* Typhimurium as a result of a 3.5-second spray using sodium hypochlorite at 20-40 ppm.

Such methods often reduce but seldom eliminate *Salmonella* on poultry carcasses because they are ineffective in relation to bacterial cells settled on or firmly attached to the skin. Hence, there is a need to test media which neutralises *Salmonella* that are firmly attached to the skin (Tamblyn & Conner, 1997; Conner & Bilgili, 1994).

The critical point in research on neutralisation of *Salmonella* is the fact that these bacteria can be firmly attached to the skin, especially when carcasses are in the initial phase of the production process. It can even be the case that *Salmonella* become irreversibly attached to the skin. In view of this, it might be the case that no currently utilized antimicrobial will be fully effective (Conner & Bilgili, 1994).

The next problem in assessing the effectiveness of media inactivating *Salmonella* is the fact that despite the use of various techniques in rinsing, washing, and multiple re-rinsing of carcasses, not all bacteria can be removed (Izat et al., 1991). Lillard (1989b) confirmed that removal of bacteria attached to poultry skin is very difficult, though repeated rinsing can lead to removal of large numbers. In many publications (Conner & Bilgili, 1994; Izat et al. 1991) it is stated that the removal of *Salmonella* is based on multiple rinsing; nevertheless, it is apparent that not all cells can successfully be removed.

3. Conclusion

1. The inhibiting influence of sodium orthophosphate in bacterial substrates was high. The unfavorable effect of this compound in relation to *Salmonella* can also be applied to poultry carcasses.
2. Among the various concentrations of solution used for neutralizing *Salmonella* on elements of turkey carcasses stored at a temperature of 4°C for 6 days, the greatest effect was shown by a 5% solution of trisodium phosphate.
3. With samples treated with a 1% solution of trisodium phosphate (E 339 iii), stored for 6 days, the number of *Salmonella* did not undergo any substantial changes, still remaining at the same level.
4. In the case of 2.5% and 5% solutions of trisodium phosphate (E 339 iii), it was noticed that, along with an extension of the storage period, their limiting influence on the number of *Salmonella* in turkey carcasses increased.

4. References

Anonymus (2005). Sodium phosphate. Code of Federal Regulations - Title 21: Food and Drugs, section 182.1778. U.S. Government Printing Office, Washington, D.C.

Anonymus (2009). Everything Added to Food in the United States (EAFUS), U.S. Departament of Health and Human Services (HHS), U.S. Food and Drug Administration (FDA). Available at: http://www.cfsan.fda.gov/~lrd/foodadd.html

Bailey J. S., Thomson J. E., Cox N. A., Shackelford A. D. (1986). Chlorine spray washing to reduce bacterial contamination of poultry processing equipment. Poult. Sci., 65(6): 1120-1123.

Benedict R. C., Schultz F. J., Jones S. B. (1991). Attachment and removal of *Salmonella* spp. on meat and poultry tissues. J. Food Safety, 11(2): 135-148.

Bender F. G., Brotsky E. (1990). Process for treating poultry carcasses to control *Salmonella* growth. U. S. Patent 5.069. 922 US 5301131.

Conner D. E., Bilgili S. F. (1994). Skin attachment model for improved laboratory evaluation of potential carcass disinfectants for their efficacy against *Salmonella* attached to broiler skin. J. Food Prot. 57(8): 684-688.

De Graft-Hanson J., Heath J. L. (1990). Effect of d-mannose on fimbriae of bacterial isolates from chicken carcasses. Poult. Sci. 69(9): 1582-1589.

Dickson J. S. 1992. Acetic acid action on beef tissue surfaces contaminated with *Salmonella* typhimurium. J. Food Sci., 57(2): 297-301.

Directive of the Ministry of Health, 18 September 2005, on permitted substances, with appendices, Journal of Statutes/2008, No. 177, item 1094, 3 October 2008.

Giese J. (1992). Press conference report: Experimental process reduces *Salmonella* in poultry. Food Technol., 46(4): 112.

Giese J. (1993). *Salmonella* reduction process receives approval. Food Technol., 47(6): 110.

Hwang C.-A., Beuchat L. R. (1995). Efficacy of selected chemicals for killing pathogenic and spoilage microorganisms on chicken skin. J. Food Prot., 58(1): 19-23.

ISO 6579: 1993(E). (1993). Microbiology - General guidance on methods for the detection of *Salmonella*.

ISO 7218: 1996(E). (1996). Microbiology of food and animal feeding stuffs - General rules for microbiological examinations.

Izat A. L., Yamaguchi W., Kaniawati S., McGinnis J. P., Raymond S. G., Hierholzer R. E., Kopek J. M. (1991). Research note: use of consecutive carcasses rinses and a most probable number procedure to estimate *Salmonella*e contamination of inoculated carcasses. Poult. Sci. 70(6): 1448-1451.

Lillard H. S. (1989a). Factors affecting the persistence of *Salmonella* during the processing of poultry. J. Food Prot., 52(11): 829-831.

Lillard H. S. (1989b). Incidence and recovery of *Salmonella*e and other bacteria from commercially processed poultry carcasses at selected pre- and post-evisceration steps. J. Food Prot., 52(11): 888-891.

Mikołajczyk A., Radkowski M. (2002a). *Salmonella* spp. on chicken carcasses in processing plants in Poland. Journal of Food Protection 65: 1475 - 1479.

Mikołajczyk A., Radkowski M. (2002b). The occurrence of *Salmonella* spp. in turkeys investigation results from a slaughter and after-slaughter dressing line in Poland. Fleischwirtschaft 32: 52-54.

Official Journal of the European Communities (1995): Council Directive No. 95/2/EC of 20 February 1995 on food additives other than colourings and sweeteners L61 (L61, 18.3).

Official Journal of the European Union (2008): Regulation of the European Parliament and of the Council No. 1333/2008/ EC of 16 December 2008 on food additives L 354/16.

PN-A-82055-3. (1994). Meat and meat products. Microbiological research. Preparation of samples and dilutions.

PN-ISO 6579. (1998). Microbiology. General principles of methods of detecting Salmonella bacteria.

Popoff M.Y. and Le Minor L. 1997. Antigenic Formulas of the Salmonella Serovars. WHO Collaborating Center for Reference and Research on Salmonella, Institue Pasteur, Paris, France

Tamblyn K. C., Conner D. E. (1997). Bactericidal activity of organic acids against *Salmonella* typhimurium attached to broiler chicken skin. J. Food Prot., 60(6): 629-633.

Tamblyn. K. C., Conner D. E., Bilgili S. F., Hall G. S. (1997). Utilization of the skin attachment model (SAM) to determine the antimicrobial activity of potential carcass treatmens. Poult. Sci., 76(9): 1318-1323.

8

Bacteriophage PPST1 Isolated from Hospital Wastewater, A Potential Therapeutic Agent Against Drug Resistant *Salmonella enterica* subsp. *enterica* serovar Typhi

Pongsak Rattanachaikunsopon and Parichat Phumkhachorn
Faculty of Science, Ubon Ratchathani University
Thailand

1. Introduction

Salmonella enterica subsp. *enterica* serovar Typhi (hereafter referred to as *Salmonella* Typhi) is a Gram-negative enteric bacillus belonging to the family *Enterobacteriaceae*. It is a facultative anaerobe that is motile by peritrichous flagella. The bacterium is catalase positive, oxidase negative. It produces no gas when grown in Triple Sugar Iron (TSI) broth, which is used to differentiate it from other *Enterobacteriaceae* (Murray, 1994).

The bacterium is restricted to humans and is not known to have a reservoir in animals. Thus, the transmission of *S.* Typhi has only been shown to occur from person to person via fecal-oral route. Infection of *S.* Typhi leads to the development of typhoid, or enteric fever. This disease is characterized by the sudden onset of a sustained and systemic fever, severe headache, nausea, and loss of appetite. Other symptoms include constipation or diarrhea, enlargement of the spleen, possible development of meningitis, and/or general malaise. The disease has caused many deaths in developing countries where sanitation is poor and is spread through contamination of water and undercooked food (Murray, 1994).

Treatment of typhoid fever relies mainly on such antibiotics as chloramphenicol, ampicillin and trimethoprim-sulfamethoxazole (Rowe et al., 1997; Trung et al., 2007); however, the success of the antibiotic based therapeutic approach has currently been limited because of the emergence of multidrug resistant strains of *S.* Typhi. Owing to the development of bacterial resistance to chloramphenicol during the 1970s and 1980s, treatment with this drug was widely replaced by ampicillin and trimethoprim-sulfamethoxazole; however, by the 1980s and 1990s, *S.* Typhi developed resistance simultaneously to all drugs used for first-line treatment, namely, chloramphenicol, ampicillin and trimethoprim-sulfamethoxazole (Trung et al., 2007). These multidrug resistant *S.*Typhi strains have been found to be responsible for numerous outbreaks in many countries in the Indian subcontinent, Southeast Asia, and Africa (Rowe et al., 1997). In light of the evidence of the rapid global spread of drug resistant *S.* Typhi strains, the need to find new antibiotics to treat diseases caused by the bacteria is of paramount importance. However, the past record of rapid emergence of resistance to newly introduced antibiotics indicates that even new families of antibiotics will have a short life expectancy (Coates et al., 2002). For this reason, researchers are increasingly turning their attention to alternative therapeutic approaches to combat drug resistant *S.* Typhi. One of the promising approaches is bacteriophage therapy or phage therapy.

Bacteriophages or phages are viruses that infect bacteria. Lytic or virulent bacteriophages have been considered to be a new class of antibacterial agents because they undergo rapid growth, disrupt bacterial metabolism and reproduction, and lyse the bacterial cells. They have been used for therapeutic purposes since the 1920s. Several studies have shown that bacteriophages could be used successfully for therapeutic purposes both in humans and animals (Bruttin & Brussow, 2005; Chhibber et al., 2008; Deresinski, 2009; Nakai & Park, 2002). In addition, there have been several reports showing the ability of lytic bacteriophages to kill drug resistant bacteria (Capparelli et al., 2007; Thamniamton et al., 2010; Vinodkumar et al., 2005). Therefore, it is of interest to find a bacteriophage for use as a therapeutic agent to control drug resistant *S.* Typhi.

In this study, a bacteriophage specific to drug resistant *S.* Typhi was isolated from hospital wastewater. It was also characterized with respect to host range, adsorption, thermal and pH sensitivity, one step growth, and morphology, genome and protein composition. The bacteriophage from this study may be useful as a potential therapeutic agent for controlling drug resistant *S.* Typhi infections.

2. Materials and methods

2.1 Bacterial strains and culture conditions

The bacterial strain used as the indicator strain for the isolation, propagation, and characterization of the bacteriophage named PPST1 was drug resistant *Salmonella enterica* subsp. *enterica* serovar Typhi strain SSH1 (hereafter referred to as *S.* Typhi SSH1) which was kindly donated by Sappasitiprasong Hospital, Ubon Ratchathani, Thailand. The bacterial strain was confirmed as *S.* Typhi by the API 20 E test kit (bioMerieux Industry, Hazelwood, MO, USA). Antibiotic susceptibility testing by Kirby-Bauer's method revealed that *S.* Typhi SSH1 was resistant to most of the commonly-used drugs including chloramphenicol, ampicillin, trimethoprim, tetracycline, streptomycin, sulfanilamideand ciprofloxacin. Bacterial strains used to test the host range of the bacteriophage PPST1 are listed in Table 1. All of them were obtained from the American Type Culture Collection (ATCC).

All bacteria were maintained on Brain Heart Infusion (BHI) agar (Oxoid, Wesel, Germany). Fresh colonies were cultured and subcultured in BHI broth at 37°C. Stock cultures of all bacteria were stored as a frozen culture at -80°C in BHI broth containing 20% glycerol (vol/vol).

2.2 Bacteriophage isolation and purification

The water sample for bacteriophage isolation was collected from wastewater treatment tank located at Sappasitiprasong Hospital, Ubon Ratchathani, Thailand. The sample was stored at 4°C overnight to allow larger suspended sediments to settle out. The crudely clarified sample was centrifuged at 4,500 xg for 10 min to remove bacterial cells and debris. The supernatant was passed through a 0.22-μm-pore-size membrane filter (SartoriusAG, Gottingen, Germany). For bacteriophage enrichment, the filtrate was added to an equal volume of double strength BHI broth containing log phase *S.* Typhi SSH1 cells (final concentration of 10^6 CFU/ml). After incubation at 37°C overnight, the culture was centrifuged at 4,500 xg for 10 min and the supernatant was filtered through a 0.22-µm-pore-size membrane filter. The presence of a lytic phage in the filtrate was examined by using the double layer method with some modifications (Paterson et al., 1969). One hundred µl of the filtrate was mixed with 400 µl of a log phase culture of *S.* Typhi SSH1 and incubated at 37°C for 30 min. The mixture was added into 4.5 ml of molten BHI soft agar (0.7% agar) which was already cooled down to 50°C, mixed gently, and poured onto a BHI agar plate (1.5% agar). The plate was left to stand at room temperature for 30 min to allow the top agar to solidify. The presence of a lytic bacteriophage in the form of plaques was detected after incubation of the plate at 37°C overnight.

For bacteriophage purification, a single plaque was picked with a sterile glass Pasteur pipette, and put into a log phase culture of *S.* Typhi SSH1. After incubated at 37°C overnight, the bacteriophage-host mixture was centrifuged at 4,500 xg for 10 min and filtered through a 0.22-µm-pore-size membrane filter. The filtrate was subjected to the double layer method as mentioned above. Three repeated rounds of single plaque isolation and re-inoculation were performed. The bacteriophage was eluted from the final resulting plate by adding 5 ml of SM buffer (50 mM Tris-HCl, pH 7.5, 99 mM NaCl, 8 mM $MgSO_4$, 0.01% gelatin) on top of the plate and incubated at room temperature for 4 h with shaking. The bacteriophage containing buffer retrieved from the plate was centrifuged at 4,500 xg for 10 min and filtered through a 0.22-µm-pore-size membrane filter. The resulting filtrate was called bacteriophage suspension.

2.3 Bacteriophage titer determination

The bacteriophage containing solution was serially diluted in SM buffer. Each dilution was subjected to plaque assay using the double layer method as mentioned earlier. Plaques were counted in the plate containing 50-300 plaques and expressed as plaque forming unit per milliliter (PFU/ml).

2.4 Bacteriophage host range determination

The spot test method described by Chang et al. (2005) was used for bacteriophage host range determination using the bacteria listed in the Table 1 as hosts. Each bacterial strain was grown overnight in BHI broth. One hundred µl of the culture was mixed well with 4 ml of BHI soft agar (0.7% agar) and then overlaid on the surface of the BHI agar (1.5% agar). After solidication, 10 µl of the bacteriophage suspension was spotted onto the top agar layer, which was then incubated at 37°C overnight. Bacterial sensitivity to the bacteriophage was notified by a clear zone at the spot where the phage suspension was deposited.

2.5 Bacteriophage adsorption study

The bacteriophage adsorption was studied according to the protocol of Lu et al. (2003) with some modifications. A *S.* Typhi SSH1 culture with the concentration of 10^8 CFU/ml was infected with the bacteriophage suspension to give a multiplicity of infection (MOI) of 0.01 and incubated at 37°C. Aliquots were taken at 5 min intervals (up to 30 min) after infection and immediately centrifuged at 4,500 xg for 10 min to sediment the bacteriophage-adsorbed cells. filtered through a 0.22-µm-pore-size membrane filter. Filtrates were subjected to determination of titer of unadsorbed bacteriophages (residual titer) by the double layer method as mentioned earlier. BHI broth containing only bacteriophage was used as a control. The percentage of adsorption was calculated as follows: [(control titer-residual titer)/control titer] x 100%.

2.6 Thermal and pH sensitivity test

The sensitivity of bacteriophage PPST1 to temperature was examined as follows. Nine hundred µl of sterile deionized water was preheated to a desirable temperature, ranging from 50°C to 90°C. One hundred µl of the bacteriophage suspension was added to the preheated water to obtain the final bacteriophage concentration of about at 10^6 PFU/ml. After heating at the assigned temperatures for 30 min, the solutions were placed in an ice bath. Surviving bacteriophage titer was assayed by the double layer method.

The sensitivity of bacteriophage PPST1 to pH was also examined. The bacteriophage (at the final concentration of 10^6 PFU/ml) was incubated overnight at 37°C in phosphate buffered saline (135 mM NaCl, 1.3 mM KCl, 0.5 mM KH_2PO_4, 3.2 mM Na_2HPO_4, pH 7.4), adjusted in steps of 1 pH unit from pH 2 to 12 using HCl or NaOH as required. Upon re-adjustment to pH 7, the double layer method was performed to determine bacteriophage titer.

2.7 Study of one-step growth kinetics

One step growth experiment was performed as described by (Caso et al., 1995) with some modifications. Briefly, 10 ml of log phase culture of *S.* Typhi SSH1 was harvested by centrifugation at 4,500 xg for 10 min and resuspended in 5 ml of fresh BHI broth in order to obtain a final concentration of 10^8 CFU/ml. To this suspension, 5 ml of the bacteriophage suspension was added in order to have a MOI of 0.01 and the bacteriophage was allowed to adsorb for 30 min at 37°C. The mixture was centrifuged at 4,500 × g for 10 min, and the pellets containing infected cells were resuspended in pre-warmed (37°C) BHI broth, followed by incubation at 37°C. Samples were taken at 10-min intervals (up to 3 h) and immediately diluted, and bacteriophage titers were determined by the double layer method.

2.8 Examination of bacteriophage morphology

The morphology of bacteriophage PPST1 was examined by transmission electron microscopy. Bacteriophage particles were fixed by mixing 25 µl of the bacteriophage suspension with 25 µl of 50% glutaraldehyde in 4% paraformaldeyde. A 5-µl aliquot of this mixture was placed on a carbon Formvar-coated copper grid (Proscitech, Brisbane, Queenland, Australia) and allowed to adsorb for 5 min at room temperature. The bacteriophage was negatively stained with 0.5% uranyl acetate for 2 min then inspected with a Philips EM 300 electron microscope (Philips, Eindhoven, the Netherlands) operated at 60 kV. The bacteriophage size was determined from the average of five independent measurements.

2.9 Analysis of bacteriophage proteins

The protein composition of bacteriophage PPST1 was examined by sodium dodecyl sulfate-polyacrylamide gel eectrophoresis (SDS-PAGE) using NuPAGE Novex gel system

(Invitrogen, Carlsbad, CA, USA). A 26-µl aliquot of the bacteriophage suspension was mixed with 10 µl of sample buffer and 4 µl of reducing agent. The mixture was heated in boiling water for 10 min and then subjected to electrophoresis on a 4-12% Bis-Tris gel at 200 V and 120 mA for 35 min. The protein bands were stained with Coomassie blue G-250 (Sigma-Aldrich, St. Louis, MO, USA), followed by destaining with a solution containing 50% methanol and 1% acetic acid.

2.10 Analysis of bacteriophage nucleic acid

Bacteriophage nucleic acid was extracted by using PureLink Viral RNA/DNA Mini Kit (Invitrogen, Carlsbad, CA, USA) according to the protocol provided by the manufacturer. The purified nucleic acid was tested for sensitivity to Ribonuclease A, Nuclease S_1 and restriction enzyme *Pst*I (all from Sigma-Aldrich, St. Louis, MO, USA), according to the supplier's recommendations. The results were analyzed by 0.8% agarose gel electrophoresis.

The genome size of the bacteriophage PPST1 was determined by pulse-field gel electrophoresis (PFGE) of the purified bacteriophage nucleic acid. The electrophoresis was carried out with 0.8% agarose gel in 0.5x Tris-borate-EDT buffer at 15°C for 15 h, using switch time ramped from 1 to 12 s and a voltage of 6 V/cm. The PFGE size standard used was Low range PFG marker (New England Biolabs, Ipswich, MA, USA).

3. Results

3.1 Bacteriophage isolation

A bacteriophage was isolated from the hospital wastewater by the double layer method using *S.* Typhi SSH1 as a host bacterial strain. The bacteriophage produced clear plaques on the lawn of the host bacterial strain, indicating that it was a lytic or virulent bacteriophage. The plaques were small with an average diameter of 1 mm (Fig. 1), and the isolated bacteriophage was designated PPST1.

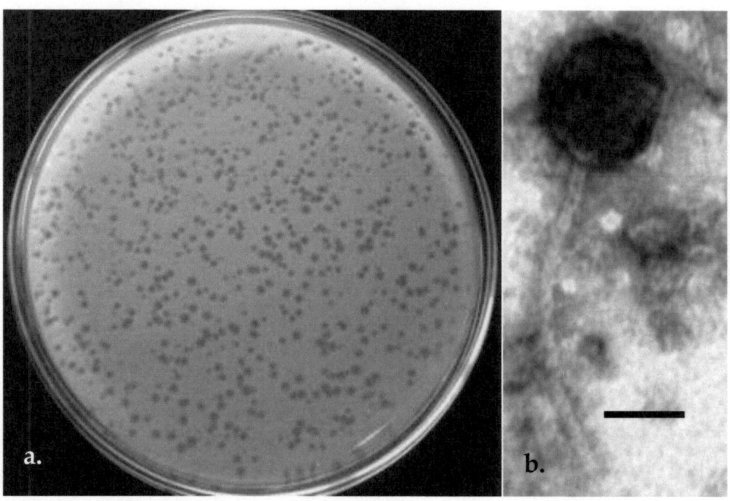

Fig. 1. Plaques on *S.* Typhi SSH1 lawn (a) and transmission electron micrograph (b) of bacteriophage PPST1. Bar = 50 nm

3.2 Bacteriophage host range

Specifictity of bacteriophage PPST1 to a variety of bacteria was examined by the spot test method. Of all 23 bacterial strains used in this experiment, only *S.* Typhi SSH1, *S.* Typhi ATCC 19430, *S.* Typhi ATCC 19214 were susceptible to the bacteriophage as shown in Table 1. On the other hand, the rest of the tested bacterial strains used in this study were not sensitive to the bacteriophage. Among the three sensitive bacterial hosts, two of them, *S.* Typhi SSH1 and *S.* Typhi ATCC 19214, are drug resistant strains. These results suggested that the bacteriophage had a broad host range with specificity to *S.* Typhi and the specificity of the bacteriophage was not influenced by the drug-resistance properties of the hosts.

Bacteria	Lysis[a]
Campylobacter jejuni ATCC 29428	-
Enterobacter aerogenes ATCC 13048	
Enterococcus faecalis ATCC 51575 (vancomycin resistant)	-
Escherichia coli ATCC 11229	-
Escherichia coli O157:H7 ATCC 35150	-
Klebsiella pneumoniae ATCC 4352	-
Listeria monocytogenes ATCC 19111	-
Pseudomonas aeruginosa ATCC 15442	-
Salmonella enterica serovar Choleraesuis ATCC 6958	-
Salmonella enterica serovar Derby ATCC 6960	-
Salmonella enterica serovar Enteritidis ATCC 4931	-
Salmonella enterica serovar Heidelberg ATCC 8326	-
Salmonella enterica serovar Paratyphi A ATCC 9150	-
Salmonella enterica serovar Typhi SSH1 (multidrug resistant)	+
Salmonella enterica serovar Typhi ATCC 19430	+
Salmonella enterica serovar Typhi ATCC 19214 (multidrug resistant)	+
Salmonella enterica serovar Typhimurium ATCC 6994	-
Salmonella enterica serovar Typhimurium ATCC 700408 (multidrug resistant)	-
Salmonella enterica serovar Typhisuis ATCC 8321	-
Shigella flexneri ATCC 29903	-
Staphylococcus aureus ATCC 6538	-
Staphylococcus aureus ATCC 33592 (methicillin resistant)	-
Streptococcus pyogenes ATCC 19615	-

[a] + = clear zone form, - = no clear zone formed

Table 1. Bacterial strains used in this study and their sensitivity to bacteriophage PPST1

3.3 Bacteriophage adsorption

The adsorption rate of bacteriophage PPST1 on *S.* Typhi ST1 is shown in Fig 2. Most of the bacteriophage particles were rapidly adsorbed to host cells within the first 10 minutes of the observation period; after which, the bacteriophage particles were adsorbed into the host cells at a relatively slow rate. Almost all of the bacteriophage particles were adsorbed into the host cells within 30 minutes. The results demonstrated that ca. 80%, 90% and 98% of bacteriophage PPST1 particles adsorbed to the host cells within 10 min, 20 min and 30 min, respectively.

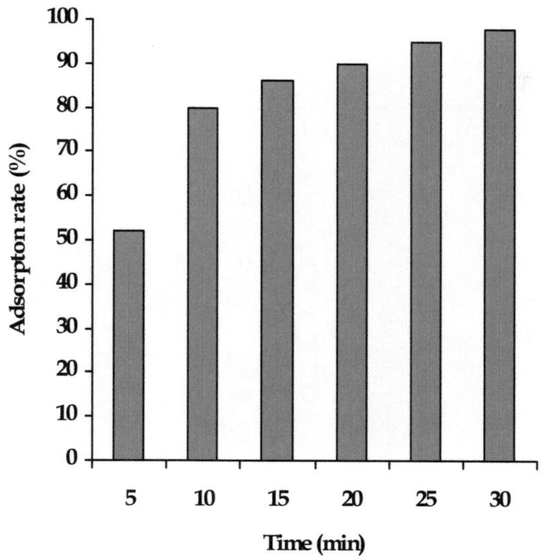

Fig. 2. Adsorption of bacteriophage PPST1 on *S.* Typhi SSH1 cells

3.4 Thermal and pH sensitivity

Thermal lability of bacteriophage PPST1 was investigated by thermal treatments at 50, 60, 70, 80 and 90°C for 30 min (Table 2). At 50°C, only a small reduction of the bacteriophage was observed. In contrast, the bacteriophage titers decreased considerably at 60 and 70°C. The higher temperature resulted in fewer bacteriophage titers. Heating at 80 and 90°C for 30 min completely inactivated the bacteriophage, thus phage titer could not be detected in the samples.

The stability of bacteriophage PPST1 was also investigated by incubating the bacteriophage overnight in a phosphate buffered saline solution at pH ranging from 2 to 12. The bacteriophage maintained its infectivity when incubated in a pH range of from 4 to 10. In contrast, the bacteriophage lost its infectivity completely at pH 3 or below as well as at pH 11 or above. The highest stability of bacteriophage was observed at pH 7 (Table 2).

3.5 One step growth kinetics

Multiplication parameters of the lytic cycle of bacteriophage PPST1 including latent period, burst period and burst size were determined from the dynamic change in the number of bacteriophage during one replicative cycle (Fig. 3). It was determined that bacteriophage PPST1 had latent and burst periods of ca. 30 and 150 min, respectively. The burst size estimated from the one-step growth curve was about 79 PFU/infected cell (Fig. 3).

3.6 Morphology, genome and protein composition

Morphological characterization of bacteriophage PPST1 was examined by transmission electron microscopy. It was shown that the bacteriophage had an icosahedral head (64 ± 2.4 nm in diameter) with a noncontractile tail of 157 ± 8.6 nm long and 12 ± 0.6 nm wide. No collar or tail appendages were observed (Fig. 1).

Treatment	Initial bacteriophage concentration (log PFU/ml)	Final bacteriophage concentration (log PFU/ml)[a]
Heat (for 30 min)		
50 °C	6.09	5.57
60 °C	6.04	3.62
70 °C	5.97	2.46
80 °C	6.08	-
90 °C	6.00	-
pH (for 1 h)		
2	6.02	-
3	5.98	-
4	6.08	3.96
5	6.00	3.51
6	6.02	4.83
7	6.04	5.89
8	5.99	4.93
9	6.03	3.73
10	6.02	2.67
11	5.97	-
12	6.00	-

a = undetectable

Table 2. Sensitivity of bacteriophage PPST1 to temperature and pH.

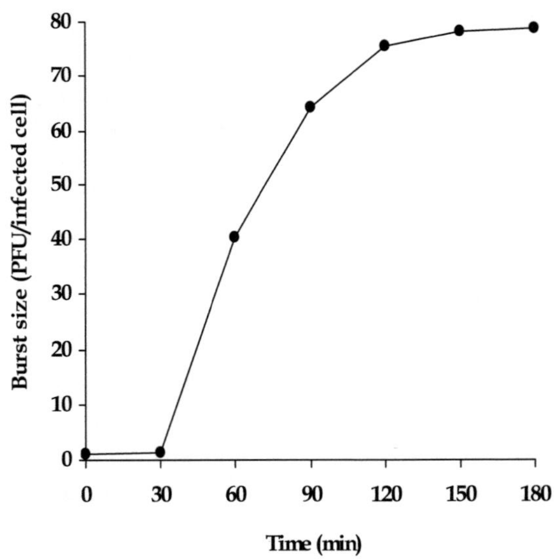

Fig. 3. One-step growth curve of bacteriophage PPST1.

The nucleic acid extracted from bacteriophage PPST1 was examined for its sensitivity to different nucleic acid digesting enzymes. It was found that the nucleic acid could not be digested either by Ribonuclease A or Nuclease S_1; however, it was sensitive to the restriction enzyme *Pst*I (Fig. 4). The size of the nucleic acid as revealed by the pulsed-filed gel electrophoresis was ca. 70 kb.

The protein composition of bacteriophage PPST1 was analyzed by SDS-PAGE and the result is shown in Fig. 5. Four protein bands were clearly detected in the SDS-PAGE gel. Based on sizes of protein standard SeeBlue Plus 2 (Invitrogen, Carlsbad, CA, USA), their estimated molecular masses were 81, 32, 24 and 15 kDa.

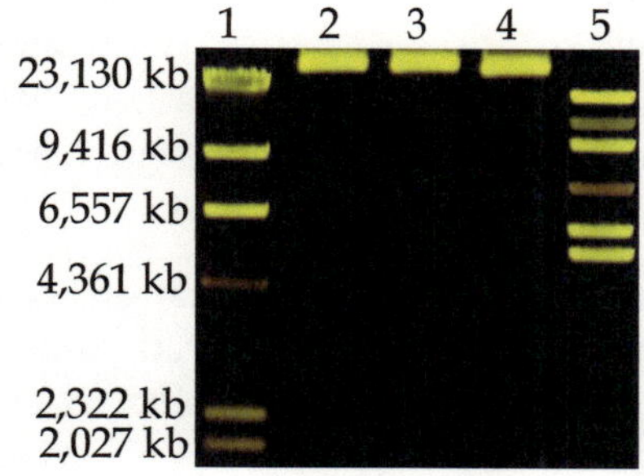

Fig. 4. Agarose gel electrophoresis of bacteriophage PPST1 nucleic acid. Lane 1, lambda DNA digested with *Hin*dIII marker; lane 2 uncut PPST1 nucleic acid; lane 3, PPST1 nucleic acid digested with Ribonuclease A; lane 4, PPST1 nucleic acid digested with Nuclease S_1, lane 5, PPST1 nucleic acid digested with *Pst*I.

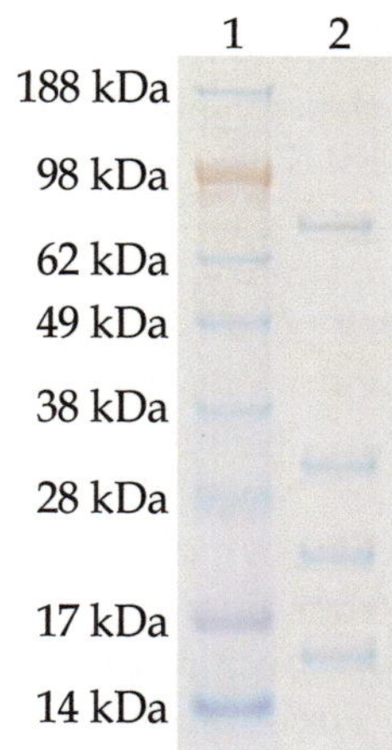

Fig. 5. SDS-PAGE analysis of bacteriophage PPST1 proteins. Lane 1, the protein standard SeeBlue Plus2, lane 2, proteins of bacteriophage PPST1.

4. Discussion

Typhoid fever caused by *S.* Typhi is a major pubic health problem worldwide, especially in developing countries. Although its incidence in the developed countries has been declining, the disease is still a frequent cause of death in parts of the world with poor sanitation (Murray, 1994). Until just recently, antibiotics were widely used to control *S.* Typhi infections; however, the emergence of antibiotic resistant *S.* Typhi in reducing drug efficacy has led to a need for alternatives to antibiotics in controlling infections as a result of the pathogenic bacteria. Bacteriophage therapy is one of the promising alternatives to control infections caused by drug resistant bacteria. This may be due to the fact that bacteriophages and antibiotics have different mechanisms of action (McAuliffe et al., 2007). Besides the ability to inhibit the growth of drug resistant bacteria, many attributes of bacteriophages make them more favorable than antibiotics for therapeutic purposes. They infect only their specific hosts, having no harm on normal microflora, and because of their host dependent multiplication, bacteriophages increase their numbers at the sites of infection, thereby increasing therapeutic efficacy. After their hosts are inactivated, bacteriophages tend to be rapidly cleared from bodies of treated organisms (Carlton, 1999; Matsuzaki et al., 2005) by innate immune mechanisms. Therefore, bacteriophage therapy may be considered an effective and safe therapeutic approach.

Bacteriophages generally reside in environments that are habitats for their host bacteria (McLaughlin et al., 2006; Sundar et al., 2009). Wastewater from Sappasitthiprasong hospital, Ubon Ratchathani, Thailand was ideal for isolation of bacteriophages in this study since the drug resistant *S.* Typhi strain SSH1 used as the main host in the present bacteriophage screening is a clinical strain isolated from a patient admitted to the hospital. When screening for bacteriophages to be used in bacteriophage therapy, bacteriophages with a broad host range spectrum within a species are more preferable because they can be effective against a large variety of a particular species. The narrow host specificity of bacteriophages can cause complexity in preparation of therapeutic phages. In some cases, combinations of several bacteriophages are required for therapeutic application. In this study, bacteriophage PPST1 was showed to be lytic to all of the tested *S.* Typhi strains, but not any other tested bacteria. Furthermore, among the sensitive bacterial strains, two were multi-drug resistant. *S* Typhi SSH1 is resistant to chloramphenicol, ampicillin, trimethoprim, tetracycline, streptomycin, sulfanilamide and ciprofloxacin while *S* Typhi ATCC 19214 is resistant to chloramphenicol, tetracycline and streptomycin. These results suggest that bacteriophage PPST1 is a potential candidate for use as a therapeutic agent to control infectious diseases caused by drug resistant *S.* Typhi. Finding a lytic bacteriophage with a broad host range is not unusual. A number of studies have reported the isolation of lytic bateriophages with a broad host range. Vinod et al. (2006) isolated a *Vibrio harveyi* bacteriophage from shrimp farm water, which was virulent to all 50 strains of *V. harveyi* tested that were originally isolated from different sources such as seawater, hatchery water, shrimp farm water and sediment. Moreover, some bacteriophages were reported to be lytic to bacteria in more than one genera. For example, phage KPO1K2 infected several strains of *Klebsiella pneumoniae* and *Escherichia coli* (Verma et al., 2009).

From previous studies, *Salmonella* bacteriophages were found to be heterogeneous, comprising all of the three families of tailed bacteriophages, including *Siphoviridae, Myoviridae* and *Podoviridae* (Demczuk et al., 2004; McLaughlin, 2006; De Lappe et al., 2009). The criteria commonly used for the classification of bacteriophages to a particular group are bacteriophage genetic and morphological characteristics. The genome of bacteriophage PPST1 was double stranded DNA because it was resistant to Nuclease S_1, a single stranded DNA digesting enzyme, and Ribonuclease A, a RNA digesting enzyme, but sensitive to the restriction enzyme *Pst*I, a double stranded DNA digesting enzyme. Transmission electron microscopy revealed that the bacteriophage was a tailed bacteriophage with an icosahedral head and a long noncontractile tail. Based on these characteristics, bacteriophage PPST1 can be tentatively classified as a member of the family *Siphoviridae,* according to the International Committee on Taxonomy of Viruses (Ackermann, 2005). There are several previously studied *S.* Typhi bacteriophages that have never been classified into a particular family due to the lack of genetic or morphological characteristics. The lytic bacteriophage specific to *S.* Typhi DMS 5784 was found to have an icosahedral head that was ca. 44 to 47 x 43 to 51 nm in diameter and a very short tail. Since its genomic characteristic has been studied, no classification of the bacteriophage has ever been reported (Neukdee, 2007). The *S.* Typhi bacteriophage j2 studied by Mise et al. (1981) is a DNA lysogenic bacteriophage. The lack of its morphological information has impeded the classification of the bacteriophage.

Variations in nucleic acid sequence and numbers of genes and proteins of bacteriophages in the family *Siphoviridae* have been reported (Rohwer and Edwards, 2002). In this study, four proteins with molecular masses ranging from 15 to 81 kDa were identified by SDS-PAGE analysis. However, their amino acid sequences and functions are still unknown. A detailed nucleic acid sequence analysis and identification of the open reading frames corresponding to the observed structural proteins are the subjects of future research.

Several studies have demonstrated that thermal and pH stability of bacteriophages varied depending on types of bacteriophage; therefore, it is of interest to investigate the stability of bacteriophage PPST1 in a wide temperature and pH range. These results demonstrate that bacteriophage PPST1 is stable in a broad pH range (4-10) and at a temperature as high as 70°C for at least 3 min. These morphological characteristics may be useful in broad applications of bacteriophage therapy.

In conclusion, the data obtained from the present study clearly indicates that the bacteriophage PPST1 is a lytic bacteriophage capable of killing several strains of *S.* Typhi, including drug resistant strains. This property of the bacteriophage, together with its stability at a high temperature and over a wide pH range, makes bacteriophage PPST1 a potential alternative to antibiotics as a therapeutic agent for infections of drug resistant *S.* Typhi. Future research is needed to elucidate the most suitable condition for the application of this characterized bacteriophage in treating experimentally-induced drug resistant *S.* Typhi infection in animal models.

5. Summary

The emergence of drug resistant *Salmonella* Typhi has limited the efficacy of antibiotic based therapeutic approach. Bacteriophage therapy has recently been considered a promising approach to control infections caused by drug resistant bacteria. In this study, a lytic bacteriophage, specific to drug resistant *S.* Typhi strain SSH1, was isolated from hospital wastewater. The bacteriophage, designated PPST1, had broad host range within the species *S.* Typhi. It was lytic against all of the tested *S.* Typhi strains, but not any other tested bacteria. The bacteriophage was completely inactivated at 80 and 90°C for 30 min but was stable at 50 °C for 30 min and over a wide pH range (4 to 10). Approximately 80%, 90% and 98% of bacteriophage particles adsorbed to the host cells within 10, 20 and 30 min after infection, respectively. One-step growth kinetics of the bacteriophage showed that the latent and burst periods were 30 and 150 min, respectively, and the burst size was about 79

PFU/infect cell. As shown by transmission electron microscopy, the bacteriophage had an icosahedral head of ca. 64 nm in diameter and a long noncontractile tail of ca. 157 nm long and 12 nm wide. Its genome was double stranded DNA, 70 kb in size. It was classified as a member of the family *Siphoviridae*. A total of 4 bacteriophage proteins with molecular masses of 15, 24, 32 and 81 kDa were detected by sodium dodcyl sulfate-polyacrylamide gel electrophoresis. Knowledge of the properties of bacteriophage PPST1 may be useful for the development of the bacteriophage to use as therapeutic agents against infections as a result of drug resistant *S.* Typhi

6. References

Ackermann, H.W. (2005). Bacteriophage classification, In: *Bacteriophages: Biology and applications*, E. Kutter & A. Sulakvelidze, (Ed.), 67-90, CRC Press, ISBN 978-0-8493-1336-3, Boca Raton, FL, USA

Bruttin, A. & Brussow, H. (2005). Human volunteers receiving *Escherichia coli* phage T4 orally: a safety test of phage therapy. *Antimicrobial Agents and Chemotherapy*, Vol. 49, No. 7, (July 2005), pp. 2874-2878, ISSN 1098-6596

Capparelli, R., Parlato, M., Borriello, G., Salvatore, P. & Iannelli, D. (2007). Experimental phage therapy against *Staphylococcus aureus* in mice. *Antimicrobial Agents and Chemotherapy*, Vol.51, No.8, (August 2007), pp. 2765-2773, ISSN 1098-6596

Carlton, R.M. (1999). Phage therapy: past history and future prospects. *Archivum Immunologiae et Therapiae Experimentalis*, Vol. 47, No.5, (September 1999), pp. 267-274, ISSN 1661-4917

Caso, J.L., De Los Reyes-Gavilan, C.G., Herrero, M., Montilla, A., Rodriguez, A. & Suarez, J.E. (1995). Isolation and characterization of temperate and virulent bacteriophages of *Lactobacillus plantarum*. *Journal of Dairy Science*, Vol.78, No.4, (April 1995), pp. 741-750, ISSN 1525-3198

Chang, H.C., Chen, C.R., Lin, J.W., Shen, G.H., Chang, K.M., Tseng, Y.H. & Weng, S.F. (2005). Isolation and characterization of novel giant *Stenotrophomonas maltophilia* phage ΦSMA5. *Applied and Environmental Microbiology*, Vol.71, No.3, (March 2005), pp. 1387-1393, ISSN 1098-5336

Chhibber, S., Kaur, S. & Kumari, S. (2008). Therapeutic potential of bacteriophage in treating *Klebsiella pneumoniae* B5055-mediated lobar pneumonia in mice. *Journal of Medical Microbiology*, Vol.57, No.12, (December 2008), pp. 1508-1513, ISSN 1473-5644

Coates, A., Hu, Y., Bax, R. & Page, C. (2002). The future challenges facing the development of new antimicrobial drugs. *Nature Reviews Drug Discovery*, Vol.1, No.11, (November 2002), pp. 895-910, ISSN 1474-1776

De Lappe, N., Doran, G., O'Connor, J., O'Hare, C. & Cormican, M. (2009). Characterization of bacteriophages used in the *Salmonella enterica* serovar Enteritidis phage-typing scheme. *Journal of Medical Microbiology*, Vol.58, No.1, (January 2009), pp. 86-93, ISSN 1473-5644

Demczuk, W., Ahmed, R. & Ackermann, H.W. (2004). Morphology of *Salmonella enterica* serovar Heidelberg typing phages. *Canadian Journal of Microbiology*, Vol.50, No.10, (October 2004), pp. 873-875, ISSN 1480-3275

Deresinski, S. (2009). Bacteriophage therapy: exploiting smaller fleas. *Clinical Infectious Diseases*, Vol.48, No.8, (April 2009), pp. 1096-1101, ISSN 1058-4838

Lu, Z., Breidt, F., Fleming, H.P., Altermann, E. & Klaenhammer, TR. (2003). Isolation and characterization of a *Lactobacillus plantarum* bacteriophage, ΦJL-1, from a cucumber fermentation. *International Journal of Food Microbiology*, Vol.84, No.2, (July 2003), pp. 225-235, ISSN 0618-1605

Matsuzaki, S., Rashel, M., Uchiyama, J., Sakurai, S., Ujiara, T., Kuroda, M., Ikeuchi, M., Tani, T., Fujieda, M., Wakiguchi, H. & Imai, S. (2005). Bacteriophage therapy: a revitalized therapy against bacterial infectious diseases. *Journal of Infection and Chemotherapy*, Vol.11, No.5, (October 2005), pp. 211-219, ISSN 1437-7780

McAuliffe, O., Ross, R.P. & Fitzgerald, GF. (2007). The New Phage Biology: From Genomics to Applications, In: *Bacteriophage: Genetics and Molecular Biology*, S. McGrath & D. van Sinderen, (Ed.), 1-42, Caister Acadamic Press, ISBN 978-1-904455-14-1, Norfolk, UK

McLaughlin, M.R., Balaa, M.F., Sims, J. & King, R. (2006). Isolation of Salmonella bacteriophages from swine effluent lagoons. *Journal of Environmental Quality*, Vol.35, No.2, (February 2006), pp. 522-528, ISSN 0047-2425

Mise, K., Kawai, M., Yoshida, Y. & Nakamura, A. (1981). Characterization of bacteriophage j2 of *Salmonella typhi* as a generalized transducing phage closely related to coliphage P1. *Journal of General Microbiology*, Vol.126, No.2, (October 1981), pp. 321-326, 0022-1287

Murray, P.R. (1994). Enterobacteriaceae, In: *Medical Microbiology*, R. Farrell, (Ed.), 227-240, Mosby Year Book Inc., ISBN 0723420106, London, UK

Nakai, T. & Park, S.C. (2002). Bacteriophage therapy of infectious diseases in aquaculture. *Research in Mirobiology*, Vol.153, No.1, (January 2002), pp. 13-18, ISSN 0923-2508

Nuekdee, K. (2007). Isolation and partial characterization of *Salmonella typhi*-specific bacteriophage. *Khon kaen University Science Journal*, Vol.35, No.3, (July 2007), pp. 162-169, ISSN 0125-2364

Paterson, W.D., Douglas, R.J., Grinyer, I. & McDermott, L.A. (1969). Isolation and preliminary characterization of some *Aeromonas salmonicida* bacteriophages. *Journal of the Fisheries Research Board of Canada*, Vol.26, No.3, (March 1969), pp. 629-632, ISSN 0015-296x

Rohwer, F. & Edwards, R. (2002). The Phage Proteomic Tree: a genome-based taxonomy for phage. *The Journal of Bacteriology*, Vol.184, No.16, (Auguat 2002), pp. 4529-4535, ISSN 1098-5530.

Rowe, B., Ward, L.R. & Threlfall, EJ. (1997). Multidrug-resistant *Salmonella typhi*: a worldwide epidemic. *Clinical Infectious Diseases*, Vol.24, Suppl. 1, (January 1997), pp. S106-S109, ISSN 1058-4838

Sundar, M.M., Nagananda, G.S., Das, A., Bhattacharya, S. & Suryan, S. (2009). Isolation of host-specific bacteriophages from sewage against human pathogens. *Asian Journal of Biotechnology*, Vol.1, No.4, (October 2009), pp. 163-170, ISSN 1996-0700

Thamniamton, W., Boonsarn, V., Phumkhachorn, P. & Rattanachaikunsopon, P. (2010). Isolation and characterization of a bacteriophage specific to drug resistant *Klebsiella pneumoniae* DR1. *International Journal of Current Research and Review*, Vol.2, No.4, (April 2010), pp. 30-43, ISSN 0975-5241

Trung, N.D., Suthisarnsuntorn, U., Kalambaheti, T., Wonglumsom, W. & Tunyong, W. (2007). Antimicrobial susceptibility patterns and phage types of *Salmonella typhi* from Vietnam. *Southeast Asian Journal of Tropical Medicine & Public Health*, Vol.38, No.3, (May 2007), pp. 487-492, ISSN 0038-3619

Verma, V., Harjai, K. & Chhibber, S. (2009). Characterization of a T7-like lytic bacteriophage of *Klebsiella pneumoniae* B5005: a potential therapeutic agent. *Current Microbiology*, Vol.59, No.3, (September 2009), pp. 274-281, ISSN 1432-0991

Vinod, M.G., Shivu, M.M., Umesha, K.R., Rajeeva, B.C., Krohne, G., Karunasagar, I. & Karunasagar, I. (2006). Isolation of *Vibrio harveyi* bacteriophage with a potential for biocontrol of luminous vibriosis in hatchery enviroments. *Aquaculture*, Vol.255, No.1-4, (May 2006), pp. 117-124, ISSN 0044-8486

Vinodkumar, C.S., Neelagund, Y.F. & Kalsurmath, S. (2005). Bacteriophage in the treatment of experimental septicemic mice from a clinical isolate of multidrug resistant *Klebsiella pneumoniae*. *Journal of Communicable Diseases*, Vol.37, No.1, (March 2005), pp. 18-29, ISSN . 0019-5138

9

The Seasonal Fluctuation of the Antimicrobial Activity of Some Macroalgae Collected from Alexandria Coast, Egypt

Mohamed E.H. Osman*, Atef M. Abu-Shady and Mostafa E. Elshobary
Botany Department, Faculty of Science, Tanta University, Tanta, Egypt

1. Introduction

Infectious diseases are a major cause of morbidity and mortality worldwide (WHO 2004). Synthetic drugs are not only expensive but are also often with adulterations and side effects. Therefore, there is a need to search for new strategies to control microbial infections (Sieradzki and Tomasz 1999). Pharmaceutical industries are increasingly recognizing the importance of compounds derived from soil plants and other sources such as marine organisms (McGee 2006).

The biodiversity of the marine ecosystem provides an important source of chemical compounds, which have many therapeutic applications such as antiviral, antibacterial, antifungal and anticancer activities (Caccamese and Azzolina 1979; Perez *et al.* 1990; Harada and Kamei 1997; Siddhanta *et al.* 1997; Pereira *et al.* 2004). The ability of seaweeds to produce secondary metabolites of potential interest has been extensively documented (Faulkner 1993). There are numerous reports concerning compounds derived from macroalgae with a broad range of biological activities, such as antibiotics (antibacterial and antifungal properties), as well as characteristics pertaining antiviral effects (Trono 1999), antitumors and anti-inflammator mechanisms (Scheuer 1990) as well as protections against neurotoxins (Kobashi 1989).

Transplant experiments suggest that environmental conditions are able to alter the concentrations of secondary metabolites although the types of compounds are genetically fixed (Hay 1996). Also, physical stress such as desiccation, UV and visible light and nutrient availability are able to alter secondary metabolites in seaweeds (Watson and Cruz-Rivera 2003).

Alexandria, Egypt has an extensive coast where seaweeds from virtually all groups are present. In our previous work (Osman *et al.* 2010) we tested in vitro the antimicrobial activity of some seaweed collected from Alexandria coast with special reference to the type of solvent used for extraction. In the present work, we aimed to study the seasonal fluctuation in production of the antimicrobial active substances from the collected seaweeds.

---

* Corresponding Author

2. Materials and methods

2.1 Collection of algae

In our study, 13 species of seaweeds (6 Rhodophyceae, 4 Chlorophyceae and 3 Phaeophyceae) were collected seasonally at depths of 0.2 m or less for Chlorophyceae and 1 m for Rhodophyceae and Phaeophyceae from Rocky Bay of Abu Qir (N 31° 19` E 030° 03`) (Plate 1). All samples were brought to the laboratory in plastic bags containing sea water to prevent evaporation. Algae were then cleaned from epiphytes and rock debris and given a quick fresh water rinse to remove surface salts. The collected seaweeds were preserved for identification. All seaweeds were identified following the methods of Abbott and Hollenberg (1976), Taylor (1960), and Aleem (1993). The collected species were identified as *Jania rubens* (Linnaeus) Lamouroux, *Corallina elongata* Ellis and Solander *Pterocladia capillacea* (Gmelin) Bornet *ex* Bornet and Thuret, *Galaxaura fragilis* (Ellis et Solanoer) Lamouroux), *Laurencia obtusa* (Hudson) Lamouroux and *Hypnea valentiae* (Turner)Montagne from Rhodophyceae, *Ulva fasciata* Agardh , *Ulva lactuca* (Linnaeus), *Enteromorpha compressa* (Linnaeus) Greville and *Enteromorpha linza* (Linnaeus) Agardh from Chlorophyceae, and *Sargassum vulgare* Agardh, *Padina pavonica* (Linnaeus) Thivy and *Colpomenia sinuosa* (Mertens ex Roth) Derbes and Solier from Phaeophyceae.

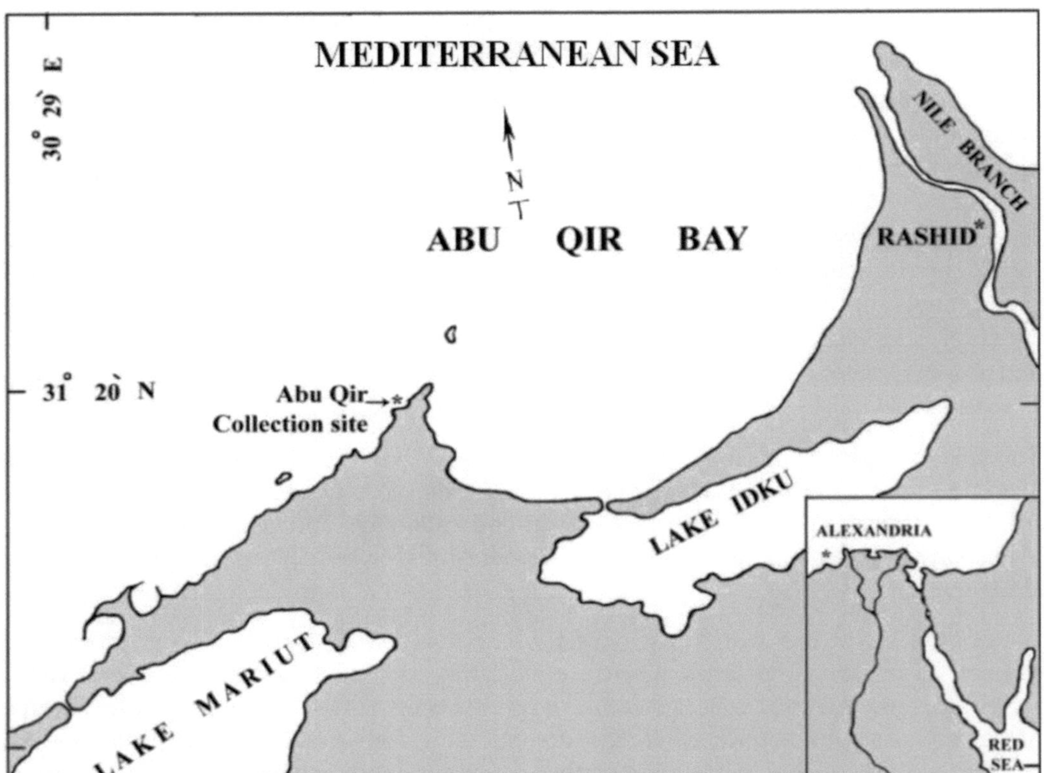

Plate 1. Location of study area

2.2 Test microorganisms

Seven pathogenic microorganisms were isolated from different patients at Tanta university hospital, and primary identified it in microbiology section in Botany Department, Faculty of Science, Tanta University, Egypt. They included (*Bacillus subtilis, Staphylococcus aureus* and *Streptococcus sp.*) as Gram-positive bacteria, (*Escherichia coli, Salmonella typhi and Klebsiella pneumoniae*) as Gram-negative bacteria and one yeast strain *Candida albicans.*

2.3 Determination of the optimum solvent for extraction the antagonistic material from collected seaweeds

Nine seaweeds listed in Table 1 were collected randomly and clean materials were air dried in the shade at room temperature 25°C -30°C on absorbent paper, then ground to fine powder in an electrical coffee mill. Extraction was carried out with different solvents (i.e., 70% ethanol, 70% methanol and 70% acetone) by soaking in the respective solvents (1:15 v/v) on a rotary shaker at 150 rpm at room temperature (25°C-30°C) for 72h. Varying solvent extractions were carried out individual samples. Extracts from three consecutive soakings were pooled and filtered using filter paper (Whatman No. 4), and the obtained filtrate was freed from the solvent by evaporation under reduced pressure. The residues (crude extracts) obtained were suspended in the respective solvents to a final concentration of 100mg/ml, then stored at -20°C in an airtight bottle.

2.4 Seasonal variation of the antimicrobial activity

To evaluate the possible influence of sampling season on antimicrobial activity, the maximum possible number of different tested seaweeds in each season (winter, spring, summer and autumn) were collected. Seaweeds were collected by hand every 3 months in (viz.,October-2007, January-2008, April-2008 and July-2008), then cleaned, air-dried, ground to a fine powder and extracted for 72 h as previously described using the suitable solvent. Residues were concentrated to 100 mg/ml and stored at -20°C in an airtight bottle until used. Seasonal variations in air temperature, water temperature and pH value were also measured at the time of each collection.

2.5 Antimicrobial activity test

Fifteen ml of the sterilized media (nutrient agar (Oxoid, Basingstoke, U.K.)) for bacteria and Sabouraud dextrose agar (for yeast) were poured into sterile capped test tubes. Test tubes were allowed to cool to 50°C in a water bath and 0.5 ml of a uniform mixture of inocula (10^8 CFU for bacteria and yeast) were added. Tubes were mixed using a vortex mixer vibrating at 1500-2000 revolutions min^{-1} for 15-30 seconds. Contents from each test tube was then poured into sterile 100 mm diameter Petri dishes for solidification (Mtolera and Semesi 1996).

The antimicrobial activity was evaluated using a well-cut diffusion technique (El-Masry *et al.* 2000). Wells were punched out using a sterile 0.7 cm cork borer in suitable media agar plates inoculated with the test microorganism. Approximately 50 µL of various algal extracts were transferred into each well. For each microorganism, controls were maintained where pure solvents were used instead of the extract. All plates were subjected to 4°C incubation for 2 hours. To prevent drying, plates were covered with sterile plastic bags and later incubated at 37°C for 24 hours (Mtolera and Semesi 1996). Result was obtained by measuring the inhibition zone diameter for each well expressed in millimeters. The experiment was carried out three times and mean values were recorded.

Seaweeds		Solvents (70%)	*B. subtilis*	*Staph. aureus*	*Strept. sp*	*E. coli*
Rhodophyta	*J. rubens*	Ethanol	^{a}12.2±0.3	^{a}11.3±0.3	^{a}11.5±0.5	12.0±1.0
		Methanol	^{ab}12.8±0.7	^{ab}11.8±0.3	^{ab}12.5±0.5	14.0±0.0
		Acetone	^{b}14.0±0.1	^{b}12.1±0.1	^{b}13.0±0.0	16.0±0.0
	F-Value		**11.45***	**7.72**$^{(n.s)}$	**10.5***	**36****
	Cor. elongata	Ethanol	^{a}13.8±0.3	13.2±0.3	^{a}13.0±0.0	^{a}13.0±1.0
		Methanol	^{cb}15.3±0.5	13.7±0.2	^{a}14.0±1.0	^{a}14.3±0.5
		Acetone	^{b}16.2±0.3	15.0±0.0	^{a}14.3±0.5	^{b}19.8±0.1
	F-Value		**23.6****	**53.6****	**3.3**$^{(n.s)}$	**88.6****
	Ptero. capillacea	Ethanol	^{a}11.6±0.5	^{a}10.5±0.5	^{a}11.3±0.5	^{a}13.0±0.0
		Methanol	^{a}13.0±1.0	^{ab}13.0±0.0	^{a}11.8±0.7	^{a}13.6±0.5
		Acetone	^{a}13.3±0.2	^{b}13.5±0.5	^{b}13.0±0.0	^{a}17.0±0.0
	F-Value		**5.3**$^{(n.s)}$	**46.5****	**124****	**3.11**$^{(n.s)}$
Chlorophyta	*U. fasciata*	Ethanol	15.3±0.5	^{a}16.2±0.2	^{a}16.0±1.0	^{a}17.6±1.2
		Methanol	18.0±1.0	^{a}17.0±0.0	^{a}18.6±0.6	^{a}19.2±0.3
		Acetone	22.2±0.2	^{b}19.3±1.1	^{a}20.0±1.0	^{b}24.6±0.5
	F-Value		**78.02****	**16.8***	**6.8**$^{(n.s)}$	**69.8****
	U. lactuca	Ethanol	^{a}14.6±1.7	^{a}12.2±0.7	^{a}13.0±1.0	^{a}13.0±0.0
		Methanol	^{a}16.0±0.0	^{a}12.6±0.5	^{a}13.5±0.5	^{a}13.5±0.5
		Acetone	^{b}19.0±0.0	^{b}17.6±0.7	^{b}15.5±0.5	^{b}15.6±0.5
	F-Value		**14.4****	**55.5****	**10.5***	**31****
	E. compressa	Ethanol	^{a}14.3±0.3	^{a}12.0±0.0	^{a}13.5±0.3	^{a}14.6±0.5
		Methanol	^{cb}16.5±0.8	^{cb}15.5±0.5	^{a}14 ±1.8	^{a}16.5±0.0
		Acetone	^{c}17.1±0.3	^{c}16.0±1.4	^{b}16.6±0.5	^{a}16.6±0.5
	F-Value		**19.8****	**34.2****	**93****	**4.04**$^{(n.s)}$
	E. linza	Ethanol	^{a}14.0 ±1.7	^{a}13.0±1.0	^{a}13.5±0.5	^{a}11.8±0.3
		Methanol	^{a}15.0±0.0	^{a}14.5±0.5	^{a}15.0±1.0	^{ab}12.6±0.5
		Acetone	^{a}17.0±0.0	^{a}15.3±1.2	^{a}15.6±1.5	^{a}13.6±0.5
	F-Value		**99999****	**4.44**$^{(n.s)}$	**3.09**$^{(n.s)}$	**10.1***
Phaeophyceae	*Col. sinuosa*	Ethanol	^{a}11.3±1.5	^{a}11.0±1.1	^{a}11.5±0.5	^{a}11.6±1.5
		Methanol	^{a}11.6±0.5	^{ab}12.0±1.0	^{a}11.8±0.7	^{a}13.0±1.0
		Acetone	^{a}12.5±1.5	^{b}14.0±0.0	^{a}13.0±1.0	^{a}14.0±1.0
	F-Value		**0.6**$^{(n.s)}$	**10.50***	**3.05**$^{(n.s)}$	**2.85**$^{(n.s)}$
	Sar. vulgare	Ethanol	^{a}10.3 ±0.5	^{a}11.0±0.5	^{a}10.2±0.7	^{a}10.0±0.0
		Methanol	^{a}11.0±1.0	^{a}11.2±0.7	^{a}10.5±0.5	^{ab}11±0.5
		Acetone	^{a}12.0±1.0	^{b}15.6±0.3	^{a}11.5±0.5	^{b}12.0±1.0
	F-Value		**2.7**$^{(n.s)}$	**68.8****	**4**$^{(n.s)}$	**9***

Means with the same letter are insignificant using one way analysis of variance (ANOVA).
* Significant at $P \leq 0.01$,** Significant at $P \leq 0.001$ and (ns) Non-significant at $P \leq 0.01$ using one way analysis of variance (ANOVA).

Table 1. Antimicrobial activity of different seaweeds extracted with different solvents. (±) standard deviation of the means (n=3)

2.6 Purification of the most active crude extract

The most active crude extract was partially purified using the TLC technique with glass plates (20x20 cm). The flow rate of the active material was determined using different eluent systems. The elution of the active material was made using of the following eluents.

1. Ethyl acetate: methanol: hexane (2:1.5:0.5 v/v) (Wagner and Bladt 1996)
2. Hexane: ethyl acetate (3:2 v/v) (Wendy and Diana 2007)
3. Benzene: ethyl acetate (3:1 v/v) (Sastry and Rao 1995)
4. Butanol: acetic acid: water (4:1:5 v/v) (Partridge 1948)

The developed spot was scrapped off and dissolved in pure acetone. The solution was centrifuged to remove the silica gel and the supernatant was dried under reduced pressure to dryness and stored at 4°C. The developed spot was examined for the antimicrobial activity using well-cut diffusion technique.

2.7 Statistical analysis

Results are presented as mean ± SD (standard deviation) for three replicates. The statistical analyses were carried out using SAS programming (1989-1996) version 6.12. Data obtained were analyzed statistically to determine the degree of significance between treatments using one, two, and three way analysis of variance (ANOVA) at $P \leq 0.01$ and $P \leq 0.001$ levels of significance.

3. Results

Results of the antimicrobial activity of different organic crude extracts are summarized in Table 1. Acetone (70%) extracts showed the strongest inhibitory effect against the tested microorganisms relative to other solvents with inhibition activity percentage* on 36.7%, followed by 70% methanol extracts with inhibition activity percentage 32.9%, whereas, 70% ethanol extracts showed the weakest inhibition with inhibition activity percentage 30.2% of all tested microorganisms.

$$\text{*Inhibition activity percentage} = \frac{\text{Average diameter of inhibition zone of each solvent}}{\text{Average diameter of inhibition zone of all solvents}} \text{ X } 100$$

The statistical analyses using one way ANOVA confirm that the effect of antimicrobial activities for most treatments were significant (Table 1). Three-way ANOVA confirmed that the variation in the antimicrobial activity in relation to seaweeds, microorganisms, solvents and their interactions were significant at $P \leq 0.001$ (Table 2).

Source	DF	F Value	P-value	R2
Seaweeds	8	325.3	0.0001	95.5%
Microorganisms	6	20.4	0.0001	
Solvents	2	387.2	0.0001	
Seaweeds*Microorganisms	48	6.7	0.0001	
Seaweeds*Solvents	16	4.5	0.0001	
Microorganisms*Solvents	12	3.9	0.0001	
Microorganisms*Solvents* Seaweeds	96	1.73	0.0002	

Table 2. Three-way analysis of variance (ANOVA) of different seaweeds extracts against different microorganisms using different solvents.

The results for the acetone extracts from each season are summarized in Figure 1, 2, 3 and 4. However, data of environmental parameters are reported in Table 3.

Environmental Parameters	**Seasons**			
	Autumn (2007)	**Winter (2008)**	**Spring (2008)**	**Summer (2008)**
Air temperature in °C	26.3	19	24	31.3
Water temperature in °C	20.4	14	14	21.5
pH value	8.0	7.9	7.5	8.1

Table 3. Environmental parameters of the sampling site in each collection time.

In autumn (October, 2007) four seaweeds samples were collected (2 Rhodophyceae *and* 2 Chlorophyceae). The results show that the red seaweeds extract exhibited stronger antimicrobial activity than the green. For red seaweeds, *Cor. elongata* was most active and exhibited the most inhibition *for K. pneumoniae with* an inhibition zone of 15.7 mm. With respect to green seaweeds, *U. fasciata* showed the strongest activity which exhibited most inhibition for *Strept. sp* with inhibition zone of 15 mm (Fig. 1).

In winter (January, 2008) five samples of seaweeds were collected (3 Rhodophyceae and 2 Chlorophyceae). Results demonstrated that extract of green seaweeds was more active than red seaweeds. The highest antimicrobial activity of the collected green seaweeds species was observed in *U. fasciata,* which had the strongest inhibition against *K. pneumoniae* with an inhibition zone diameter of 24.6 mm. *However, the red seaweeds, Cor. elongate* showed the highest antimicrobial activity than others. *The most sensitive microorganism for Cor. elongate was K. pneumoniae* showing an inhibition zone of 19.8 mm *(Fig.* 2)

In spring (April, 2008) nine seaweeds samples were collected (3 Rhodophyceae, 4 Chlorophyceae and 2 Phaeophyceae). The obtained data show that the extract of tested red seaweeds was more active than green and brown seaweeds, respectively. The most active specie was *Cor. elongata. Sensitivity responses showed that K. pneumoniae* exhibited the *highest sensitivity for Cor. elongata* extract *with* an inhibition zone of 21.6 mm. Among the green seaweeds, obtained results show that *U. fasciata* has the strongest antimicrobial action. *K. pneumoniae* exhibited *higher sensitivity for U. fasciata* with an inhibition zone of 17.2 mm. Concerning brown seaweeds, results show that *Sar. vulgare extract showed higher antimicrobial activity* than *Col. sinuosa,* where *Staph. aureus* exhibited *higher sensitivity for Sar. vulgare* with an inhibition zone of 15.6 mm. (Fig. 3)

In the summer (June, 2008) ten seaweeds were collected (5 Rhodophyceae, 3 Chlorophyceae and 2 Phaeophyceae). The extracts of collected green seaweeds exhibited the strongest antimicrobial activity followed by red and brown species. The results show that the most active one was that from *U. fasciata*. The most sensitive microorganism for *U. fasciata* extract was *Strept. sp.* with an inhibition zone of 14.5 mm. With regard to red seaweeds, the obtained data show that the most active one was *Gal. fragilis;* however, *Can. albicans* exhibited *higher sensitivity for Gal. fragilis* with an inhibition zone of 12.0 mm. Concerning brown seaweeds, the obtained results showed that *P. pavonia was the strongest* antimicrobial activity which exhibited the highest inhibitory effect against *Sal. typhi* with an inhibition zone of 12 mm. (Fig. 4). The statistical analyses using two-way ANOVA confirmed that the variation in antimicrobial activities in relation to seaweeds, microorganisms and their interactions were significant at $Pr \geq 0.001$ for all treatments (Table 4).

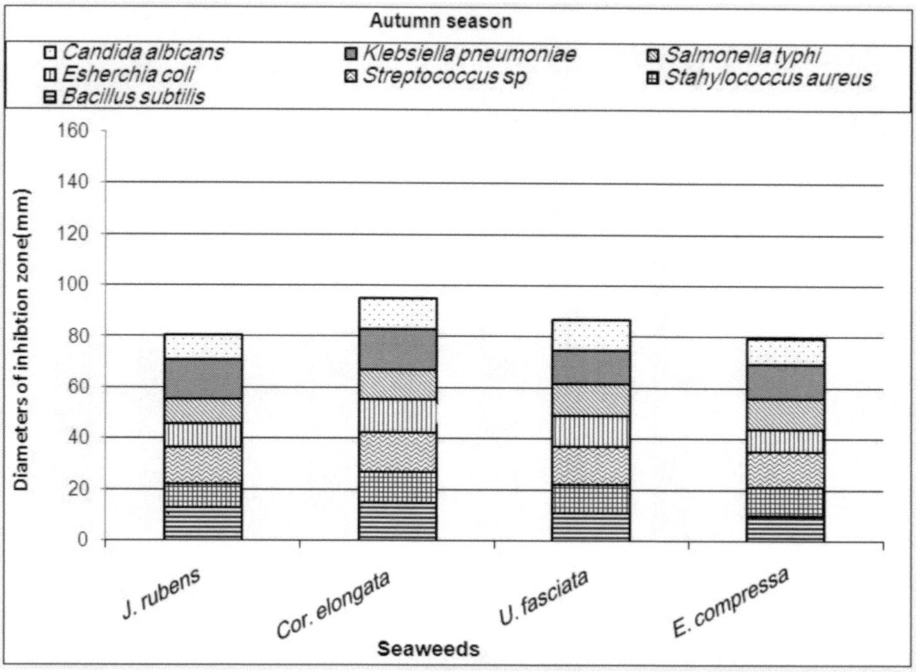

Fig. 1. Diameter of inhibition zone of autumn collected seaweeds against each tested microorganism.

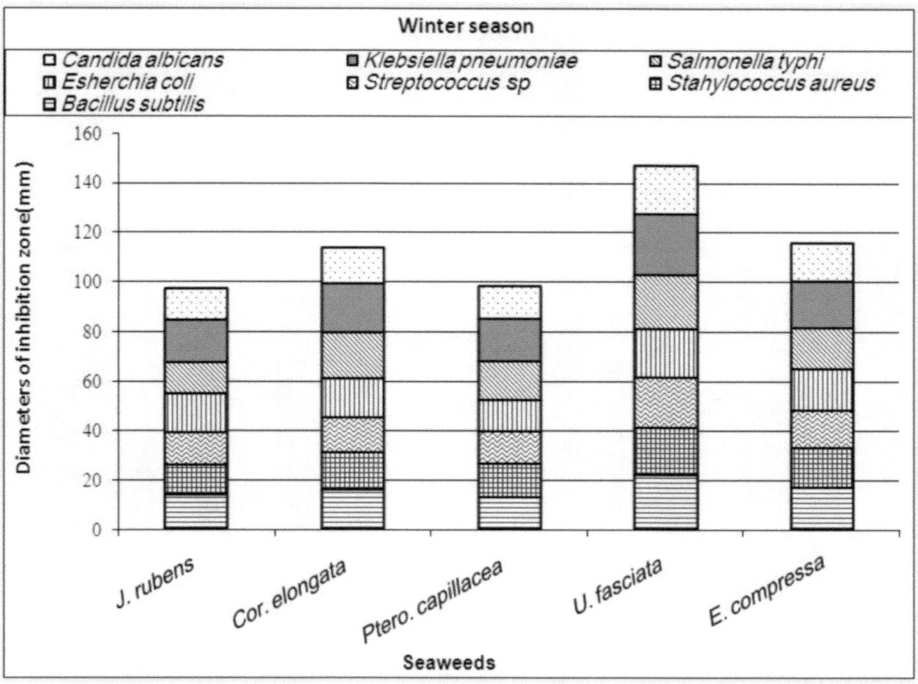

Fig. 2. Diameter of inhibition zone of winter collected seaweeds against each tested microorganism.

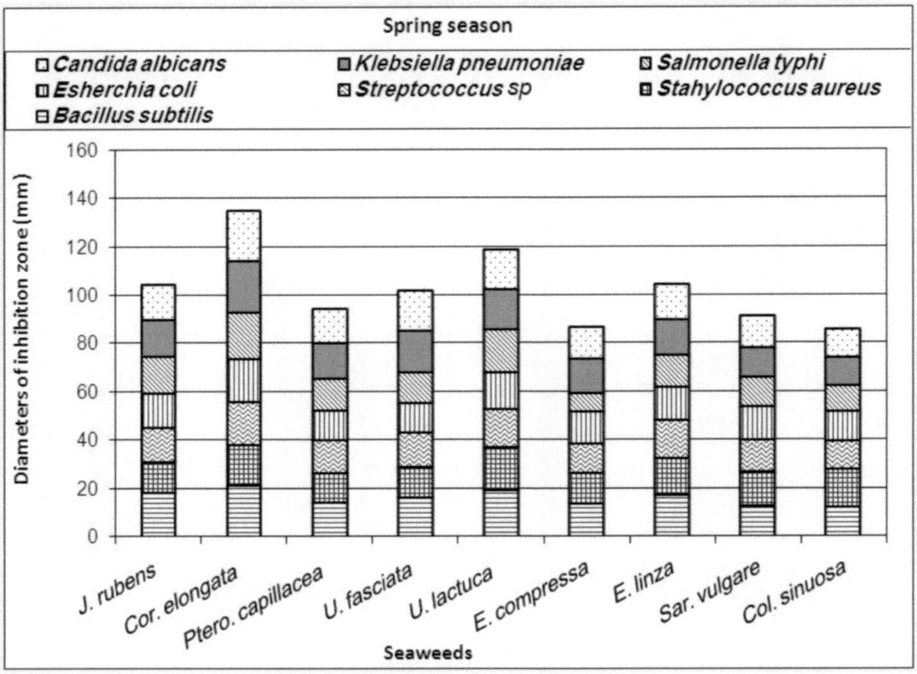

Fig. 3. Diameter of inhibition zone of spring collected seaweeds against each tested microorganism.

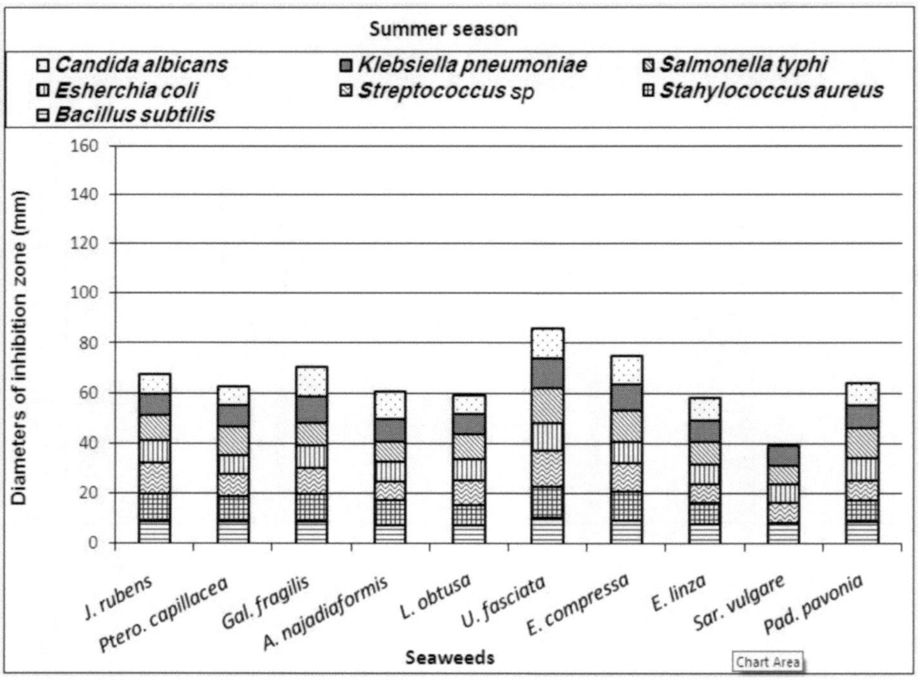

Fig. 4. Diameter of inhibition zone of summer collected seaweeds against each tested microorganism.

Seasons	Source	DF	F Value	P-value	R2
Autumn	Seaweeds	3	44.1	0.0001	92.7%
	Microorganisms	6	72.1	0.0001	
	Seaweeds*Microorganisms	18	8.3	0.0001	
Winter	Seaweeds	4	528.9	0.0001	97.7%
	Microorganisms	6	112.7	0.0001	
	Seaweeds*Microorganisms	24	9.3	0.0001	
Spring	Seaweeds	8	145.3	0.0001	93.0%
	Microorganisms	6	26.0	0.0001	
	Seaweeds*Microorganisms	48	7.7	0.0001	
Summer	Seaweeds	9	206.3	0.0001	96.2%
	Microorganisms	6	42.1	0.0001	
	Seaweeds*Microorganisms	54	26.8	0.0001	

Table 4. Two-way analysis of variance (ANOVA) of seasonal collected seaweeds extracts against different microorganisms

3.1 Seasonal variation of antimicrobial activity

Species of green and red seaweeds were found and collected in four seasons whereas brown seaweeds were collected only in spring and summer. The highest activity of the different seaweeds extracts were those collected in spring, followed by winter, summer and autumn, respectively (Fig. 5). According to the taxonomic group level, the most active extracts were

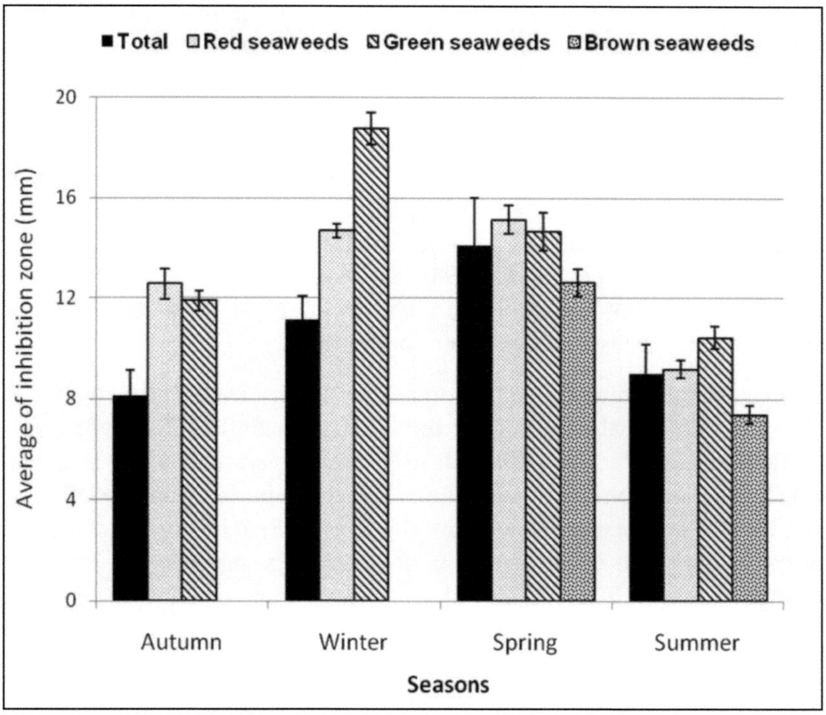

Fig. 5. Seasonal variation of antimicrobial activity of different seaweeds extracts.

the green seaweeds. The antimicrobial activity of the different species with respect to different seasons could be arranged in the following order, green seaweeds in winter > spring > autumn > summer followed by red seaweeds in spring > winter > autumn > summer and brown seaweeds in spring > summer. The above-mentioned results indicate that the promising seaweed for production of antimicrobial antagonistic material was winter-collected *U. fasciata* (Chlorophyceae).

The suitable solvent system used in the TLC technique was ethyl acetate: methanol: hexane (2:1.5:0.5 v/v). The obtained result show that there are three spots formed with different R_f values (0.5, 0.6, 0.6 and 0.7). All spots were examined against *K. pneumoniae* and the most active one had an R_f value of 0.53 with an inhibition zone of 30 mm. This spot is currently undergoing further analysis to determine the nature and identify of the active constituents.

The statistical analyses conducted using three-way ANOVA confirmed that the effects of different seasons, seaweeds, microorganisms and their interactions on antimicrobial activity were highly significant.

4. Discussion

The present study showed that 70% acetone could be considered a good solvent for extracting the bioactive substance in the studied seaweeds against the tested microorganisms. However, Tüney *et al.* (2006) reported that diethyl ether was the best solvent for extracting the bioactive compounds of 11 seaweeds species from the coast of Urla, which agreed with Wefky and Ghobrial (2008) and Fareed and Khairy (2008).

Macroalgae are already well-documented as possess antibacterial activities against pathogenic bacteria (Kumar and Rengasamy 2000; Lipton 2004; Tüney *et al.* 2006; Karabay-Yavasoglu *et al.* 2007; Salvador *et al.* 2007; Chiheb *et al.* 2009). The results reported by the above-mentioned authors are in accordance with our data, which demonstrated that the collected seaweeds have antimicrobial activity against the tested microorganisms. In contrast to our results, Salvador *et al.* (2007) detected that some seaweeds such as *Ptero. capillacea* showed no antimicrobial activity in any seasons. Gonzalez del Val (2001) also demonstrated that the extract of *Enter. compressa* showed no antimicrobial activity against the tested microorganisms. Perez *et al.* (1990) observed that the extract of *U. lactuca* had no antibacterial activity. These differences in activity may be due to different seaweeds developmental stages, locality and extraction methods, *etc.*

In relation to taxonomic groups, Reichelt and Borowitzka (1984) and Salvador *et al.* (2007) screened many species of algae for their antibacterial activity. They reported that the members of the red algae family exhibited high antibacterial activity. In contrast, in our study, green algae (Chlorophyceae) were the most active species. The present results agreed with the results of Kandhasamy and Arunachalam (2008) who reported that green algae (Chlorophyceae) were more active taxa than others and also agreed with Fareed and Khairy (2008) who showed that *U. lactua* (Chlorophyceae) were more active when compared with *J. rubens* (Rhodophyceae).

Some pure compounds from algae have been identified as natural antimicrobial; however, the relationship between their ecologic role and their antimicrobial activity is not fully understood in many studies which were based on the screening of antimicrobial activities from macroalgae. These studies determined that the range of chemical defenses can differ from narrow to broad spectrum, depending on the extraction method, the algae species, the collected season of the algae, algal growth phases, *etc.* The variation in the production of secondary metabolites has been reported for a variety of marine algae (Hay 1996). In the present study, we focused on the possibility that antimicrobial activity will fluctuate seasonally. Abu Qir (Alexandria, Egypt) was chosen as a sample site, so geographical and spatial variation was eliminated.

As regards seasonal variation of bioactivity, for all of the tested subdivisions, spring was the season with the highest activity against test microorganisms, followed by winter. These results are in accordance with those obtained from Atlantic samples by Hornsey and Hide (1974), from Mediterranean samples by Khaleafa *et al.* (1975) and Stirk and Reinecke (2007) who reported that seasonal variation in antibacterial activity was observed with extracts which have antibacterial activity in late winter and early spring. This is in contrast to studies carried out by Rao and Parekh (1981), and Arun, Kumar and Rengasamy (2000) using Indian samples, and from Mediterranean samples by Martí *et al.* (2004) who demonstrated the most active season was autumn. Salvador *et al.* (2007), nevertheless, demonstrated that autumn and spring were the seasons with the highest percentage of active taxa against at least one test microorganism (69% and 67% respectively), followed by winter (56%) and summer (50%).

It is worthy to mention that Abu Qir Bay is a very important productive area of the Mediterranean Sea on the Egyptian coast, since it receives nutrient-rich brackish water from Lake Edku as well as the El-Tabia pump station. The obtained data in this study demonstrated that environmental parameters (air and water temperature and pH) showed insignificant correlations with antimicrobial activities of tested seaweeds. Moreover, Shams El-Din *et al.* (2007) studied the nutrient concentration in Abu Qir and found that the correlation coefficient between nutrients and the natural components in some seaweeds were not significant, which may be due to the water deterioration, resulting from the acute eutrophication and the increase of pollution stress in the bay.

In the present study *U. fasciata* (green seaweeds) was the most effective seaweeds species, having antibacterial activity throughout the year compared to other seaweeds screened for antibacterial activity. *Ulva fasciata* inhibited the growth of all tested microorganisms, which agreed with Selvin and Lipton (2004) reported that the green alga *U. fasciata* exhibited broad-spectrum antibacterial activity.

These results show that *U. fasciata* extracts of the winter collection exhibited stronger antimicrobial effects followed by spring season (more so than summer or autumn) which agrees with Stirk and Reinecke (2007) who demonstrated that *U. fasciata* collected in winter and spring seasons were more active against tested organisms when compared to other seasons. This may be influenced by the seasonal variation as extracts of *U. fasciata* from winter and spring collection were more potent as compared to the summer and autumn collection, the former representing the peak growing and reproductive season, while the later is the stasis and senescence period for *U. fasciata* growth. The better antimicrobial action of winter collection is possibly due to the elevated biochemical constituents during the growing and reproductive phase of the *U. fasciata*. This hypothesis is further strengthened by Hornsey and Hide (1974), Daly and Prince (1981), Moreau *et al.* (1984) and Rao and Indusekhar (1989)

Finally, we conclude that macroalgae from Abu Qir coast in Alexandria are potential sources of bioactive compounds. The production of these compounds could be affected by seasonal variation and should be investigated for natural antimicrobial properties. Furthermore, *U. fasciata* collected in the winter could be considered the most active species for production of antagonistic materials. Thus, the suitable season for collection of seaweeds producing antimicrobial activity must be taken in consideration.

5. References

Abbott I.A. & Hollenberg I.G. (1976). Marine algae of California Stanford University press. pp. 827.

Aleem A.A. (1993). Marine algae of Alexandria, Egypt. Alexandria: Privately published.pp. [i-iv], [1]-135.

Caccamese S. & Azzolina R. (1979). Screening for antimicrobial activities in marine algae from eastern Sicily. Planta Med. 37:333–339.

Chiheb I.; Riadi H.; Martinez-Lopez J.; Dominguez S.J.F.; Gomez V.J.A.; Bouziane H.& Kadiri M. (2009). Screening of antibacterial activity in marine green and brown macroalgae from the coast of Morocco. Afr. J. Biotechnol. 8 (7):1258-1262.

Daly J.E.L. & Prince J.S. (1981). The ecology of Sargassum pteropleuron Grunow (Phaeophyceae, Fucales) in the waters off South Florida. III, Seasonal variation in alginic acid concentration. Phycologia. 20: 352–357.

El-Masry H.A.; Fahmy H.H. & Abdelwahed A.S.H. (2000). Synthesis and antimicrobial activity of some new benzimidazole derivatives. Molecules. 5:1429-1438.

Fareed M.F. & Khairy H.M. (2008). In vitro antimicrobial activities of seaweeds collected from Abu Qir bay Alexandria, Egypt. World App. Sci. J. 5 (4):389-396.

Faulkner D.J. (1993). Marine natural products chemistry: introduction. Chem. Rev. 93:1671–1673.

Gonzalez del Val A.; Platas G. & Basilio A. (2001). Screening of antimicrobial activities in red, green and brown macroalgae from Gran Canaria (Canary Islands, Spain). Int. Microbiol. 4:35-40.

Harada H. & Kamei Y. (1997). Selective cytotoxicity of marine algae extracts to several human leukemic cell lines. Cytotechnology. 25:213–219.

Hay M.E. (1996). Marine chemical ecology: what's known and what next? J. Exp. Mar. Biol. Ecol. 200:103–134.

Hornsey I.S. & Hide D. (1974). The production of antimicrobial substances by British marine algae I. Antibiotic producing marine algae. Br. Phycol. J. 9:353–361.

Kandhasamy M. & Arunachalam K.D. (2008). Evaluation of in vitro antibacterial property of seaweeds of southeast coast of India. Afr. J. Biotechnol. 7(12):1958-1961.

Karabay-Yavasoglu N.U.; Sukatar A.; Ozdemir G. & Horzum Z. (2007). Antimicrobial activity of volatile components and various extracts of the red alga Jania rubens. Phytother. Res. 21: 153-156.

Khaleafa A.F.; Kharboush A.M.; Metwalli A.A.; Mohsen F. & Serwi A. (1975). Anitibiotic fungicidal action from extracts of some seaweeds. Bot. Mar. 18: 163-165.

Kobashi K. (1989). Pharmacologically active metabolites from symbiotic microalgae in Okinawan marine invertebrates. J. Nat. Prod. 52:225-238.

Kumar K.A. & Rengasamy R. (2000). Evaluation of antibacterial potential of seaweeds occurring along the coast of Tamil Nadu, India against the plant pathogenic bacterium Xanthomonas oryzae pv. oryzae (Ishiyama) Dye Bot. Mar. 5(43): 409-415.

Martí R.; Uriz M.J. & Turon X. (2004). Seasonal and spatial variation of species toxicity in Mediterranean seaweeds communities: correlation to biotic and abiotic factors. Mar. Ecol. Prog. Ser. 282:73-85.

McGee P. (2006). Natural products re-emerge. Drug Disc. Develop. 9:18–26.

Moreau J.; Pesando D. & Bernad P. (1988). Seasonal variations in the production of antifungal substances by some Dictyotales (brown algae) from French Mediterranean coast. Hydrobiology, 162:157-162.

Mtolera M. S.P. & Semesi A.K. (1996). Antimicrobial activity of extracts from six green algae from Tanzania. In: Current Trends in Marine Botanical Research in the East African Region. Uppsala, Sweden, Gotab AB. pp. 211-217.

Osman M.E.H.; Abushady A.M. & Elshobary M.E. (2010). In vitro screening of antimicrobial activity of extracts of some macroalgae collected from Abu Qir bay Alexandria, Egypt. African Journal of Biotechnology 9(12): 7203-7208.

Ozdemir G.; Horzum Z.; Sukatar A. & Karabay-Yavasoglu N.U. (2006). Antimicrobial activity of volatile component and various extracts of Enteromorpha linza (Linnaeus) J. Agardh from the coast of Izmir, Turkey Annals of Microbiology, 56(3): 275-279

Partridge S.M. (1948). Filter paper Partition Chromatography of Sugars. I. General Description and Application to the Qualitative Analysis of Sugars in Apple Juice, Egg White and Foetal Blood of Sheep. Bioehem. 42:238-250.

Pereira HS.; Lea˜o-Ferreira L.R.; Moussatche ´N.; Teixeira V.L.; Cavalcanti D.N.; Costa L.J.; Diaz R. & Frugulhetti I.C. (2004). Antiviral activity of diterpenes isolated from the Brazilian marine alga Dictyota menstrualis against human immunodeficiency virus type 1 (HIV-1). Antiviral Res. 64:69–76.

Perez R.M.; Avila J.G.; Perez S.; Martinez A. & Martinez G. (1990). Antimicrobial activity of some American algae. J. Ethnopharmacol. 29:111–116.

Rao C.K. & Indusekhar V.K. (1989). Seasonal variation in chemical constituents of certain brown seaweeds and seawater from Saurashtra coast. I. Carbon, nitrogen and phosphorus. Mahasagar. 22: 63–72.

Rao P.S. & Parekh K.S. (1981). Antibacterial activities of Indian seaweeds extracts. Bot. Mar. 24:577–582.

Reicheltl J.L. & Borowitzka M.A. (1984). Antimicrobial activity from marine algae: Results of a large-scale screening programme. Hydrobiologia. 116/117 158-168.

SAS (1996). Copyright (c) 1989-1996 by SAS Institute Inc., Cary, NC, USA. SAS (r) Proprietary Software Release 6.12 TS020.

Salvador N.; Gomez-Garreta A.; Lavelli L. & Ribera M.A. (2007). Antimicrobial activity of Iberian macroalgae. Sci. Mar. 71:101-113.

Sastry V.M.V.S. & Rao G.R.K. (1995). *Dioctyl phthalate,* and antibacterial compound from the marine brown alga *Sargassum wightii*. J. Appl. Phycol. 7:185-186.

Scheuer P.J. (1990). Some marine ecological phenomena: chemical basis and biomedical potential. Science. 248:173-177.

Selvin J. & Lipton A.P. (2004). Biopotentials of *U. fasciata* and *hypnea musciformis* collected from the peninsular coast of india J. Mar. Sci. Technol. 12: (1)1-6.

Shams El-Din N.G.; Amer A.M. & Abdallah M.A. (2007). Study of natural components in some marine macroalgae in relation to nutrients along Alexandria coast, Egypt. Egyptian Journal of Aqu. Res. 33(2): 87-112.

Siddhanta A.K.; Mody K.H.; Ramavat B.K.; Chauhan V.D.; Garg H.S.; Goel A.K.; Doss M.J.; Srivastava M.N.; Patnaik G.K. & Kamboj V.P. (1997). Bioactivity of marine organisms: Part VIII–Screening of some marine flora of western coast of India. Indian J. Exp. Biol. 35:638–643.

Sieradzki K.W.S.W. & Tomasz A. (1999). Inactivation of the methicillin resistance gene mecA in vancomycin-resistant Staphylococcus aureus. Micro. Drug. Resist. 5: 253-257.

Stirk W.A. & Reinecke D.L. (2007). Seasonal variation in antifungal, antibacterial and acetylcholinesterase activity in seven South African seaweeds J. Appl. Phycol. 19:271–276.

Taylor W.R. (1960). Marine algae of the easterntropical and subtrobical coasts of Americas. ANN Arbor the University of Michigan press. pp. 870.

Trono J.G.C. (1999). Diversity of the seaweeds flora of the Philippines and its utilization. Hydrobiologia, 398/399, 1–6.

Tüney I.; Çadirci B.H.; Ünal D. & Sukatar A. (2006). Antimicrobial Activities of the Extracts of Marine Algae from the Coast of Urla (Üzmir, Turkey) Turk. J. Biol., 30:171-175.

Wagner H. & Bladt S. (1996). Plant drug analysis: a thin layer chromatography atlas. Springer-Verlag, Berlin. pp. 349-354.

Watson S.B. & Cruz-Rivera E. (2003). Algal chemical ecology: an introduction to the special issue. Phycologia. 42:319–323.

Wefky S. & Ghobrial M. (2008). Studies on the Bioactivity of Different Solvents Extracts of Selected Marine Macroalgae Against Fish Pathogens. Res. J. Microbiol. 3 (12):673-682.

Wendy A.S. & Diana L.R. (2007). Seasonal variation in antifungal, antibacterial and acetyl cholinesterase activity in seven South African seaweeds. J. Appl. Phycol. 19:271–276.

WHO (World Health Organization) (2004). The world health report. Changing history. Statistical annex. Death by cause, sex and mortality stratum in WHO regions, estimates for 2002. Geneva, Switzerland, pp. 120-121.

10

The Role of Proteomics in Elucidating Multiple Antibiotic Resistance in *Salmonella* and in Novel Antibacterial Discovery

Rui Pacheco[1-4], Susana Correia[1-4], Patrícia Poeta[3,4], Luís Pinto[1-4] and Gilberto Igrejas[1,2,*]

[1]*Institute for Biotechnology and Bioengineering, Center of Genomics and Biotechnology University of Trás-os-Montes and Alto Douro*
[2]*Department of Genetics and Biotechnology, University of Trás-os-Montes and Alto Douro*
[3]*Center of Studies of Animal and Veterinary Sciences*
[4]*Veterinary Science Department, University of Trás-os-Montes and Alto Douro*
Portugal

1. Introduction

Salmonellae are Gram-negative facultative anaerobes that have been divided into two species: *S. enterica*, which is subdivided into over 2,500 serovars, and *Salmonella bongori*. Some serovars of *S. enterica*, such as *S.* Typhi, cause systemic infections and typhoid fever, whereas others, such as *S.* Typhimurium, cause gastroenteritis. Nontyphoidal *Salmonella* are a major cause of food poisoning being Salmonellosis one of the most common and widely distributed foodborne diseases. Millions of human cases are reported worldwide every year and the disease constitutes a major public health burden, causing significant morbidity and mortality in several countries. Since the beginning of the 1990s, strains of *Salmonella* which are resistant to a range of antimicrobials, including first-choice agents for human treatment, have emerged and are threatening to become a serious public health problem. Multidrug-resistant strains of *Salmonella* are now frequently encountered and the rates of multidrug-resistance (MDR) have been increasing considerably in recent years [World Health Organization (WHO, 2005)].

Strains of *Salmonella* spp. with resistance to antimicrobial drugs are now widespread in both developed and developing countries. Effective antimicrobial agents are essential for human and animal health and welfare. However, infections caused by resistant microorganisms often fail to respond to standard treatment, resulting in prolonged illness and greater risk of death. Hence, the increasing antimicrobial resistance is considered a public health problem at a global level (Musgrove et al., 2006; Võ, 2007). A diversity of foods and environmental sources harbor bacteria that are resistant to antimicrobial drugs used in medicine and in food-animal production (Bager & Helmuth, 2001; Schroeder et al., 2004). Also the misuse and/or excessive use of antibiotics in human and veterinary medicine are in certain cases

---

* Corresponding author

responsible for the increase and spread of resistance seen among the bacterial population. Antimicrobial agents are known to be clinically prescribed in situations where there is no bacterial infection or the illness event is a viral infection. In other cases, the treatment of an infection is made with the incorrect antibiotic combinations, doses or durations that are sometimes excessive. Antimicrobial resistance reduces the effectiveness of treatment as patients remain infected for longer, thus potentially spreading resistant microorganisms to others. The achievements of modern medicine are also at risk since, without effective antimicrobials for care and prevention of infections, the success of treatments such as organ transplantation, cancer chemotherapy and major surgery would be compromised. In addition, the growth of global trade and travel allows resistant microorganisms to be spread rapidly to distant countries and continents; this represents a threat to health security, and damages trade and economies (WHO, 2011).

Bacterial antibiotic resistance can be classified in five different main mechanisms, involving the antibiotic molecules or its targets in the cell (Figure 1).

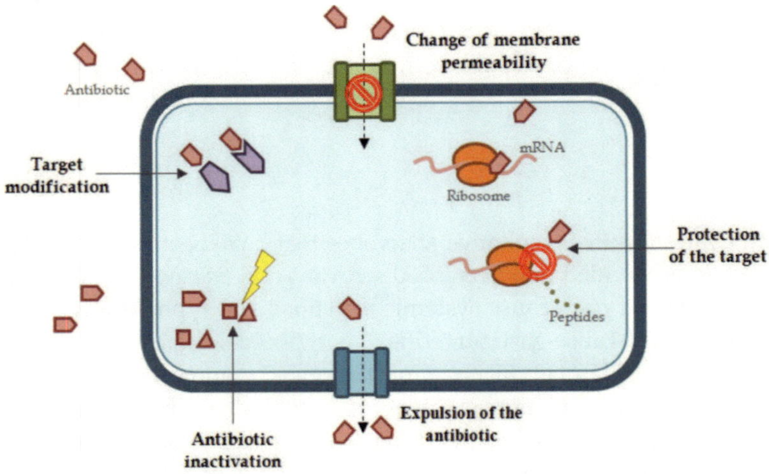

Fig. 1. Antibiotic resistance mechanisms. Adapted from Yao & Moellering, 2003. Antibacterial Agents American Society for Microbiology, Washington.

Although genes encoding efflux pumps can be found on plasmids, the carriage of efflux pump genes on the chromosome gives the bacterium an intrinsic mechanism that allows survival in a hostile environment (e.g. the presence of antibiotics), and so mutant bacteria that over-express efflux pump genes can be selected without the acquisition of new genetic material (Webber & Piddock, 2003). Before the development of genomics, the scientific community focused investigations on single or small groups of genes or proteins. The genome-sequencing projects of the late 1990's yielded entire genome sequences of many bacteria, leading to a large amount of genetic data. These new platforms of the so-called "omic" technologies allow the analysis and characterization of biological systems and promised to facilitate our understanding of normal cellular function and dysfunction by permitting simultaneous monitoring of thousands of molecular components. There are currently 1587 complete bacterial genomes and 4901 bacterial genomes in-progress at NCBI (http://www.ncbi.nlm.nih.gov/genomes/lproks.cgi). Even though the number of encoding entities (open reading frames, ORFs) can be predicted from the genome, the number of different proteins that an organism is capable of generating cannot directly be deduced - a global protein analysis is needed to define the protein composition of a given cell under a certain circumstance (Brotz-Oesterhelt et al., 2005).

Proteomics, defined as the global analysis of cellular proteins, is a key area of research that is developing in the post-genome era (Osman et al., 2009). The term proteome, in analogy to the term genome, was coined to describe the complete set of proteins that an organism has produced under a defined set of conditions (Wasinger et al., 1995). In the last few years proteomics has become a powerful tool for the investigation of complex biochemical processes, the discovery of new proteins and investigation of protein-protein interactions. The proteome is highly dynamic and much more complex than the genome - the number of encoding entities can be predicted from the genome, but the number of different proteins that an organism is capable of generating cannot be directly deduced. Hence, a global protein analysis is needed to define the protein composition of a given cell under a specific circumstance (Brotz-Oesterhelt et al., 2005). Moreover, the evaluation of protein profiles in response to multiple stress mechanisms, such as sensitivity to antibiotics or modifications related to antibiotic resistance, could represent a valid and integrating approach for the development of new therapeutic strategies. In complement, Mass Spectrometry (MS)-based proteomics and bioinformatics were shown to be suitable for evaluation of the effect of protein extracts, whole cell versus outer membrane proteome (OMP), on the identification of Gram-negative organisms. Different numbers of distinguishing, unique proteins were obtained by the bioinformatics procedure between the two protein extraction methods.

This chapter will present an overview of the major achievements of proteomic approaches to study *Salmonella* and its adaptation networks that are crucial for bacteria. Furthermore the published efforts to exploit the knowledge derived from the proteomic studies directly for the antibacterial drug discovery process will be reviewed. Special focus will be placed on antibiotic treatment induced stress and particular stressful environments. Finally, recent developments related to the *Salmonella* proteome and technological determinants used as biomarkers will be discussed.

2. Proteomics in practice

In the mid-1990's, two factors arose that substantially simplified proteomic analysis. For the first time, DNA sequences of whole bacterial genomes became available and allowed the prediction of the approximate total number of encoded ORFs (Brotz-Oesterhelt et al., 2005). At the same time, progress in MS facilitated the analysis of peptides and small proteins, and the accuracy of the measured peptide masses was sufficient to allow protein identification. The introduction of user-friendly, browser-based bioinformatics tools to extract information from these databases constituted a key of the post-genomic era. It is now possible to search entire genome sequences for specific nucleic acid or protein sequences to have a global view of living organisms through *in silico* analysis. Proteome informatics tools span today a large panel of very diverse applications ranging from simple tools to compare protein amino acid compositions to sophisticated software for large-scale protein structure determination (Palagi et al., 2006). The application of proteomics provides major opportunities to elucidate disease mechanisms and to identify new diagnostic markers and therapeutic targets. Significant progress has been made in the characterisation of bacterial pathogens using a combination of genomic and proteomic technologies. Pathogenic determinants are identified through comparative proteomics between virulent and avirulent isolates whereas complex disease phenotypes can be correlated with specific proteomic signatures identified through the analysis of large collections of natural isolates (Osman et al., 2009).

Proteomics is used to describe any large-scale investigation of proteins and can be approached in many ways but in principle it consists in three steps (Figure 2): (1) protein extraction, (2) separation and (3) identification. Most of the approaches require MS and database searching for protein identification but differ in the way the proteins are separated and isolated (Westermeier & Naven, 2002). In the extraction process, depending on the source, the proteins have to be brought into solution by breaking the tissue or cells containing them. Several methods like repeated freezing and thawing, sonication, homogenization by high pressure, filtration, or permeabilization by organic solvents are used to achieve this purpose. The methodology used depends on how fragile the protein is and how sturdy the cells are.

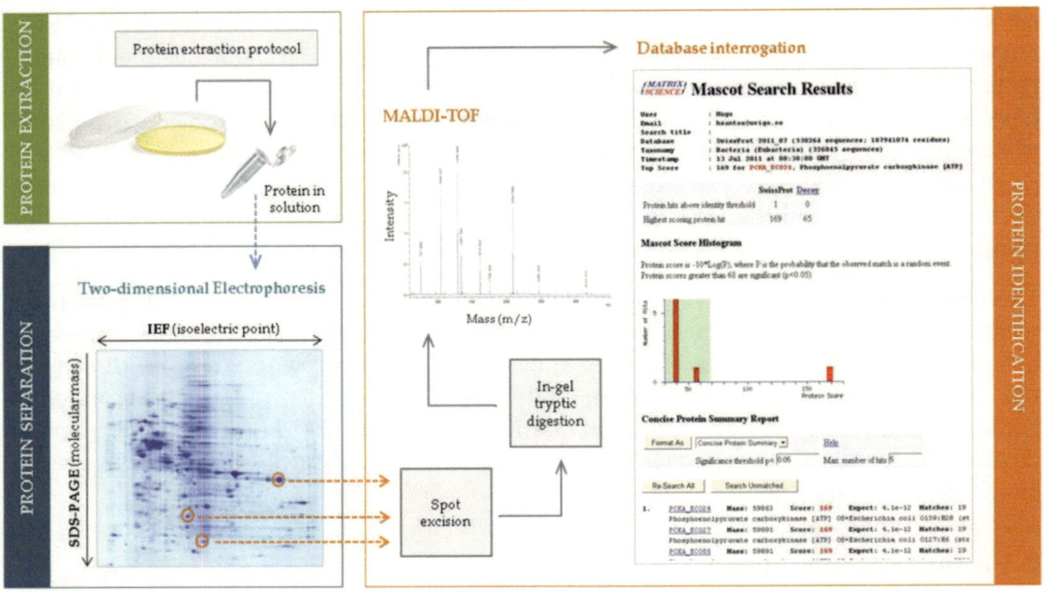

Fig. 2. Typical proteomic workflow representing the classical components of protein identification. Proteins are extracted and then separated according to isoelectric point and molecular mass (two-dimensional gel electrophoresis, 2-DE). Spots of interest are excised, digested and then proteins are identified by MS followed by data interrogation against genomic or proteomics databases using bioinformatic tools.

One of the most important ways that proteins are separated is by electrophoresis, including two-dimensional gel electrophoresis (2-DE) and capillary electrophoresis (Mishra, 2010). The latter involves the separation of proteins and peptides carried in a thin glass tube under high voltage before injection into the mass spectrometer for their identification. Thin tubes have the advantage of dissipating heat by high voltage, and separated proteins can be visualized and monitored by ultraviolet (UV) light during the eletrophoretic run. However, protein separation by 2-DE is the most commonly used method in proteomics. Proteins are separated according to isoelectric point (pI) in the first dimension and to molecular mass (M*r*) in the second. The gels are stained to visualize the resolved proteins using a dye that can contain zinc or copper, Coomassie Blue, silver or a fluorescent dye (Mishra, 2010). Zinc or copper staining is a negative staining because it stains the gel and not the protein spots; this method is inexpensive and has a sensitivity to detect spots containing 6-12 ng of protein, but it has difficulty in handling thin gels. Coomassie Blue is an easy and an inexpensive stain that is used to identify proteins by mass spectrometry; it has a sensitivity of 36-45 ng of protein per spot in the gel. Silver staining is expensive and time consuming but with high sensitivity as it can detect 0.5-1.2 ng of protein per spot in the gel. 2D Differential Gel Electrophoresis (DIGE) is a modification of 2D gel electrophoresis to avoid any differences that are usually encountered when samples are run on different gels even under identical conditions. In this method, multiple protein samples are separately labelled with different fluorescent dyes and then co-electrophoresed on the same 2-DE gel. Fluorescent dyes come in a variety of choices; they are quick and easy to use and are highly sensitive like silver staining but not compatible to subsequent techniques of protein identification by MS (Mishra, 2010).

After staining, the spots of interest are excised, either manually or automatically. An in-gel tryptic digestion of the gel spot is conducted and the protein is identified by MS analysis of the resultant peptides followed by data interrogation against genomic or proteomics databases using bioinformatic tools. This technique was initiated by Stegemann (1970) (as cited in Westermeier & Naven, 2002), combining isoelectric focusing (IEF) and SDS polyacrylamide gel electrophoresis (SDS-PAGE). 2-DE resolution was considerably increased when O'Farrell, in 1975, introduced denaturating conditions during sample preparation and IEF. This modification gave wide acceptance to the method but the technique only became reproducible enough for proteome analysis in 1982, with the application of immobilized pH gradients for the first dimension (Bjellqvist et al., 1982). 2-DE/MS provides a direct method to separate proteins and to visualize changes between complex proteome samples and it is able to resolve thousands of proteins. Many technological improvements have made 2-DE relatively inexpensive and accessible to most biomedical research labs but criticisms such as the inability of 2D-PAGE to resolve membrane proteins and its lack of reproducibility have been to some extent tempered by the development of better reagents, techniques, and gel alignment software. Even though 2-DE is still limited in sensitivity and dynamic range (Veenstra, 2007), it is still the most widely used method for protein separation. Nonetheless, liquid chromatography methods which includes gel filtration, affinity chromatography, ion exchange chromatography, Reverse-Phase (RP) and High-Performance Liquid Chromatography (HPLC), and multidimensional chromatography are also used for protein separation in proteomic analysis (Mishra, 2010).

For protein identification one can use an approach that is not based on spectrometry (determination of the amino acid sequence from the DNA sequence or the identification of one amino acid at a time from the N-terminus of the peptide - Edman Degradation) or a MS approach which allows protein identification based on their amino acid sequence (Mishra, 2010). Peptide mass fingerprinting (PMF) is the easiest and fastest way to identify proteins (Westermeier & Naven, 2002). In this method, the protein of interest is digested with a proteolytic enzyme, commonly trypsin, inside a gel plug and the cleavage products (peptides) are eluted and submitted to MS analysis. MALDI-TOF (Matrix-assisted laser desorption/ionization – Time-of-flight) instruments are preferably used because they are easier to handle than electrospray systems (ESI-TOF). The mass spectrum with the accurately measured peptide masses is matched with theoretical peptide spectra in various databases using adequate bioinformatic tools. Even though this procedure works very well for protein identification, the method can be compromised for several reasons. In these circumstances, more specific information is needed for unambiguous protein identification and so the amino acid sequence is determined. During MS analysis a peptide can be selected from the spectrum and fragmented inside the instrument, termed tandem MS (MS/MS). The resultant fragment ion masses are indicative of amino acid sequence that can be used to search not only protein databases but also Expressed Sequence Tag (EST) databases and used for *de novo* sequencing when necessary.

The evolution of MS-based proteomic technologies has advanced our understanding of the complex and dynamic nature of proteomes while simultaneously revealing that no proteomic strategy can be used alone to address all biological questions. Figure 3 depicts a typical proteomic workflow with examples of commonly used techniques that may be

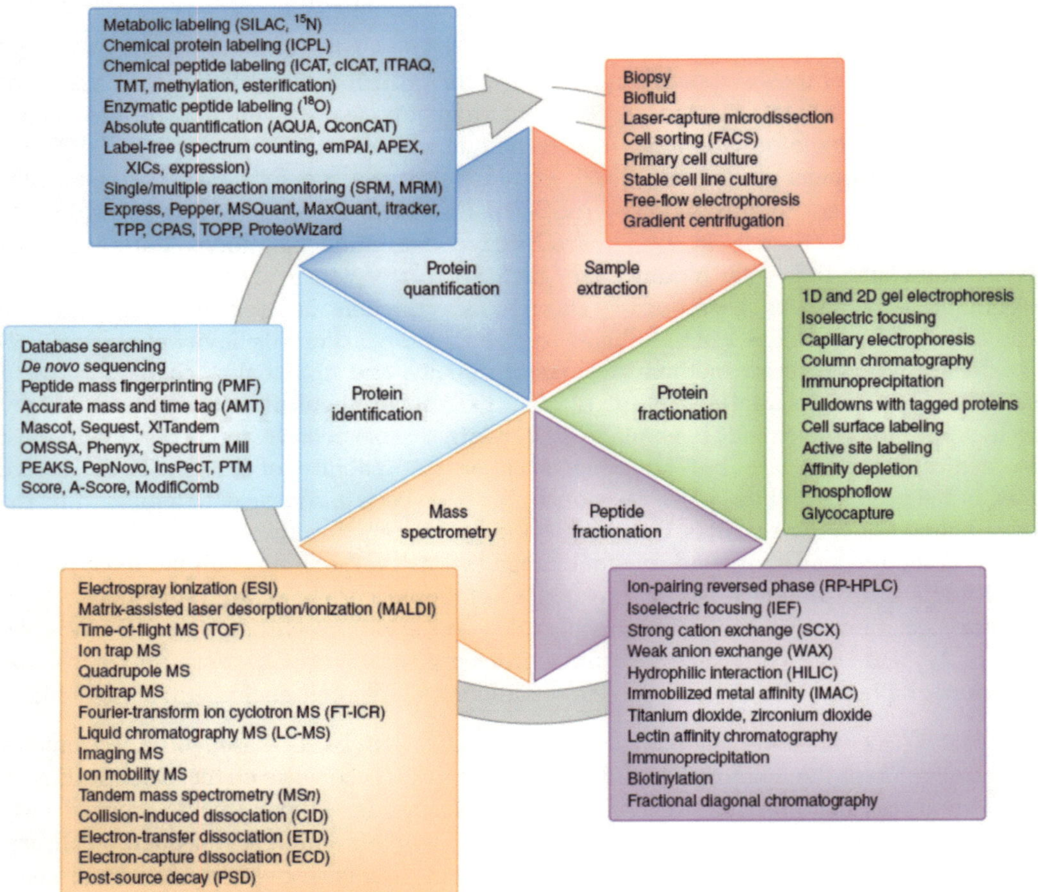

Fig. 3. Technologies for proteomics. This figure depicts the proteomic workflow from sample extraction to protein quantification. For each step in the workflow, the text boxes give examples of commonly used techniques, many of which may be combined in any one study. Reprinted by permission from Macmillan Publishers Ltd: [Nature Biotechnology] (Proteomics: A Pragmatic Perspective., 28(7): 695-709), copyright (2010) (Mallick & Kuster, 2010).

applied in most types of proteomics studies. Several tools are available to help quantify and interpret data generated through specific applications of MS. MS-based quantitative approaches include tagging or chemical modification methods, such as isotope-coded affinity tags (ICAT), isobaric tag for relative and absolute quantitation (iTRAQ) or stable isotope labelling by amino acids in cell culture (SILAC). A further detailed description of proteomic techniques can be consulted in Hamacher et al., 2011; Mallick & Kuster, 2010; Mishra, 2010; Parker et al., 2010; Veenstra, 2007; Westermeier & Naven, 2002.

Despite the variation in proteomics approaches, all techniques generate large quantities of data. Bioinformatics approaches appear as an essential mean for analysis, storage and retrieval of all that information. In 2-DE, there are several software available for image analysis that allow the comparison of different gels. 2-DE gels are not exactly identical; different factors may cause variation between analysis, such as preparation methods, staining, and unequal mobility in the different gels' regions and variations in electrophoretic conditions, even when studying the same sample. Automatic gel matching methods include features like spot detection, gel warping and auto-matching; this matching is the starting point for deeper analysis and statistical studies. Through MS, integrated systems allow protein identification, based on comparison of peptide fingerprints with proteins in databases (Vihinen, 2003). Bioinformatics not only helps the interpretation of results but it also may guide the course of new investigations since results and new discoveries from laboratories from all over the world can be stored in online databases, available to any researcher.

Due to the wide diversity of proteins and properties in complex proteomes, it is anticipated that no single proteome analysis technology will be able to effectively address all proteome analysis requirements. 2-DE gels will probably remain the "gold standard" within the foreseeable future to which any competing method should be compared, and to which it should display clear advantages of 2-DE with IPGs (Görg et al., 2009). In contrast to the 2-DE approaches, information about protein abundances is initially unavailable in the non-gel-based technologies, unless stable isotope labelling is applied. Moreover, 2-DE is highly parallel and unsurpassed for its ability to run as far as 20 2-D gels at a time with thousands of proteins per gel. Post-translationally modified (PTM) proteins can be readily located in 2-DE gels because they appear as distinctive spot clusters, which can be subsequently identified by MS analysis. For a global view, post-translational modifications (PTMs) (e.g. glycosylation or phosphorylation) can be visualized with specific fluorescent dyes (Hecker et al., 2008; Zong et al., 2008). However, there are challenges, in particular, with respect to detection of low-abundance proteins and, particularly, of integral membrane proteins, whereas non-gel-based methods are unsurpassed by their potential to cover the whole proteome (de Godoy et al., 2008).

3. Antimicrobial resistance in *Salmonella*

An alarming increase in the incidence of antibiotic resistant strains of *Salmonella* was pointed out by the World Health Organization more than 20 years ago (Brisabois et al., 1997). Multiple antibiotic resistance in *Salmonella* has also been increasing; about 45% of the isolates of *Salmonella* Typhimurium reported to the Enter-net surveillance network in recent years presented a MAR phenotype (International surveillance network for the enteric infections Salmonella and VTEC O157, 2008).

Salmonella commonly show resistance to ampicillin, chloramphenicol, streptomycin/ spectinomycin, sulphonamides and tetracyclines (R-type ACSSuT), with additional resistance to third-generation cephalosporins mediated by the CMY-2 beta-lactamase gene (Antunes et al., 2006; Threlfall, 2002; Threlfall, 2008). The increasing number of infections with R-type ACSSuT *Salmonella,* with extended-spectrum ß-lactamase (ESBL)-producing *Salmonella* and with quinolone-resistant *Salmonella* strains, have emerged as a global health problem and deserve special attention (Antunes et al., 2006; Threlfall, 2008).

Infections due to antibiotic-resistant *Salmonella* may have different consequences. People treated with antimicrobial drugs for unrelated reasons, such as upper respiratory tract infections, are at increased risk of infection with *Salmonella* that are resistant to the given antibiotic. Infections by resistant *Salmonella* have been proven to be more severe than infections with susceptible strains and resistance is directly associated with increased frequency of treatment failures, mainly when there is a prolonged duration of illness, associated with increased hospitalization (WHO, 2005).

The emergence of MDR *Salmonella* strains with resistance to fluoroquinolones and third-generation cephalosporins is also a serious development, which results in severe limitation of the possibilities for effective treatment of human infections. Ceftiofur and ceftriaxone are two of the most common antimicrobials used for treatment of infections caused by *Salmonella*, especially invasive ones, but there are already records of strains containing the bla_{CMY-2} cephalosporine-resistance gene (Dunne et al., 2000; Fey et al., 2000; Winokur et al., 2000). The concern rises from the fact that third generation cephalosporins are drugs of choice in invasive infections caused by strains with resistance to ciprofloxacin (Threlfall, 2002). Also, mobile genetic elements allow and have been associated to resistance transmission as they may contain one or more resistance-associated genes (White et al., 2001). This spread of resistances has led to a predominance of resistant strains in several countries. In the United States of America, United Kingdom, France and Germany, the predominant *Salmonella* type is resistant to at least five drugs: ampicillin, chloramphenicol, streptomycin, sulfonamides and tetracycline (Helms et al., 2002).

While resistance to fluoroquinolones often emerges as a result of mutations in the bacterial genome (DNA), resistance to other antimicrobials often spread by DNA transfer between bacterial strains through plasmids. Nalidixic acid was the first quinolone antibacterial agent licensed for use in the United States. Since introduction of nalidixic acid in the 1960s, subsequent generations of fluoroquinolones have been licensed by the US Food and Drug Administration (FDA). Fluorination of quinolone compounds resulted in the introduction of norfloxacin in 1986 and ciprofloxacin in 1987, followed by other second-generation fluoroquinolones. Additional modifications resulted in third- and fourth-generation fluoroquinolones. Some fluoroquinolones are no longer available, and others are of limited use clinically. Currently, ciprofloxacin, levofloxacin, gatifloxacin, and moxifloxacin are the most widely used fluoroquinolones. When fluoroquinolones were first licensed for human therapy, no immediate rise in *Salmonella* resistance was observed (WHO, 2005). In contrast, when fluoroquinolones were subsequently licensed for use in food animals, the rates of fluoroquinolone-resistant *Salmonella* in animals and food, and then subsequently in human infections, rapidly increased in several countries (WHO et al., 2003). Even worse than the increasing rates of drug-resistant *Salmonella* is the fact that some variants of *Salmonella* have developed MDR as an integral part of the genetic material of the organism, and are therefore likely to retain their drug-resistant genes even when antimicrobial drugs are no longer used, a situation where other resistant strains would typically lose their resistance (WHO, 2005).

Evidence from many countries supports the role of agricultural antimicrobial use and increasing prevalence of resistance among commensal and pathogenic bacteria isolated from food animals, humans, the food supply, and the environment. First, a mass flow concept of antimicrobial pressure and resistance evolution supports the importance of controlling the agricultural use of antimicrobials because this is the primary category of use worldwide; and second, the problem must be redefined as one of resistance and gene flow, thus challenging the basis of policies that respond to or prioritize specific drug/bug combinations (Silbergeld et al., 2008). In developed countries the existence of *Salmonella* organisms resistant to antibiotics is an almost inevitable consequence of the use of antimicrobial drugs in food-producing animals. Although legislation targeted at controlling the overall usage of antimicrobials in livestock, in recent years there have been significant increases in the occurrence of resistance in non-typhoidal *Salmonella*. Selective pressure from the use of antimicrobials in food animals may be a major driving force behind the emergence of resistance but other factors must also be considered; some *Salmonella* serotypes are more prone to develop resistance than others and major shifts in the occurrence of *Salmonella* serotypes in food animal and humans are regularly seen. An example is the global spread of a multidrug-resistant *S.* Typhimurium phage type DT104 in animals and humans that may not only have been facilitated by the use of antimicrobials, but also worsened by international and national trade of infected animals.

In the past, studies on *Salmonella* isolates from human infection cases and clinical animal samples showed low resistance levels (Seyfarth et al., 1997). Nevertheless, it has been shown that the occurrence of resistant *Salmonella* strains in domestic animals is associated with the continuing use of antimicrobial agents in animal herds (van Leeuwen et al., 1979; Threlfall et al., 1993, as cited in Seyfarth et al., 1997). The routine practice of giving antimicrobial drugs to domestic livestock as a mean of preventing and treating diseases, as well as promoting growth, is an important factor in the emergence of antibiotic-resistant bacteria that are subsequently transferred to humans by the food chain (Angulo et al., 2004, as cited in Miko et al., 2005). Even indirect contact between animals, humans and ecosystems may lead to the transference of bacteria and/or resistance genes from one microorganism to another (Radhouani et al., 2010), making resistant *Salmonella* strains a cross-species problem. Hence, the emergence and dissemination of antimicrobial-resistant pathogens such as *Salmonella* has become a serious health hazard worldwide. The comparison between the genomes of different serovars revealed that despite their similarities, each serovar has many insertions and deletions in relation to the others, which vary in size from 1 to 50 kB (Edwards et al., 2002). However, the observed differences at the DNA level proved to be unrelated to protein expression. Therefore, it is of great importance to determine if the observed genomic difference could impact its expressed protein outcome. Taoka et al. (2004) found that the majority of horizontally transferred genes in the genome of *E. coli* are not translated into proteins. Recent data from transcriptomic and/or proteomic profiling suggest that marker panels derived from transcriptomic or proteomic profiling are superior to single genes or markers, in differentiating non-infectious from sepsis-associated systemic inflammation, and thus may overcome some of the limitations of procalcitonin (Johnson et al., 2007; Tang et al., 2009).

The use of biomarkers might help to avoid antibiotic misuse and overuse and to curb the rising incidence of microbial resistance. Increasing rates of bacterial resistance among common pathogens are threatening the effectiveness of even the most potent antibiotics. Through proteome analysis we showed how mechanisms of antimicrobial resistance can affect other important characteristics, like virulence, possibly resulting in low dissemination of such strains. Further work focusing on the interactions between antimicrobial resistance and virulence mechanisms is important. There is also a need for further epidemiological studies to determine whether different kinds of disinfectants contribute to the emergence of antibiotic resistance in order to establish the best practices to prevent or minimize the selection of antibiotic resistance (Karatzas et al., 2008).

4. The potential role of proteomics in *Salmonella* research

Functional genomics allows identification of complex pathways and interactions between gene expression products that provides insight into processes beyond their clinical appearance. Single cell signaling stimuli can define complex cellular pathways but multicellular and whole organism systems require an understanding of complex interrelationships, both structurally and temporally. These complex interrelationships are based on numerous individual components, diffuse interconnectivity between components, differences in spatio-temporal relations, and complexity in signaling network control interactions. Together, comparative proteomics, MS and bioinformatics contributed to the achievement of significant progress on the characterization of bacterial pathogens (Osman et al., 2009). MALDI has been used for the identification of bacteria since 1996 (Holland et al., 1996; Krishnamurthy & Ross, 1996) and this technique can be used for determining the causes of infection in patients, for the detection of bioterrorism agents, for the detection of toxic molds and bacteria in indoor air and for the detection of infectious agents in water (Parker et al., 2010).

Nevertheless, a broader definition states that proteomics deals with the large-scale analysis of proteins, including identification, measure of expression levels and partial characterization by the analysis of pre-, co-, and post-translational modifications, their structures, functions and interactions. Proteomics has four main objectives: (i) to identify all proteins from a proteome creating a catalogue of information; (ii) to analyze differential protein expression associated to a disease, different cell states, sample treatments and drug targets; (iii) to characterize proteins by discovering their function, cellular localization, PTMs, etc. and (iv) to describe and understand protein interaction networks (Palagi et al., 2006).

Proteomic profiling is a useful approach to obtain an overview of the proteins present in a bacterial system under differing conditions (DelVecchio et al., 2002; Lipton et al., 2002). Additionally, it can aid in understanding the molecular determinants involved with pathogenesis, which is essential for the development of effective strategies to combat infection and revealing new therapeutic targets (Lucas & Lee, 2000). Therefore, proteomics presents one of the best ways to investigate changes in the genome expression profile (Leverrier et al., 2004). Protein profiles can reveal the complexity of expressed proteins in bacteria, representing phenotypic characteristics, but they can also provide an excellent approximation of a microorganism's genome information. Also, proteomic methodologies contribute to the determination of antimicrobial resistance mechanisms, through the capacity to analyze global changes of bacteria (Radhouani et al., 2010). The use of *Salmonella* reference protein maps may be helpful in the identification of proteins in different *Salmonella* strains. In addition, these maps can facilitate the determination of different growth conditions (Qi et al., 1996). Studying the proteome of *Salmonella* with its small genome (with an estimated coding potential of 4000 gene products) makes it theoretically simple to determine if a certain protein is known or novel. Further, the close evolutionary relationship between *E. coli* and *Salmonella*, in which protein homologues usually have similar sequences, allows a reliable assignment of proteins and PTMs which appears to be relatively rare. Also, the availability of decreased-virulence-strains, as a result of mutations in key regulatory proteins, allows the comparison of protein expression profiles between strains, which permits the identification of proteins under the control of a specific regulator (O'Connor et al., 1997).

Because *Salmonella* need to invade a specific host cell to initiate the disease process, the characterization of the *Salmonella* proteins that are induced during and following invasion of different types of mammalian cells is of particular interest (O'Connor et al., 1997), particularly in the development of new antimicrobial approaches. Studies performed by our research group have proven the capability of proteomics to provide results that allow the comparison between *Salmonella* strains, as long as the detection of proteins related to antibiotic resistance, pathogenesis and virulence in this species (Pinto et al., 2010). Therefore, our group developed an integrated genomic and proteomic evaluation of antibiotic resistance in *Salmonella* strains with different serotypes and antibiotic resistance phenotypes, recovered from faecal samples of wild rabbits and wild boars from the North of Portugal. All strains used in the referred study are listed in Table 1, which shows the resistance profiles of the different samples of *Salmonella* serotypes displayed in the 1-D gel. Analysis of different strains by SDS-PAGE gave reproducible whole-cell protein patterns which allowed differentiation among the serovars included in this study (Figure 4). The genetic characterization of antimicrobial resistance genes as well as their location and diversity is important in identifying factors involved in resistance, understanding the diversity of multi-drug resistant strains, identifying genetic linkages among markers, understanding potential transfer mechanisms, and developing efficient detection methods.

Cell wall changes that result in reduced permeability can also be responsible for resistance to biocides and antibiotics. These common mechanisms of resistance to biocides and antibiotics should be a public health concern, and prevention of the dissemination of antibiotic-resistant strains in the environment and animal hosts, including farm animals and humans, is important (Karatzas et al., 2008). The application of proteomics to the antibiotic-discovery process, technically spoken, requires the same methodological approaches as those applied to study the physiological response to environmental stresses. Nevertheless, there are many potential questions to be asked that are specific for drug-discovery applications. Antibiotics exert their antibacterial activity via binding to and inhibition of certain molecular targets, thereby usually blocking a function essential for microbial survival. Therefore, one application of proteomics in drug discovery is the identification of novel antibacterial targets. Target identification will critically rely either on the availability of similar protein expression profiles for comparison or on the detailed investigation of proteome signatures induced by the compound tested. For target validation, proteome analysis of mutants may be helpful if an inhibitor of a novel target of interest is not yet available. For certain groups of inhibitors it might be beneficial to extend the analysis to different pI ranges or to include different protein fractions to increase the number of marker proteins. For instance, it would be interesting to identify marker proteins in the membrane fraction that help differentiate between membrane-active antibacterial compounds (Apfel et al., 2001; Bandow et al., 2003; Evers et al., 2001; Gmuender et al., 2001; Gray & Keck, 1999; Singh et al., 2001).

Sample	Serotype	Resistance profile
J27(1)	*S.* Typhimurium	AMP; TET; STR; CHL
J32(2)	*S.* Typhimurium	AMP; TET; STR; CHL
C71(1)	*S.* Typhimurium	AMP; TET; STR; CHL
P40(a)	*S.* Typhimurium	AMP; TET; STR; CHL
P16(1)	*S.* Typhimurium	AMP; TET; STR; CHL
P20(2)	*S.* Enteritidis	AMP; TET; STR; NAL; CHL
P29(2)	*S.* Rissen	AMP; TET; STR; NAL; SXT
J45(1)	*S.* Rissen	AMP; TET; SXT
P1(1)	*S.* Enteritidis	AMP; TET; NAL; SXT
AVT14(1)	ND	TET; SXT
C12(1)	*S.* Rissen	AMC; AMP; TET; STR; SXT
C16(1)	*S.* Typhimurium	AMP; TET; AK; STR; CHL
C40(2)	*S.* Typhimurium	AMP; STR; CHL
P57(c)	*S.* Enteritidis	TOB; STR
C37(1)	*S.* Enteritidis	-
J15(2)	*S.* Typhimurium	AMP; STR; CHL

J—wild boars; C—wild rabbit; P—swine; AVT—ostrich; AK—amikacin; AMC—amoxicillin-clavulanic acid; AMP—ampicillin; CHL—chloramphenicol; NAL—nalidixic acid; STR—streptomycin; SXT—sulfamethoxazole-trimethoprim; TET—tetracycline; TOB—tobramycin; ND—not determined. Adapted from Journal of Proteomics, 73 (8), (Pinto et al., 2010), Genomic and proteomic evaluation of antibiotic resistance in *Salmonella* strains, 1535-1541, Copyright (2010), with permission from Elsevier.

Table 1. Resistance profiles of the different samples of *Salmonella* serotypes displayed in the 1-D gel.

According to these patterns, two different serotypes were chosen based on differences in serotypification and antibiotic resistance to proceed to a full proteomic study: the wild boar *S.* Typhimurium J15(2) strain, which demonstrated resistance to three antimicrobial agents (ampicillin, streptomycin and chloramphenicol) and *S.* Enteritidis C37(1), recovered from a wild rabbit, where no antibiotic resistance was found. 2-DE (Figure 5) combined with MS (MALDI-TOF/TOF) and then the correlation with web databases allowed the exact identification and characterization of proteins related to antibiotic resistance, pathogenesis and virulence in both *Salmonella* strains (Table 2). In *S.* Enteritidis isolated from a wild rabbit [C37(1)], the protein "Virulence transcriptional regulatory protein phoP" was detected in spot 47 and was previously reported in three different *Salmonella* strains: *S.* Typhi (accession number Q8Z7H2), *S.* Typhimurium (P14146) and *S.* Choleraesuis (Q57QC3). Protein phoP is a member of the two-component regulatory system phoQ/phoP that regulates the gene expression involved in virulence and resistance to host defensive antimicrobial peptides, promoting intramacrophage survival of *S.* Typhimurium (Miller et al., 1989). Transcriptional regulatory protein basR/pmrA (P36556) was also found in C37(1), and is related to *S.* Typhimurium where it is involved with processes of antibiotic resistance and pathogenesis, more exactly in the resistance to polymyxin (McClelland et al., 2001).

Isolates	Spot	Protein Description	*Salmonella* serovar	Protein Name	Accession Number	Protein MW	Protein PI	Peptide Count	Protein Score	Protein Score C.I. %	References
C37(1)	6	Superoxide dismutase [Mn]	*S.* Typhimurium	sodA	P43019	23064,68945	6.45	7	323	100	McClelland et al., 2001; Tsolis et al., 1995
	6	Superoxide dismutase [Mn]	*S.* Typhi	sodA	Q8Z2V9	23092,68945	6.23	8	419	100	Deng et al., 2003; Parkhill et al., 2001
	18	Chaperone protein dnaJ	*S.* Paratyphi B	dnaJ	A9MXI3	41286,62891	8.42	11	159	100	McClelland et al., 2007
	18	Chaperone protein dnaJ	*S. arizonae*	dnaJ	A9MR76	40909,53125	8.67	8	136	100	McClelland et al., 2007
	47	Virulence transcriptional regulatory protein phoP	*S.* Typhi	phoP	Q8Z7H2	25607,26953	5.28	9	270	100	Deng et al., 2003; Parkhill et al., 2001; van Velkinburgh & Gunn, 1999
	47	Virulence transcriptional regulatory protein phoP	*S.* Choleraesuis	phoP	Q57QC3	25661,32031	5.28	7	244	100	Chiu et al., 2005
	47	Virulence transcriptional regulatory protein phoP	*S.* Typhimurium	phoP	P14146	25617,28906	5.28	9	313	100	Miller et al., 1989; van Velkinburgh & Gunn, 1999
	91	Transcriptional regulatory protein basR/pmrA	*S.* Typhimurium	pmrA	P36556	25019,03906	5.79	2	75.6	100	McClelland et al., 2001
	106	Superoxide dismutase [Mn]	*S.* Typhimurium	sodA	P43019	23064,68945	6.45	6	123	100	McClelland et al., 2001; Tsolis et al., 1995
J15(2)	5	Superoxide dismutase [Mn]	*S.* Typhimurium	sodA	P43019	23064,68945	6.45	8	240	100	McClelland et al., 2001; Tsolis et al., 1995
	46	Superoxide dismutase [Mn]	*S.* Typhi	sodA	Q8Z2V9	23092,68945	6.23	1	65.7	100	Deng et al., 2003; Parkhill et al., 2001
	47	Superoxide dismutase [Mn]	*S.* Typhimurium	sodA	P43019	23064,68945	6.45	1	84.8	100	McClelland et al., 2001; Tsolis et al., 1995
	51	Superoxide dismutase [Mn]	*S.* Typhimurium	sodA	P43019	23064,68945	6.45	7	318	100	McClelland et al., 2001; Tsolis et al., 1995
	66	Chaperone protein dnaJ	*S.* ParaTyphi B	dnaJ	A9MXI3	41286,62891	8.42	7	178	100	McClelland et al., 2007
	66	Chaperone protein dnaJ	*S. arizonae*	dnaJ	A9MR76	40909,53125	8.67	5	155	100	McClelland et al., 2007
	93	Transcriptional regulatory protein basR/pmrA	*S.* Typhimurium	pmrA	P36556	25019,03906	5.79	2	50.9	100	McClelland et al., 2001

Adapted from Journal of Proteomics, 73 (8), (Pinto et al., 2010), Genomic and proteomic evaluation of antibiotic resistance in *Salmonella* strains, 1535-1541, Copyright (2010), with permission from Elsevier.

Table 2. Protein spots identification and sequencing results from *Salmonella* spp. isolates C37(1) and J15(2) 2-DE gels, by MALDI-TOF.

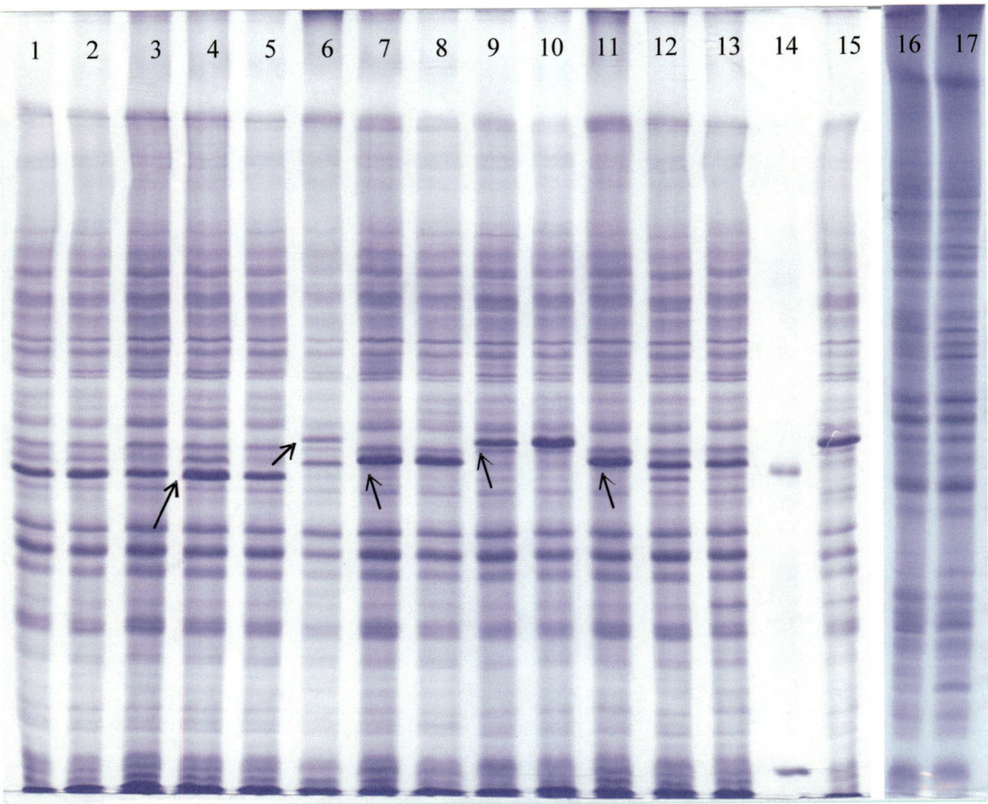

Fig. 4. SDS-PAGE of total protein extracts from *Salmonella* serotypes. 1-J27(1); 2-J32(2); 3-C71(1); 4-P40(a); 5-P16(1); 6-P20(2); 7-P29(2); 8-J45(1); 9-P1(1); 10-AVT14(1); 11-C12(1); 12-C16(1); 13-C40(2); 14- Marker; 15-P57(c); 16-C37(1); 17-J15(2). Arrows indicate the clearest differences between protein samples. Reprinted from Journal of Proteomics, 73 (8), (Pinto et al., 2010), Genomic and proteomic evaluation of antibiotic resistance in *Salmonella* strains, 1535-1541, Copyright (2010), with permission from Elsevier.

Since horizontal gene transfer among bacteria is a common mechanism of antibiotic resistance transmission within different bacteria, the presence of this protein in *Salmonella* carried in a faecal sample of a wild animal represents a concern, in the event of contact with domestic or commercial animals, or even humans. In *S.* Typhimurium J15(2), recovered from the faecal sample of a wild boar, the transcriptional regulatory protein basR/pmrA (P36556) was also found. Protein Superoxide dismutase [Mn] (sodA) was found in both isolates and is known to be responsible for the destruction of radicals that are normally produced within the cells and that are toxic to biological systems. The presence of this protein allows these bacteria to prevent an early killing by J774 cells and thus play a minor role in *Salmonella* pathogenesis (Tsolis et al., 1995). Chaperone protein dnaJ was also identified and is important for its relationship with the stress response mechanism towards heat, a very important reaction for the survival of bacteria such as *Salmonella* and its contribution to antibiotic resistance capability. This work, albeit preliminary in nature, reveals the complexity of expressed proteins in bacteria or different serotypes and profiles of antibiotic resistance. Bearing in mind that serotypes are related to infectious processes in humans and animals, it is important to explore the proteome of new strains which might serve as protein biomarkers for biological activity.

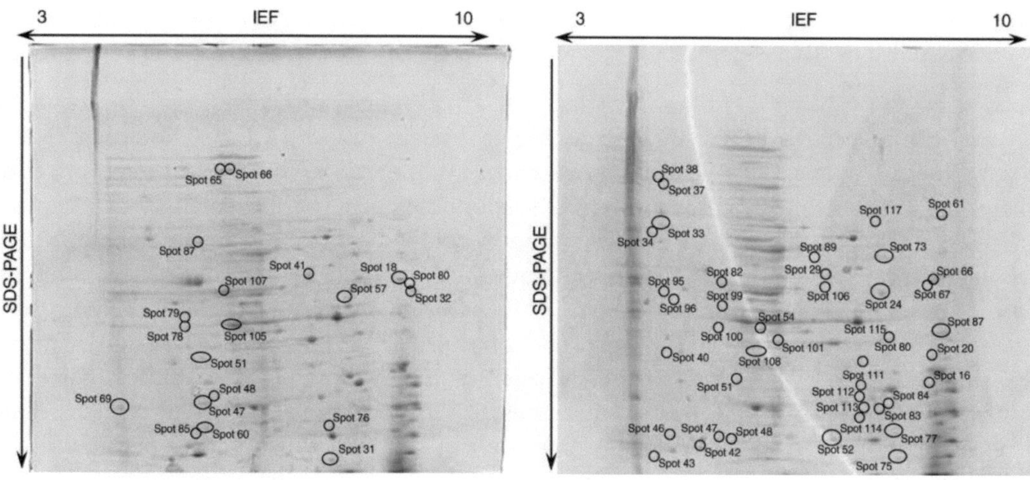

Fig. 5. 2-DE gel image of *Salmonella* samples with IPG strips pH3–10. Left: Serotype C37(1); Right: Serotype J15(2). Reprinted from Journal of Proteomics, 73 (8), (Pinto et al., 2010), Genomic and proteomic evaluation of antibiotic resistance in *Salmonella* strains, 1535-1541, Copyright (2010), with permission from Elsevier.

4.1 Proteomic mapping analysis and proteomic signatures

Proteomics already allowed substantial progress in elucidating the basic regulatory networks that form the basis for the extraordinary capacity of bacteria to adapt to a diversity of lifestyles and external stress factors. The application of this method for antibacterial drug-discovery purposes, however, is still in its early days. One reason for this phenomenon is the fact that the discovery of novel targets, which is one of the most important applications of proteome studies in other areas of drug discovery, is not so much a bottleneck in antibiotic research, because the pathophysiology of most bacterial infections is relatively well-understood and simple: killing the bacterium or interfering with its growth and, possibly, its virulence is usually all it takes. The term "proteomic signature" is defined by a subset of proteins, whose expression levels are characteristic for a defined condition (VanBogelen et al., 1999). To spot a proteomic signature, it is essential to recognize the connection between the expression levels of specific proteins and a particular physiological state. The establishment of protein signatures can be extremely helpful in the interpretation of a protein expression profile obtained under an unprecedented growth condition (Brotz-Oesterhelt et al., 2005).

Since its inception, the goal of proteomics has been the complete characterization of all proteins. However, considering the proteome of an organism as all protein forms expressed, including splice isoforms and PTMs, this goal consists of a considerably complex amount of information that needs to be gathered. Whereas the genome of an organism generally does not vary from cell to cell, the proteome will change in response to different stimuli, even for a single cell (Han et al., 2008). When grown under moderate stress conditions, bacteria may develop an adaptive response, allowing them to cope with subsequent more severe stresses. In general, this adaptation phenomenon appears to involve multiple genes encoding stress proteins, which can be specifically induced by a particular stress factor or induced by several conditions (Rince et al., 2002).

Protein maps associate a protein spot from a 2D gel to its corresponding ORF and also provide the respective knowledge pertaining to protein function (Brotz-Oesterhelt et al., 2005). 2D-PAGE, as already referred, is the most used technique for protein mapping and analysis. However, there are by now published studies proving the potential of non-gel-based technologies, like liquid chromatography coupled with ion-trap tandem MS. The number of proteins identified in both techniques may be quite similar, but it is possible to detect some different types of proteins (Brotz-Oesterhelt et al., 2005). Analyzing the proteome of a human pathogen like *Salmonella* has proven to be crucial. The establishment of protein reference maps is a significant point for many physiological studies that may follow. Nevertheless, protein maps only represent virtual compilations of all proteins ever detected or identified in an organism; they do not disclose which subset of proteins is expressed under specific growth conditions. In order to obtain such information, protein-expression profiles must be generated (Brotz-Oesterhelt et al., 2005).

The adaptation status of each organism to a specific ecological niche is reflected by the different types of proteins encoded and variations in their amino acid sequences. That adaption is achieved by differences in post-transcriptional and post-translational regulation that mediate the adaptation on the protein level. Thus, proteins that constitute a proteomic signature for a specific condition in one organism do not necessarily belong to the proteomic signature for the same physiological state in another organism.

Genomic and proteomic technologies have revolutionized the way we design and conduct current biological experiments. Our ability to rapidly analyze hundreds of expressed proteins and identify which gene encodes a specific protein generates a vast amount of information essential in examining different but interrelated pathways within the organism. Knowing which proteins are phosphorylated, for instance, may explain the differential expression of certain genes responsible for attenuating virulence or conferring host specificity. Beyond these, results of proteomics studies may be used in the development of a more potent vaccine, rapid detection methodology and fingerprinting, and novel antimicrobial drugs (DelVecchio et al., 2002; Lipton et al., 2002). Proteomic technologies have been greatly refined during the past decade and have been applied to investigate differences in the protein expression profiles of cells grown under a broad spectrum of growth conditions and with different stress factors including some antibiotics inhibiting protein synthesis or gyrase function.

4.2 Comparative proteomics and antibacterial drug discovery process

Evaluation of protein profiles in response to multiple stress mechanisms, such as sensitivity to antibiotics or modifications related to antibiotic resistance, could represent a valid and integrating approach for the development of new therapeutic strategies (Roncada et al.,

2009). It is widely recognized that the development of novel antibacterial agents without cross-resistance to existing antibiotics should have high priority on any meaningful public health agenda. Therefore, it is not surprising that proteome analysis of the consequences of antimicrobial treatment for bacteria has recently gained increasing interest. This approach provides a deeper insight into bacterial response to a certain antimicrobial treatment and benefits are expected in many other aspects of modern drug development such as the identification of novel target areas and the elucidation of the molecular mechanisms of action of novel drug candidates.

Antibiotics exert their antibacterial activity by binding to and inhibiting certain molecular targets, thereby usually blocking a function essential for microbial survival. Thus, one application of proteomics in drug discovery is the identification of novel antibacterial targets. Some available studies in which proteomics was performed with clear emphasis on antibacterial drug discovery focus on either target validation or mode of action, including those that aim at a better molecular understanding of the mechanisms of action of existing drugs (Apfel et al., 2001; Bandow et al., 2003; Evers et al., 2001; Gmuender et al., 2001; Gray & Keck, 1999; Singh et al., 2001). In these studies, the proteome of bacteria grown *in vitro* under standardized conditions in the presence and absence of the antibiotic of interest is analyzed with respect to changes in the protein-expression pattern.

Thus, significant progress has been made on the characterization of bacterial pathogens through comparative proteomics correlated with MS and bioinformatics (Pinto et al., 2010). In comparative proteomic studies, proteins from different biological states are quantitatively compared to obtain a complete understanding of the biological processes affecting their expression and/or in which they are involved (Renzone et al., 2005). This is a two-step process in which proteins within cellular extracts are first fractionated to reduce sample complexity, and then the proteins are identified by MS (Minden, 2007). Two-dimensional electrophoresis is the long-time standard for protein separation as it provides a direct method to visualize changes in proteins between complex proteome samples and is able to resolve thousands of proteins; however, it has suffered from poor reproducibility and limited sensitivity (Minden, 2007; Veenstra, 2007). DIGE was developed to overcome the reproducibility and sensitivity limitations and provides a reliable and sensitive platform to discover proteome changes in a boundless variety of circumstances (Minden, 2007). Discovery proteomics also involves multi-dimensional separation steps and liquid chromatography-tandem mass spectrometry (LC-MS/MS) with long gradients (Qi et al., 1996).

According to Brotz-Oesterhelt et al. (2005) successful exploitation of those technologies for the antibacterial drug discovery process depends on further progress in three main areas: i) data collection, which should be expanded to comprise as many antibacterial compounds with diverse mechanisms of action as possible, to ideally cover all relevant targets (for novel targets, where such reference antibiotics are not always available, the analysis of conditional mutants should be included); ii) the data analysis tools, which should be optimized or developed to efficiently handle the enormous datasets and to facilitate data evaluation in terms of mechanism-specific signatures (by including clustering, chemometric, and artificial intelligence approaches, for example); and iii) further methodological progress in order to increase the speed, throughput, and reproducibility of 2D gel-based as well as non-gel-based techniques. In comparative proteomics, data analysis in most cases concentrates on listing the proteins with significantly altered expression levels, which are subsequently discussed with respect to the current knowledge of the antibiotic's mode of action. It is known that antibiotics such as β-lactams, glycopeptides, D-cycloserine and fosfomycin, act at different stages of bacterial cell wall synthesis and that compounds such as quinolones inhibit DNA gyrase. For all proteins with an altered expression in response to a particular stimulus, the term "stimulon" was coined (Neidhardt et al., 1990) to describe the changes in protein expression on a phenotypic level. Therefore, if antibiotics with known activity in a certain metabolic pathway are investigated, the data can be exploited to define a pathway-specific stimulon or a proteomic signature that is indicative of the inhibition of a specific target, which might prove to be useful later in identifying and characterizing novel antibiotics that act within that pathway. Another application for proteomic studies within the drug-discovery process is the verification that a compound, which inhibits the activity of a desired isolated protein in a biochemical target assay, acts indeed as expected when tested against whole bacterial cells, and does not kill the cell due to other, not target-related, possibly undesired and non-specific activities such as general membrane perturbation or intercalation into nucleic acids.

Gene-expression analysis is increasingly important in many fields of biological research. Understanding patterns of expressed genes is expected to provide insight into complex regulatory networks and will most probably lead to the identification of genes relevant to new biological processes, or implicated in disease. Real-time PCR provides the simultaneous measurement of gene expression in many different samples for a limited number of genes, and is especially suitable when only a small number of cells are available (Fink et al., 1998). Many changes in the protein synthesis patterns in response to the antibiotics were consistent with existing knowledge on the modes of action and on the cellular responses to changes in environmental conditions. Inhibition of Ile-tRNA synthetase induced the stringent response, and protein synthesis inhibitors that interfere with translation accuracy induced class I heat shock proteins known to be induced by misfolded proteins. Each response, however, also yielded new information, for example, the expression of proteins with unknown function, a shift in the pIs of proteins newly synthesized after actinonin treatment, or the good correlation of the protein expression profiles of nitrofurantoin and diamide (Bandow et al., 2003). The NCBI-matched proteins that show overregulation were then further confirmed on the mRNA level by quantitative real time PCR. Identified proteins were representing diverse functional activities including energy production, metabolism, and nucleic acid synthesis. Interestingly, some recognized proteins have some relevance to bacterial virulence e.g. *Salmonella* pathogenicity island 1 effector protein, T-cell inhibitor protein, response regulator protein, paratose synthetase protein (RfbS) and heat shock protein 90. Comparative proteomics analysis of the cytosolic proteins of *S.* Gallinarum and *S.* Enteritidis isolated from poultry was performed and revealed the presence of some proteins of unknown function, which raise the speculation for their importance in either host adaptation or pathogenicity among *S.* Gallinarum serovars (Osman et al., 2009).

Current strategies for the discovery of novel antibacterial agents can be categorized as being either directed against a specific molecular target or based on reverse genomics. In the target-based approach, a certain molecular target is carefully selected and then compound libraries are screened specifically for inhibitors of its function. In the "reverse-genomics" approach, a compound is selected for its promising antibacterial activity and the target is determined in a second step.

In antibiotic drug discovery two major strategies are used (Bandow et al., 2003): the evaluation of structural variations among existing antibiotic classes in order to find compounds which hit the same targets by similar molecular mechanisms and the evaluation of novel antibiotic substances arising either from high-throughput target-based assays, or from antibacterial activity screening. If, through its antibacterial activity alone, a novel compound class arouses interest, its molecular target needs to be identified so that undesirable side effects on eukaryotic cells can be minimized (target identification). In addition, for structurally modified antibiotics or compounds derived from the target-based assays it is necessary to prove that interaction with the cellular target is indeed the direct cause for bacterial cell death (target validation).

Bandow et al. (2003) used a proteomic approach to study the responses of bacteria to antibacterial compounds and demonstrated that proteome analysis is useful for both target identification and target validation. They began building a database from 2D protein analysis of bacterial responses to antibiotic treatment, considering all important established and emerging antibiotic classes as well as some substances causing generalized cell damage. *Bacillus subtilis* was the chosen organism because its genome is fully sequenced and earlier proteome studies focusing on the description of protein signatures of environmental stimuli were accessible in the Sub2D database. Therefore, 30 antimicrobial compounds were studied, most of which have been well characterized in terms of their mechanisms of action and by comparison with known antibiotics, and they were able to predict the mode of action of the structurally new antibacterial BAY 50-2369. This study also provided a better understanding of nitrofurantoin's mode of action, which has been used for decades in the treatment of urinary tract infections. Hence, Bandow et al. (2003) showed that, by mirroring the complex molecular reactions of bacteria, proteomics is able to enlarge the view of known antibiotics and assist in the discovery of new drugs.

5. Effects of external stress on the *Salmonella* proteome

The capability of growing many bacterial species in well-defined artificial culture media has been a pre-requisite for the current in-depth understanding of bacterial physiology. Repeatedly, those culture media provide the most advantageous growth conditions that allow maximal and uniform logarithmic bacterial growth until some components of the medium become exhausted and logarithmic growth ceases. Under such optimal conditions, the protein composition of the cell is usually quite constant and tuned to support the special conditions of rapid growth. However, on the external environment, outside the laboratory, bacteria face much less supportive and highly variable growth conditions, with respect to temperature, pH, osmolarity, nutrient availability, host interactions, etc. Those stress situations do not principally differ from the stresses induced by antibiotic attack. Antibiotics are frequently encountered by many bacteria in their natural habitats, because many microorganisms produce them to suppress the growth of competitors. Hence, even antibiotic classes that stem from purely synthetic approaches and are never encountered by bacteria during evolution can, to a certain extent, mimic "natural" processes for which bacteria have developed regulatory mechanisms (Brotz-Oesterhelt et al., 2005).

It is critical for survival that the protein composition of a cell is constantly adjusted to meet the challenges of changing environmental conditions. Thus, bacteria respond to their environment with programmed changes in gene expression and their evolutionary success is strongly dependent on their ability to respond to external adverse conditions through a set of behavioural responses (Brotz-Oesterhelt et al., 2005). Proteomic technologies appear to be the natural tools to study the consequences of these regulatory processes on protein composition since a large number of external and internal signal molecules and signal transduction processes are present in bacteria to adapt their protein composition to the changing requirements of their environment (Armitage et al., 2003). During the past decade, proteomic technologies have been greatly refined and have been applied to investigate differences in the protein expression profiles of cells grown under a broad spectrum of growth conditions and with different stress factors, including some antibiotics (Bandow et al., 2003).

The number of detected proteins in response to stress mechanisms represents only a small proportion of the predicted proteome, as many genes may only be induced and expressed under certain conditions. Coldham et al. (2006) evaluated the effect of fluoroquinolone exposure on the proteome of *S. enterica* serovar Typhimurium using strain SL1344 and a MAR mutant. Broth cultures of strain SL1344 were treated with ciprofloxacin and enrofloxacin. Then, protein expression was determined by two-dimensional HPLC-MS^n and also, after exposure to ciprofloxacin, by two-dimensional gel electrophoresis (Figure 6).

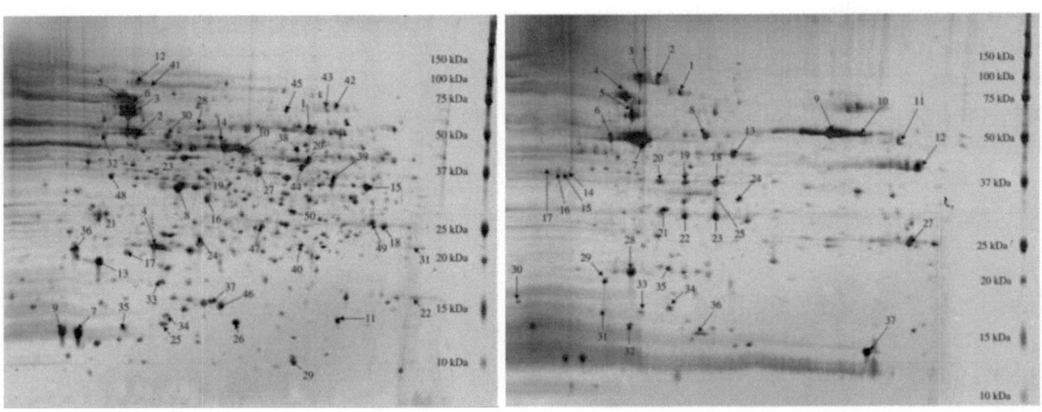

Fig. 6. Silver-stained second-dimension electrophoretogram of the proteome of S. Typhimurium extracted from untreated cultures (left) and from a culture following treatment with ciprofloxacin (right). Coldham et al., 2006, Effect of fluoroquinolone exposure on the proteome of *S. Enterica* serovar Typhimurium. Journal of Antimicrobial Chemotherapy, 2006, 58 (6): 1145-1153, by permission of Oxford University Press.

Coordinated regulation of protein effector expression is a key feature of innate reduced susceptibility to multiple antibiotics (Randall & Woodward, 2002). The chromosomal MAR locus of *E. coli,* in cooperation with other regulatory loci, plays a pivotal role in innate reduced susceptibility (circa 4-fold) to some unrelated antibiotics and certain disinfectants (Levy, 2002). Overexpression of the AcrAB-TolC efflux pump contributes to multiple antibiotic resistance in *E coli,* and has also been associated in conjunction with mutations in gyrA with resistance to fluoroquinolones in *S. enterica.* The AcrAB efflux pump of *E. coli* and *S. enterica* belongs to the resistance/nodulation/cell division (RND) family and consists of a proton antiporter (AcrB) and a membrane fusion protein (AcrA) (Borges-Walmsley & Walmsley, 2001; Zgurskaya & Nikaido, 2000). These two proteins associate with an outer membrane channel protein, such as TolC, to form a functional efflux pump unit providing selective molecular translocation of solutes from the periplasm to the external environment. Reduced expression of porin proteins located in the outer cell membrane may act synergistically with efflux pumps to reduce penetration of antibiotic into the bacterial periplasm. Whilst much is understood about the mechanisms of efflux, little is known of the secondary responses enabling the physiological adaptation of *Salmonella* to fluoroquinolones. This study demonstrated an increased and decreased expression of a wide range of proteins on the proteome of *S. enterica* serovar Typhimurium after fluoroquinolone exposure; the basal expression of the efflux system AcrAB/TolC, which contributes to antibiotic resistance, was elevated in the multiple antibiotic resistant mutant when compared with the untreated wild-type and also increased following treatment with ciprofloxacin. Therefore, an amplified expression of AcrAB/TolC was associated with resistance while other increases, such as in F_1F_0-ATP synthase and Imp, were a response to fluoroquinolone exposure (Coldham et al., 2006).

Proteomic analysis of triclosan resistance in *S. enterica* serovar Typhimurium by proteomics identified a set of proteins with commonly altered expression in all triclosan-resistant mutants. According to the authors, this 'triclosan resistance network' included nine proteins involved in the production of pyruvate or fatty acid. This may represent a mechanism by which the triclosan-resistant mutants have increased throughput of fatty acid biosynthesis by increased pyruvate production or have altered metabolic pathways in order to produce fatty acid via a different pathway (conversion of glycerol to hexadecanoate or increased citrate production to feed acetyl-CoA production). Proteomic data revealed specific patterns of protein expression in each mutant as well as the 25 proteins that constitute a common metabolic resistance network in all mutants studied. These data show that triclosan resistance is multifactorial and a number of resistance mechanisms act in synergy to achieve high-level resistance. This indicates that triclosan is likely to act on multiple targets within the cell rather than being exclusively an inhibitor of fabI (Webber et al., 2008). The physiological status of supercritical carbon dioxide (SC-CO_2) treated *S. enterica* serotype Typhimurium was analyzed by using gas chromatography mass spectrometry (GC–MS) analysis of fatty acids with principal component analysis and two-dimensional electrophoresis for protein profiling. From the results of these systemic analyses, it was revealed that SC-CO_2 caused significant alterations to the profiles of fatty acids and proteins of the cells (Kim et al., 2009). This data and other results of stress induced/repressed proteins obtained by proteomics in *Salmonella spp.* are summarized in Table 3.

Stress	Differential expression	Identified Proteins	Relevant Protein Function	Reference
Acid	Overexpression	fliC	Virulence during infection	Jindal et al., 2011
Anaerobiosis	Overexpression	38 proteins, more importantly Mdh, PflI, FrdA, AckA, AdhE	Metabolism (mixed-acid fermentation)	Encheva et al., 2009
	Underexpression	42 proteins, more importantly ArgT, HisJ, GlnQ, GltI, OppA, DppA, SodA, SuhB, DnaK, GroS, SspA, PspA, OsmC, UspG	Transport, stress-response and chaperone function	
Fluoroquinolone	Overexpression	43 proteins, more importantly AtpA, AtpC, AtpD, AtpH, Imp, TolC, AcrB	Mechanisms of resistance	Coldham et al., 2006
Hydrogen Peroxide (H_2O_2)	Over- and underexpression	76 proteins, more importantly SipC, SopB, SipA	Survival and replication under oxidative stress and during infection	Kim et al., 2010
Propionate (PA)	Overexpression	Dps, CpxR, RplE, RplF, SodA	PA-induced acid resistance, virulence and pathogenesis	Calhoun et al., 2010
Thymol	Over- and underexpression	45 proteins, more importantly Trx1, FtsZ, CheW, GroEL, DnaK	Antioxidant and chaperon function	Di Pasqua et al., 2010
Triclosan	Overexpression	25 proteins, more importantly ArcA, GcvP, MdH, MaeB, GapA, PpS, FadB, GltA, GlpK	Pyruvate or fatty acid production (Metabolic triclosan resistance network)	Webber et al., 2008

Table 3. Summary of some results on stress induced/repressed proteins obtained by proteomics in *Salmonella spp.*

6. Remarks on proteomics as a biomarker search tool

After its steep rise in the late 1970s and the early 1980s after O'Farrell's outstanding publication, there was a slow decline of the application of 2-DE in the late 1980s due to the inability to identify the gel-separated proteins of interest on a large scale. However, after the introduction of large-scale genome sequencing, the development of MS methods for the analysis of proteins and peptides, progress in bioinformatic tools and the rise of proteomics in general has experienced a revival and is today by far the most commonly applied protein separation technology in proteome research (Görg et al., 2009). Recent advances in biological and analytical sciences have led to an unprecedented interest in the discovery and quantification of endogenous molecules which serve as indicators of drug safety, mechanism of action, efficacy, and disease state progression. By allowing better decision-making, these indicators, referred to as biomarkers, can dramatically improve the efficiency of drug discovery and development (Ackermann et al., 2006).

Comparative genomics and several genomic tools have been used to identify virulence factors and genes involved in environmental persistence of pathogens. Proteomics has been contributing to a wide-range of scientific disciplines, but perhaps no area is more critical than the discovery of novel biomarkers. The extraordinary developments made in proteomic technologies in the past decade have enabled investigators to search for biomarkers by scanning complex proteome samples using unbiased methods (Veenstra, 2007). Currently, the search for protein biomarkers has been dominated by the employment of MS. Its high mass accuracy, resolution, dynamic range, sensitivity and even more importantly the speed at which MS/MS is performed, allowing thousands of proteins to be unambiguously identified, have made MS an invaluable tool for biomarker discovery (Blonder et al., 2011).

To identify novel diagnostic and therapeutic biomarkers, investigators focus on the discovery of proteins that are more or less abundant in samples obtained from patients with a specific disease compared to those acquired from healthy-matched control patients. There are a number of different MS-based methods to conduct these studies such as 2-DE/MS, proteomic profiling, stable-isotope proteome tagging and subtractive proteomics (for detailed description of each method see Veenstra, 2007).

Recent data suggests that marker panels derived from transcriptomic or proteomic profiling are superior to single genes or markers in differentiating non-infectious from sepsis-associated systemic inflammation (Johnson et al., 2007). Early and adequate antibiotic therapy is mandatory for successful sepsis therapy; hence a rapid diagnosis of infection and sepsis is of great significance. Diagnostic uncertainty is usually compensated by the liberal use of broad-spectrum antibiotics which leads to increased drug resistance. Therefore, the use of these biomarkers might help to avoid antibiotic misuse and overuse and to curb the rising incidence of microbial resistance (Reinhart & Hartog, 2010).

With the advent of large-scale proteomic sequencing, the general belief was that biomarkers would be obvious within the data sets but unfortunately the results showed numerous background proteins that are routinely identified but have little value as biomarkers and numerous proteins that show a difference in comparative studies but their value as a reliable biomarker is extremely difficult to determine (Blonder et al., 2011). Having too many potential biomarkers is considered a problem when examining the workflow required to validate a biomarker for clinical use (Figure 7). In this scheme, thousands of analytes are measured in a few samples and when potential biomarkers are found, a more direct approach is taken to specifically measure these potential biomarkers again in a small number of samples to qualify the results from the discovery stage. The analytes that pass the qualification stage are then specifically measured in a larger number of samples to verify their utility as biomarkers. Those that pass the verification stage are then measured in a very large number of clinical samples to provide final validation that these proteins can function reliably (Blonder et al., 2011).

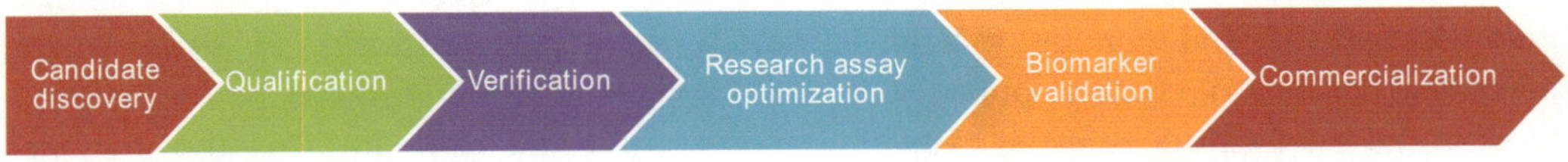

Fig. 7. The six essential process components in the biomarker pipeline: candidate discovery, qualification, verification, research assay optimization, biomarker validation and commercialization. Based on Rifai et al., 2006: Protein biomarker discovery and validation: The long and uncertain path to clinical utility. Nat Biotechnol, 24(8): 971-983.

The advances made in proteomic technology, primarily in the field of MS, allowed to scrutinize proteome samples to a far greater extent than previously possible. There are many options available to measure the relative abundance of proteins but unfortunately the number of biomarkers that have ultimately been successfully validated using these discovery approaches is discouraging - between 2003 and 2008, only 7 protein biomarkers were approved by the US FDA (Qi et al., 1996). In fact, MS-based studies are able to come up with very large numbers of "potential" biomarkers but the challenge relies on how to identify those that have the highest chance of being validated in a well-controlled clinical trial. Validation of a single biomarker is expensive in terms of money and time and so it is impossible to graduate a large number of potential biomarkers to a validation phase. Unfortunately, it is difficult to inherently recognize those proteins identified in the discovery phase that may turn out to be the best biomarker. Nevertheless, encouragement can be found in the progress that has been made in the past years, allowing investigators to attempt the types of biomarker studies that are being conducted today (Veenstra, 2007). On the other hand, the current proteomic technology still does not allow studying the full genomic equivalent of all proteins, whereas transcriptome analyses cover the whole genomic sequence and are also able to produce data at a much higher pace. Nevertheless, transcript expression profiling is unable to distinguish between different gene products derived from the same coding region on the genome (due to, e.g., modifications, truncations, or splice variants). It should also be kept in mind that none of these technologies alone will be able to deliver novel drugs.

7. Outlook

The genomics revolution has changed the paradigm for the comprehensive analysis of biological processes. The genomic era began in the year 1995 when the first complete bacterial genomic sequence of *Haemophilus influenzae* was published. Since that moment, a distinct change in the quality of microbial genetic studies can be observed. Analyses of single genes leads presently to global analyses of microbial cells, while analyses of full genetic sequences, whole transcriptomes as well as total protein content or networks of protein-protein interactions is directed to the genome, transcriptome, proteome and interactome, respectively. The word Proteome describes the ensemble of protein forms expressed in a biological sample at a given point in time and in a given situation. Proteomics has seen the increasing creation of new useful techniques, but the study of proteomes is still based on 2-DE, allied with MS analysis. Among the proteomic techniques commonly used for analysis of protein expression in biological samples, 2D-PAGE is a popular technique for the separation of proteins. However, 2-DE still has some drawbacks, like excluding the smallest and the largest proteins, those which are extremely acidic and those extremely basic (Gygi et al., 2000). Furthermore, some proteins cannot be detected due to the low sensitivity of the system (Washburn et al., 2001; Wu & Han, 2006). On the other hand, there are certain limitations to the universal use of this technology, such as low detection sensitivity and linearity, poor solubility of membrane proteins, limited loading capacity of gradient pH strips, gel reproducibility, relatively low throughput and low linear range of visualisation procedures (López et al., 2004). RNA profiling, which is capable of addressing the expression of all genes in an organism, can be used to complement proteome analysis. An increase in sensitivity can be achieved through modifications or additions to the common proteomic methods. Loading higher amounts of proteins onto a 2-DE gel can help in the identification of low-expressed proteins, despite the fact that, in this case, these can be "hidden" by high-abundance proteins. Also, the use of different protein extraction buffers and detergents can improve the sensitivity and resolution of the 2-DE profiles. IPG strips provide reproducibility, increased resolution and loading capacity and simplicity to isoelectric focusing of 2-DE. With this technique, a higher number of different proteins can be resolved where previously a single spot was present in the gel (Fey & Larsen, 2001; Wildgruber et al., 2000). Non-equilibrium pH gel electrophoresis (NEPHGE) is another method that allows a better resolution of protein spots; the resulting peptides are then separated through multi-dimensional chromatography and analyzed using tandem-MS, and if combined with stable isotope labeling experiment methods, it can be a very powerful tool for proteome characterization. Protein arrays and antibody microarrays can create proteomic maps, revealing the proteome (Souza et al., 2008; Wingren & Borrebaeck, 2004).

Substantial progress has already been made in elucidating the basic regulatory networks that form the basis for the extraordinary capacity of bacteria to adapt to a diversity of lifestyles and external stress factors. A database of these results will be able to facilitate the identification of more comprehensive signatures for treatment with antimicrobial agents and support functional analysis by combined protein and RNA profiling. However, since classical proteomic approaches alone mainly provide information on the relative amounts of protein species and only rarely provides information on the activity of these protein species, it is necessary to complement these findings with metabolomics and interaction studies to determine the true functional level of biological systems. Proteomics and genomics technologies offer more sensitive and specific methods for identification of microbial food contaminants and their toxins. Classical antibiotics are characterized as compounds which influence microbial life processes without harming the host's cells. Their main mechanism of action is based on blocking cell wall synthesis and replication or translation inhibition. Metagenomic techniques, based on direct cloning of DNA present in natural environments, allow the identification of several new antibiotics. The increasing resistance of bacterial pathogens to present day antibiotics and the lack of a robust pipeline of innovative antimicrobial substances demand innovative and more efficient approaches towards the development of anti-infective drugs.

8. References

Ackermann, B. L., Hale, J. E. & Duffin, K. L. (2006). The Role of Mass Spectrometry in Biomarker Discovery and Measurement. *Curr Drug Metab*, Vol. 7, No. 5, (Jun, 2006), pp. (525-539), ISSN 1389-2002

Angulo, F., Nargund, V. & Chiller, T. (2004). Evidence of an association between use of anti-microbial agents in food animals and anti-microbial resistance among bacteria isolated from humans and the human health consequences of such resistance. *Journal of Veterinary Medicine B. Infectious Diseases and Veterinary Public Health.* No. 51, pp. 374-379

Antunes, P., Machado, J. & Peixe, L. (2006). Characterization of Antimicrobial Resistance and Class 1 and 2 Integrons in Salmonella Enterica Isolates from Different Sources in Portugal. *J Antimicrob Chemother*, Vol. 58, No. 2, (Aug, 2006), pp. (297-304), ISSN 0305-7453

Apfel, C. M., Locher, H., Evers, S., Takacs, B., Hubschwerlen, C., Pirson, W., Page, M. G. & Keck, W. (2001). Peptide Deformylase as an Antibacterial Drug Target: Target Validation and Resistance Development. *Antimicrob Agents Chemother*, Vol. 45, No. 4, (Apr, 2001), pp. (1058-1064), ISSN 0066-4804

Armitage, J. P., Dorman, C. J., Hellingwerf, K., Schmitt, R., Summers, D. & Holland, B. (2003). Thinking and Decision Making, Bacterial Style: Bacterial Neural Networks, Obernai, France, 7th-12th June 2002. *Mol Microbiol*, Vol. 47, No. 2, (Jan, 2003), pp. (583-593), ISSN 0950-382X

Bager, F. & Helmuth, R. (2001). Epidemiology of Resistance to Quinolones in Salmonella. *Vet Res*, Vol. 32, No. 3-4, (May-Aug, 2001), pp. (285-290), ISSN 0928-4249

Bandow, J. E., Becher, D., Buttner, K., Hochgrafe, F., Freiberg, C., Brotz, H. & Hecker, M. (2003). The Role of Peptide Deformylase in Protein Biosynthesis: A Proteomic Study. *Proteomics*, Vol. 3, No. 3, (Mar, 2003), pp. (299-306), ISSN 1615-9853

Bandow, J. E., Brotz, H., Leichert, L. I., Labischinski, H. & Hecker, M. (2003). Proteomic Approach to Understanding Antibiotic Action. *Antimicrob Agents Chemother*, Vol. 47, No. 3, (Mar, 2003), pp. (948-955), ISSN 0066-4804

Bjellqvist, B., Ek, K., Righetti, P. G., Gianazza, E., Gorg, A., Westermeier, R. & Postel, W. (1982). Isoelectric Focusing in Immobilized Ph Gradients: Principle, Methodology and Some Applications. *J Biochem Biophys Methods*, Vol. 6, No. 4, (Sep, 1982), pp. (317-339), ISSN 0165-022X

Blonder, J., Issaq, H. J. & Veenstra, T. D. (2011). Proteomic Biomarker Discovery: It's More Than Just Mass Spectrometry. *Electrophoresis*, Vol. 32, No. 13, (Jun, 2011), pp. (1541-1548), ISSN 1522-2683

Borges-Walmsley, M. I. & Walmsley, A. R. (2001). The Structure and Function of Drug Pumps. *Trends Microbiol*, Vol. 9, No. 2, (Feb, 2001), pp. (71-79), ISSN 0966-842X

Brisabois, A., Cazin, I., Breuil, J. & Collatz, E. (1997). Surveillance of Antibiotic Resistance in Salmonella. *Euro Surveill*, Vol. 2, No. 3, (Mar, 1997), pp. (19-20), ISSN 1560-7917

Brotz-Oesterhelt, H., Bandow, J. E. & Labischinski, H. (2005). Bacterial Proteomics and Its Role in Antibacterial Drug Discovery. *Mass Spectrom Rev*, Vol. 24, No. 4, (Jul-Aug, 2005), pp. (549-565), ISSN 0277-7037

Calhoun, L. N., Liyanage, R., Lay, J. O., Jr. & Kwon, Y. M. (2010). Proteomic Analysis of Salmonella Enterica Serovar Enteritidis Following Propionate Adaptation. *BMC Microbiol*, Vol. 10, No. 2010), pp. (249), ISSN 1471-2180

Chiu, C. H., Tang, P., Chu, C., Hu, S., Bao, Q., Yu, J., Chou, Y. Y., Wang, H. S. & Lee, Y. S. (2005). The Genome Sequence of Salmonella Enterica Serovar Choleraesuis, a Highly Invasive and Resistant Zoonotic Pathogen. *Nucleic Acids Res*, Vol. 33, No. 5, 2005), pp. (1690-1698), ISSN 1362-4962

Coldham, N. G., Randall, L. P., Piddock, L. J. & Woodward, M. J. (2006). Effect of Fluoroquinolone Exposure on the Proteome of Salmonella Enterica Serovar Typhimurium. *J Antimicrob Chemother*, Vol. 58, No. 6, (Dec, 2006), pp. (1145-1153), ISSN 0305-7453

de Godoy, L. M., Olsen, J. V., Cox, J., Nielsen, M. L., Hubner, N. C., Frohlich, F., Walther, T. C. & Mann, M. (2008). Comprehensive Mass-Spectrometry-Based Proteome Quantification of Haploid Versus Diploid Yeast. *Nature*, Vol. 455, No. 7217, (Oct 30, 2008), pp. (1251-1254), ISSN 1476-4687

DelVecchio, V. G., Wagner, M. A., Eschenbrenner, M., Horn, T. A., Kraycer, J. A., Estock, F., Elzer, P. & Mujer, C. V. (2002). Brucella Proteomes--a Review. *Vet Microbiol*, Vol. 90, No. 1-4, (Dec 20, 2002), pp. (593-603), ISSN 0378-1135

Deng, W., Liou, S. R., Plunkett, G., 3rd, Mayhew, G. F., Rose, D. J., Burland, V., Kodoyianni, V., Schwartz, D. C. & Blattner, F. R. (2003). Comparative Genomics of Salmonella Enterica Serovar Typhi Strains Ty2 and Ct18. *J Bacteriol*, Vol. 185, No. 7, (Apr, 2003), pp. (2330-2337), ISSN 0021-9193

Di Pasqua, R., Mamone, G., Ferranti, P., Ercolini, D. & Mauriello, G. (2010). Changes in the Proteome of Salmonella Enterica Serovar Thompson as Stress Adaptation to Sublethal Concentrations of Thymol. *Proteomics*, Vol. 10, No. 5, (Mar, 2010), pp. (1040-1049), ISSN 1615-9861

Dunne, E. F., Fey, P. D., Kludt, P., Reporter, R., Mostashari, F., Shillam, P., Wicklund, J., Miller, C., Holland, B., Stamey, K., Barrett, T. J., Rasheed, J. K., Tenover, F. C., Ribot, E. M. & Angulo, F. J. (2000). Emergence of Domestically Acquired Ceftriaxone-Resistant Salmonella Infections Associated with Ampc Beta-Lactamase. *JAMA*, Vol. 284, No. 24, (Dec 27, 2000), pp. (3151-3156), ISSN 0098-7484

Edwards, R. A., Olsen, G. J. & Maloy, S. R. (2002). Comparative Genomics of Closely Related Salmonellae. *Trends Microbiol*, Vol. 10, No. 2, (Feb, 2002), pp. (94-99), ISSN 0966-842X

Encheva, V., Shah, H. N. & Gharbia, S. E. (2009). Proteomic Analysis of the Adaptive Response of Salmonella Enterica Serovar Typhimurium to Growth under Anaerobic Conditions. *Microbiology*, Vol. 155, No. Pt 7, (Jul, 2009), pp. (2429-2441), ISSN 1350-0872

Evers, S., Di Padova, K., Meyer, M., Langen, H., Fountoulakis, M., Keck, W. & Gray, C. P. (2001). Mechanism-Related Changes in the Gene Transcription and Protein Synthesis Patterns of Haemophilus Influenzae after Treatment with Transcriptional and Translational Inhibitors. *Proteomics*, Vol. 1, No. 4, (Apr, 2001), pp. (522-544), ISSN 1615-9853

Fey, P. D., Safranek, T. J., Rupp, M. E., Dunne, E. F., Ribot, E., Iwen, P. C., Bradford, P. A., Angulo, F. J. & Hinrichs, S. H. (2000). Ceftriaxone-Resistant Salmonella Infection Acquired by a Child from Cattle. *N Engl J Med*, Vol. 342, No. 17, (Apr 27, 2000), pp. (1242-1249), ISSN 0028-4793

Fey, S. J. & Larsen, P. M. (2001). 2d or Not 2d. Two-Dimensional Gel Electrophoresis. *Curr Opin Chem Biol*, Vol. 5, No. 1, (Feb, 2001), pp. (26-33), ISSN 1367-5931

Fink, L., Seeger, W., Ermert, L., Hanze, J., Stahl, U., Grimminger, F., Kummer, W. & Bohle, R. M. (1998). Real-Time Quantitative Rt-Pcr after Laser-Assisted Cell Picking. *Nat Med*, Vol. 4, No. 11, (Nov, 1998), pp. (1329-1333), ISSN 1078-8956

Gmuender, H., Kuratli, K., Di Padova, K., Gray, C. P., Keck, W. & Evers, S. (2001). Gene Expression Changes Triggered by Exposure of Haemophilus Influenzae to Novobiocin or Ciprofloxacin: Combined Transcription and Translation Analysis. *Genome Res*, Vol. 11, No. 1, (Jan, 2001), pp. (28-42), ISSN 1088-9051

Görg, A., Drews, O., Lück, C., Weiland, F. & Weiss, W. (2009). 2-De with Ipgs. *Electrophoresis*, Vol. 30, No. S1, 2009), pp. (122-132), ISSN 1522-2683

Gray, C. P. & Keck, W. (1999). Bacterial Targets and Antibiotics: Genome-Based Drug Discovery. *Cell Mol Life Sci*, Vol. 56, No. 9-10, (Nov 30, 1999), pp. (779-787), ISSN 1420-682X

Gygi, S. P., Corthals, G. L., Zhang, Y., Rochon, Y. & Aebersold, R. (2000). Evaluation of Two-Dimensional Gel Electrophoresis-Based Proteome Analysis Technology. *Proc Natl Acad Sci U S A*, Vol. 97, No. 17, (Aug 15, 2000), pp. (9390-9395), ISSN 0027-8424

Hamacher, M. Eisenacher, M. & Stephan, C. (2011). *Data Mining in Proteomics from Standards to Applications,* Springer, ISBN 978-1-60761-986-4, Germany

Han, X., Aslanian, A. & Yates, J. R., 3rd. (2008). Mass Spectrometry for Proteomics. *Curr Opin Chem Biol*, Vol. 12, No. 5, (Oct, 2008), pp. (483-490), ISSN 1367-5931

Hecker, M., Antelmann, H., Buttner, K. & Bernhardt, J. (2008). Gel-Based Proteomics of Gram-Positive Bacteria: A Powerful Tool to Address Physiological Questions. *Proteomics*, Vol. 8, No. 23-24, (Dec, 2008), pp. (4958-4975), ISSN 1615-9861

Helms, M., Vastrup, P., Gerner-Smidt, P. & Molbak, K. (2002). Excess Mortality Associated with Antimicrobial Drug-Resistant Salmonella Typhimurium. *Emerg Infect Dis*, Vol. 8, No. 5, (May, 2002), pp. (490-495), ISSN 1080-6040

Holland, R. D., Wilkes, J. G., Rafii, F., Sutherland, J. B., Persons, C. C., Voorhees, K. J. & Lay, J. O., Jr. (1996). Rapid Identification of Intact Whole Bacteria Based on Spectral Patterns Using Matrix-Assisted Laser Desorption/Ionization with Time-of-Flight Mass Spectrometry. *Rapid Commun Mass Spectrom*, Vol. 10, No. 10, 1996), pp. (1227-1232), ISSN 0951-4198

International surveillance network for the enteric infections Salmonella and VTEC O157. 10 January 2008, Available from: http://www.hpa.org.uk/hpa/inter/enternet_menu.htm

Jindal, T., Mandal, S. N., Kamal, M. R., Das, A. K. & Karmakar, D. (2011). Occult Mucin Secreting Adenocarcinoma of Gall Bladder with Metastasis to Urinary Bladder. *Updates Surg*, Vol. No. (Jul 1, 2011), pp. ISSN 2038-131X

Johnson, S. B., Lissauer, M., Bochicchio, G. V., Moore, R., Cross, A. S. & Scalea, T. M. (2007). Gene Expression Profiles Differentiate between Sterile Sirs and Early Sepsis. *Ann Surg*, Vol. 245, No. 4, (Apr, 2007), pp. (611-621), ISSN 0003-4932

Karatzas, K. A., Randall, L. P., Webber, M., Piddock, L. J., Humphrey, T. J., Woodward, M. J. & Coldham, N. G. (2008). Phenotypic and Proteomic Characterization of Multiply Antibiotic-Resistant Variants of Salmonella Enterica Serovar Typhimurium Selected Following Exposure to Disinfectants. *Appl Environ Microbiol*, Vol. 74, No. 5, (Mar, 2008), pp. (1508-1516), ISSN 1098-5336

Kim, K., Yang, E., Vu, G. P., Gong, H., Su, J., Liu, F. & Lu, S. (2010). Mass Spectrometry-Based Quantitative Proteomic Analysis of Salmonella Enterica Serovar Enteritidis Protein Expression Upon Exposure to Hydrogen Peroxide. *BMC Microbiol*, Vol. 10, No. 2010), pp. (166), ISSN 1471-2180

Kim, S. R., Kim, H. T., Park, H. J., Kim, S., Choi, H. J., Hwang, G. S., Yi, J. H., Ryu do, H. & Kim, K. H. (2009). Fatty Acid Profiling and Proteomic Analysis of Salmonella Enterica Serotype Typhimurium Inactivated with Supercritical Carbon Dioxide. *Int J Food Microbiol*, Vol. 134, No. 3, (Sep 15, 2009), pp. (190-195), ISSN 1879-3460

Krishnamurthy, T. & Ross, P. L. (1996). Rapid Identification of Bacteria by Direct Matrix-Assisted Laser Desorption/Ionization Mass Spectrometric Analysis of Whole Cells. *Rapid Commun Mass Spectrom*, Vol. 10, No. 15, 1996), pp. (1992-1996), ISSN 0951-4198

Leverrier, P., Vissers, J. P., Rouault, A., Boyaval, P. & Jan, G. (2004). Mass Spectrometry Proteomic Analysis of Stress Adaptation Reveals Both Common and Distinct Response Pathways in Propionibacterium Freudenreichii. *Arch Microbiol*, Vol. 181, No. 3, (Mar, 2004), pp. (215-230), ISSN 0302-8933

Levy, S. B. (2002). Active Efflux, a Common Mechanism for Biocide and Antibiotic Resistance. *J Appl Microbiol*, Vol. 92 Suppl, No. 2002), pp. (65S-71S), ISSN 1364-5072

Lipton, M. S., Pasa-Tolic, L., Anderson, G. A., Anderson, D. J., Auberry, D. L., Battista, J. R., Daly, M. J., Fredrickson, J., Hixson, K. K., Kostandarithes, H., Masselon, C., Markillie, L. M., Moore, R. J., Romine, M. F., Shen, Y., Stritmatter, E., Tolic, N., Udseth, H. R., Venkateswaran, A., Wong, K. K., Zhao, R. & Smith, R. D. (2002). Global Analysis of the Deinococcus Radiodurans Proteome by Using Accurate Mass Tags. *Proc Natl Acad Sci U S A*, Vol. 99, No. 17, (Aug 20, 2002), pp. (11049-11054), ISSN 0027-8424

López, J.A., Bernard, A. & Albar, J. P. (2004). Protein expression profiling analysis in hematopoietic stem cells: phenotypic characterization of mesenchymal stem cells, In: *Biomedical Applications of Proteomics*, Sanchez, J. C., Corthals, G. & Hochstrasser, D. F., pp. (155–171), WILEY-VCH Verlag, Weinheim, Germany.

Lucas, R. L. & Lee, C. A. (2000). Unravelling the Mysteries of Virulence Gene Regulation in Salmonella Typhimurium. *Mol Microbiol*, Vol. 36, No. 5, (Jun, 2000), pp. (1024-1033), ISSN 0950-382X

Mallick, P. & Kuster, B. (2010). Proteomics: A Pragmatic Perspective. *Nat Biotechnol*, Vol. 28, No. 7, (Jul, 2010), pp. (695-709), ISSN 1546-1696

McClelland, M., Sanderson, K. E., Spieth, J., Clifton, S. W., Latreille, P., Courtney, L., Porwollik, S., Ali, J., Dante, M., Du, F., Hou, S., Layman, D., Leonard, S., Nguyen, C., Scott, K., Holmes, A., Grewal, N., Mulvaney, E., Ryan, E., Sun, H., Florea, L., Miller, W., Stoneking, T., Nhan, M., Waterston, R. & Wilson, R. K. (2001). Complete Genome Sequence of Salmonella Enterica Serovar Typhimurium Lt2. *Nature*, Vol. 413, No. 6858, (Oct 25, 2001), pp. (852-856), ISSN 0028-0836

McClelland, M., Sanderson, E. K., Porwollik, S., Spieth, J., Clifton, S. W., Fulton, R., Chunyan, W., Wollam, A., Shah, N., Pepin, K., Bhonagiri, V., Nash, W., Johnson, M., Thiruvilangam, P. & Wilson, R. K. (2007). Submited to the Embl/Genbank/Ddbj Databases. (November, 2007)

Miko, A., Pries, K., Schroeter, A. & Helmuth, R. (2005). Molecular Mechanisms of Resistance in Multidrug-Resistant Serovars of Salmonella Enterica Isolated from Foods in Germany. *J Antimicrob Chemother*, Vol. 56, No. 6, (Dec, 2005), pp. (1025-1033), ISSN 0305-7453

Miller, S. I., Kukral, A. M. & Mekalanos, J. J. (1989). Atwo-Component Regulatory System (Phop-Phoq) Controls Salmonella Typhimurium Virulence. *Proc Natl Acad Sci U S A*, Vol. 86, No. 13, 1989), pp. (5054-5058),

Minden, J. (2007). Comparative Proteomics and Difference Gel Electrophoresis. *Biotechniques*, Vol. 43, No. 6, (Dec, 2007), pp. (739, 741, 743 passim), ISSN 0736-6205

Mishra, N. (2010). *Introduction to Proteomics: Principles and Applications* John Wiley & Sons Inc., ISBN 978-0-471-75402-2,

Musgrove, M. T., Jones, D. R., Northcutt, J. K., Cox, N. A., Harrison, M. A., Fedorka-Cray, P. J. & Ladely, S. R. (2006). Antimicrobial Resistance in Salmonella and Escherichia Coli Isolated from Commercial Shell Eggs. *Poult Sci*, Vol. 85, No. 9, (Sep, 2006), pp. (1665-1669), ISSN 0032-5791

Neidhardt, F. C., Ingraham, J. L. & Schaechter, M. (1990). *Physiology of the Bacterial Cell: A Molecular Approach* Sunderland, MA: Sinauer Associates Inc, ISBN 0878936084,

O'Connor, C. D., Farris, M., Fowler, R. & Qi, S. Y. (1997). The Proteome of Salmonella Enterica Serovar Typhimurium: Current Progress on Its Determination and Some Applications. *Electrophoresis*, Vol. 18, No. 8, (Aug, 1997), pp. (1483-1490), ISSN 0173-0835

O'Farrel, P. H. (1975) High resolution two-dimensional electrophoresis of proteins. *J Biological Chemistry*, Vol. 250. No. 10, pp. 4007-4021, ISSN 0021-9258

Osman, K. M., Ali, M. M., Radwan, M. I., Kim, H. K. & Han, J. (2009). Comparative Proteomic Analysis on Salmonella Gallinarum and Salmonella Enteritidis Exploring Proteins That May Incorporate Host Adaptation in Poultry. *J Proteomics*, Vol. 72, No. 5, (Jul 21, 2009), pp. (815-821), ISSN 1876-7737

Palagi, P. M., Hernandez, P., Walther, D. & Appel, R. D. (2006). Proteome Informatics I: Bioinformatics Tools for Processing Experimental Data. *Proteomics*, Vol. 6, No. 20, (Oct, 2006), pp. (5435-5444), ISSN 1615-9853

Parker, C. E., Pearson, T. W., Anderson, N. L. & Borchers, C. H. (2010). Mass-Spectrometry-Based Clinical Proteomics--a Review and Prospective. *Analyst*, Vol. 135, No. 8, (Aug, 2010), pp. (1830-1838), ISSN 1364-5528

Parkhill, J., Dougan, G., James, K. D., Thomson, N. R., Pickard, D., Wain, J., Churcher, C., Mungall, K. L., Bentley, S. D., Holden, M. T., Sebaihia, M., Baker, S., Basham, D., Brooks, K., Chillingworth, T., Connerton, P., Cronin, A., Davis, P., Davies, R. M., Dowd, L., White, N., Farrar, J., Feltwell, T., Hamlin, N., Haque, A., Hien, T. T., Holroyd, S., Jagels, K., Krogh, A., Larsen, T. S., Leather, S., Moule, S., O'Gaora, P., Parry, C., Quail, M., Rutherford, K., Simmonds, M., Skelton, J., Stevens, K., Whitehead, S. & Barrell, B. G. (2001). Complete Genome Sequence of a Multiple Drug Resistant Salmonella Enterica Serovar Typhi Ct18. *Nature*, Vol. 413, No. 6858, (Oct 25, 2001), pp. (848-852), ISSN 0028-0836

Pinto, L., Poeta, P., Vieira, S., Caleja, C., Radhouani, H., Carvalho, C., Vieira-Pinto, M., Themudo, P., Torres, C., Vitorino, R., Domingues, P. & Igrejas, G. (2010). Genomic and Proteomic Evaluation of Antibiotic Resistance in Salmonella Strains. *J Proteomics*, Vol. 73, No. 8, (Jun 16, 2010), pp. (1535-1541), ISSN 1876-7737

Qi, S. Y., Moir, A. & O'Connor, C. D. (1996). Proteome of Salmonella Typhimurium Sl1344: Identification of Novel Abundant Cell Envelope Proteins and Assignment to a Two-Dimensional Reference Map. *J Bacteriol*, Vol. 178, No. 16, (Aug, 1996), pp. (5032-5038), ISSN 0021-9193

Radhouani, H., Poeta, P., Pinto, L., Miranda, J., Coelho, C., Carvalho, C., Rodrigues, J., Lopez, M., Torres, C., Vitorino, R., Domingues, P. & Igrejas, G. (2010). Proteomic Characterization of Vana-Containing Enterococcus Recovered from Seagulls at the Berlengas Natural Reserve, W Portugal. *Proteome Sci*, Vol. 8, No. 2010), pp. (48), ISSN 1477-5956

Randall, L. P. & Woodward, M. J. (2002). The Multiple Antibiotic Resistance (Mar) Locus and Its Significance. *Res Vet Sci*, Vol. 72, No. 2, (Apr, 2002), pp. (87-93), ISSN 0034-5288

Reinhart, K. & Hartog, C. S. (2010). Biomarkers as a Guide for Antimicrobial Therapy. *Int J Antimicrob Agents*, Vol. 36 Suppl 2, No. (Dec, 2010), pp. (S17-21), ISSN 1872-7913

Renzone, G., D'Ambrosio, C., Arena, S., Rullo, R., Ledda, L., Ferrara, L. & Scaloni, A. (2005). Differential Proteomic Analysis in the Study of Prokaryotes Stress Resistance. *Ann Ist Super Sanita*, Vol. 41, No. 4, 2005), pp. (459-468), ISSN 0021-2571

Rifai, N., Gillette, M. A. & Carr, S. A. (2006). Protein Biomarker Discovery and Validation: The Long and Uncertain Path to Clinical Utility. *Nat Biotechnol*, Vol. 24, No. 8, (Aug, 2006), pp. (971-983), ISSN 1087-0156

Rince, A., Uguen, M., Le Breton, Y., Giard, J. C., Flahaut, S., Dufour, A. & Auffray, Y. (2002). The Enterococcus Faecalis Gene Encoding the Novel General Stress Protein Gsp62. *Microbiology*, Vol. 148, No. Pt 3, (Mar, 2002), pp. (703-711), ISSN 1350-0872

Roncada, P., Deriu, F., Gaviraghi, A., Martino, P. A. & Bonizzi, L. (2009). Proteomic Study of Antibiotic Resistance in Escherichia Coli Strains. *Vet Res Commun*, Vol. 33 Suppl 1, No. (Sep, 2009), pp. (157-160), ISSN 1573-7446

Schroeder, C. M., White, D. G. & Meng, J. (2004). Retail Meat and Poultry as a Reservoir of Antimicrobial-Resistant *Escherichia Coli*. *Food Microbiology*, Vol. No. 21, 2004), pp. (249-255), ISSN

Seyfarth, A. M., Wegener, H. C. & Frimodt-Moller, N. (1997). Antimicrobial Resistance in Salmonella Enterica Subsp. Enterica Serovar Typhimurium from Humans and Production Animals. *J Antimicrob Chemother*, Vol. 40, No. 1, (Jul, 1997), pp. (67-75), ISSN 0305-7453

Silbergeld, E. K., Graham, J., Price, L. B. (2008). Industrial Food Animal Production, Antimicrobial Resistance, and Human Health. *Annu. Rev. Public Health* Vol. 29, pp. (151–69).

Singh, V. K., Jayaswal, R. K. & Wilkinson, B. J. (2001). Cell Wall-Active Antibiotic Induced Proteins of Staphylococcus Aureus Identified Using a Proteomic Approach. *FEMS Microbiol Lett*, Vol. 199, No. 1, (May 15, 2001), pp. (79-84), ISSN 0378-1097

Souza, D. M., Oliveira, B. M., Castro-Dias, E., Winck, F. V., Horiuchi, R. S. O., Baldasso, P. A., Caetano, H. T., Pires, N. K. D., Marangoni, S. & Novello, J. C. (2008). The Untiring Search for the Most Complete Proteome Representation: Reviewing the Methods. *Brief Funct Genomic Proteomic*, Vol. 7, No. 4, 2008), pp. (312-321)

Stegemann, H. (1970). Proteinfraktionierungienn polyacrylamid und die anwendung auf die genetische analyse bei pflanzen. *Angew. Chem.* Vol. 82, pp. (640).

Tang, B. M., McLean, A. S., Dawes, I. W., Huang, S. J. & Lin, R. C. (2009). Gene-Expression Profiling of Peripheral Blood Mononuclear Cells in Sepsis. *Crit Care Med*, Vol. 37, No. 3, (Mar, 2009), pp. (882-888), ISSN 1530-0293

Taoka, M., Yamauchi, Y., Shinkawa, T., Kaji, H., Motohashi, W., Nakayama, H., Takahashi, N. & Isobe, T. (2004). Only a Small Subset of the Horizontally Transferred Chromosomal Genes in Escherichia Coli Are Translated into Proteins. *Mol Cell Proteomics*, Vol. 3, No. 8, (Aug, 2004), pp. (780-787), ISSN 1535-9476

Threlfall, E. J., Rowe, B. & Ward, L. R. (1993). A comparison of multiple drug resistance in salmonellas from humans and food animals in England and Wales, 1981 and 1990. *Epidemiology and Infection*, No. 111, pp. 189-197

Threlfall, E. J. (2002). Antimicrobial Drug Resistance in Salmonella: Problems and Perspectives in Food- and Water-Borne Infections. *FEMS Microbiol Rev*, Vol. 26, No. 2, (Jun, 2002), pp. (141-148), ISSN 0168-6445

Threlfall, E. J. (2008). Transmission of Antimicrobial-Resistant *Salmonella* from Food Animals to Humans, *Proceedings of Antimicrobial Resistance in Zoonotic Bacteria and Foodborne Pathogens*,Washington, DC, June 2008

Tsolis, R. M., Baumler, A. J. & Heffron, F. (1995). Role of Salmonella Typhimurium Mn-Superoxide Dismutase (Soda) in Protection against Early Killing by J774 Macrophages. *Infect Immun*, Vol. 63, No. 5, (May, 1995), pp. (1739-1744), ISSN 0019-9567

van Leeuwen, W. J., van Embden, J., Guinée, P., Kampelmacher, E. H., Manten, A., van Schothorst, M. (1979). Decrease of drug resistance in salmonella in the Netherlands. *Antimicrobial Agentes and Chemotherapy*. No. 16, pp. 237-239

van Velkinburgh, J. C. & Gunn, J. S. (1999). Phop-Phoq-Regulated Loci Are Required for Enhanced Bile Resistance in Salmonella Spp. *Infect Immun*, Vol. 67, No. 4, (Apr, 1999), pp. (1614-1622), ISSN 0019-9567

VanBogelen, R. A., Schiller, E. E., Thomas, J. D. & Neidhardt, F. C. (1999). Diagnosis of Cellular States of Microbial Organisms Using Proteomics. *Electrophoresis*, Vol. 20, No. 11, (Aug, 1999), pp. (2149-2159), ISSN 0173-0835

Veenstra, T. D. (2007). Global and Targeted Quantitative Proteomics for Biomarker Discovery. *J Chromatogr B Analyt Technol Biomed Life Sci*, Vol. 847, No. 1, (Feb 15, 2007), pp. (3-11), ISSN 1570-0232

Vihinen, M. (2003). Bioinformatics in Proteomics, In: *Handbook of Proteomic Methods*, P. Michael Conn, pp. Humana Press Inc.

Võ, A. T. T. (2007). Antibiotic Resistance in *Salmonella* - Thesis. Ultrecht University

Washburn, M. P., Wolters, D. & Yates, J. R., 3rd. (2001). Large-Scale Analysis of the Yeast Proteome by Multidimensional Protein Identification Technology. *Nat Biotechnol*, Vol. 19, No. 3, (Mar, 2001), pp. (242-247), ISSN 1087-0156

Wasinger, V. C., Cordwell, S. J., Cerpa-Poljak, A., Yan, J. X., Gooley, A. A., Wilkins, M. R., Duncan, M. W., Harris, R., Williams, K. L. & Humphery-Smith, I. (1995). Progress with Gene-Product Mapping of the Mollicutes: Mycoplasma Genitalium. *Electrophoresis*, Vol. 16, No. 7, (Jul, 1995), pp. (1090-1094), ISSN 0173-0835

Webber, M. A. & Piddock, L. J. (2003). The Importance of Efflux Pumps in Bacterial Antibiotic Resistance. *J Antimicrob Chemother*, Vol. 51, No. 1, (Jan, 2003), pp. (9-11), ISSN 0305-7453

Webber, M. A., Coldham, N. G., Woodward, M. J. & Piddock, L. J. (2008). Proteomic Analysis of Triclosan Resistance in Salmonella Enterica Serovar Typhimurium. *J Antimicrob Chemother*, Vol. 62, No. 1, (Jul, 2008), pp. (92-97), ISSN 1460-2091

Westermeier, T. & Naven, T. (2002). *Proteomics in Practice: A Laboratory Manual of Proteome Analysis* Wiley

White, D. G., Zhao, S., Sudler, R., Ayers, S., Friedman, S., Chen, S., McDermott, P. F., McDermott, S., Wagner, D. D. & Meng, J. (2001). The Isolation of Antibiotic-Resistant Salmonella from Retail Ground Meats. *N Engl J Med*, Vol. 345, No. 16, (Oct 18, 2001), pp. (1147-1154), ISSN 0028-4793

Wildgruber, R., Harder, A., Obermaier, C., Boguth, G., Weiss, W., Fey, S. J., Larsen, P. M. & Gorg, A. (2000). Towards Higher Resolution: Two-Dimensional Electrophoresis of Saccharomyces Cerevisiae Proteins Using Overlapping Narrow Immobilized Ph Gradients. *Electrophoresis*, Vol. 21, No. 13, (Jul, 2000), pp. (2610-2616), ISSN 0173-0835

Wingren, C. & Borrebaeck, C. A. (2004). High-Throughput Proteomics Using Antibody Microarrays. *Expert Rev Proteomics*, Vol. 1, No. 3, (Oct, 2004), pp. (355-364), ISSN 1744-8387

Winokur, P. L., Brueggemann, A., DeSalvo, D. L., Hoffmann, L., Apley, M. D., Uhlenhopp, E. K., Pfaller, M. A. & Doern, G. V. (2000). Animal and Human Multidrug-Resistant, Cephalosporin-Resistant Salmonella Isolates Expressing a Plasmid-Mediated Cmy-2 Ampc Beta-Lactamase. *Antimicrob Agents Chemother*, Vol. 44, No. 10, (Oct, 2000), pp. (2777-2783), ISSN 0066-4804

WHO - World Heath Organization, FAO - Food and Agriculture Organization & OIE - The World Organization for Animal Health (2003). Joint FAO/OIE/WHO Expert

Workshop on Non-Human Antimicrobial Usage and Antimicrobial Resistance: Scientific assessment

WHO - World Health Organization (2005). Drug-resistant *Salmonella* - Fact Sheet N° 139

WHO - World Health Organization (2011). Antimicrobial resistance - Fact Sheet N° 194

Wu, L. & Han, D. K. (2006). Overcoming the Dynamic Range Problem in Mass Spectrometry-Based Shotgun Proteomics. *Expert Rev Proteomics*, Vol. 3, No. 6, (Dec, 2006), pp. (611-619), ISSN 1744-8387

Yao, J. & Moellering, R. (2003). Antibacterial Agents, In: *Manual of Clinical Microbiology*, P. Murray, E. Baron, J. Jorgenses, M. Pfaller and R. Yolken, pp. American Society for Microbiology Press, Washington

Zgurskaya, H. I. & Nikaido, H. (2000). Multidrug Resistance Mechanisms: Drug Efflux across Two Membranes. *Mol Microbiol*, Vol. 37, No. 2, (Jul, 2000), pp. (219-225), ISSN 0950-382X

Zong, C., Young, G. W., Wang, Y., Lu, H., Deng, N., Drews, O. & Ping, P. (2008). Two-Dimensional Electrophoresis-Based Characterization of Post-Translational Modifications of Mammalian 20s Proteasome Complexes. *Proteomics*, Vol. 8, No. 23-24, (Dec, 2008), pp. (5025-5037), ISSN 1615-9861

11

Use of Integrated Studies to Elucidate Potential Benefits from Genetic Resistance to *Salmonella* Carrier State in Fowl

Beaumont Catherine, Thanh-Son Tran,
Zongo Pascal, Viet Anne-France and Magal Pierre
French National Institute for Agricultural Research
UR083 Recherche Avicole, Nouzilly
UMR1300 Bio-agression Epidémiologie et Analyse de Risques, Nantes
LUNAM Université, Oniris, Nantes
Victor Segalen Bordeaux 2 University, Mathematics Institute of Bordeaux, Bordeaux
France

1. Introduction

Salmonella, and especially *Salmonella* enteritidis, are one of the major causes of human toxi-infections (Humphrey, 1990), even if the trend is decreasing (European Food Safety Agency [EFSA], 2011). Many prophylactic means have thus been investigated to control the incidence of *Salmonella* in poultry flocks, including vaccination (Zhang-Barber et al., 1999, Curtiss et al, 2010), competitive exclusion (Nurmi & Rantala, 1973), acidification of feed and genetic resistance. More precisely, animals' ability to clear bacteria was considered. Indeed, the absence of clinical symptoms (which is the most classical definition of resistance) does not preclude human contamination since some animals may remain contaminated for weeks or even months without showing any symptoms. Such silent carriers cannot be identified as dangerous and may therefore enter the food chain. At the opposite spectrum, animals' ability to clear bacteria will reduce the risk of transmission, first to other animals and second to humans. It will thereafter be denoted as resistance to carrier-state.

The feasibility of selection for an improved resistance to asymptomatic carriers has been demonstrated by a divergent selection experiment (§2). Thanks to development of genomics, many results were obtained in the past 10 years: several genome regions controlling different traits were identified and the role of other genes was suggested. It will dramatically increase the efficiency of selection. With traditional selection, it is necessary to perform experimental inoculations and to slaughter animals to register the level of contamination. With marker-assisted selection and furthermore genomic selection, it will be possible to directly choose the future breeders. In addition to improved selection efficiency, it will discard the need for artificial infections.

However, even if numerous data are currently available, strategy for application of these results are still questionable: genetic relations between resistance traits are complex and the choice of selection criteria deserves more investigations. Therefore, the whole process, leading from fowl contamination to transmission to other animals or humans was described in an integrated approach, combining genetics and other means. First results showed possible synergy between resistance and at least one another mode of prevention, vaccination. Other studies are required to compare different combinations of prophylactic means and identify new strategies for eradication of Salmonellosis, in coherence with new regulation implemented by the European Commission. They aim at reducing *Salmonella* prevalence in poultry flocks at less than 2% while a recent study estimated it at 29.7 and 23.7%, respectively, of laying and broiler flocks, respectively, with large differences between countries (EFSA, 2007a, 2007b)

The goal of this chapter is to make a review of data currently available on the possibility of reduction of fowl carrier-state through genetic selection. It will enhance the benefits that may be obtained from an integrated approach of genetics of resistance in hens to improve the control of the incidence of *Salmonella* within a flock.

2. Main results on genetics of resistance to *Salmonella*

First studies were achieved very early (Lambert & Knox, 1928; DeVolt et al., 1941) at a time when many animals died from acute salmonellosis. They thus focussed on the reduction of mortality. No experimental inoculation was needed to observe diseased animals and experiments could be achieved directly on the field. Studies focussed on serotypes pathogenic for birds (*Salmonella* Pullorum, *Salmonella* Gallinarum and *Salmonella* Typhimurium). Later on, the incidence of those diseases dramatically reduced with the reinforcement of preventive measures in poultry breeding. The same held for studies of resistance to *Salmonella*. But, in the end of the 1980's, many outbreaks of human toxi-infections due to *Salmonella* Enteritidis occurred, resulting in new developments in genetics of resistance to *Salmonella*. As in former studies, feasibility of such an approach was considered through selection experiment; genetic parameters were estimated to appreciate the response that could be expected. However, with the beginnings of molecular genetics, the research of genes controlling these traits was also addressed.

2.1 Development of protocols of measures and identification of genetic models

One main feature of studies of genetic resistance to *Salmonella* is the very large number of resistance-related traits that were considered (see Calenge et al., (2010) for a review). They differ in many factors. Inoculation by the oral route is more representative of what occurs in the field but less reproducible than the intravenous or intramuscular route. According to the *Salmonella* serotype, carrier-state (mostly observed after inoculation with *Salmonella* Enteritidis) or acute disease (mostly observed after inoculation with *Salmonella* Typhimurium) will be studied, but to an extent also depending, among others, on the number of inoculated bacteria. The animal's age at infection is a very important parameter. The interval between infection and observation will also be of importance, especially with reference to long-term carrier-state. Animals' conditions of rearing also influence the outcome of the infection. The susceptibility of egg to *Salmonella* multiplication may also be considered as described by Sellier et al. (2007).

Many studies involve both the development of a protocol of measure of resistance and the identification, with this protocol, of lines differing in resistance. Identifying such genotypes is of great importance: their existence strongly suggests the role of genetics in the control of resistance-related traits that are measured. Genetic models for resistance or susceptibility are needed for research of genome regions controlling those traits. The first study was achieved by Bumstead & Barrow (1988). They considered resistance to acute disease due to *Salmonella* Typhimurium and observed difference between partially inbred lines that are especially interesting for QTL research. Other studies addressed carrier-state and focussed on *Salmonella* Enteritidis. Guillot et al., (1995) observed differences in response to inoculation of chickens with a high bacterial dose. To mimic carrier-state in chicks, Duchet-Suchaux et al., (1995) developed a protocol of experimental inoculation where animals were orally infected with a low dose, showed no symptom but remained infected for several weeks. They could thus identify genetic models for further research, both outbred (Duchet-Suchaux et al., 1997) and partially inbred lines (Tilquin et al., 2005). It is to notice that the former study focussed on the same lines as in Bumstead & Barrow, (1988). Other protocols of inoculation were developed to study persistence for a shorter term (Lamont et al., 2002; Kramer et al., 2003; Hasenstein & Lamont, 2007).

Studies on resistance to carrier-state in adults were less numerous, in spite of importance of laying hens for the risk of human contamination. Protais et al., (1996) orally contaminated hens at the peak of lay and bacteria were searched in caeca, spleen, liver and ovary four weeks later. They observed differences between outbred poultry lines. Later on, Sadeyen et al., (2006) identified differences between inbred lines using the same protocol while Lindell et al., (1994) used a slightly different protocol.

2.2 Response to selection

The first selection experiment for resistance to salmonellosis after an experimental inoculation was undertaken in 1932; it proved to be efficient (Lambert, 1932). A higher resistance was observed for some breeds, among which White Leghorns (Robert and Card, quoted by Hutt & Scholes (1941)). But De Volt et al., (1941) showed that the former were less resistant than selected Rhode Island Red hens. This result and others contributed to the development of selection for a higher resistance (see Beaumont et al., 2003a, for a review).

These results are coherent with the estimations of heritability of resistance to death (0.15 and 0.12) obtained respectively by Beaumont et al., (1999) after intramuscular inoculation of day-old chicks and by Janss & Bolder (2000) after inoculation at two weeks of age. It is to notice that, according to genetic parameters estimated by the latter, more resistant animals would survive longer, contributing to a higher risk for consumers if they were still carriers. This emphasizes the importance of an increase in genetic resistance to carrier-state. An experiment of divergent selection on this trait was achieved by Beaumont et al., (2009; 2010). The base population was issued from a layer-type line. Two series of divergent lines were selected, for increased or decreased resistance at a younger age (as in Duchet-Suchaux et al., 1995) or at the peak of lay (using the protocol described by Protais et al., 1996). In adults, selection was on an all-or-none trait called global contamination, coded "1" if at least one organ (i.e. spleen, liver, caeca or ovary) was found positive and "0" in the other cases. Resistance of chicks was assessed by the logarithm of the number of colonies forming units (c.f.u.) per gram of caeca measured 5 weeks after inoculation (i.e. contamination level). A total of 3817 animals were thus measured (1408 adults and 2409 chicks). Clear and significant differences were observed in lines selected on adult performance, with difference in prevalence of about 20%. Selection may be efficient in reducing the level of *Salmonella* carrier-state in hens. Differences between the "chicken" lines were, at least until now, smaller. This may be due to lower heritability but also smaller selection pressure and family sizes, due to experimental constraints and to variations in responses to infections. Indeed, in two hatches out of eight, only a small proportion of animals were still contaminated by *Salmonella* at slaughter; others could not be measured for level of contamination, which also slowed down selection.

Values of estimated genetic parameters were the main information from this experiment. Heritability of resistance was estimated at 0.16 in chicks while it varied from 0.14 to 0.23 with analysed organ in adult hens. It was higher in caeca (0.23) while heritability of ovarian contamination was estimated at a lower value (0.11). Heritability of adult global contamination was found at 0.18.

All genetic correlations between contamination rates of individual organs were positive, ranging from 0.46 to 0.67. Genetic correlations between adult global contamination and contamination in individual organs were very high (from 0.75 for liver to 0.85 for spleen and caeca), except for ovary (0.32). These results are related to the central role of intestine in carrier-state of gastro-intestinal bacteria: bacteria pass through it when inoculated or after recontamination; at the opposite, contamination of other organs is dependent on translocation of intestinal barrier. Contamination of ovaries is especially rare: in this experiment only 6% of them were found contaminated versus 49%, 21% and 62%, respectively, for spleens, livers and caeca, respectively (resulting in a percentage of contaminated adults equal to 76%). This low rate of ovarian infection further reduced the expected response to direct selection against ovarian contamination. An indirect selection on another criterion should be more efficient. This result and the positive values of genetic correlations between contamination rates of individual organs reinforce the interest of the overall adult contamination: it is more precisely assessed and combines several traits, all of which being positively correlated.

All genetic correlations between carrier-state in chicks and production traits (egg numbers, egg weights and body weights at various ages) were small and positive (ranging from 0 to 0.37) except for the number of eggs laid between 18 and 24 weeks of age, which was slightly but negatively correlated with *Salmonella* load (0.17). These results suggest that selection for increased resistance may be achieved without much detrimental effect on production traits. Unlike what was observed for resistance at a younger age, genetic correlation between adult carrier-state (global contamination) and egg numbers laid at the beginning of lay (between 18 and 24 weeks of age) was positive. At the opposite, those with laying intensity at older ages were negative or very close to 0 (ranging between -0.33 and 0.01). Correlation with body weight at 17 weeks of age was close to 0. These differences in genetic correlations between production traits and resistance at a younger or an older age are consistent with the negative genetic correlation observed between chicken and adult resistance.

The latter was estimated at a quite high and negative value (-0.50) and the probability of the true correlation being positive was estimated at only 5%. This major result holds whether overall contamination is considered or different organs distinguished and whatever the method of estimation. It is probably linked to differences in mechanisms of resistance between chicks, whose immune system is not mature, and hens, who may also benefit from adaptive immune response. The variation with animals' age in genetic control of adult and chicken resistance was suspected, because of differences in relative resistance of poultry lines to resistance to carrier-state at a younger (Duchet-Suchaux et al., 1997) or an older age (Protais et al., 1996). This result implies that most results obtained at a younger age are expected to be irrelevant in adults, if not of opposite sign. They may not be extrapolated to hens without experimental validation. Indeed, differences in expression of gallinacins observed by Sadeyen et al., (2004) and Sadeyen et al. (2006) were found to be associated, in young chicken, with increased susceptibility but, in adults, with resistance. Similar variations with age should also be the case of a large proportion of genes or genome regions found to be involved in resistance (for a review, see Calenge et al., 2010). This result also implies that increasing genetic resistance of hens should reduce resistance in chicks. This holds for marker-assisted or genomic selection.

2.3 Towards identification of genes or genome regions involved in the control of resistance

Though promising these results may seem, large-scale selection for increased resistance is very difficult to implement since experimental infections, which are both very expensive and time consuming, are required. Identifying the underlying genes of genetic markers could make it possible to alleviate the need of such experiments.

The major drawback of such genomic studies is the numbers of both phenotypes and genotypes which are required. Studying crosses between inbred lines, following the pioneer studies of Bumstead & Barrow, (1988; 1993) is of great relevance, as it makes it possible to identify QTLs with much less animals than with crosses between outbred lines. Backcross (Mariani et al., 2001; Lamont et al., 2002; Fife et al., 2011), F2 cross (Tilquin et al., 2005) or, more recently, advanced intercross lines (AIL) were considered (Hasenstein et al., 2007; Ghebremichael et al., 2008) .

Candidate genes, i.e. genes chosen according to an a priori knowledge of their effect in *Salmonella* resistance were first investigated. That was in particular the case for two genes, SLC11A1 and TLR4, known to be involved in resistance to *Salmonella* in mouse. The first one corresponds to the formerly called Nramp1 (natural resistance-associated macrophage protein) gene. It is responsible for resistance of mice to inoculation with *Salmonella* Typhimurium, Mycobacterium bovis and Leishmania donovani (Vidal et al., 1993). Later, Nramp1 has been described as a member of a solute carrier family and hence renamed Slc11a1. It is involved in the control of the intracellular replication of parasites in phagosomes. An homologue of Nramp1 was mapped on the chicken chromosome 7 (Hu et al., 1995; Girard-Santosuosso, 1997) and subsequently cloned (Hu et al., 1996).

The second candidate gene, TLR4 (Toll-like receptor 4), previously named Lps, belongs to the large family of Toll-like receptors involved, among others, in the recognition of LPS (lipo-polysaccharides), a component specific of Gram negative bacteria (among which *Salmonella*). Its mutation results in a lack of response to LPS and a higher susceptibility to Gram negative bacteria. The positional cloning of Lps led to the identification of TLR4 as a positional candidate. It was mapped to the chicken micro-chromosome 17 and cloned (Leveque et al., 2003).

Hu et al., (1997) observed that both genes explained together up to 33% of the difference in survival of young chicks during the first week after an intra-muscular inoculation at one day of age with *Salmonella* Typhimurium. This difference was smaller when survival during the whole experiment was considered. The effect of the NRAMP1 gene was shown in many other experiments: in early stages of systemic *Salmonella* infection in meat-type chicks (Kramer et al., 2003) and layer-type hens (Lamont et al., 2002; Liu et al., 2002) or in spleen infection after intravenous inoculation of pullets (Girard-Santossuoso et al. 2002) or hens (Beaumont et al., 2003b). It is interesting to note that Caron et al., (2002) showed that the NRAMP1 allele coding for a better resistance of mice to an early and acute infection was also responsible for a higher excretion rate in later stages. This result has not yet been investigated in fowls. If it held, it could imply that selecting for the NRAMP1 allele coding for higher resistance to disease would result in a more intense excretion of *Salmonella* in the environment and thus quicker and more important transmission between animals. At the opposite, only the study of Beaumont et al (2003b) suspected a role of the TLR4 gene. Other candidate genes involved in the immune response were investigated using either polymorphisms within the gene or genetic markers (for a review, see Calenge et al (2010).

Searching for Quantitative Trait Loci (QTLs) is another way to identify genome regions involved in resistance. It is based on a systematic research of effects, on resistance, of anonymous genetic markers, chosen to cover as regularly as possible the whole genome. A first genome scan was achieved by Mariani et al., (2001) on resistance to disease due to *Salmonella* typhimurium. A major QTL controlling spleen bacterial load was identified on chromosome 5 and named SAL1. A 6th generation backcross allowed confirming and refining the QTL (Fife et al., 2009). It also suggested two very promising functional candidate genes, which should lead to the identification of the gene(s) underlying the QTL. Tilquin et al., (2005) identified QTL for resistance to both disease and carrier-state. One genome-wise significant QTL and five chromosome-wise significant QTL were observed on chromosomes 2, 1, 5, 11 and 16, respectively. This genome scan used selective genotyping (i.e. genotyping of only a subset of animals, chosen as particularly informative, because of extreme phenotypic values); two of those QTLs (on chromosomes 2 and 16) were confirmed after targeted genotyping of all animals (Calenge et al., 2009) while the QTLs on chromosomes 1 and 16 were also observed in the lines issued from the experiment of divergent selection on resistance to carrier-state described by Beaumont et al., (2010) (Calenge et al., 2009). More recently, the development of a new generation of genetic markers, Single Nucleotide Polymorphisms (SNP) allowed a denser coverage of the genome and the identification of new QTLs (Calenge et al., 2011; Fife et al., 2011) one of which is close to the zone observed on chromosome 2 by Fife et al. (2011). The results of all publications of QTL research are shown on Table 1.

Functional genomics compares the levels of expression (i.e. of activity) of genes at the genome-wide level. It allows the identification of genes involved in the mechanisms of resistance and may also lead to the identification of the genes controlling resistance, provided that the mutations responsible for differences in resistance also result in variations in the levels of expression. Studies compared levels of expression before and after infection, on animals from the same genotypes, or between animals issued from resistant and susceptible poultry lines (for a review, see Calenge et al., 2010). Focussing on the expression of candidate immune genes allows a better understanding of their role (as in Sadeyen et al., 2004; Sadeyen et al., 2006; Swaggerty et al., 2006) in relation with the type of cells as shown by Chausse et al., (2011), when comparing results obtained on the whole caeca by Sadeyen et al. (2004) to observations obtained on sorted cells from this organ.

Chromosome	Position (in cM or Mb)	Reference
1	85, 207 cM 509 cM	Tilquin et al., 2005 Calenge et al., 2011
2	87 cM 20 Mb	Tilquin et al., 2005 Fife et al., 2011
3	123 cM 96 Mb	Calenge et al., 2011 Fife et al., 2011
4	158, 242 cM	Calenge et al., 2011
5	157 cM 100, 111 cM 38 cM	Mariani et al., 2001 Tilquin et al., 2005 Calenge et al., 2011
6	8 cM	Calenge et al., 2011
9	68 cM	Calenge et al., 2011
11	18 cM 63 cM	Tilquin et al., 2005 Calenge et al., 2011
12	15 Mb	Fife et al., 2011
14	72, 74, 80 cM	Calenge et al., 2011
16	2 cM	Tilquin et al., 2005
18	12, 14 cM	Calenge et al., 2011
22	29 cM	Calenge et al., 2011
24	41 cM	Calenge et al., 2011
25	1 Mb cM	Fife et al., 2011
27	37, 54, 68 cM	Calenge et al., 2011

Table 1. Position of QTLs for resistance to *Salmonella* in chicken already published.

2.4 Potential efficiency of marker assisted or genomic selection

Using results currently available makes it possible to use marker-assisted selection. A first experiment of SNP-assisted selection was achieved by Legarra et al., (2011). A total of 600 animals were genotyped for 831 SNP; these markers explained a large proportion of genetic variance, even if no reduction in residual variance could be observed. This drawback will no doubt be alleviated when a larger number of SNP will be considered, leading to genomic selection, i.e. marker-assisted selection based on genotypes assessed on a very large number of anonymous markers, most often SNP (Meuwissen et al., 2001). Genomic selection investigates the whole genome at least as far as the markers cover it. Even if no application of this procedure to selection of commercial fowls is known yet, that should be the case in the near future. That should especially hold for traits whose measure is expensive and heritability low, as resistance related traits. It should also make it possible to select for several resistance related traits, even if genetic correlations are negative.

However, even with genomic selection, the choice of selection criteria remains a main issue. Whatever the method, it is not possible to consider the numerous resistance-related traits that might be measured using the different protocols of experimental infection described in subsection 2.1. It is necessary to find out the most important ones. Modelling will no doubt be of great interest for such studies. It will consider current knowledge on genetic resistance and other prophylactic means and investigate what may be expected from different methods of selection and prevention as well as from their combination.

3. Mathematical modelling: A way to integrate genetic results for a better understanding of *Salmonella* propagation within a flock of hens

A few models have already been proposed to study *Salmonella* spread within hens (Leslie, 1996, Thomas et al., 2009; Prévost et al., 2006; Zongo et al, 2010a). In two models (Leslie, 1996; Thomas et al., 2009), the transmission of the *Salmonella* is determined by direct contact between animals and the density of bacteria in environment neglected. Prévost et al. (2006, 2007, 2008) and Zongo et al. (2010a) took into account the effect of the bacterial load of the environment. Variability in animal genetic resistance was introduced by Prévost et al, (2008). They distinguished two subpopulations of hens, with a lower or higher resistance to *Salmonella* carrier-state, as the model is a deterministic compartmental model (i.e. the population is divided into categories). In Zongo et al (2010a), individuals are represented, which makes it possible to model the contamination of each hen and to assume them to have varying degrees of resistance. In particular, effects of animal's capacity of defense on the evolution of the individual bacterial load were considered. Since the model is stochastic, the impact of this variability on propagation within the flock can be investigated.

3.1 Model at the population level

Classically, for a large population (as a flock), compartmental deterministic models are defined and the numbers of animals in each category are modelled. Prévost et al., (2006) developed such a model. These authors considered four categories of hens. Naïve (also called susceptible) birds have no protection against *Salmonella*: they are at risk of becoming infected. For hens' contamination, three steps were distinguished. The first is digestive contamination, when the bacteria are located in the digestive tract. Systemic infection occurs after translocation of bacteria through the digestive barrier; it results in contamination of systemic organs, such as liver or spleen, and sometimes also in egg contamination. Afterwards, bacterial clearance leads to recovery (see figure 1).

First contamination depends on the environmental bacterial load. Indeed, propagation of the infection may occur through aerosols from one contaminated animal to another animal, especially when they are reared in the same cage, or indirectly because of environmental contamination, mainly through water and feed. It is to note that this model neglected vertical transmission though transovarian route (Humphrey et al., 1989). Once contaminated at the digestive level, animals will become infected to a systemic level then get immunised. Thus, the rates of transition to the systemic level and, afterwards, the recovered status are constant.

Numerical analyses give hints for developing control measures as they highlight the influence of factors contributing to the variation of egg contamination and thus to the risk of human contamination. The recovery rate, representing the ability of hens to eliminate *Salmonella*, influences both maximal prevalence and duration of the epizooty. The rate of return to the susceptible state, i.e. the loss of protective immunity, is also of major importance. These results could be related to biological mechanisms. The mechanisms explaining the response to selection for a lower or higher contamination level were not the same. Selection on higher resistance had mostly modified the hen's clearance ability while a higher rate of return to the susceptible state was responsible for the higher level of contamination of the other line, which had a shorter immune protection time. This is coherent with results on immune response of lines differing (among other resistance traits) in resistance to carrier state, whether inbred (Sadeyen et al., 2006), or outbred (Proux et al., 2002; Protais et al., 2003).

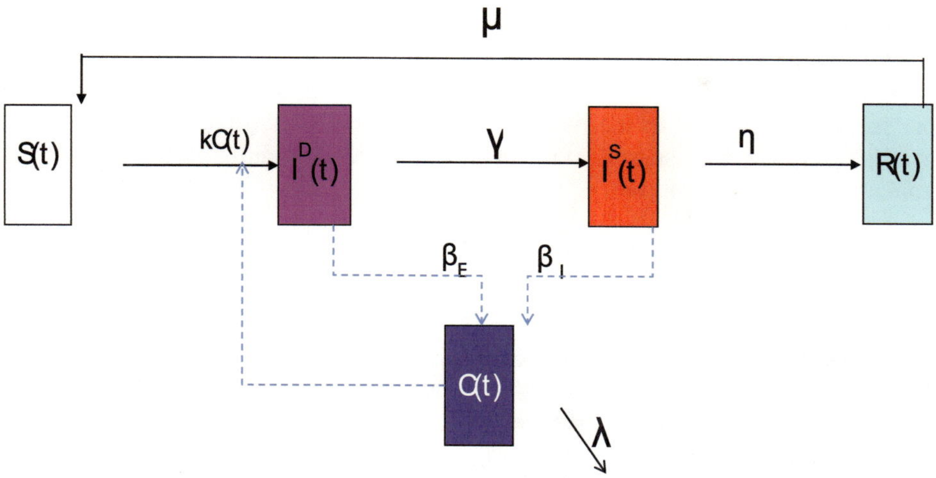

Fig. 1. Diagrammatic representation of the evolution of health status for an individual at a given time t: individual may be susceptible (S), infected at the digestive level (I^D) or at the systemic level (I^S) or recovered (R). β_E and β_I are the rates of excretion of infected animals at the digestive or systemic levels. They contribute to the increase in the number of bacteria in the environment. The rate of transition (k C(t)) from the susceptible (S) to the infected at the digestive level (I^D) status depends on the number of bacteria in the environment (C(t)). Parameters γ, η and μ, respectively, are the rates of transition from one status to another (i.e. from infected at the digestive (I^D) to infected at the systemic level (I^S), from infected at the systemic level I^S to recovered (R) and from recovered to susceptible (S), respectively).

The effect of the introduction of a proportion of more resistant animals among the population was investigated. It reduces the peak of infection (i.e. the maximal percentage of infected animals), because the more resistant animals excrete less bacteria in the environment, reducing cross contamination. But it also delays the extinction of the epizooty as a higher proportion of animals are still naïve and infected later. Increasing genetic resistance to a greater extent but in a proportion of the population or increasing it to a lesser extent but in all animals will lead to different results. Inversely, results of genotype comparisons will not be the same when animals with different degrees of bacterial clearance are reared together or not. This point should be further studied in practice.

The effect of vaccination on flocks with different levels of genetic ability to clear bacteria was also investigated. The vaccine was more efficient in more resistant animals, in relation with the differences in the persistence of immunity. These differences are coherent with observations made by Protais et al. (2003). It is important to note that the combination of vaccination and genetic selection resulted in a percentage of contamination similar to what the European community is asking for.

3.2 Taking into account the variability at the animal level

A stochastic individual-based model was developed for a finer modelling of the variability of hen's response to contamination (Zongo et al., 2010a). Such models are largely used in ecology (Grimm et al., 2006) and were already used to model the growth and migration of *Salmonella* enteritidis in hens' eggs (Grijspeerdt et al., 2005). The model extends the model previously derived by Prévost et al. (2006).

The variation over time (that is the derivative) of the individual bacterial load B(τ,x) was modelled as resulting from bacterial multiplication within the individual (i.e. growth rate), and from contamination by environmental bacteria. The latter was dependant on the number of bacteria present in the neighbourhood of the individual, that is the density of bacteria. It is to note that such a more precise modelling could also be derived using a deterministic approach as follows:

$$\underbrace{\partial B(\tau, x) / \partial \tau}_{\textit{Variation within individual}} = \underbrace{B(\tau, x))}_{\textit{Growth rate}} + \underbrace{I_P(t, x)}_{\substack{\textit{Inhaled or ingested} \\ \textit{within environment}}}$$

Equation 1: Derivative, according to time, of individual bacterial load (B(t,x) at time t and position x is equal to the sum of growth rate, g, of B(t,x) and of contamination through ingestion or inhalation of bacteria present in in the neighbourhood, that is $I_p(C(t,x))$. This derivative is computed at each time step and position.

Contrary to Prévost et al. (2008), two steps in digestive contamination were distinguished (Figure 2): a transient contamination and a long term one. When in the transient status, animals may overcome the contamination and get rid of the bacteria, provided that their bacterial load (thereafter denoted B) remains lower than a threshold D. Once the hen is contaminated at a bacteria load higher than D, its capacities of defence are overwhelmed and it will become systematically infected.

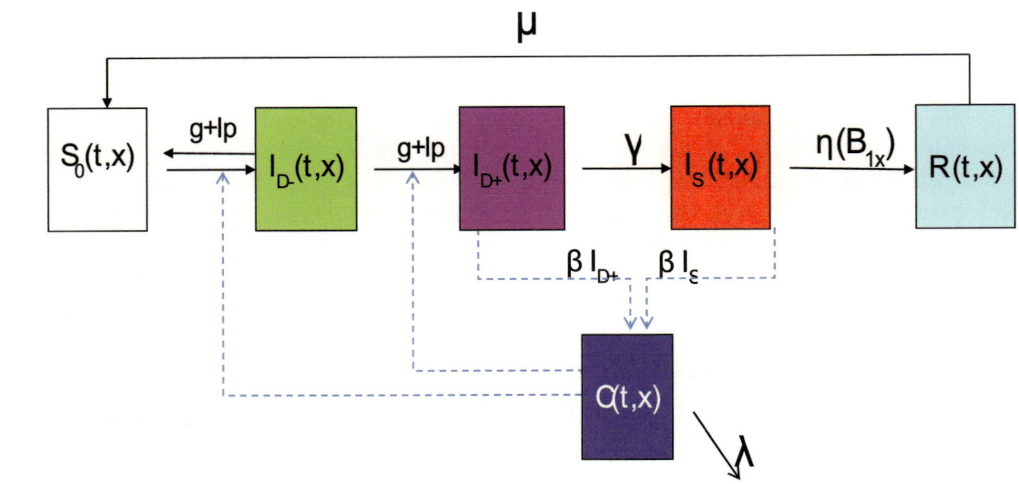

Fig. 2. Diagrammatic representation of the evolution of health status for an individual at time t and position x and its interaction with the level of environmental contamination at this position, C(t,x). The individual may be susceptible (S_0), infected at the digestive level with a low dose of contamination (I_{D-}), suffering from a long term digestive contamination (I_{D+}), contaminated at the systemic level (I_S) or recovered (R). The number of bacteria carried by an individual in the I_{D-} status depends on the growth rate g of its bacterial load and of the quantity of ingested bacteria; the latter depends on the level of environmental contamination in the neighbourhood ($I_{p(t,x)}$). The individual bacterial load regulates transitions from S_0 to I_{D-} (reciprocally from I_{D-} to S_0) and from I_{D-} to I_{D+}. Parameters γ, η and μ, respectively, regulates durations of status I_{D+}, I_S and R, respectively. β_{D+} and β_I are the rates of excretion of infected animals at respectively the transient digestive and systemic level.

Transitions from susceptible to digestive contamination status (both I_{D-} and I_{D+}) are regulated by the individual bacterial load, which is computed at each time step and for each animal. When it is greater than zero and lower that the individual threshold, D(x), individual status changes from S_0 to I_{D-}. The individual may go back in S_0-state unless $B(t_{n+1},x)$ becomes greater than D(x) and individual status changes from I_{D-} to I_{D+}. Other transitions are stochastic with average durations equal to $1/\gamma$, $1/\eta(B_{1x})$ and $1/\mu$, respectively, for the transitions from I_{D+} -state to I_S-state, I_S- -state to R-state and from R state to S_0 respectively.

The threshold D(x) is assumed to vary from an animal to another as it depends on many factors: the bacterial strain (as can be seen for example from Bumstead and Barrow, 1993), gut flora (Nurmi & Rantala, 1973), animals' genetic resistance (§ 1). This variability and the differences in initial contamination result in a variability in bacterial load as can be seen in Figure 3.

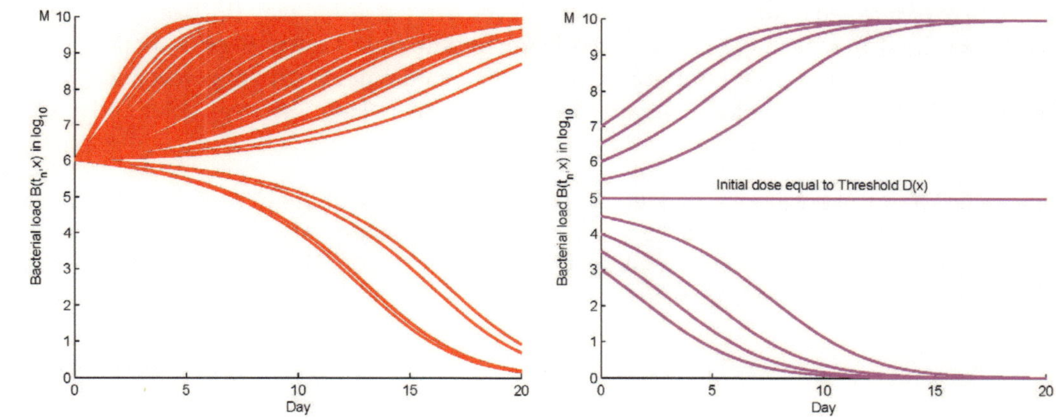

Fig. 3. Evolution of individual bacterial load (B(t,x)) within an individual at the position x and time t according to the number of bacteria ingested by the animal and the threshold for animals' ability to overcome the contamination (D(x)). M is the maximal bacterial load that an animal may carry (set here at 10 log10 c.f.u.). In (a), D(x) is set to the same value for each animal (5 log10 c.f.u.). Four initial doses are above the threshold, one equal to it and four doses below it. In (b), the thresholds D are random, leading to different thresholds for each animal so that, for the same initial dose (set here at 6log10 c.f.u.), there is individual variability in evolution of the bacteria load.

The density of bacteria (C(t,x)) in the environment at time t and position x depends on the rate of diffusion of bacteria, on the natural rate of mortality of bacteria, λ, as well as on the density of bacteria excreted by infectious individuals close to position x.

As the model is spatial, Zongo et al (2010a) show that the position of the first contamination influences both the kinetics of infection and the maximal percentages of infected animals (see figure 4).

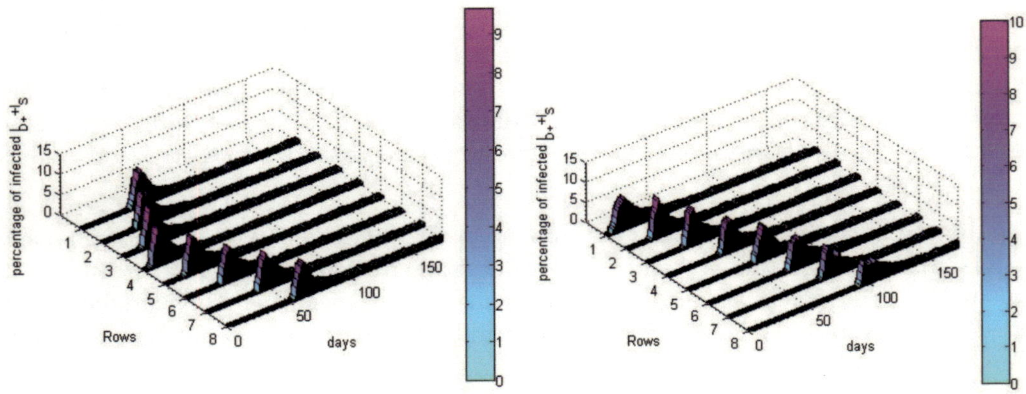

Fig. 4. Influence of the position of the first infection on the evolution over time of the percentage of infected animals (at the digestive level, in a persistent way (I_{D+}), or systematically (I_S)), when (a) infection starts in the middle (row 4 out of 8) or (b) in the corner of the hen house (row 1 out of 8). Only median values of the sum of percentages of infected animal are represented. The color bars indicate the relation between color and percentage of infected animals.

One investigation considered two levels of excretion, since it may vary between hens (Ishola, 2009). As can be seen on figure 5, both the propagation speed and the maximum level of infection are strongly influenced (Zongo et al, 2010b). But more studies are still needed to investigate this question.

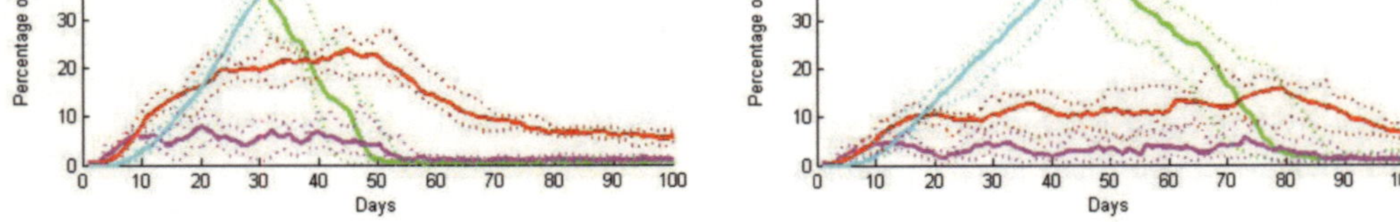

Fig. 5. Evolution of status of individuals (susceptible (S_0), infected at the digestive level with a low dose of contamination (I_{D-}), suffering from a long term digestive contamination (I_{D+}), contaminated at the systemic level (I_S) or recovered (R)), according to days after the first contamination, when (a) all individuals in the I_{D+} or I-state excrete (b) half of individuals at I_{D+}-state or I_S-state excrete. Median values obtained on 100 simulations are shown by solid lines curves, while the 5th and 95th percentiles are shown by dotted lines.

3.3 Perspectives

First, the relative effects of animals' capacity of bacterial clearance and level of excretion should be studied. Both have important effects and most probably interact with each other and with the animals' capacities to overcome transient digestive contamination (threshold D). Since, in hen houses, bacterial doses are most often rather small, it will be important to study the effects of both average values and variability of these factors.

Second, interactions between animals may be more precisely modelled. The model derived by Zongo et al. (2010a) assumes that all hens within a cage are contaminated at the same time and carry the same bacterial load. When the number of hens within cage becomes large, this major hypothesis does not totally hold. Moreover, new systems of rearing should be considered, such as aviaries, extensive rearing or enriched cages. They should be more and more frequent with the European commission banning of traditional cages after 2012. They no doubt interact with sanitary risks. *Salmonella* propagation should also be considered in flocks of younger animals.

Rearing together animals with different profiles of resistance should also be considered. It is worth comparing whether it is more efficient to select one type of resistance (as for example capacity of bacterial clearance or low level of excretion) or several resistance-related traits. In particular, flocks composed of several lines selected on different resistance related traits or performance should be considered. At a longer term, such studies should integrate the links between immune capacities and performance, as investigated by Van der Most et al. (2010). Complementary studies should also consider egg yolk's genetic ability to resist bacterial infection as evidenced by Sellier et al., (2007).

4. Conclusion

Selection for higher resistance to carrier-state may be an efficient way to control *Salmonella* propagation within a flock. It might profitably be used as an additional mean of prevention of human food poisoning. The choice of the selection criteria must be considered carefully as it will have a strong influence on the results of selection. Other means of prevention must also be considered to choose the best strategy of prevention according to its impact on the level of animal contamination and then on the *Salmonella* propagation. Modelling will contribute to integrate genetic and experimental data at individual level to evaluate the propagation at the population level. It will allow the comparison of the impact of different scenarios on the propagation within a flock with, for example, different profiles of resistance or different prophylactic measures. Reversely, these studies will ask new questions and necessitate new experiments to confirm results or give values of some parameters. In particular, if the resistance and the propagation are different according to *Salmonella* strains, different models can be developed, providing there are sufficient data to define them. For other pathogenic agents, such as Campylobacter, integrated studies should also be envisaged.

5. Acknowledgment

The grants Aliment Demain SF20 from French Ministries of Research and of Agriculture, RESISAL from French National Agency for Research, as well the help of the Region Centre and of the EADGENE Network of Excellence are greatly acknowledged. Pascal Zongo benefited from a post-doctoral scholarship from the INRA direction. The authors are grateful to all those who contributed to these studies, in particular to experimental units Pole d'Expérimentation Avicole de Tours et Plate-Forme d'Infectiologie Expérimentale who reared animals. The help of Nathaele Wacrenier for literature review is acknowledged.

6. References

Beaumont, C.; Protais, J.; Guillot, J.; Colin, P.; Proux, K.; Millet, N. & Pardon, P. (1999). Genetic Resistance to Mortality of Day-Old Chicks and Carrier-Sate of Hens after Inoculation with *Salmonella* Enteritidis. *Avian Pathology,* Vol. 28, No. 2, (Avril 1999.), pp. (131-135), ISSN 0307-9457

Beaumont, C.; Dambrine, G.; Chaussé, A.-M. & Flock, D. (2003a). Selection for Disease Resistance: Conventional Breeding for Resistance to Bacteria and Viruses, In: *Poultry Genetics, Breeding and Biotechnology,* W. Muir & S. Aggrey (Eds.), pp. (357-382), CAB International, ISBN 0-85199-660-4, Oxon, UK

Beaumont, C.; Protais, J.; Pitel, F.; Leveque, G.; Malo, D.; Lantier, F.; Plisson-Petit, F.; Colin, P.; Protais, M.; Roy, P. L.; Elsen, J.; Milan, D.; Lantier, I.; Neau, A.; Salvat, G. & Vignal, A. (2003b). Effects of Two Candidate Genes on the *Salmonella* Carrier-State in Fowl. *Poultry Science,* Vol. 82, No. 5, (May 2003.), pp. (721-726), ISSN 0032-5791

Beaumont, C.; Chapuis, H.; Sellier, N.; Calenge, F.; Zongo, P.; Velge, P. & Protais, J. (2009). Selection for Increased Resistance to Salmonella Carrier-State. World Poultry Science Association (WPSA), 6th European Poultry Genetics Symposium, Bedlewo, Poland, 30 September - 2 October, 2009, pp.(26-35)

Beaumont, C.; Chapuis, H.; Sellier, N.; Calenge, F.; Zongo, P.; Velge, P. & Protais, J. (2010). Selection for Increased Resistance to Salmonella Carrier-State. Worlds Poultry Science Journal, Vol. 66, No. 2, (June 2010), pp. (251-259), ISSN 0043-9339

Bumstead, N. & Barrow, P. (1988). Genetics of Resistance to Salmonella Typhimurium in Newly Hatched Chicks. British Poultry Science, Vol. 29, No. 3, (September 1988), pp. (521-529), ISSN 0007-1668

Bumstead, N. & Barrow, P. (1993). Resistance to Salmonella Gallinarum, S. Pullorum and S. Enteritidis in Inbred Lines of Chickens. Avian Diseases, Vol. 37, No. 1, (January 1993.), pp. (189-193), ISSN 0005-2086

Calenge, F.; Lecerf, F.; Demars, J.; Feve, K.; Vignoles, F.; Pitel, F.; Vignal, A.; Velge, P.; Sellier, N. & Beaumont, C. (2009). Qtl for Resistance to Salmonella Carrier State Confirmed in Both Experimental and Commercial Chicken Lines. Animal Genetics, Vol. 40, No. 5, (April 2009), pp. (590-597), ISSN 0268-9146

Calenge, F.; Kaiser, P.; Vignal, A. & Beaumont, C. (2010). Genetic Control of Resistance to Salmonellosis and to Salmonella Carrier-State in Fowl: A Review. Genetics Selection Evolution, Vol. 42, No. 11, (April 2010), doi:10.1186/1297-9686-42-11, ISSN 0999-193X

Calenge, F.; Vignal, A.; Demars, J.; Feve, K.; Menanteau, P.; Velge, P. & Beaumont, C. (2011). New Qtl for Resistance to Salmonella Carrier-State Identified on Fowl Microchromosomes. Molecular Genetics and Genomics, Vol. 285, No. 3, pp. (237-243), ISSN 1617-4615

Caron, J.; Loredo-Osti, J.; Laroche, L.; Skamene, E.; Morgan, K. & Malo, D. (2002). Identification of Genetic Loci Controlling Bacterial Clearance in Experimental Salmonella Enteritidis Infection: An Unexpected Role of Nramp1 (Slc11a1) in the Persistence of Infection in Mice. Genes and Immunity, Vol. 3, No. 4, (June 2002), pp. 196-204, ISSN 1466-4879

Chaussé, A. M.; Grépinet, O.; Bottreau, E.; Le Vern, Y.; Menanteau, P.; Trotereau, J.; Robert, V.; Kaiser, P.; Kerboeuf, D.; Beaumont, C. & Velge, P. (2011). Expression of TLR4 and downstream effectors in selected caecal cell sub-populations of chicks resistant or susceptible to Salmonella carrier-state. Infection and Immunity, Vol.79, No. 8, (August 2011), pp (3445-3454), ISSN : 0019-9567

Curtiss, R. III; Xin, W.; Li Y.; Kong, W.; Wanda, S.Y. ; Gunn, B. & Wang, S.F. (2010). New Technologies in Using Recombinant Attenuated *Salmonella* Vaccine Vectors. Criticial reviews in immunology. Vol. 30, No. 3, pp (255-270), ISSN: 1040-8401.

DeVolt, H.; Quigley, G. & Byerly, T. (1941). Studies of Resistance to Pullorum Diseases in Chickens. *Poultry Science,* Vol. 20, No. 4, pp. (339-341), ISSN 0032-5791

Duchet-Suchaux, M.; Léchopier, P.; Marly, J.; Bernardet, P.; Delaunay, R. & Pardon, P. (1995). Quantification of Experimental *Salmonella* Enteritidis Carrier State in B13 Leghorn Chicks. *Avian Diseases,* Vol. 39, No. 4, (October-December 1995) pp. (796-803), ISSN 0005-2086

Duchet-Suchaux, M.; Mompart, F.; Berthelot, F.; Beaumont, C.; Léchopier, P. & Pardon, P. (1997). Differences in Frequency, Level and Duration of Cecal Carriage between Four Outbred Chicken Lines Infected Orally with *Salmonella Enteritidis. Avian Diseases,* Vol. 41, No. 3, (July-September 1997), pp. (559-567), ISSN 0005-2086

EFSA. (2007a). *The Community Summary Report on Trends and Sources of Zoonoses, Zoonotic Agents, Antimicrobial Resistance and Foodborne Outbreaks in the European Union in 2005,* EFSA, Retrieved from http://www.efsa.europa.eu/EFSA/efsa_locale-1178620753812_1178620767319.htm

EFSA. (2007b). Report of the Task Force on Zoonoses Data Collection on the Analysis of the Baseline Survey on the Prevalence of *Salmonella* in Broiler Flocks of Gallus Gallus, in the Eu, 2005-2006. *The EFSA Journal,* Vol. 98, No 2, (April 2007.), pp. (1-85) ISSN 1831-4732

EFSA. (2011). The European Union Summary Report on Trends and Sources of Zoonoses, Zoonotic Agents and Food-borne Outbreaks in 2009. The EFSA Journal, Vol. 9, No. 3, (March 2010), pp. (2090-2367), ISSN 1831-4732

Fife, M.; Salmon, N.; Hocking, P. & Kaiser, P. (2009). Fine Mapping of the Chicken Salmonellosis Resistance Locus (Sal1). *Animal Genetics,* Vol. 40, No. 6, (December 2009), pp. (871-877), ISSN 0268-9146

Fife, M.; Howell, J.; Salmon, N.; Hocking, P.; van Diemen, P.; Jones, M.; Stevens, M. & Kaiser, P. (2011). Genome-Wide Snp Analysis Identified Major Qtl for *Salmonella* Colonization in the Chicken. *Animal Genetics,* Vol. 42, No. 2, (April 2011), pp. (134-140), ISSN 0268-9146

Ghebremicael, S.B.; Hasenstein, J.R.& Lamont, S. (2008). Association of interleukin-10 cluster genes and *Salmonella* response in the chicken. Poultry Science, Vol. 87, No. 1, (January 2008), pp (22-26), ISSN 0043-9339

Girard-Santosuosso, O. (1997). Partial Conservation of the Mammalian Nramp1 Syntenic Group on Chicken Chromosome 7. *Mammalian Genome,* Vol. 8, (August 2007), pp. (614-616) ISSN 0938-8990

Girard-Santosuosso, O.; Lantier, F.; Lantier, I.; Bumstead, N.; Elsen, J.-M. & Beaumont, C. (2002). Heritability of Susceptbility to *Salmonella Enteritidis* Infection in Fowls and Test of the Role of the Chromosome Carrying the Nramp1 Gene. *Genetic Selection Evolution,* Vol. 342, (April 2002), pp. (211-219), ISSN 0999-193X

Grijspeerdt, K.; Kreft, J. U. & Messens, W. (2005). Individual-Based Modelling of Growth and Migration of *Salmonella Enteritidis* in Hens' Eggs. *International Journal of Food Microbiology,* Vol. 100, No. 1-3, (April 2005), pp. (323-333), ISSN 0168-1605

Grimm, V.; Berger, U.; Bastiansen, F.; Eliassen, S.; Ginot, V.; Giske, J.; Goss-Custard, J.; Grand, T.; Heinz, S. K.; Huse, G.; Huth, A.; Jepsen, J. U.; Jorgensen, C.; Mooij, W. M.; Müller, B.; Pe'er, G.; Piou, C.; Railsback, S. F.; Robbins, A. M.; Robbins, M. M.; Rossmanith, E.; Rüger, N.; Strand, E.; Souissi, S.; Stillman, R. A.; Vabo, R.; Visser, U. & DeAngelis, D. L. (2006). A Standard Protocol for Describing Individual-Based and Agent-Based Models. *Ecological Modelling,* Vol. 198, No. 1-2, (June 2006), pp. 115-126), ISSN 0304-3800

Guillot, J.; Beaumont, C.; Bellatif, F.; Mouline, C.; Lantier, F.; Colin, P. & Protais, J. (1995). Comparison of Resistance of Various Poultry Lines to Infection by *Salmonella Enteritidis. Veterinary Research,* Vol. 26, No. 2, pp. (81-86), ISSN 0928-4249

Hasenstein, J. R. & Lamont, S. J. (2007). Chicken Gallinacin Gene Cluster Associated with *Salmonella* Response in Advanced Intercross Line. *Avian Diseases,* Vol. 51, No. 2, (June 2007), pp. (561-567), ISSN 0005-2086

Hu, J.; Bumstead, N.; Burke, D.; FA, P. d. L.; Skamene, E.; Gros, P. & Malo, D. (1995). Genetic and Physical Mapping of the Natural Resistance-Associated Macrophage Protein 1 (Nramp1) in Chicken. *Mammalian Genome,* Vol. 6, No. 11, (November 1995), pp. (809-815), ISSN 0938-8990

Hu, J.; Bumstead, N.; Skamene, E.; Gros, P. & Malo, D. (1996). Structural Organization, Sequence, and Expression of the Chicken Nramp1 Gene Encoding the Natural Resistance-Associated Macrophage Protein 1. *DNA Cell Biol,* Vol. 15, No. 2, (February 1996), pp. (113-123), ISSN 1044-5498

Hu, J.; Bumstead, N.; Barrow, P.; Sebastiani, G.; Olien, L.; Morgan, K. & D, M. (1997). Resistance to Salmonellosis in the Chicken Is Linked to Nramp1 and Tnc. *Genome Research,* Vol. 7, No. 7, (July 1997), pp. (693-704), ISSN 1088-9051

Humphrey, T.J.; Baskerville, A.; Mawer, S.; Rowe, B, & Hopper, S. (1989). *Salmonella* Enteritidis Phage Type 4 From The Contents Of Intact Eggs: A Study Involving Naturally Infected Hens. *Epidemiology and Infection,* Vol. 103, No. 3, (December 1989), pp.(415-423), ISSN 0950-2688

Humphrey, T. J. (1990). Public Health Implications of Infection of Egg-Laying Hens with *Salmonella* Enteretidis Phage Type 4. World Poultry Science Association Journal, Vol. 46, No. 1, (March 1990), pp. 5-13, ISSN 0043-9339

Hutt, F. & Scholes, J. (1941). XIII. Breed Differences in Susceptibility to *Salmonella* Pullorum. Poultry Science, Vol. 20, No. 4, (July 1941), pp. 342-352, ISSN 0032-5791

Ishola, O. O. (2009) Effects Of Challenge Dose On Faecal Shedding Of *Salmonella* Enteritidis In Experimental Infected Chickens. African Journal of Biotechnology , Vol. 8, No. 7, (April 2009), pp. (1343–1346), ISSN 1684-5315

Janss, L. L. G. & Bolder, N. M. (2000). Heritabilities of and Genetic Relationships between *Salmonella* Resistance Traits in Broilers. Journal of Animal Science, Vol. 78, No. 9, (September 2000), pp. (2287-2291), ISSN 0021-8812

Kramer, J.; Malek, M. & Lamont, S. (2003). Association of Twelve Candidate Gene Polymorphisms and Response to Challenge with *Salmonella* Enteritidis in Poultry. *Animal Genetics,* Vol. 34, No. 5, (October 2003), pp. (339-348), ISSN 0268-9146

Lambert, W. & Knox, C. (1928). The Inheritance of Resistance to Fowl Typhoid in Chickens. *Iowa State Journal of Science,* Vol. 2, pp. (179-187)

Lambert, W. V. (1932). Natural Resistance to Disease in the Chicken. Natural Resistance to disease in the chickens. III The Comparative Resistance of Different Breeds. *Journal of Immunology,* Vol. 23, No.3, (September 1932), pp. (253–259) , ISSN 0022-1767

Lamont, S.; Kaiser, M. & Liu, W. (2002). Candidate Genes for Resistance to *Salmonella* Enteritidis Colonization in Chickens as Detected in a Novel Genetic Cross.

Veterinary Immunology and Immunopathology, Vol. 87, No. 3-4, (September 2002), pp. (423-428), ISSN 0165-2427

Legarra, A.; Calenge, F.; Mariani, P.; Velge, P. & Beaumont, C. (2011). Use of a Reduced Set of Single Nucleotide Polymorphisms for Genetic Evaluation of Resistance to *Salmonella* Carrier State in Laying Hens. *Poultry Science,* Vol. 90, No. 4, (April 2011), pp. (731-736), ISSN 0032-5791

Leslie, J. (1996). Simulation of the Transmission of *Salmonella* Enteritidis Phage Type 4 in a Flock of Laying Hens. *Veterinary Record,* Vol. 139, No. 16, (October 1996), pp. (388-391), ISSN 0042-4900

Leveque, G.; Forgetta, V.; Morroll, S.; Smith, A.; Bumstead, N.; Barrow, P.; Loredo-Osti, J.; Morgan, K. & Malo, D. (2003). Allelic Variation in *Tlr4* Is Linked to Susceptibility to *Salmonella Enterica* Serovar Typhimurium Infection in Chcickens. *Infection and Immunity,* Vol. 71, No. 3, (March 2003), pp. (1116-1124), ISSN 0019-9567

Lindell, K.; Saeed, A. & McCabe, G. (1994). Evaluation of Resistance of Four Strains of Commercial Laying Hens to Experimental Infection with *Salmonella* Enteritidis Phage Type Eight. *Poultry Science,* Vol. 73, No. 6, (June 1994), pp. (757-762), ISSN 0032-5791

Liu, W.; Miller, M. & Lamont, S. (2002). Association of Mhc Class I and Class I Gene Polymorphisms with Vaccine or Challenge Response to *Salmonella Enteritidis* in Young Chicks. *Immunogenetics,* Vol. 54, No. 8, (November 2002), pp. (582-590), ISSN 0093-7711

Mariani, P.; Barrow, P.; Chang, H.; Groenen, M.; Negrini, R. & Bumstead, N. (2001). Localization to Chicken Chromosome 5 of a Novel Locus Determining Salmonellosis Resistance. *Immunogenetics,* Vol. 53, No. 9, (December 2001), pp. (786-791), ISSN 0093-7711

Meuwissen, T.; Hayes, B. & Goddard, M. (2001). Prediction of Total Genetic Value Using Genome Wide Dense Marker Maps. *Genetics,* Vol. 157, No. 4, (April 2001), pp. (1819-1829), ISSN 0016-6731

Nurmi, E. & Rantala, M. (1973). New Aspects of *Salmonella* Infection in Broiler Production. *Nature,* Vol. 241, No. 5386, (January 1973), pp. (210-211), ISSN 0028-0836

Prévost, K.; Magal, P. & Beaumont, C. (2006). A Model of *Salmonella* Infection within Industrial House Hens. *Journal of Theoretical Biology,* Vol. 242, No. 3, (October 2006), pp.(755-763), ISSN: 0022-5193

Prévost, K, ; Magal, P.; Protais, J. & Beaumont, C. (2008), Effect of hens' genetic resistance to *Salmonella* carrier-state on incidence of bacterial contamination: synergy with vaccination, *Veterinary Research,* Vol. 39, No. 2, (March-April 2008), doi: 10.1051/vetres:2007058, ISSN 0928-4249

Prévost, K. ; Beaumont, C. & Magal, P. (2007), Asymptotic behavior in a *Salmonella* Infection Model, Mathematical Modelling of Natural Phenomena, Vol. 2, No. 1, (January 2007), pp. (1-22), ISSN: 0973-5348

Protais, J.; Nagard, B.; Boscher, E.; Queguiner, S.; Beaumont, C. & Salvat, G. (2003). Changes in *Salmonella Enteritidis* Contamination in Two Layer Lines Vaccinated During the Rearing Period. *British Poultry Science,* Vol. 44, No. 5, (December 2003), pp. (827-828), ISSN 0007-1668

Protais, J.; Colin, P.; Beaumont, C.; Guillot, J.; Lantier, F.; Pardon, P. & Bennejean, G. (1996). Line Differences in Resistance to *Salmonella Enteritidis* Pt4 Infection, *Poultry Science,* Vol. 37, No. 2, (May 1996), pp.(329-339), ISSN 0007-1668

Proux, K.; Jouy, E.; Houdayer, C.; Protais, J.; Dibb-Füller, M.; Boscher, E.; Gillard, A.; Gracieux, P.; Gilbert, F.; Beaumont, C. & Duchet-Suchaux, M. (2002). Reliable Elisas Showing Differences between Resistant and Susceptible Lines in Hens Orally

Inoculated with *Salmonella Enteritidis*. *Veterinary Research*, Vol. 33, No. 1, (January-February 2002), pp. (23-33), ISSN 0928-4249

Sadeyen, J.-R.; Trotereau, J.; velge, P.; Marly, J.; Beaumont, C.; Barrow, P.; Bumstead, N. & Lalmanach, A.-C. (2004). *Salmonella* Carrier State in Chicken: Comparison of Expression of Immune Response Genes between Susceptible and Resistant Animals. *Microbes and Infection*, Vol. 6, No. 14, (November 2004), pp. (1278-1286), ISSN 1286-4579

Sadeyen, J.-R.; Trotereau, J.; Protais, J.; Beaumont, C.; Sellier, N.; Salvat, G.; Velge, P. & Lalmanach, A.-C. (2006). *Salmonella* Carrier-State in Hens: Study of Host Resistance by a Gene Expression Approach. *Microbes and Infection*, Vol. 8, No. 5, (April 2006), pp. (1308-1314), ISSN 1286-4579

Sellier, N.; Vidal, M. L.; Baron, F.; Michel, J.; Gautron, J.; Protais, M.; Beaumont, C.; Gautier, M. & Nys, Y. (2007). Estimations of Repeatability and Heritability of Egg Albumen Antimicrobial Activity and of Lysozyme and Ovotransferrin Concentrations. *British Poultry Science*, Vol. 48, No. 5, (October 2007), pp. (559-566), ISSN 0007-1668

Swaggerty, C.; Kaiser, P.; Rothwell, L.; Pevzner, I. & Kogut, M. (2006). Heterophil Cytokine Mrna Profiles from Genetically Distinct Lines of Chickens with Differential Heterophil-Mediated Innate Immune Responses. *Avian Pathology*, Vol. 35, No. 2, (April 2006), pp. (102-109), ISSN 0307-9457

Thomas, M. E.; Klinkenberg, D.; Ejeta, G.; Knapen, F. V.; Bergwerff, A. A.; Stegeman, J. A. & Bouma, A. (2009). Quantification of Horizontal Transmission of *Salmonella Enterica* Serovar Enteritidis Bacteria in Pair-Housed Groups of Laying Hens. *Applied and Environmental Microbiology*, Vol. 75, No. 19, (October 2009), pp. (6361-6366), ISSN 0099-2240

Tilquin, P.; Barrow, P.; Marly, J.; Pitel, F.; Plisson-Petit, F.; Velge, P.; Vignal, A.; Baret, P.; Bumstead, N. & Beaumont, C. (2005). A Genome Scan for Quantitative Trait Loci Affecting the *Salmonella* Carrier-State in the Chicken. *Genetics Selection Evolution*, Vol. 37, No. 5, (September-October 2005), pp. 539-561, ISSN 0999-193X

Van der Most, P. J.; De Jong, B.; Parmentier, H. K. & Verhulst, S. (2010) Ecological immunology Trade-Off Between Growth And Immune Function: A Meta-Analysis Of Selection Experiments. *Functional Ecology*. Vol. 25, No. 1, (February 2011), pp. (74-80), doi: 10.1111/j. pp. 1365-2435. 2010.01800.x, ISSN 0269-8463

Vidal, S.; Tremblay, M.; Govoni, G.; Gauthier, S.; Sebastiani, G.; Malo, D.; Skamene, E.; Olivier, M.; Jothy, S. & Gros, P. (1993). The Ity/Lsh/Bcg Locus: Natural Resistance to Infection with Intracellular Parasites Is Abrogated by Disruption of the Nramp1 Gene. *Journal of Experimental Medicine,*, Vol. 182, No. 3, (September 1995), pp. (655-666), ISSN 0022-1007

Zhang-Barber, L.; Turner, A. K. & Barrow, P. A. (1999). Vaccination for Control of *Salmonella* in Poultry. *Vaccine*, Vol. 17, No. 20-21, (June 1999), pp. (2538-2545), ISSN 0264-410X

Zongo, P.; Viet, A.-F.; Magal, P. & Beaumont, C. (2010a). A Spatio-Temporal Model to Describe the Spread of *Salmonella* within a Laying Flock. *Journal of Theoretical Biology*, Vol. 267, No. 4, (December 2010), pp. (595-604), ISSN 0022-5193

Zongo, P.; Viet, A.F.; Magal, P. & Beaumont, C. (2010b). A Model Of Spatio-Temporal Propagation Of *Salmonella* Considering The Animal Immune Response, *European Poultry Conference*, Tours, France, August 24-26, 2010.

12

16S rRNA Methyltransferases: An Emerging Resistance Mechanism Against Aminoglycosides in *Salmonella*

Katie L. Hopkins[1] and Bruno Gonzalez-Zorn[2]
[1]*Health Protection Agency Microbiology Services Colindale*
[2]*Universidad Complutense de Madrid*
[1]*United Kingdom*
[2]*Spain*

1. Introduction

Infections with non-typhoidal *Salmonella* are the second most common cause of bacterial gastroenteritis in developed countries, with the incidence of multidrug-resistant non-typhoidal Salmonella increasing considerably in the last two decades. Non-typhoidal salmonellosis in otherwise healthy individuals usually results in mild, self-limiting diarrhoea, but treatment with an appropriate antimicrobial can be life-saving in vulnerable patient groups such as the elderly, immunocompromised patients or those with underlying disease, and in cases of invasive disease such as *Salmonella* bacteraemia, osteomyelitis and meningitis.

Aminoglycosides are often used in combination with broad-spectrum ß-lactams for the treatment of life-threatening infections due to both Gram-positive and Gram-negative bacteria due to their potent concentration-dependent bactericidal activity and postantibiotic effect, and their ability to act synergistically with many other antimicrobials (Lacy et al., 1998). They have been classified as critically important antimicrobials in human medicine (World Health Organisation, 2007). By binding irreversibly to the highly-conserved aminoacyl (A-site) of the 16S ribosomal subunit they inhibit bacterial protein synthesis, thereby leading to cell death (Kotra et al., 2000). The most common mechanism for resistance to aminoglycosides results from production of aminoglycoside-modifying enzymes (phosphotransferases, nucleotidyltranferases and acetyltransferases), which compromise the binding of the aminoglycoside to the target site. Resistance may also result from reduced intracellular drug uptake and accumulation (likely to be due to changes in membrane permeability) or mutation of ribosomal proteins or rRNA (Mingeot-Leclercq et al., 1999). However, recent years have seen the emergence of several 16S rRNA methyltransferases in clinical isolates of Gram-negative bacteria in Europe, the Far East, and North and South America.

2. Aminoglycoside resistance mediated by 16S rRNA methylation

Aminoglycoside-producing actinomycetes are intrinsically resistant to very high levels (MIC >512 mg/L) of the aminoglycoside they produce due to rRNA methyltransferase enzymes, but until recently no clinical isolate that was resistant to aminoglycosides as a result of an rRNA methyltransferase had been identified (Davies & Wright, 1997). The first reported 16S rRNA methyltransferase gene *armA* (*a*minoglycoside *r*esistance *m*ethyltransferase) was identified in a multiresistant *Klebsiella pneumoniae* isolated in France (Galimand et al., 2003). A further seven enzymes have been associated with 16S rRNA methylation: *rmtA* (Yokoyama et al., 2003), *rmtB* (Doi et al., 2004), *rmtC* (Wachino et al., 2006a), *rmtD* (now renamed as *rmtD1*) (Doi et al., 2007), *rmtD2* (shares 96.4% amino acid identity with *rmtD1*) (Tijet et al., 2011), *rmtE* (Davis et al., 2010) and *npmA* (Wachino et al., 2007). The deduced amino acid sequences show homology with 16S rRNA methyltransferases produced by *Actinomycetales*, including *Streptomyces* and *Micromonospora* spp. (Fig. 1). However, the degree of identity shared overall between the 16S rRNA methyltransferase genes is less than 30%, which suggests that this is not a recent transfer event.

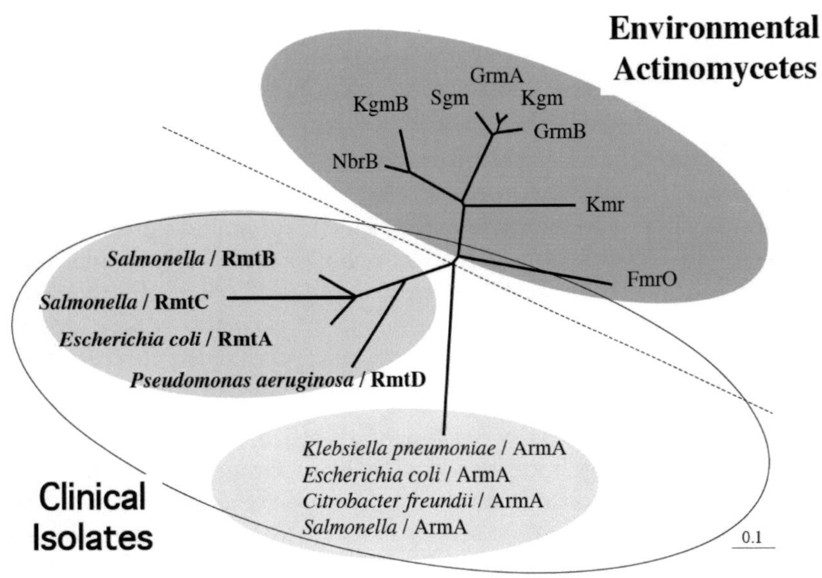

Fig. 1. 16S rRNA methyltransferases conferring high-level resistance to aminoglycosides identified to date.

3. Clinical relevance of 16S rRNA methyltransferases

Unlike the aminoglycoside-modifying enzymes, which vary in their substrate specificity, 16S rRNA methyltransferases *armA* and *rmtA-E* confer high-level resistance to all clinically-important aminoglycosides used for systemic therapy except streptomycin; *npmA* confers high-level resistance mainly to 4,5, disubstituted deoxystreptamines like apramycin. These genes are linked with mobile genetic elements and usually confirmed as located on large conjugative plasmids, allowing potential spread among bacterial populations. In addition, they have been commonly associated with other genes encoding resistance to clinically relevant antimicrobials such as ß-lactams (bla_{SHV}, bla_{CTX-M}, plasmid-mediated AmpC), carbapenems (bla_{SPM-1}, bla_{NDM-1}, bla_{KPC-2}) and fluoroquinolones (plasmid-mediated *qepA*, *aac(6')-Ib-cr* and *qnr* family), thereby allowing potential co-selection and maintenance of resistance by use of other antimicrobial agents. 16S rRNA methyltransferases have been identified in glucose non-fermentative Gram-negative bacilli and enterobacteria, including *Salmonella enterica,* isolated from clinical, veterinary and food sources.

4. Detection of 16S rRNA methyltransferases

4.1 Phenotypic detection

armA and *rmtA-E* confer resistance to 4,6-disubstituted deoxystreptamines such as amikacin, kanamycin, tobramycin and gentamicin by methylation at position A1405 within the A-site of the 16S rRNA, whilst *npmA* confers panaminoglycoside resistance due to methylation at position A1408 (Liou et al., 2006; Wachino et al., 2007). 16S rRNA methyltransferase producers characteristically demonstrate aminoglycoside MICs ≥256 mg/L and are unique in expressing high-level resistance to the semisynthetic aminoglycoside arbekacin (Doi & Arakawa, 2007). Production of a 16S rRNA methyltransferase should be expected in enterobacteria exhibiting resistance to multiple aminoglycosides according to Clinical and Laboratory Standards Institute (CLSI) guidelines and demonstrating little or no inhibitory zones when using gentamicin, amikacin and arbekacin disks. Although arbekacin may not be readily available Doi & Arakawa (2007) noted that inclusion of an arbekacin disk was preferable as this increased the positive predictive value of this method to ≥90%, compared to only *ca.* 60% when using amikacin alone (Lee et al., 2006). Alternatively, using aminoglycoside MICs ≥256 mg/L as a screen has been reported to have an excellent positive predictive value (Lee et al., 2006; Doi & Arakawa; 2007).

4.2 Molecular detection and characterization

With the exception of *npmA*, phenotypic resistance traits cannot be used to differentiate between the 16S rRNA methyltransferase variants. Instead PCR amplification and comparison of the amplicon sequence to previously reported gene sequences must be used for confirmation. The published literature contains many PCR protocols for detection of these genes (Doi & Arakawa, 2007; Fritsche et al., 2008; Granier et al., 2011).

5. 16S rRNA methyltransferases in *Salmonella enterica*

Although all eight 16S rRNA methyltransferase genes have now been identified in enterobacteria; *armA* and *rmtB* are the most commonly identified and have spread worldwide. The first reported 16S rRNA methyltransferase gene in *Salmonella enterica* was *armA* in *S. enterica* serovar Enteritidis isolated in a hospital in Bulgaria (Galimand et al., 2005). Transfer of high-level aminoglycoside resistance to an Escherichia coli recipient led to transconjugants expressing resistance to 4,6-disubstituted deoxystreptamines due to *armA*, to ß-lactams due to acquisition of *bla*$_{TEM-1}$ and *bla*$_{CTX-M-3}$, to streptomycin-spectinomycin because of *ant"9*, to sulphonamides because of *sul1* and to trimethoprim because of *dfrXII*. All these resistance genes were located on a *ca.* 90-kb plasmid of incompatibility group IncL/M previously identified in Poland in *Citrobacter freundii* as pCTX-M3 (GenBank accession number AF550415; Gobiewski et al., 2007). Plasmid pCTX-M3 is responsible for the extensive spread of the extended-spectrum ß-lactamase (ESBL) *bla*$_{CTX-M-3}$ in enterobacteria in Poland (including within *S. enterica* serovars Typhimurium, Enteritidis, Mbandaka and Oranienburg expressing very high-level resistance to aminoglycosides)

(Baraniak et al., 2002; Gierczynski et al., 2003a; Gierczynski et al., 2003b). The *ant"9, sul1, dfrXII* and *armA* genes were part of a 16.6-kb composite element flanked by two direct copies of IS*6*, which was designated Tn*1548*. Tn*1548* has been identified on plasmids of other incompatibility groups and in enterobacteria of human and animal origin from several countries, thereby indicating its importance in the dissemination of *armA* (Galimand et al., 2005; González-Zorn et al., 2005a; González-Zorn et al., 2005b).

armA was also identified on a plasmid identical, or very similar to pCTX-M3 in a single isolate of *S. enterica* serovar Virchow among 1,078 non-typhoidal *Salmonella* isolates from patients hospitalized with gastroenteritis in Saint Petersburg, Russia between 2002-2005 (Egorova et al., 2007). The *armA* gene associated with Tn*1548* was also identified in one isolate of *S. enterica* serovar Stanley submitted in 1999 among a collection of 18,261 non-typhoidal *Salmonella* isolated between 1996-2006 at the Centers for Disease Control and Prevention, USA (Folster et al., 2009).

In 2004 an outbreak of diarrhoea occurred in the neonatology unit of the Hospital of Constantine in Algeria. Stool cultures yielded *S. enterica* serovar Senftenberg, which were resistant to amoxicillin, ticarcillin, piperacillin, cefalothin, extended-spectrum cephalosporins, trimethoprim-sulfamethoxazole, amikacin, gentamicin, netilmicin, tobramycin and streptomycin (Naas et al., 2005). Whilst *Salmonella* infections in hospitals are usually food-associated, in this instance spread of infection was likely to be due to horizontal transmission as the commercially prepared milk was fed to other babies that did not become infected. A subsequent screening of 12 representative ESBL-producing serovar Senftenberg isolates isolated from the ward between 1982-2005 that expressed resistance to aminoglycosides was performed (Naas et al., 2009). Only one isolate from 1998 that expressed resistance to all clinically-relevant aminoglycosides was found positive for *armA*; all other isolates were negative for 16S rRNA methyltransferase genes and showed variable levels of resistance to aminoglycosides. As before, *armA* was located within Tn*1548* on a $bla_{\text{CTX-M-3}}$-encoding IncL/M plasmid.

Another outbreak occurred on the neonatology ward of the same hospital between September 2008 to January 2009 (Naas et al., 2011). *S. enterica* serovar Infantis isolates were obtained from 138 patients (mostly from stool cultures but two neonates had positive blood cultures and another had positive gastric fluid). All but two isolates were resistant to all ß-lactams (except cephamycins and carbapenems), kanamycin, netilmicin, tobramycin, amikacin, gentamicin, rifampicin and trimethoprim/sulfamethoxazole. Molecular typing by pulsed-field gel electrophoresis (PFGE) of representative isolates indicated that they were genetically related. The presence of *armA* associated with Tn*1548*, together with $bla_{\text{CTX-M-15}}$ and $bla_{\text{TEM-1}}$ was confirmed, with the 16S rRNA methyltransferase and ß-lactamase determinants co-located on a 140-kb self-transferable IncL/M plasmid. This suggests that 12 years on, a plasmid similar to that identified in serovar Senftenberg was still present on the ward and may have transferred to serovar Infantis with the $bla_{\text{CTX-M-3}}$ evolving to $bla_{\text{CTX-M-15}}$ via a single amino acid substitution (Asp-240→Gly) that has been associated with increased activity to ceftazidime (Poirel et al., 2002). Other enterobacterial species harbouring both *armA*, and $bla_{\text{CTX-M-3}}$ or $bla_{\text{CTX-M-15}}$ were isolated from Algerian patients transferred to Belgium (Bogaerts et al., 2007), and have been identified in *Klebsiella* spp. in Taiwan and China (Ma et al., 2009; Zhang et al., 2008), indicating that the Infantis plasmid may also have been acquired from a different bacterial species. Implementation and strengthening of hygiene and infection control measures brought the outbreak under control but was insufficient to prevent further sporadic cases in 2009. These may have occurred after re-hospitalisation of colonised patients or from re-introduction of the strain onto the ward by colonised members of staff.

S. enterica serovars Typhimurium (*n*=13), 4,12:-:1,2 (*n*=1) and Enteritidis (*n*=4) co-harbouring both *bla*$_{CTX-M-15}$ and *armA* were identified in another study investigating the prevalence of 16S rRNA methyltransferase genes among ESBL-producing *S. enterica* isolates recovered in Annaba, Algeria between 2008-2009 (Bouzidi et al., 2011). Of the 18 isolates, 13 belonging to serovars Typhimurium (*n*=12) and 4,12:-:1,2 (*n*=1) harboured *bla*$_{CMY-2}$ and *bla*$_{TEM}$ in addition to *bla*$_{CTX-M-15}$ and *armA*. PFGE analysis revealed these 12 Typhimurium isolates shared an identical profile, indicating probable spread of an epidemic clone, whilst the four Enteritidis isolates shared three distinct profiles, suggesting horizontal transfer of the resistance determinants.

The continuing spread of pCTX-M3-like plasmids in the *Salmonella* population was highlighted in the recent identification of serovar Gambia strains harbouring a *ca.* 80-kb IncL/M plasmid bearing *armA* and CTX-M-3 together with sulphonamide and trimethoprim resistance determinants in France (Moissenet et al., 2011). The strains isolated from two babies in the intensive care unit of a Paris hospital in 2005 shared identical resistance profiles (resistance to cefotaxime, ceftazidime, gentamicin, tobramycin, amikacin and co-trimoxazole) and indistinguishable PFGE patterns. Given the rarity of serovar Gambia it was concluded that the second baby acquired the strain via cross-infection. Both babies had underlying disease and whilst the first baby was successfully treated with imipenem and ciprofloxacin, the second baby developed further complications and died despite broad-spectrum therapy with imipenem, gentamicin, metronidazole and vancomycin. This was the first report of a fatality associated with non-typhoidal *Salmonella* harbouring a 16S rRNA methyltransferase gene.

6. Enhanced surveillance for 16S rRNA methyltransferases in *Salmonella enterica*

Between March 2006 and December 2009 a retrospective screen to identify 16S rRNA methyltransferase-producing enterobacteria among the strain collections of veterinary, medical and food science research institutes in ten European Union (EU) countries was performed under the auspices of the European-funded MED-VET-NET Network of Excellence. Isolates were selected for further study from nearly one million bacterial isolates from all sources along the food chain, including the environment, food-production animals, food products and humans based on expression of high-level resistance (MIC >256 mg/L) to amikacin or gentamicin. PCR using a harmonized protocol was used to screen selected isolates for the presence of *armA*.

Among 46 *S. enterica* isolates selected from the culture collection of the Health Protection Agency (HPA), UK, five serovar Oranienburg isolates received in 2002 from Poland were positive for *armA* (Hopkins et al., 2007). A *ca.* 90-kb IncL/M conjugative plasmid, which harboured both *armA* and *bla*$_{CTX-M-3}$ was isolated, with *armA* borne by Tn*1548* as previously described. Transposon mapping using PCR producing overlapping amplicons along the length of the transposon indicated that the transposon structure was identical to that of pCTX-M3 (Fig. 2).

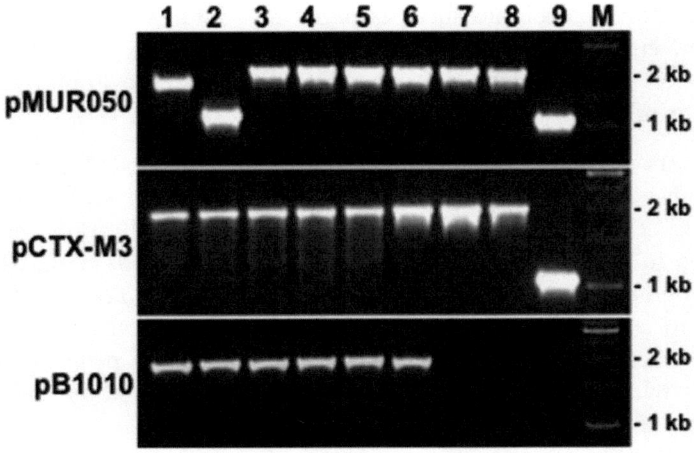

Fig. 2. PCR-mapping of Tn1548, the genetic platform of *armA*. Note that pB1010 has been identified in *Salmonella* from food (Granier et al, 2011).

S. enterica serovar Oranienburg harbouring $bla_{CTX\text{-}M\text{-}3}$ and expressing resistance to aminoglycosides has previously been isolated in Poland, where *armA* is estimated to be present in *ca.* 1.6% of human clinical isolates of enterobacteria (Gierczynski et al., 2003a; Gierczynski et al., 2007). These five isolates were part of an outbreak of enteritis associated with an orphanage for infants and children below two years of age in central Poland. The orphanage was reported to provide poor living conditions (due to a high concentration of children) and sanitary standards (i.e. overuse of antimicrobials). Infected children were hospitalised in three separate hospitals in central Poland (Table 1). In total, 52 related isolates were obtained as reported by a local sanitary and epidemiological unit. Until recently this was the only report of involvement of an *armA*-positive *Salmonella* strain in a hospital outbreak (Naas et al., 2009).

Strain identifier	Patient age (months)	Patient symptomatic?	Other information
9/01	7	Y	living at the orphanage; hospitalised in Unit A
11/01	3	Y	living at the orphanage; hospitalised in Unit B
36/01	11	Y	living with parents - no known link to the orphanage
57/01	7	N	living in the orphanage
79/01	11	Y	living with parents - no known link to the orphanage; hospitalised in Unit C.

Table 1. Epidemiological data on *S. enterica* serovar Oranienburg strains

A further 13 isolates of non-typhoidal *Salmonella* were selected based on high-level resistance to amikacin from 81,632 HPA non-typhoidal *Salmonella* isolated between 2004-

2008 (Hopkins et al., 2010). All isolates belonged to serovar Virchow of phage types 25 (*n*=6), 30 (*n*=5) or 31 (*n*=1). PCR was negative for *armA*; however screening for *rmtA*, *rmtB*, *rmtC* and *rmtD* identified *rmtC* (Doi & Arakawa, 2007). RmtC has previously been identified in *Proteus mirabilis* strain ARS68 from an inpatient in Japan (Wachino et al., 2006a) and *P. mirabilis* strain JIE273 from a patient recently returned from India to Australia (Zong et al., 2008), therefore this was the first report of *rmtC* in Europe. Twelve of the 13 strains were isolated from patients between 2005-2008, of which seven had reported recent travel abroad (four to India). *S. enterica* serovar Virchow expressing *rmtC* has also been reported in the United States in a child with a history of travel to India (Folster et al., 2009), suggesting that 16S rRNA methyltransferases may be relatively common in India. The remaining isolate was obtained from frozen produce. This was the first report of a 16S rRNA methyltransferase gene being identified in a bacterial strain isolated from food. Interestingly, a survey in Northern India identified *S. enterica* in 3.6% of vegetable samples; however >30% of isolates were resistant to amikacin (Singh et al., 2007). PFGE revealed the 13 isolates were highly related, showing only one to two band differences; the isolate from frozen produce was indistinguishable from those isolated from patients. Attempts to isolate *rmtC* by conjugation and electroporation experiments were unsuccessful and the gene was eventually discovered located on the chromosome in association with an IS*Ecp1*-like element, which has previously been shown to play a role in the expression and transposition of *rmtC* (Wachino et al., 2006b). The *rmtC* gene was localised on a *ca.* 100-kb non-conjugative plasmid in *P. mirabilis* ARS68, but attempts to transfer *rmtC* from *P. mirabilis* JIE273 to a donor were unsuccessful. This contrasts with *armA* and *rmtB*, which are commonly localised on plasmids (Doi & Arakawa, 2007) and may explain at least in part the higher prevalence and increased dissemination of these genes in comparison to *rmtC*. *rmtC*-positive strains of *S. enterica* serovar Virchow belonging to the same phage types are still being received at the HPA from patients reporting recent return from India, suggesting persistence of this multidrug-resistant clone (Hopkins, unpublished observation).

Further evidence for food being a possible vehicle of infection for bacterial strains harbouring 16S rRNA methyltransferase genes was provided by a recent study reporting the identification of *armA* in a *S. enterica* serovar 4,12:i:- isolate recovered from chicken meat in La Réunion, a French island in the Indian Ocean (Granier et al., 2011). This was the first report of *armA* in a bacterial isolate originating from food. As well as *armA*, the isolate harboured $bla_{CTX\text{-}M\text{-}3}$, bla_{TEM}, the *Salmonella* Genomic Island-1 (as previously associated with multidrug-resistant *Salmonella enterica* serovar Typhimurium definitive phage type (DT) 104 (Boyd et al., 2000)), and acquired AmpC ß-lactamase $bla_{CMY\text{-}2}$. Conjugation experiments indicated that *armA*, $bla_{CTX\text{-}M\text{-}3}$ and bla_{TEM} were located on the same plasmid. However, further characterisation revealed that, in contrast to previous studies, these genes were located on a *ca.* 110-kb incompatibility group IncP plasmid. IncP plasmids have a broad host range, including *Pseudomonas* spp. and Gram-positive bacteria, therefore association with an IncP plasmid may further broaden the dissemination of *armA*. Transposon mapping using PCR also suggested a deletion event downstream of *armA* and insertion of an IS*26* element, which knocked out genes encoding a macrolide resistance efflux pump and macrolide phosphotransferase gene (Fig. 2 and Fig. 3). Investigation of other *S. enterica* serovar 4,12:i:- isolates recovered from broiler chickens failed to identify any expressing high-level resistance to aminoglycosides, therefore it is likely that this strain was present in the chicken meat sample as a consequence of cross-contamination by a food-handler.

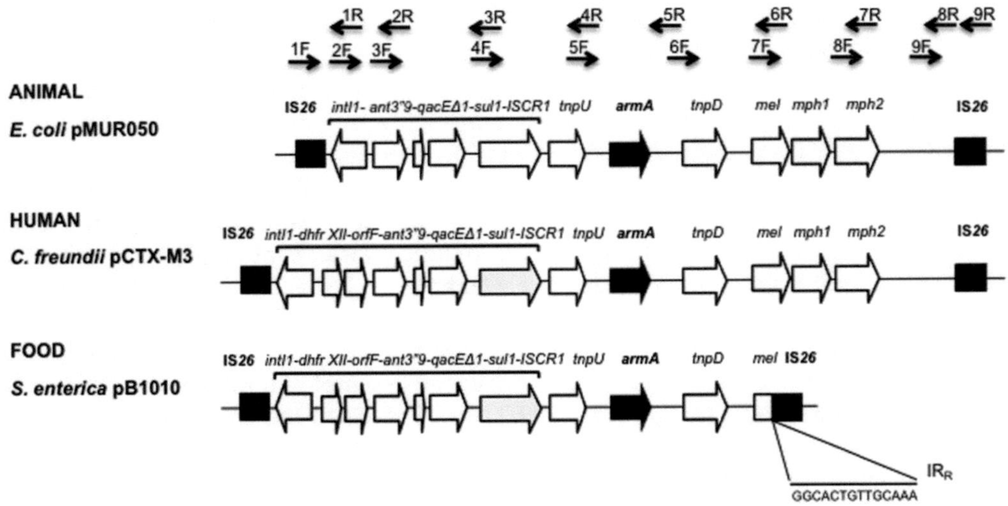

Fig. 3. Schematic representation of the genetic structure of Tn1548 reported from an animal isolate (pMUR050), a human isolate(pCTX-M-3), and a food isolate of Salmonella enterica (pB1010). Blackarrows in the upper part of the panel represent pairs of primers designed for the mapping of Tn1548. (Granier et al., 2011)

7. Conclusion

The worldwide prevalence of *S. enterica* harbouring 16S rRNA methyltransferase genes is very low; however within the EU, Poland appears to represent a major reservoir of these genes. The majority of *S. enterica* isolates have been from nosocomial diarrhoeal outbreaks, with the occurrence of these genes in aminoglycoside-resistant strains from community patients relatively rare. Interestingly, veterinary use of aminoglycosides in food-production animals does not appear to be involved greatly in the spread of 16S rRNA methyltransferase genes as had previously been hypothesized in the literature (González-Zorn et al., 2005a). Food products have recently been identified as a source of *S. enterica* harbouring 16S rRNA methyltransferase genes (Hopkins et al., 2010; Granier et al., 2011), though whether this is an indication of an animal source of these genes, or cross contamination by food handlers has yet to be elucidated. Further evolution and dissemination of these genes may be limited to environments such as hospitals, and countries in which antimicrobial usage is unregulated where a strong selective pressure results from high-level use of a diverse range of aminoglycosides. This is compounded by their common association with other resistance genes, leading to potential co-selection and maintenance of resistance by use of extended-spectrum ß-lactams, carbapenems and fluoroquinolones (Cantón, 2009). Spread of 16S rRNA methyltransferase genes in association with these resistance genes would seriously compromise use of aminoglycosides for treatment of life-threatening infections caused by Gram-negative bacteria such as *S. enterica* and raises the possibility of untreatable *Salmonella* infections. Ongoing surveillance of aminoglycoside resistance in *S. enterica* isolated from humans, animals and food products is therefore crucial to delay the spread of resistance to these classes of antimicrobial agents.

8. References

Baraniak, A., Sadowy, E., Hryniewicz, W. & Gniadkowski, M. (2002). Two Different Extended-Spectrum ß-Lactamases (ESBLs) in One of the First ESBL-Producing Salmonella Isolates in Poland. *Journal of Clinical Microbiology*, Vol.40, No.3, (March 2002), pp.1095-1097, ISSN 0095-1137.

Bogaerts, P., Galimand, M., Bauraing, C., Deplano, A., Vanhoof, R., De Mendonca, R., Robriguez-Villabos, H., Struelens, M. & Glupczynski, Y. (2007). Emergence of ArmA and RmtB Aminoglycoside Resistance 16S rRNA Methylases in Belgium. *The Journal of Antimicrobial Chemotherapy*, Vol.59, No.3, (March 2007), pp.459-464, ISSN 0305-7453.

Bouzidi, N., Aoun, L., Dekhil, M., Granier, S., Poirel, L., Brisabois, A., Nordmann, P. & Millemann, Y. (2011). Co-occurrence of Aminoglycoside Resistance Gene *armA* in Non-Typhi *Salmonella* Isolates Producing CTX-M-15 in Algeria. *The Journal of Antimicrobial Chemotherapy*, published in September edition of JAC (Sep;66(9):2180-1).

Boyd, D., Peters, G., Ng, L. & Mulvey, M. (2000). Partial Characterization of a Genomic Island Associated with the Multidrug Resistance Region of *Salmonella enterica* Typhymurium DT104. *FEMS Microbiology Letters*, Vol.189, No.2, (August 2000), pp.285-291, ISSN 0378-1097.

Cantón, R. (2009). Antibiotic Resistance Genes from the Environment: a Perspective Through Newly Identified Antibiotic Resistance Mechanisms in the Clinical Setting. *Clinical Microbiology and Infection*, Vol.15, Suppl.s1, (January 2009), pp.20-25, ISSN 1469-0691.

Davies, J & Wright, G. (1997). Bacterial Resistance to Aminoglycoside Antibiotics. *Trends in Microbiology*, Vol.5, No.6, (June 1997), pp.234-240, ISSN 0966-842X.

Davis, M., Baker, K., Orfe, L., Shah, D., Besser, T. and Call, D. (2010). Discovery of a Gene Conferring Multiple-Aminoglycoside Resistance in *Escherichia coli*. *Antimicrobial Agents and Chemotherapy*, Vol.54, No.6, (June 2010), pp.2666-2669, ISSN 0066-4804.

Doi, Y., Yokoyama, K., Yamane, K., Wachino, J., Shibata, N., Yagi, T., Shibayama, K., Kato, H. & Arakawa, Y. (2004). Plasmid-Mediated 16S rRNA Methylase in *Serratia marcescens* Conferring High-Level Resistance to Aminoglycosides. *Antimicrobial Agents and Chemotherapy*, Vol.48, No.2, (February 2004), pp.491-496, ISSN 0066-4804.

Doi, Y. & Arakawa, Y. (2007). 16S Ribosomal Methylation: Emerging Resistance Mechanism Against Aminoglycosides. *Clinical Infectious Diseases*, Vol.45, No.1, (January 2007), pp.88-94, ISSN 1058-4838.

Doi, Y., de Oliveira Garcia, D., Adams, J. & Paterson, D. (2007). Coproduction of Novel 16S rRNA Methylase RmtD and Metallo-Beta-Lactamase SPM-1 in a Panresistant *Pseudomonas aeruginosa* Isolate from Brazil. *Antimicrobial Agents and Chemotherapy*, Vol.51, No.3, (March 2007), pp.852-856, ISSN 0066-4804.

Egorova S, Kaftyreva L, Grimont PA, Weill FX. Prevalence and characterization of extended-spectrum cephalosporin-resistant nontyphoidal Salmonella isolates in adults in Saint Petersburg, Russia (2002-2005). Microb Drug Resist. 2007 Summer;13(2):102-7.

Fritsche, T., Castanheira, M., Miller, G., Jones, R. & Armstrong, E. (2008). Detection of Methyltransferases Conferring High-Level Resistance to Aminoglycosides in Enterobacteriaceae from Europe, North America and Latin America. *Antimicrobial Agents and Chemotherapy*, Vol.52, No.5, (May 2008), pp.1843-1845, ISSN 0066-4804.

Folster, J., Rickert, R., Barzilay, E. & Whichard, J. (2009). Identification of the Aminoglycoside Resistance Determinants *armA* and *rmtC* among Non-Typhi *Salmonella* Isolates from Humans in the United States. *Antimicrobial Agents and Chemotherapy*, Vol.53, No.10, (October 2009), pp.4563-4564, ISSN 0066-4804.

Galimand, M., Courvalin, P. & Lambert, T. (2003). Plasmid-Mediated High-Level Resistance to Aminoglycosides in *Enterobacteriaceae* Due to 16S rRNA Methylation. *Antimicrobial Agents and Chemotherapy*, Vol.47, No.8, (August 2003), pp.2565-2571, ISSN 0066-4804.

Galimand, M., Sabtcheva, S., Courvalin, P. & Lambert, T. (2005). Worldwide Disseminated *armA* Aminoglycoside Resistance Methylase Gene is Borne by Composite Transposon Tn*1548*. *Antimicrobial Agents and Chemotherapy*, Vol.49, No.7, (July 2005), pp.2949-2953, ISSN 0066-4804.

Gierczyński, R., Szych, J., Cieślik, A., Rastawicki, W. & Jagielski, M. (2003a). The Occurrence of the First Two CTX-M-3 and TEM-1 Producing Isolates of *Salmonella enterica* Serovar Oranienburg in Poland. *International Journal of Antimicrobial Agents*, Vol.21, No.5, (May 2003), pp.497-499, ISSN 0924-8579.

Gierczyński, R., Szych, J., Rastawicki, W. & Jagielski, M. (2003b). The Molecular Characterisation of the Extended-Spectrum ß-Lactamase (ESBL) Producing Strain of *Salmonella enterica* Serovar Mbandaka Isolated in Poland. *Acta Microbiologica Polonica*, Vol. 52, No.2, pp.183-190, ISSN 0137-1320.

Gierczynski, R., Szych, J., Lawrynowicz-Paciorek, M. & Wardak, S. (2007). Occurrence of the 16S rRNA Methylase *armA* in Human Clinical Isolates of *Enterobacteriaceae* in Poland. In: *3rd Annual Scientific Meeting Abstract Book*, Abstract D&C07, p.23, Med-Vet-Net, Lucca, Italy, June 2007.

Gobiewski, M., Kern-Zdanowicz, I., Zienkiewicz, M., Adamczyk, M., Żylinska, J., Baraniak, A., Gniadkowski, M., Bardowski, J. & Cegłowski, P. (2007). Complete Nucleotide Sequence of the pCTX-M3 Plasmid and Its Involvement in Spread of the Extended-Spectrum ß-Lactamase Gene *bla*$_{CTX-M-3}$. *Antimicrobial Agents and Chemotherapy*, Vol.51, No.11, (November 2007), pp.3789-3795, ISSN 0066-4804.

González-Zorn, B., Teshager, T., Casa, M., Porrero, M., Moreno, M., Courvalin, P. & Domínguez, L. (2005a). *armA* and Aminoglycoside Resistance in *Escherichia coli*. *Emerging Infectious Diseases*, Vol.11, No.6, (June 2005), pp.954-955, ISSN 1080-6040.

González-Zorn, B., Catalan, A., Escudero, J., Domínguez, L., Teshager, T., Porrero, C. & Moreno, M. (2005b). Genetic Basis for Dissemination of *armA*. *The Journal of Antimicrobial Chemotherapy*, Vol.56, No.3, (September 2005), pp.583-585, ISSN 0305-7453.

Granier, S., Hidalgo, L., San Millan, A., Escudero, J., Gutierrez, B., Brisabois, A. & González-Zorn, B. (2011). ArmA Methyltransferase in a Monophasic *Salmonella enterica* Isolated from Food. *Antimicrobial Agents and Chemotherapy*, published in November edition of AAC (Nov;55(11):5262-6).

Hopkins, K., Catalan, A., Szych, J., Cieslik, A., Gierczyński, R., Threlfall, E. & González-Zorn, B. (2007). Characterisation of *Salmonella* Oranienburg Bearing the 16S rRNA Methylase *armA* from an Enteritis Outbreak in a Polish Hospital. In: *Abstracts of the 47th Interscience Conference on Antimicrobial Agents and Chemotherapy*, Abstract C2-1531, American Society for Microbiology, Chicago, IL, September 2007.

Hopkins, K., Escudero, J., Hidalgo, L & González-Zorn, B. (2010). 16S rRNA Methyltransferase RmtC in *Salmonella enterica* Serovar Virchow. *Emerging Infectious Diseases*, Vol.16, No.4, (April 2010), pp.712-715, ISSN 1080-6040.

Kotra, L., Haddad, J. & Mobashery, S. (2000). Aminoglycosides: Perspectives on Mechanisms of Action and Resistance and Strategies to Counter Resistance. *Antimicrobial Agents and Chemotherapy*, Vol.44, No.12, (December 2000), pp.3249-3256, ISSN 0066-4804.

Lacy, M., Nicolau, D., Nightingale, C. & Quintiliani, R. (1998). The Pharmacodynamics of Aminoglycosides. *Clinical Infectious Diseases*, Vol.27, No.1, (January 1998), pp.23-27, ISSN 1058-4838.

Lee, H., Yong, D., Yum, J., Roh, K., Lee, K., Yamane, K., Arakawa, Y. & Chong, Y. (2006). Dissemination of 16S rRNA Methylase-Mediated Highly Amikacin-Resistant Isolates of *Klebsiella pneumoniae* and *Acinetobacter baumannii* in Korea. *Diagnostic Microbiology and Infectious Disease*, Vol.56, No.3, (November 2006), pp.305-312, ISSN 0732-8893.

Liou, G., Yoshizawa, S., Courvalin, P & Galimand, M. (2006). Aminoglycoside Resistance by ArmA-Mediated Ribosomal Methylation in Human Bacterial Pathogens. *Journal of Molecular Biology*, Vol.359, No.2, (June 2006), pp.358-364, ISSN 0022-2836.

Ma, L., Lin, C., Chen, J., Fung, C., Chang, F., Lai,Y., Lin, J., Siu, L. and the Taiwan Surveillance of Antimicrobial Resistance Project. (2009). Widespread Dissemination of Aminoglycoside Resistance Genes *armA* and *rmtB* in *Klebsiella pneumoniae* Isolates in Taiwan Producing CTX-M-Type Extended-Spectrum β-Lactamases. *Antimicrobial Agents and Chemotherapy*, Vol.53, No.1, (January 2009), pp.104-111, ISSN 0066-4804.

Mingeot-Leclercq, M.-P., Glupczynski, Y. & Tulkens, P. (1999). Aminoglycosides: Activity and Resistance. *Antimicrobial Agents and Chemotherapy*, Vol.43, No.4, (April 1999), pp.727-737, ISSN 0066-4804.

Moissenet, D., Weill, F.-X., Arlet, G., Harrois, D., Girardet, J. & Vu-Thien, H. (2011). *Salmonella enterica* Serotype Gambia with CTX-M-3 and *armA* Resistance Markers: Nosocomial Infections with a Fatal Outcome. *Journal of Clinical Microbiology*, Vol.49, No.4, (April 2011), pp.1676-1678, ISSN 0095-1137.

Naas, T., Lezzar, A., Bentchouala, C., Smati, F., Scheftel, J.-M., Monteil, H. & Nordmann, P. (2005). Multidrug-Resistant *Salmonella enterica* Serotype Senftenberg Isolates Producing CTX-M ß-Lactamases from Constantine, Algeria. *The Journal of Antimicrobial Chemotherapy*, Vol.56, No.2, (August 2005), pp.439-440, ISSN 0305-7453.

Naas, T., Bentchouala, C., Lima, S., Lezzar, A., Smati, F., Scheftel, J.-M. & Nordmann, P. (2009). Plasmid-Mediated 16S rRNA Methylases among Extended-Spectrum- ß-Lactamase-Producing *Salmonella enterica* Senftenberg Isolates from Algeria. *The Journal of Antimicrobial Chemotherapy*, Vol.64, No.4, (April 2009), pp.866-867, ISSN 0305-7453.

Naas, T., Bentchouala, C., Cuzon, G., Yaou, S., Lezzar, A., Smati, F & Nordmann, P. (2011). Outbreak of *Salmonella enterica* Serotype Infantis Producing ArmA 16S RNA Methylase and CTX-M-15 Extended-Spectrum ß-Lactamase in a Neonatology Ward in Constantine, Algeria. *International Journal of Antimicrobial Agents*, Vol.38, No.2, (August 2011), pp.135-139, ISSN 0924-8579.

Poirel, L., Gniadkowski, M. & Nordmann, P. (2002). Biochemical Analysis of the Ceftazidime-Hydrolysing Extended-Spectrum ß-Lactamase CTX-M-15 and of its

StructurallyRrelated ß-Lactamase CTX-M-3. *The Journal of Antimicrobial Chemotherapy*, Vol.50, No.6, (June 2002), pp.1031-1034, ISSN 0305-7453.

Singh, B., Singh, P., Agrawal, S., Teotia, U., Verma, A., Sharma, S., Chandra, M., Babu, N. & Agarwal, R. (2007). Prevalence of Multidrug Resistant *Salmonella* in Coriander, Mint, Carrot, and Radish in Bareilly and Kanpur, Northern India. *Foodborne Pathogens and Disease*, Vol.4, No.2, (Summer 2007), pp.233-240, ISSN 1535-3141.

Tijet, N., Andres, P., Chung, C., Lucero, C., WHONET-Argentina Group, Low, D., Galas, M., Corso, M., Petroni, A. & Melano, R. (2011). *rmtD2*, a New Allele of a 16S rRNA Methylase Gene, Has Been Present in Enterobacteriaceae Isolates from Argentina for More than a Decade. *Antimicrobial Agents and Chemotherapy*, Vol.55, No.2, (February 2011), pp.904-909, ISSN 0066-4804.

Wachino, J., Yamane, K., Shibayama, K., Kurokawa, H., Shibata, N., Suzuki, S., Doi, Y., Kimura, K., Ike, Y. & Arakawa Y. (2006a). Novel Plasmid-Mediated 16S rRNA Methylase, RmtC, Found in a *Proteus mirabilis* Isolate Demonstrating Extraordinary High-Level Resistance Against Various Aminoglycosides. *Antimicrobial Agents and Chemotherapy*, Vol.50, No.1, (January 2006), pp.178-184, ISSN 0066-4804.

Wachino, J., Yamane, K., Kimura, K., Shibata, N., Suzuki, S., Ike, Y. & Arakawa, Y. (2006b). Mode of Transposition and Expression of 16S rRNA Methyltransferase Gene *rmtC* Accompanied by IS*Ecp1*. *Antimicrobial Agents and Chemotherapy*, Vol.50, No.9, (September 2006), pp.3212-3215, ISSN 0066-4804.

Wachino, J., Shibayama, K., Kurokawa, H., Kimura, K., Yamane, K., Suzuki, S., Shibata, N., Ike, Y. & Arakawa, Y. (2007). Novel Plasmid-Mediated 16S rRNA m^1A1408 Methyltransferase, NpmA, Found in a Clinically Isolated *Escherichia coli* Strain Resistant to Structurally Diverse Aminoglycosides. *Antimicrobial Agents and Chemotherapy*, Vol.51, No.12, (December 2007), pp.4401-4409, ISSN 0066-4804.

World Health Organisation (2007). Critically Important Antimicrobials for Human Medicine: Categorization for the Development of Risk Management Strategies to Contain Antimicrobial Resistance Due to Non-Human Antimicrobial Use: Report of the Second WHO Expert Meeting, 29-31 May 2007, Copenhagen, Denmark. 04.07.2011, Available from http://www.who.int/foodborne_disease/resistance/antimicrobials_human.pdf

Yokoyama, K., Doi, Y., Yamane, K., Kurokawa, H., Shibata, N., Shibayama, K., Yagi, T., Kato, H. & Arakawa, Y. (2003). Acquisition of 16S rRNA Methylase Gene in *Pseudomonas aeruginosa*. *The Lancet*, Vol.362, No.9399, (December 2003), pp.1888-1893, ISSN 0140-6736.

Zhang, Y., Zhou, H., Shen, X., Shen, P., Yu, Y. & Li, L. (2008). Plasmid-borne *armA* Methylase Gene, Together with $bla_{CTX\text{-}M\text{-}15}$ and $bla_{TEM\text{-}1}$, in a *Klebsiella oxytoca* Isolate from China. *Journal of Medical Microbiology*, Vol.57, No.10, (October 2008), pp.1273-1276, ISSN 0022-2615.

Zong, Z., Partridge, S. & Iredell, J. (2008) 16S rRNA Methyltransferase in Australia. *Antimicrobial Agents and Chemotherapy*, Vol.52, No.2, (February 2008), pp.794-794, ISSN 0066-4804.

13

The Phosphoinositides: Key Regulators of *Salmonella* Containing Vacuole (SCV) Trafficking and Identity

M.C. Kerr, N.A. Castro, S. Karunaratne and R.D. Teasdale
Institute for Molecular Bioscience, The University of Queensland
Australia

1. Introduction

Derived from the base of membrane ruffles in response to growth factor stimulation (Haigler, McKanna et al., 1979), the macropinosome is a large (diameters >0.2μm) phase-bright endocytic organelle that is readily labelled with fluid-phase markers. It is the primary means by which macrophages sample their immediate environment for antigens, is essential for proper renal function, is intrinsically linked to cellular migration and has a major role in the down-regulation of signalling from cell surface receptors (Kerr and Teasdale, 2009; Swanson and Watts, 1995). To promote invasion and survival, *Salmonella* subverts the host cell's normal macropinocytic machinery to gain entry into the non-phagocytic epithelial cells of the intestinal wall. Upon binding to the host cell surface the pathogen utilises a specialised apparatus called the type III secretion system (T3SS) to deliver a suite of bacterial virulence proteins directly into the host cell's cytoplasm. *Salmonellae* encode two distinct T3SSs within *Salmonella* Pathogenicity islands 1 and 2 (SPI1 and SPI2) that function at discrete stages of the infection. Whilst SPI1-T3SS is predominantly active on contact with the host cell's surface and serves to translocate virulence proteins across the plasma membrane, driving cytoskeletal rearrangements and signalling events that promote the uptake of the pathogen, SPI2-T3SS is active within intracellular compartments during the later stages of infection to generate a replicative niche (Haraga, Ohlson et al., 2008). As the environment of the encompassing macropinosome, also called the *Salmonella* Containing Vacuole (SCV) acidifies and matures, losing markers of the early endosomal system like transferrin receptor, EEA1 and Rab5, *Salmonellae* undergo extensive bacterial surface remodelling and expression and assembly of SPI2-T3SS is induced. The SPI2-T3SS enables the translocation of virulence factors across the SCV membrane into the host cell's cytoplasm. These virulence factors initiate a dramatic alteration in the host cell's vesicular trafficking pathways leading to the accumulation of late endosomal markers like Rab7 and LAMP1 and 2 on the SCV and the formation of long filamentous membrane structures. These *Salmonella*-induced filaments (SIFs) originate from the SCV, are LAMP1-positive, and function to increase the size of the SCV in a specific and directional fashion to accommodate bacterial replication during systemic infection as well as provide nutrients to the isolated pathogen (Garcia-del

Portillo and Finlay, 1995; Garcia-del Portillo, Zwick et al., 1993a, b; Haraga, Ohlson et al., 2008). What is clear from the literature is that this entire process reflects a carefully choreographed interaction between the bacterial virulence factors and the molecular machinery of the host cell.

2. Phosphoinositides and their effectors, tightly controlled regulators

Phosphoinositides (PI), the phosphorylated derivatives of the lipid phosphatidylinositol (PtdIns), can be singly or multiply phosphorylated on the 3′, 4′, and 5′ position of the inositol headgroup to generate 7 distinct PI isoforms (Vicinanza, D'Angelo et al., 2008). Reversibly phosphorylated in a tightly regulated fashion by phosphatases and kinases that are heterogeneously localised within the cell, the PIs are consequently enriched on the cytosolic face of distinct intracellular membranes (Di Paolo and De Camilli, 2006). For example, the most abundant PIs, PI(4,5)P_2 and PI(4)P, are each constitutively present in the cytosolic leaflet of the plasma membrane and Golgi apparatus respectively whilst the 3-phosphorylated PIs, PI(3)P, PI(3,4)P_2 and PI(3,5)P_2 are found distributed throughout the endolysosomal system. The relative amounts of the PIs also vary dramatically between and within cells. Virtually undetectable in quiescent cells, PI(3,4,5)P_3 levels rapidly spike upon stimulation and during specialised membrane trafficking events through the coordinated and regulated activity of class Ia PI3-kinase phosphorylating the 3′ position of PI(4,5)P_2 (Vanhaesebroeck, Leevers et al., 2001).

Remarkably complex, PI metabolism represents a delicate equilibrium balancing the relative abundance and position of these lipids within the cell. Briefly, PtdIns is converted to PI(3)P or PI(4)P on endosomes or the Golgi through the actions of vacuolar protein sorting (Vps) 34-p150 and PI(4)KII⟨ respectively. Additionally, conversion of PI(3,4,5)P_3 to PI(3)P on nascent endocytic compartments may be the consequence of the sequential dephosphorylation of PI(3,4,5)P_3 as catalysed by 4- and 5-phosphatases. Src homology 2 domain-containing inositol 5-phosphatase (SHIP) 1 and 2 are potential 5-phosphatase candidates, dephosphorylating PI(3,4,5)P_3 to PI(3,4)P_2 at the cell surface or on newly formed endocytic structures. Type I and II 4-phosphatases may then catalyse the conversion between PI(3,4)P_2 and PI(3)P (Krauss and Haucke, 2007). Alternatively PI(3,4,5)P_3 may simply be lost from the endocytic membrane and VPS34-p150, an effector of early endosomal Rab5, could drive the *de novo* synthesis of PI(3)P from PtdIns (see Figure 1) (Zerial and McBride, 2001).

Relatively high concentrations of PI(4,5)P_2 are constitutively maintained at the plasma membrane primarily through the actions of a diverse family of PI(4)P 5-kinases and the 3-phosphatases. In addition to being intrinsic to numerous signalling, cytoskeletal and endocytic events PI(4,5)P_2 also serves as a precursor to PI(4)P contributing to the pool found predominantly within the Golgi Apparatus and in secretory granules (Levine and Munro, 2002; Panaretou, Domin et al., 1997; Wang, Wang et al., 2003). The accumulation of PI(4)P within the Golgi reflects the presence of multiple PI(4)Ks and PI(4,5)P_2 phosphatases in conjunction with relatively low levels PI(4)P 5-kinase activity.

The most recently identified of the PIs, PI(3,5)P_2, is synthesised from PI(3)P by the PI(5) kinase, PIKfyve (Shisheva, 2008). Whilst the precise role PI(3,5)P_2 plays in the mammalian

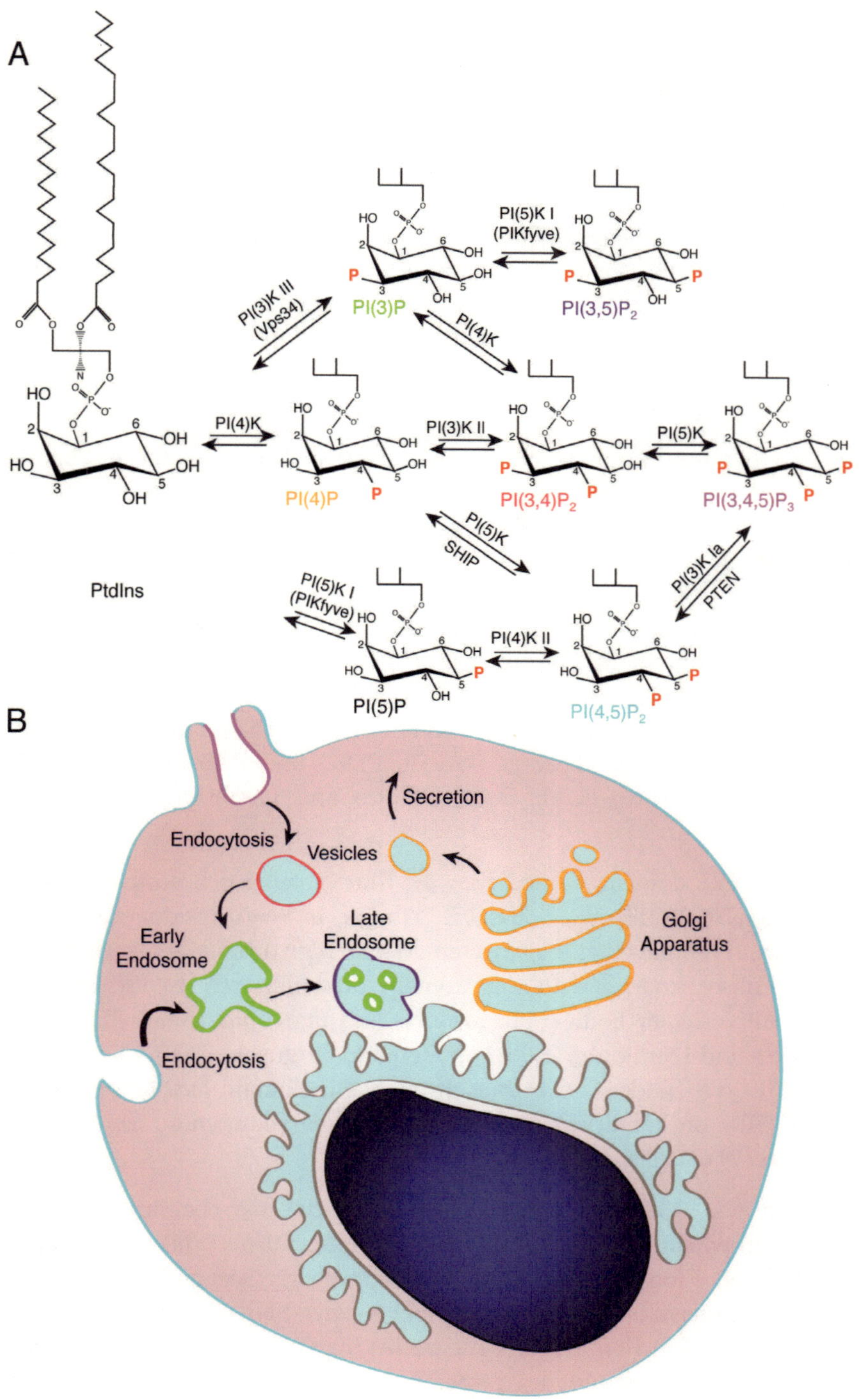

Fig. 1. PI metabolism and subcellular distribution. The phosphoinositides are phosphorylated derivatives of phosphatidylinositol. Their metabolism is regulated by kinases and phosphatases that are distributed heterogenously throughout the cell contributing to the accumulation of specific PIs in discrete intracellular membranes.

system is currently emergent, disruption of the yeast PIKfyve equivalent, Fab1p, results in a highly complex phenotype. The observation that a ΔFAB1 strain entirely devoid of PI(3,5)P_2 displays a dramatically enlarged vacuole that fails to acidify, partial defects in prevacuolar compartment (PVC; mammalian endosome equivalent) sorting, defective inheritance of vacuoles in daughter cells and a reduction in the number of intravacuolar vesicles seen by electron microscopy all suggest that PI(3,5)P_2 is integral to a number of processes essential for the maintenance of vacuolar/lysosomal system (Cooke, 2002; Cooke, Dove et al., 1998; Dove, McEwen et al., 1999; Dove, McEwen et al., 2002; Dove, Piper et al., 2004; Gary, Wurmser et al., 1998; Odorizzi, Babst et al., 1998; Yamamoto, DeWald et al., 1995). In agreement, we utilised time-lapse videomicroscopy to demonstrate that PIKfyve activity is essential for the fusion of macropinosomes with late endosomal/lysosomal membranes (Kerr, Wang et al., 2010).

The unique spatial and temporal distribution of the PIs provides the mechanism for the exquisite control with which this protein-lipid network regulates membrane trafficking and signalling events. Specifically, they serve as membrane anchors to recruit a suite of PI-binding molecules of diverse function through a variety of domains with differing PI-affinities and -specificities. The most thoroughly investigated of these, the *plekstrin homology* (PH) domain, is a ~120 residue motif found in 275 human proteins (DiNitto and Lambright, 2006; Lemmon and Ferguson, 2000). The relatively low sequence conservation between PH domains is reflected in the significant variation in specificity and affinity for individual PIs. For example, the PH domains of Grp1 and PLCδ1 each bind PI(3,4,5)P_3 and PI(4,5)P_2 respectively, whilst those of DAPP1, PDK1 and PKB bind both PI(3,4)P_2 and PI(3,4,5)P_3 (Cronin, DiNitto et al., 2004; DiNitto and Lambright, 2006; Lemmon and Ferguson, 2000).

In contrast, the *FYVE* domain, named after the four cysteine-rich proteins in which it was first identified (Fab1, YOTB, Vac1, and EEA1) after, is a ~70 residue zinc-binding finger found in 28 human proteins that displays remarkably high affinity and specificity for PI(3)P. It serves to localise proteins with this domain predominantly to PI(3)P-enriched early endosomes, multivesicular bodies, phagosomes and macropinosomes (Cronin, DiNitto et al., 2004; DiNitto and Lambright, 2006; Lemmon and Ferguson, 2000). The afore-mentioned PI(5) kinase, PIKfyve, binds its substrate through this domain facilitating the turnover of PI(3)P to PI(3,5)P_2 on maturing endocytic organelles (Ikonomov, Sbrissa et al., 2006; Rutherford, Traer et al., 2006; Shisheva, 2008).

The PX domain is a ~130 residue motif named after the two phagocyte NADPH oxidase (*phox*) subunits in which it was first described (Ponting, 1996). Whilst PI(3)P appears to be the preferred target of most PX domain containing proteins (Seet and Hong, 2006), a variety of other specificities have been reported. Sorting Nexins (SNX) 9 and 18 both bind PI(4,5)P_2 where they appear to function in endocytic trafficking events at the plasma membrane and AP1-positive endosomal membranes respectively, whilst SNX1 is reported to bind both PI(3)P and PI(3,5)$_2$ and is involved in retrograde trafficking events from early endosomes to the Golgi (Carlton, Bujny et al., 2004; Haberg, Lundmark et al., 2008; Shin, Ahn et al., 2008; Soulet, Yarar et al., 2005; Yarar, Waterman-Storer et al., 2007). Interestingly, the PX domain in isolation is often not sufficient to recruit these molecules to PI-enriched membranes.

Removal of the membrane curvature sensing and bending Bin Amphiphysin Rvs (BAR) from sorting nexin 1 (SNX1) renders it cytosolic demonstrating the necessity for the *coincident detection* of both the specific PIs and the appropriately curved membranes for recruitment to endosomes (Carlton, Bujny et al., 2005).

3. Phosphoinositides in *Salmonella* Infection

Early in the *Salmonella* invasion process cellular PI levels are reported to undergo rapid and dynamic shifts. HPLC analysis of lipids extracted from *Salmonella*-infected cells revealed remarkable elevation in the relative amounts of PI(4,5)P_2, PI(3,4)P_2 and PI(3,4,5)P_3 as well as more moderate elevation in PI(3)P when compared to control cells (Bakowski, Braun et al., 2010). Modulation of PI(4,5)P_2 and PI(3,4,5)P_2 serves to destabilise the cortical cytoskeleton leading to membrane ruffling, macropinosome formation and promoting bacterial uptake whilst the accumulation of PI(3)P on membrane ruffles and the nascent SCV promotes recruitment of the PI(3)P-binding r-SNARE VAMP8 which facilitates fusion events within the endosomal network (Dai, Zhang et al., 2007).

Shortly after formation, the enveloping macropinosome shrinks to form an adherent SCV around one or more *Salmonella*. This process is mediated, at least in part, by a suite of PI-binding effector molecules known as the sorting nexins (SNX). The SNXs represent a collection of approximately 50 human proteins with diverse domain architectures that are recruited to intracellular membranes via a common PX domain (Cullen, 2008). It was revealed that SNXs 1 and 5 form heterodimers upon the surface of maturing PI(3)P-rich macropinosomes via a conserved BAR domain within their carboxyl-terminus. This dimerisation leads to the formation of tubular carriers that retrieve large quantities of membrane from and the consequent condensation of the macropinosome as the organelle matures (Kerr, Lindsay et al., 2006). The transient nature of the SNX's recruitment to the SCV was demonstrated to reflect the subsequent phosphorylation of PI(3)P within the membrane of the macropinosome to PI(3,5)P_2 by the phosphatidylinositol 5-kinase, PIKfyve. This final PI transition is necessary for the ultimate fusion of macropinosomes with the late endosomal/lysosomal system (Kerr, Wang et al., 2010).

While the SCV appears to share properties in common with constitutive macropinosomes, including SNX-recruitment, the maturation process is significantly perturbed so that the SCV persists for hours. Hernandez *et al.* (2004) observed that unlike constitutive macropinosomes, SCVs containing wild-type *Salmonella* rapidly accumulate and maintain elevated levels of PI(3)P for up to 90mins (Hernandez, Hueffer et al., 2004). Bujney et al. demonstrated that one consequence of this was the elevated and sustained accumulation of SNX1 to the newly formed SCV. This in turn results in a grossly exaggerated tubulation event that leads to the rapid contraction of the enveloping SCV to form a tightly-wrapped adherent membrane around the bacterium (Bujny, Ewels et al., 2008). Time-lapse videomicroscopy elegantly demonstrates the precision with which the pathogen is able to manipulate its local environment as the tubulation and condensation of the SCV is not observed on the surrounding constitutive macropinosomes (see Figure 2). One might speculate that this embellished contraction may facilitate the eventual engagement of the SPI2-T3SS with the membrane of the SCV.

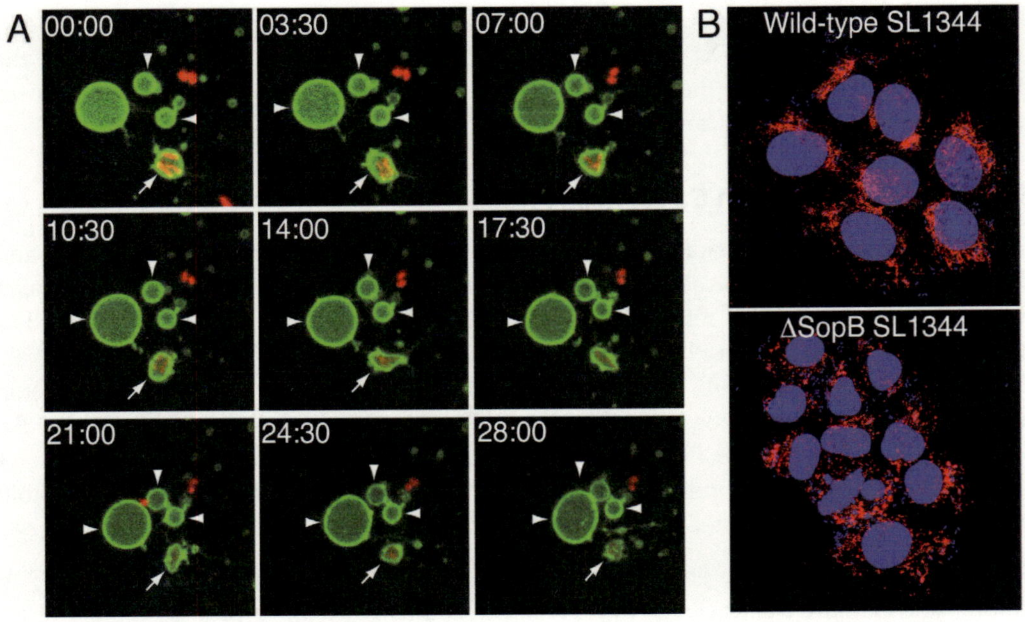

(A) A-431 cells transiently transfected with a mammalian expression construct encoding the high-affinity PI(3)P-probe $2xFYVE_{Hrs}$ fused with eGFP were infected with late-log phase wild-type *Salmonella* expressing RFP (RFP-SL1344) and imaged live using a Zeiss LSM 510 confocal scanning microscope. Initially spacious, the PI(3)P-rich SCV (arrows) is observed to undergo significant tubulation and in doing so condenses to form an adherent membrane around the bacteria (red). In contrast, surrounding constitutive macropinosomes (arrow heads) present limited tubulation and no condensation in the same time period. (B) This tubulation is mediated by SopB as evidenced by the more moderate tubulation observed in ΔSopB strain-infected cells when compared to those infected with wild-type Salmonella.

Fig. 2. SNX-mediated tubulation leads to dramatic condensation of the SCV.

3.1 SopB, a pleitropic phosphoinositide phosphatase

This striking impact upon PI metabolism and SNX recruitment is achieved, at least in part, by directly modulating the PI-composition of the SCV through the delivery of virulence factors with PI-phosphatase activity. SopB (also called SigD) is a SPI-T3SS phosphoinositide phosphatase that has diverse influence upon the pathogenesis of *S. typhimurium*. It contributes to membrane sealing at the plasma membrane and actin-rearrangement through activation of SGEF (a guanine nucleotide exchange factor for RhoG), during bacterial invasion (Patel and Galan, 2006; Terebiznik, Vieira et al., 2002). It also inhibits induction of apoptosis through activation of Akt and promotes the early recruitment of Rab5 and its effector Vps34 to the SCV (Knodler, Finlay et al., 2005; Mallo, Espina et al., 2008; Steele-Mortimer, Knodler et al., 2000).

Sharing similarity with mammalian PI 4- and 5-phosphatases, SopB is reported to hydrolyse a variety of PIs *in vitro,* including $PI(3,4)P_2$, $PI(3,5)P_2$ and $PI3,4,5P_2$, and more recently, $PI(4,5)P_2$ *in vivo* (Bakowski, Braun et al., 2010; Marcus, Wenk et al., 2001; Norris, Wilson et al., 1998). Given this apparent broad specificity and the capacity to promote Vps34 recruitment to, and presumably therefore *de novo* synthesis of PI(3)P on, the SCV, the wide ranging impact SopB has upon the infectious cycle of *Salmonella* is perhaps not surprising. Indeed, SopB was recently demonstrated to have profound affects upon the biophysical properties of the SCV itself. Bakowski *et al.* (2010) The authors used an mRFP-tagged derivative of the K-ras tail with all the serine and threonine residues mutated to alanine and the lysine residues mutated to arginine so that its recruitment to intracellular membranes was only governed by surface potential and not phosphorylation or ubiquitination. They demonstrated that by reducing the levels of negatively-charged lipids like PI(4,5)P_2 and phosphatidylserine on the nascent SCV, SopB activity orchestrates the dissociation of a number of endocytic Rab proteins and inhibits fusion of the SCV with bactericidal lysosomal compartments (Bakowski, Braun et al., 2010).

In addition to its lipid phosphatase activity, SopB was also recently revealed to interact with CDC42 suggesting an additional aspect to its contribution to the infectious process. Rodríguez-Escudero *et al.* (2011) demonstrated that a catalytically inactive SopB mutant can inhibit CDC42 but not Rac1 in a yeast model system. This interaction occurs independent of the activation state of CDC42. Interestingly, *Salmonella* strains harbouring SopB-mutations that render it unable to bind CDC42 presented similar invasion efficiencies when compared to the wild-type but reduced intracellular replication (Rodriguez-Escudero, Ferrer et al., 2011; Rodriguez-Escudero, Rotger et al., 2006). This indicates that the SopB-CDC42 association is pertinent to the intracellular adaptation of the pathogen rather than the actin-remodeling that occurs upon invasion as one might expect.

3.2 The sorting nexins coordinate *Salmonella* pathogenesis

By manipulating cellular PI metabolism, *Salmonella* effectively exaggerates and alters the function of the PI-effector molecules thereby creating a niche within the cell that supports replication and infection. In the context of SNX1, this is manifest in SopB-dependent over-recruitment and tubulation events leading to the accelerated condensation of the organelle and formation of the adherent SCV (See Figure 2). siRNA-mediated suppression of SNX1 is sufficient to inhibit SCV progression into the cell and had a moderate impact upon the intracellular replication of *Salmonella* (Bujny, Ewels et al., 2008). Similarly, knockdown of SNX3, which constitutes little more than a PX domain and is found on tubular extensions of the SCV distinct from those of SNX1, inhibits SCV maturation and intracellular replication of *Salmonella* (Braun, Wong et al., 2010). But what of the other PX proteins?

Wang *et al.* (2010) employed an ectopic screening strategy to demonstrate that a specific cohort of the SNXs, namely SNXs 1, 5, 9, 18 and 33, could significantly elevate the rate of macropinocytosis in cultured monolayers suggesting specific roles beyond the tubulation events described earlier (Wang, Kerr et al., 2010). Perhaps these SNXs have unique roles to play in *Salmonella* pathogenicity? Towards this we have initiated a detailed examination of the recruitment of the SNXs to the nascent SCV. Immunofluorescent-labelling of infected cells transiently transfected with mammalian expression constructs encoding epitope-tagged SNXs and co-labelled with endogenous SNX1 revealed 19 SNXs recruited to the SCV within the first 30mins of infection (see Figure 3).

Interestingly, significant variation in the precise distribution of these SNXs on the early SCV was observed. Those most related to SNX1, and those previous demonstrated to have a role in endosomal trafficking, namely SNXs 2, 4, 5, 6, 7 and 8, were found on the afore-mentioned SNX1-labelled tubular extensions of the SCV. mPLD2, SNX12, SNX16, SNX21, SNX23 and SNX28 were found evenly associated with the tubules and the body of the SCV proper whilst hPLD1, SNX10, SNX11, SNX15, SNX27 and p40phox were restricted to the body of the SCV only. The notable absence of SNX3 on the SCV perhaps reflects a difference in the temporal nature of the SNXs recruitment. Unlike SNX1, which is most evident on the SCV very early in the infection, SNX3 is recruited ~60mins into the infection indicating additional levels of complexity in the mechanism of recruitment within this PI-effector family (Braun, Wong et al., 2010). Indeed the PX-containing subunits of the NADPH oxidase complex represent a significant threat to intracellular *Salmonella,* providing the means to deliver a bactericidal oxidative burst to the SCV in macrophages. Virulent *Salmonella* strains avoid this through a SPI2-dependent mechanism that inhibits trafficking or targeting of NADPH oxidase-containing vesicles to the vicinity of the SCV (Vazquez-Torres, Xu et al., 2000). It will be interesting to see the likely diverse roles played by the SNXs during *Salmonella* pathogenicity emerge in the near future.

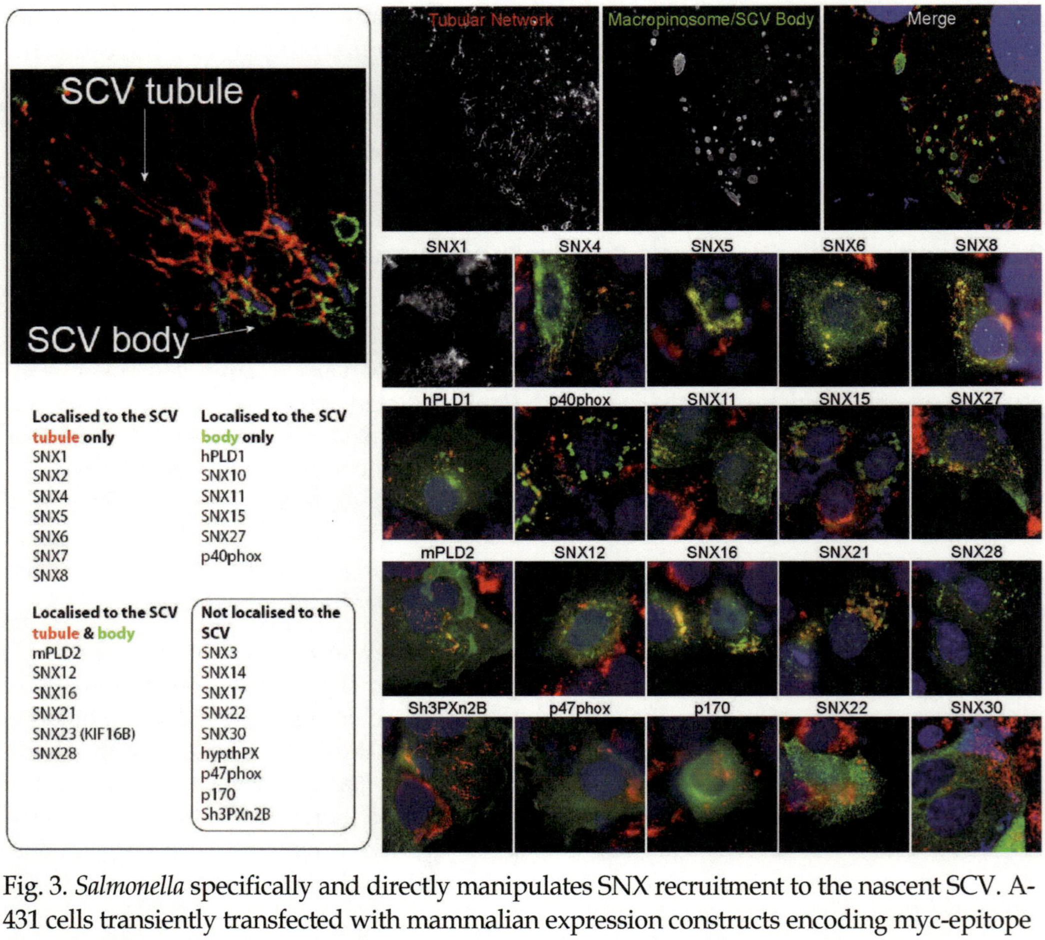

Fig. 3. *Salmonella* specifically and directly manipulates SNX recruitment to the nascent SCV. A-431 cells transiently transfected with mammalian expression constructs encoding myc-epitope tagged SNXs were infected with late-log phase *Salmonella* (SL1344) for 30mins, fixed with 4% PFA and labelled with an α-myc polyclonal antibody, a monoclonal antibody specific for SNX1, DAPI and appropriate secondary antibodies. Images were captured using a Zeiss LSM 510 confocal scanning microscope. Images were examined and the recruitment of the overexpressed SNX construct (green) was compared with that of endogenous SNX1 (red).

3.3 Targeting the phosphoinositides for therapeutic intervention

With the development of antibiotic resistance, new strategies to combat intracellular pathogens, like *Salmonella,* need to be developed. One emergent approach is to manipulate non-essential host cellular pathways required by the pathogen during its infectious cycle (Schwegmann and Brombacher, 2008). Given the frequent connections between the PIs, their effectors, and those of *Salmonella,* this protein-lipid network represents a potential opportunity for novel modes of intervention.

We recently demonstrated that disruption of $PI(3,5)P_2$-synthesis through perturbation of PIKfyve activity, be it by interfering mutant, siRNA-mediated knockdown or pharmacological means (YM201636), was led to a profound inhibition in the fusion of maturing macropinosomes with the late endosomal/lysosomal network. As mentioned earlier, these directed fusion events are necessary for the formation of SIFs during an infection with *S. typhimurium.* Remarkably, inhibition of PIKfyve was sufficient to halt SIF formation, SCV acidification, induction of the SPI2 Operon and ultimately intracellular replication of *Salmonella* whilst still maintaining the pathogen within an intracellular compartment (Kerr, Wang et al., 2010).

Of course a thorough understanding of the potential consequence of targeting PIs is required for such host-directed therapeutics to be effective. Inhibition of PI(3)P accumulation on the SCV with wortmannin is sufficient to halt recruitment of FYVE-domain containing molecules like EEA1 and even the SIF-marker LAMP1 but does not perturb intracellular replication of *Salmonella* (Scott, Cuellar-Mata et al., 2002). In fact, some have observed elevated rates of replication in host treated with wortmannin (Brumell, Tang et al., 2002). This is because, unlike those cultured in the presence of YM201626, the integrity of the SCV itself is disrupted releasing the bacteria into the cytosol, where they may freely replicate.

Aside from counteracting the evolution of bacterial antibiotic resistance, these *host-directed therapeutics* may provide broad-spectrum solutions to a variety of pathogens. Indeed, *Salmonella* is not unique in its partiality for targeting the PIs and associated molecules. *Yersinia* species activate PI(5) kinase to stimulate $PtdIns(4,5)P_2$ production at sites of bacterial invasion whilst *Listeria monocytogenes* and uropathogenic *E. coli* stimulate class I PI(3) kinase generating $PtdIns(3,4,5)P_3$ to promote uptake (Gavicherla, Ritchey et al., 2010; Ireton, 2007; Ireton, Payrastre et al., 1999; Martinez, Mulvey et al., 2000). *Mycobacterium tuberculosis* inhibits class III PI(3) kinase, Vps34, involved in the formation of PI(3)P effectively arresting phagosome maturation (Chua and Deretic, 2004). Thus by targeting the PIs, we may be able to specifically interfere with a variety of infections at different stages of there pathogenic cycle.

4. Conclusion

Despite comprising less than 1% of cellular lipids, the PIs and their effectors are key regulators of intra- and inter-cellular signalling, cell growth and survival, cytoskeletal dynamics and membrane trafficking pathways. It is perhaps not surprising that intracellular pathogens that exploit these processes directly target this remarkably complex protein-lipid network during the infectious process. Whilst the roles the PIs play directly and through their effectors like the sorting nexins during a *Salmonella* infection are only now coming to light, there is already strong evidence to consider them as viable therapeutic targets for intervention.

5. Acknowledgments

This work was supported by funding from the National Health and Medical Research Council (NHMRC) of Australia (606788). RDT is supported by NHMRC Senior Research Fellowship (511042). Microscopy was performed at the Australian Cancer Research Foundation (ACRF)/Institute for Molecular Bioscience Dynamic Imaging Facility for Cancer Biology, which was established with the support of the ACRF.

6. References

Bakowski, M.A., Braun, V., Lam, G.Y., Yeung, T., Heo, W.D., Meyer, T., Finlay, B.B., Grinstein, S., & Brumell, J.H. (2010). The phosphoinositide phosphatase SopB manipulates membrane surface charge and trafficking of the Salmonella-containing vacuole. Cell Host Microbe *7*, 453-462.

Braun, V., Wong, A., Landekic, M., Hong, W.J., Grinstein, S., & Brumell, J.H. (2010). Sorting nexin 3 (SNX3) is a component of a tubular endosomal network induced by Salmonella and involved in maturation of the Salmonella-containing vacuole. Cell Microbiol *12*, 1352-1367.

Brumell, J.H., Tang, P., Zaharik, M.L., & Finlay, B.B. (2002). Disruption of the Salmonella-containing vacuole leads to increased replication of Salmonella enterica serovar typhimurium in the cytosol of epithelial cells. Infect Immun *70*, 3264-3270.

Bujny, M.V., Ewels, P.A., Humphrey, S., Attar, N., Jepson, M.A., & Cullen, P.J. (2008). Sorting nexin-1 defines an early phase of Salmonella-containing vacuole-remodeling during Salmonella infection. J Cell Sci *121*, 2027-2036.

Carlton, J., Bujny, M., Peter, B.J., Oorschot, V.M., Rutherford, A., Mellor, H., Klumperman, J., McMahon, H.T., & Cullen, P.J. (2004). Sorting nexin-1 mediates tubular endosome-to-TGN transport through coincidence sensing of high- curvature membranes and 3-phosphoinositides. Curr Biol *14*, 1791-1800.

Carlton, J., Bujny, M., Rutherford, A., & Cullen, P. (2005). Sorting nexins--unifying trends and new perspectives. Traffic *6*, 75-82.

Chua, J., & Deretic, V. (2004). Mycobacterium tuberculosis reprograms waves of phosphatidylinositol 3-phosphate on phagosomal organelles. J Biol Chem *279*, 36982-36992.

Cooke, F.T. (2002). Phosphatidylinositol 3,5-bisphosphate: metabolism and function. Arch Biochem Biophys *407*, 143-151.

Cooke, F.T., Dove, S.K., McEwen, R.K., Painter, G., Holmes, A.B., Hall, M.N., Michell, R.H., & Parker, P.J. (1998). The stress-activated phosphatidylinositol 3-phosphate 5-kinase Fab1p is essential for vacuole function in S. cerevisiae. Curr Biol *8*, 1219-1222.

Cronin, T.C., DiNitto, J.P., Czech, M.P., & Lambright, D.G. (2004). Structural determinants of phosphoinositide selectivity in splice variants of Grp1 family PH domains. Embo J *23*, 3711-3720.

Cullen, P.J. (2008). Endosomal sorting and signalling: an emerging role for sorting nexins. Nat Rev Mol Cell Biol *9*, 574-582.

Dai, S., Zhang, Y., Weimbs, T., Yaffe, M.B., & Zhou, D. (2007). Bacteria-generated PtdIns(3)P recruits VAMP8 to facilitate phagocytosis. Traffic *8*, 1365-1374.

Di Paolo, G., & De Camilli, P. (2006). Phosphoinositides in cell regulation and membrane dynamics. Nature *443*, 651-657.

DiNitto, J.P., & Lambright, D.G. (2006). Membrane and juxtamembrane targeting by PH and PTB domains. Biochim Biophys Acta *1761*, 850-867.

Dove, S.K., McEwen, R.K., Cooke, F.T., Parker, P.J., & Michell, R.H. (1999). Phosphatidylinositol 3,5-bisphosphate: a novel lipid that links stress responses to membrane trafficking events. Biochem Soc Trans *27*, 674-677.

Dove, S.K., McEwen, R.K., Mayes, A., Hughes, D.C., Beggs, J.D., & Michell, R.H. (2002). Vac14 controls PtdIns(3,5)P(2) synthesis and Fab1-dependent protein trafficking to the multivesicular body. Curr Biol *12*, 885-893.

Dove, S.K., Piper, R.C., McEwen, R.K., Yu, J.W., King, M.C., Hughes, D.C., Thuring, J., Holmes, A.B., Cooke, F.T., Michell, R.H., Parker, P.J., & Lemmon, M.A. (2004). Svp1p defines a family of phosphatidylinositol 3,5-bisphosphate effectors. Embo J *23*, 1922-1933.

Garcia-del Portillo, F., & Finlay, B.B. (1995). Targeting of Salmonella typhimurium to vesicles containing lysosomal membrane glycoproteins bypasses compartments with mannose 6-phosphate receptors. J Cell Biol *129*, 81-97.

Garcia-del Portillo, F., Zwick, M.B., Leung, K.Y., & Finlay, B.B. (1993a). Intracellular replication of Salmonella within epithelial cells is associated with filamentous structures containing lysosomal membrane glycoproteins. Infect Agents Dis *2*, 227-231.

Garcia-del Portillo, F., Zwick, M.B., Leung, K.Y., & Finlay, B.B. (1993b). Salmonella induces the formation of filamentous structures containing lysosomal membrane glycoproteins in epithelial cells. Proc Natl Acad Sci U S A *90*, 10544-10548.

Gary, J.D., Wurmser, A.E., Bonangelino, C.J., Weisman, L.S., & Emr, S.D. (1998). Fab1p is essential for PtdIns(3)P 5-kinase activity and the maintenance of vacuolar size and membrane homeostasis. J Cell Biol *143*, 65-79.

Gavicherla, B., Ritchey, L., Gianfelice, A., Kolokoltsov, A.A., Davey, R.A., & Ireton, K. (2010). Critical role for the host GTPase-activating protein ARAP2 in InlB-mediated entry of Listeria monocytogenes. Infect Immun *78*, 4532-4541.

Haberg, K., Lundmark, R., & Carlsson, S.R. (2008). SNX18 is an SNX9 paralog that acts as a membrane tubulator in AP-1-positive endosomal trafficking. J Cell Sci *121*, 1495-1505.

Haigler, H.T., McKanna, J.A., & Cohen, S. (1979). Rapid stimulation of pinocytosis in human carcinoma cells A-431 by epidermal growth factor. J Cell Biol *83*, 82-90.

Haraga, A., Ohlson, M.B., & Miller, S.I. (2008). Salmonellae interplay with host cells. Nat Rev Microbiol *6*, 53-66.

Hernandez, L.D., Hueffer, K., Wenk, M.R., & Galan, J.E. (2004). Salmonella modulates vesicular traffic by altering phosphoinositide metabolism. Science *304*, 1805-1807.

Ikonomov, O.C., Sbrissa, D., & Shisheva, A. (2006). Localized PtdIns 3,5-P2 synthesis to regulate early endosome dynamics and fusion. Am J Physiol Cell Physiol *291*, C393-404.

Ireton, K. (2007). Entry of the bacterial pathogen Listeria monocytogenes into mammalian cells. Cell Microbiol *9*, 1365-1375.

Ireton, K., Payrastre, B., & Cossart, P. (1999). The Listeria monocytogenes protein InlB is an agonist of mammalian phosphoinositide 3-kinase. J Biol Chem *274*, 17025-17032.

Kerr, M.C., Lindsay, M.R., Luetterforst, R., Hamilton, N., Simpson, F., Parton, R.G., Gleeson, P.A., & Teasdale, R.D. (2006). Visualisation of macropinosome maturation by the recruitment of sorting nexins. J Cell Sci *119*, 3967-3980.

Kerr, M.C., & Teasdale, R.D. (2009). Defining macropinocytosis. Traffic *10*, 364-371.

Kerr, M.C., Wang, J.T., Castro, N.A., Hamilton, N.A., Town, L., Brown, D.L., Meunier, F.A., Brown, N.F., Stow, J.L., & Teasdale, R.D. (2010). Inhibition of the PtdIns(5) kinase PIKfyve disrupts intracellular replication of Salmonella. Embo J *29*, 1331-1347.

Knodler, L.A., Finlay, B.B., & Steele-Mortimer, O. (2005). The Salmonella effector protein SopB protects epithelial cells from apoptosis by sustained activation of Akt. J Biol Chem *280*, 9058-9064.

Krauss, M., & Haucke, V. (2007). Phosphoinositide-metabolizing enzymes at the interface between membrane traffic and cell signalling. EMBO Rep *8*, 241-246.

Lemmon, M.A., & Ferguson, K.M. (2000). Signal-dependent membrane targeting by pleckstrin homology (PH) domains. Biochem J *350 Pt 1*, 1-18.

Levine, T.P., & Munro, S. (2002). Targeting of Golgi-specific pleckstrin homology domains involves both PtdIns 4-kinase-dependent and -independent components. Curr Biol *12*, 695-704.

Mallo, G.V., Espina, M., Smith, A.C., Terebiznik, M.R., Aleman, A., Finlay, B.B., Rameh, L.E., Grinstein, S., & Brumell, J.H. (2008). SopB promotes phosphatidylinositol 3-phosphate formation on Salmonella vacuoles by recruiting Rab5 and Vps34. J Cell Biol *182*, 741-752.

Marcus, S.L., Wenk, M.R., Steele-Mortimer, O., & Finlay, B.B. (2001). A synaptojanin-homologous region of Salmonella typhimurium SigD is essential for inositol phosphatase activity and Akt activation. FEBS Lett *494*, 201-207.

Martinez, J.J., Mulvey, M.A., Schilling, J.D., Pinkner, J.S., & Hultgren, S.J. (2000). Type 1 pilus-mediated bacterial invasion of bladder epithelial cells. Embo J *19*, 2803-2812.

Norris, F.A., Wilson, M.P., Wallis, T.S., Galyov, E.E., & Majerus, P.W. (1998). SopB, a protein required for virulence of Salmonella dublin, is an inositol phosphate phosphatase. Proc Natl Acad Sci U S A *95*, 14057-14059.

Odorizzi, G., Babst, M., & Emr, S.D. (1998). Fab1p PtdIns(3)P 5-kinase function essential for protein sorting in the multivesicular body. Cell *95*, 847-858.

Panaretou, C., Domin, J., Cockcroft, S., & Waterfield, M.D. (1997). Characterization of p150, an adaptor protein for the human phosphatidylinositol (PtdIns) 3-kinase. Substrate presentation by phosphatidylinositol transfer protein to the p150.Ptdins 3-kinase complex. J Biol Chem *272*, 2477-2485.

Patel, J.C., & Galan, J.E. (2006). Differential activation and function of Rho GTPases during Salmonella-host cell interactions. J Cell Biol *175*, 453-463.

Ponting, C.P. (1996). Novel domains in NADPH oxidase subunits, sorting nexins, and PtdIns 3-kinases: binding partners of SH3 domains? Protein Sci *5*, 2353-2357.

Rodriguez-Escudero, I., Ferrer, N.L., Rotger, R., Cid, V.J., & Molina, M. (2011). Interaction of the Salmonella Typhimurium effector protein SopB with host cell Cdc42 is involved in intracellular replication. Mol Microbiol *80*, 1220-1240.

Rodriguez-Escudero, I., Rotger, R., Cid, V.J., & Molina, M. (2006). Inhibition of Cdc42-dependent signalling in Saccharomyces cerevisiae by phosphatase-dead SigD/SopB from Salmonella typhimurium. Microbiology *152*, 3437-3452.

Rutherford, A.C., Traer, C., Wassmer, T., Pattni, K., Bujny, M.V., Carlton, J.G., Stenmark, H., & Cullen, P.J. (2006). The mammalian phosphatidylinositol 3-phosphate 5-kinase (PIKfyve) regulates endosome-to-TGN retrograde transport. J Cell Sci *119*, 3944-3957.

Schwegmann, A., & Brombacher, F. (2008). Host-directed drug targeting of factors hijacked by pathogens. Sci Signal *1*, re8.

Scott, C.C., Cuellar-Mata, P., Matsuo, T., Davidson, H.W., & Grinstein, S. (2002). Role of 3-phosphoinositides in the maturation of Salmonella-containing vacuoles within host cells. J Biol Chem *277*, 12770-12776.

Seet, L.F., & Hong, W. (2006). The Phox (PX) domain proteins and membrane traffic. Biochim Biophys Acta *1761*, 878-896.

Shin, N., Ahn, N., Chang-Ileto, B., Park, J., Takei, K., Ahn, S.G., Kim, S.A., Di Paolo, G., & Chang, S. (2008). SNX9 regulates tubular invagination of the plasma membrane through interaction with actin cytoskeleton and dynamin 2. J Cell Sci *121*, 1252-1263.

Shisheva, A. (2008). PIKfyve: Partners, significance, debates and paradoxes. Cell Biol Int *32*, 591-604.

Soulet, F., Yarar, D., Leonard, M., & Schmid, S.L. (2005). SNX9 regulates dynamin assembly and is required for efficient clathrin-mediated endocytosis. Mol Biol Cell *16*, 2058-2067.

Steele-Mortimer, O., Knodler, L.A., Marcus, S.L., Scheid, M.P., Goh, B., Pfeifer, C.G., Duronio, V., & Finlay, B.B. (2000). Activation of Akt/protein kinase B in epithelial cells by the Salmonella typhimurium effector sigD. J Biol Chem *275*, 37718-37724.

Swanson, J.A., & Watts, C. (1995). Macropinocytosis. Trends Cell Biol *5*, 424-428.

Terebiznik, M.R., Vieira, O.V., Marcus, S.L., Slade, A., Yip, C.M., Trimble, W.S., Meyer, T., Finlay, B.B., & Grinstein, S. (2002). Elimination of host cell PtdIns(4,5)P(2) by bacterial SigD promotes membrane fission during invasion by Salmonella. Nat Cell Biol *4*, 766-773.

Vanhaesebroeck, B., Leevers, S.J., Ahmadi, K., Timms, J., Katso, R., Driscoll, P.C., Woscholski, R., Parker, P.J., & Waterfield, M.D. (2001). Synthesis and function of 3-phosphorylated inositol lipids. Annu Rev Biochem *70*, 535-602.

Vazquez-Torres, A., Xu, Y., Jones-Carson, J., Holden, D.W., Lucia, S.M., Dinauer, M.C., Mastroeni, P., & Fang, F.C. (2000). Salmonella pathogenicity island 2-dependent evasion of the phagocyte NADPH oxidase. Science *287*, 1655-1658.

Vicinanza, M., D'Angelo, G., Di Campli, A., & De Matteis, M.A. (2008). Function and dysfunction of the PI system in membrane trafficking. Embo J *27*, 2457-2470.

Wang, J.T., Kerr, M.C., Karunaratne, S., Jeanes, A., Yap, A.S., & Teasdale, R.D. (2010). The SNX-PX-BAR family in macropinocytosis: the regulation of macropinosome formation by SNX-PX-BAR proteins. PLoS One *5*, e13763.

Wang, Y.J., Wang, J., Sun, H.Q., Martinez, M., Sun, Y.X., Macia, E., Kirchhausen, T., Albanesi, J.P., Roth, M.G., & Yin, H.L. (2003). Phosphatidylinositol 4 phosphate regulates targeting of clathrin adaptor AP-1 complexes to the Golgi. Cell *114*, 299-310.

Yamamoto, A., DeWald, D.B., Boronenkov, I.V., Anderson, R.A., Emr, S.D., & Koshland, D. (1995). Novel PI(4)P 5-kinase homologue, Fab1p, essential for normal vacuole function and morphology in yeast. Mol Biol Cell *6*, 525-539.

Yarar, D., Waterman-Storer, C.M., & Schmid, S.L. (2007). SNX9 couples actin assembly to phosphoinositide signals and is required for membrane remodeling during endocytosis. Dev Cell *13*, 43-56.

Zerial, M., & McBride, H. (2001). Rab proteins as membrane organizers. Nat Rev Mol Cell Biol *2*, 107-117.

14

Searching for Outer Membrane Proteins Typical of Serum-Sensitive and Serum-Resistant Phenotypes of *Salmonella*

Bozena Futoma-Koloch[1], Gabriela Bugla-Ploskonska[1] and Jolanta Sarowska[2]
[1]*Institute of Genetics and Microbiology University of Wroclaw, Przybyszewskiego, Wroclaw*
[2]*Department of Basic Sciences Wroclaw Medical University, Chalubinskiego Poland*

1. Introduction

The pathogenesis of serum-resistance *Salmonella* infections seems to be connected with a variety of their surface structures. *Salmonella* resistance to innate immune factors aids the despersal of bacteria in host tissues and body fluids. This paper shows the natural resistance of clinical *S.* Enteritidis, *S.* Typhimurium, and *S.* Hadar strains to the antibacterial activity of human serum. Curiously, some of the pathogens modify their lipopolysaccharide (LPS) to escape host surveillance. A well-known strategy developed by bacteria is sialylation with sialic acid (NeuAc) of surface structures to mimic host tissues. It is very interesting, that even though LPS of the same chemical structure covers *Salmonella* O48, these bacteria differ in their susceptibility to the antibacterial activity of serum. Previous results indicate that the presence of sialylated LPS do not protect *Salmonella* O48 against the bactericidal activity of human and animal serum, and the presence of NeuAc in the LPS structure is not sufficient to block activation of the alternative pathway of complement in serum. Because outer membrane proteins (OMPs) are also surface virulence factors and have a significant role in pathobiology and bacterial adaptation to environmental conditions, researchers have directed their investigations through the analysis of *Salmonella* OMPs patterns and have attempted to identify among them key molecular targets of the protective immune response against *Salmonella*. This work also highlights the importance of OMPs as candidates for vaccine targets. In this review, we have collected and discussed published results, as well as new ones, shown for the first time.

2. Salmonellosis – An emerging problem

Salmonella enterica is a main ethological factor for infectious diseases worldwide (Hohmann, 2001; Rabsch et al., 2001). Serotypes, which cause disease, are divided into the following groups: typhoid species (TS) that are human specific pathogens (Typhi and Paratyphi serotypes) and non-typhoid species (NTS) spread to humans from animal sources. The most common non-typhoid *Salmonella spp.* serovars have a potential to cause two basic kinds of infections: gastroenteritis and extraintestinal infections. The host environment varies from the ubiquitous (non-host-adapted) serovars for example Typhimurium and Enteritidis, to host restricted - *S.* Dublin, *S.* Choleraesuis. Both can cause infection in cattle, pigs or humans, and host-specific ones – e.g. *S.* Pullorum, which is found in chickens only. About 5% of patients with gastrointestinal illness of non-typhoid *Salmonella* spp. serotypes develop bacteremia (Hohmann, 2001). The survival of *S.* Enteritidis in poultry products has been linked to its remarkable ability to quick respond to environmental signals and adapt to its surroundings. *S.* Enteritidis may exist naturally in poultry at low incidence but it seems to have another reservoir, rodents. Human cases of *S.* Enteritidis rapidly increased through the 1980s and 1990s. For the last few decades, *S.* Hadar has been one of the main common serotypes isolated from foodborne disease in Europe. In humans, *S.* Hadar usually causes gastroenteritis, characterized by non-bloody-diarrhea, vomiting, nausea and fever (Rowe et al., 1980). Non-typhoid *Salmonella spp.* (NTS) are broadly dispersed in the environment as well as in the gastrointestinal tracts of both domesticated and wild animals. Up to 90% of *Salmonella* infections in the United States are food-borne in origin (CDC, 2009). Regardless of the fact that non-typhoid *Salmonella spp.* gastroenteritis is most often self-limited, these bacteria cause the most food-borne disease worldwide. Among the conditions for salmonellosis to develop are: gastric hypoacidity, extremes of age, alteration of the endogenous flora, diabetes, rheumatological disorders, sickle cell disease, malaria and immunosuppression (Bronzan et al., 2007).

In developed countries, the main risk factor for acquisition of typhoid *Salmonella* bacteraemia is travel to an endemic region, however, non-typhoid *Salmonella* may more often lead to food-borne diseases in non-endemic countries (Simonsen et al., 2010; Scallan et al., 2011). Invasive NTS is endemic in sub-Saharan Africa where it is a leading cause of fatal bacteremia among African children and HIV-infected adults. Increasing levels of antibiotic resistance among African strains of NTS indicate that a vaccine is urgently needed (Siggins et al., 2011). In Malawi, MacLennan et al. (2008) recently found that NTS bacteriemia particularly affects African children between 4 months and 2 years of age, the period in which immunoglobulin levels to NTS are low or absent. Mortality for nontyphoid *Salmonella* is reported to be as high as 60% in African patients with HIV (Boyle et al., 2007).

The local inflammation of specific tissues or organs also called focal infections can cause diseases such as: pneumonia, meningitis, endocarditis, or infections of the urinary tract (Ekman et al., 2000; Tena et al., 2007; Kedzierska et al., 2008). Gastroinestinal infection due to *Salmonella* may also lead to reactive arthritis (ReA) (Yu, 1999). It has been suggested that the persistence of bacterial antigens is typical of ReA, and is a result of the ineffective elimination of microbes in patients with post infection complications (Granfors et al., 1998). Data presented by Locht et al. (1993) and Thomson et al. (1995) indicated that 1–15% of individuals infected with *Salmonella* gastroenteritis develop a postinfection ReA. Despite the fact that most *Salmonella* strains are pathogenic to humans and animals, their virulence seems to be different depending on the serovar (Threlfall, 2005). Serovars of *Salmonella* belonging to somatic antigen group O48 are clinically important bacteria causing intestinal dysfunction and diarrhoea in animals, infants and children. Table 1 includes epidemiologic data (1984-2008) of the distribution of *S. enterica* and *S. bongori* strains in animals world-wide. Note that reptiles are the hosts for the greatest number of *Salmonella* serovars producing diseases especially in children.

Salmonella isolates	Origin	Biological source	Source of occurrence in human after contact with animals/infections symptoms	References
Salmonella enterica subsp. *diarizonae*	Ireland	turtles, iguanas, snakes	*Salmonella* was detected in a 6-month-old boy who had diarrhoea and respiratory symptoms	O'Byrne and Mahon, 2008
	Japan	gecko, boa garden, python	salmonellosis	Nakadai et al., 2005
Salmonella enterica subsp. *houtenae*	Canada	turtles, iguanas, snakes	*Salmonella* was detected in blood and urine of the 11-year-old boy after contact with family pets	Woodward, 1997
Salmonella enterica subsp. *enterica* sv. Minnesota	Ireland	iguana, Persian cats, rabbits	bloody diarrhoea, fever, abdominal pain, haematuria	O'Byrne and Mahon, 2008
Salmonella enterica subsp. *enterica* sv. Enteritidis	Ireland	fish, dog, terrapin	diarrhoea, fever, abdominal pain	O'Byrne and Mahon, 2008
	Japan	gecko	salmonellosis	Nakadai et al., 2005
Salmonella enterica subsp. *enterica* sv. Pomona	Ireland	terrapins	bloody diarrhoea, vomiting	O'Byrne and Mahon, 2008
Salmonella enterica subsp. *enterica* sv. Poona	Belgium	turtles	4-month-old girl/ septicaemia	Bertrand et al, 2008
	Canada, United States (Indiana, Pensylvania)	iguana	*Salmonella* was detected in an 3-year-old boy, 3-week-old boy who died; 21-day-old girl	Woodward et al., 1997
Salmonella enterica subsp. *enterica* sv. Typhimurium	France	snakes, iguana	infection imported from China to young children	Bertrand et al., 2008
Salmonella enterica subsp. *arizonae*	Ireland	snakes, fowls, goats, swine, minks	diarrhoea	O'Byrne and Mahon, 2008
	United Kingdom	snakes	*Salmonella* was detected in the stool/gastroenteritidis with reactive arthritis	Foster and Kerr, 2005
	Japan	lizards, iguana	salmonellosis	Nakadai et al., 2005
	Italy	chameleons	-----------------	Corrente et al., 2004
Salmonella bongori	Italy	------------	*Salmonella* was detected in children/acute enteritidis	Giammanco et al., 2002
Salmonella enterica subsp. *houtenae* serovar Marina	Canada	iguanas	*Salmonella* was detected in an 11-year-old boy, twin baby brothers, and a baby boy after contact with a pet iguana	Woodward et al., 1997
	Germany	snakes	-----------------	Schröter et al., 2004

Table 1. The distribution of *Salmonella* isolates in animals, selected cases in period 1984-2008

In Poland, a total of 13,362 salmonellosis cases were reported in 2006, and 11,934 in 2007. In 2007 the incidence rate was 30.7 per 100.000 population. The most common type of outbreaks (251 recorded cases) was household outbreaks. Over seventy percent of patients were hospitalized. As in previous years, the seasonal peak of outbreak in Poland was observed in July and August. *S.* Enteritidis was the most frequently isolated serotype of *Salmonella* and constituted over 80% of cases. Two-year old children were the most affected age group (Lazinska et al., 2005; Sarowska et al., 2005). The relative high burden of *S.* Enteritidis in Europe accounts for 67% of salmonellosis, and of *S.* Typhimurium accounts for 9% of the cases (de Jong and Ekdahl, 2006). However, the proportion of *S.* Enteritidis cases from different countries varied from 25% (Iceland) to 98% (Latvia). *S.* Enteritidis is currently the second most frequently isolated serovar in the United States - accounting for nearly 15% of reported human salmonellosis cases (Callaway et al. 2008).

3. Susceptibility of *Salmonella* spp. to the bactericidal activity of serum

It is known that complement and bactericidal activity of serum may protect healthy hosts from invasion of serum sensitive microorganisms (Gondwe et al., 2010). Complement (C) is a part of the innate adaptive immune system and it consists of at least 35 proteins, mainly in pre-activated enzymatic forms. Bacterial invasion activates this defense host system in a few seconds. The complement system mainly recognizes and promotes the clearance of invading microorganisms and host cells damaged by phagocytosis. The following three mechanisms lead to complement activation: the classical pathway (CP), the alternative pathway (AP), and the lectin pathway (LP), which results in membrane attack complex (MAC, C5b-9) formation. It has been suggested that complement is necessary for protection against microbial infection. Immunoglobulins (Ab) can potentially protect against salmonellosis. Ab can protect in a cell-independent manner through complement-dependent bactericidal activity and by opsonizing bacteria for uptake and killing by phagocytic cells (Würzner, 1999; Morgan, 1999).

Resistance to complement-mediated killing is a key virulence property of microbial pathogens, such as *Salmonella* strains. Long-chain LPS has been shown to confer resistance by promoting the deposition of C components at a distance from the outer membrane (OM), thus preventing membrane disruption with MAC (Bravo et al., 2008). The surface-exposed protein, PagC has been shown to confer resistance when present in *S.* Choleraesuis (Nishio et al., 2005). The surface protease PgtE also mediates serum resistance presumably *via* its ability to cleave C components C3, C4, and C5 (Ramu et al., 2007). TraT, an OMP has been found to inhibit complement at the MAC formation stage (Pramoonjago et al., 1992). Rck is a 17-kDa protein structurally related to PagC and has been shown to inhibit MAC function. Rck belongs to a family of 17-19 kDa OMP including PagC, OmpX and Ail. Nevertheless, these proteins have been shown to confer resistance in Gram-negative bacteria to C-mediated killing. Ho and co-workers (2010) presented evidence that Rck of *S.* Typhimurium and *S.* Enteritidis expressed in *E. coli* BL21 with a defective *galE* gene binds the regulator of the AP factor H. fH binding is accociated with resistance to the AP and reduced deposition of C3b, Bb and MAC. Biedzka-Sarek and co-workers (2008) observed that Ail was not masked by distal region of LPS, such as O-antigen. Further investigations are required to determine if LPS length plays a role in fH binding to Rck. LPS with a sialic acid moiety within an O-specific chain also regulates AP amplification by binding fH, hence preventing activation of the C system through the alternative pathway.

Sialic acids present in the surface antigens of bacteria may contribute to the pathogenicity of the microorganisms by mimicking host tissue components (Vimr and Lichtensteiger, 2002). Serovars Enteritidis, Typhimurium, and Hadar do not possess sialylated O-antigens. Results presented by Cisowska et al. (2004) indicate that encapsulated *E. coli* K1 strains have different degrees of susceptibility to the bactericidal action of normal human serum (NHS). These results confirm previous observations (Mielnik et al., 2001) concerning sialylated LPS of *Salmonella spp., Escherichia spp., Citrobacter spp., and Hafnia spp.* Lipooligosaccharide sialylation in *Neisseria meningitidis* serogroup C is a critical determinant of MBL binding. Data provided by Jack et al. (2001) idicate that sialylation down-regulates the rate of MBL-mediated C activation. In nonsialylated microorganisms, MBL increased the rate of acquisition of C5b-9.

Long-term investigations carried out on *Salmonella* O48 shown that strains differ in the susceptibility to various sera, human or animal (Bugla-Ploskonska et al., 2011, 2010a, 2010b, 2009b, 2009c; Futoma et al. 2005). These authors suggest that the presense of sialylated LPSs do not play a decisive role in determining bacterial resistance to the bactericidal activity of serum, and that the presence of NeuAc in the LPS structure is not sufficient to block activation of the alternative pathway of complement in serum. Curiously, even though LPS of the same chemical structure cover *Salmonella* O48, they differ in the susceptibility to the antibacterial activity of serum. Hence we can place a question „Which feature of bacteria determines their behaviour in the serum as an environment to live?". Because OMPs are also surface virulence factors and have a significant role in pathobiology of Gram-negative bacteria and bacterial adaptation to environmental conditions, many authors have directed their investigations through the analysis of *Salmonella* OMP patterns using various molecular methods to investigate these antigens (see below). OMPs are of special interest to researchers as they can modify the susceptibility of bacteria to the bactericidal activity of serum (Alberti et al., 1993; Kustos et al., 2007).

The above-mentioned authors (Bugla-Ploskonska et al., 2011, 2010a, 2010b, 2009b, 2009c; Futoma et al. 2005) and Sarowska and co-workers (2010) described the results of *Salmonella* susceptibility to human and bovine serum. Bactericidal activity of serum was determined as described previously (Doroszkiewicz, 1997). In short, adequately prepared bacteria were incubated with diluted serum (12.5%, 25% or 30%, 50% and 75% in physiological saline) in a water bath at 37°C. The number of colony-forming units per milliliter (CFU/ml) at time 0 was taken as 100%. Strains with survival rates greater than 100% in serum after 180 min of incubation were considered resistant, and those with survival rates less than 100% were considered susceptible to the bactericidal action of the serum. The results of *Salmonella* O48 susceptibility to serum are presented in Table 2. The last column of Table 2 lists the molecular weights of OMPs, which are characteristic only for a given serovar and are characteristic for only resistant or sensitive strains.

The studies were carried out on seventeen *Salmonella* strains, which contain sialic acids in the O-specific side chains of LPSs (O48 somatic antigen group):

S. enterica subsp. *arizonae* PCM 2543, *S. enterica* subsp. *arizonae* PCM 2544, *S. enterica* subsp. *salamae* sv. Ngozi PCM 2514, *S. bongori* sv. Balboa PCM 2552, *S. enterica* subsp. *salamae* sv. Hammonia PCM 2535, *S. enterica* subsp. *salamae* sv. Hagenbeck PCM 2534, *S. enterica* subsp. *enterica* sv. Dahlem PCM 2512, *S. enterica* subsp. *enterica* sv. Djakarta PCM 2513, *S. enterica* subsp. *enterica* sv. Toucra PCM 2515, *S. enterica* subsp. *enterica* sv. Hisingen PCM 2536, *S. enterica* subsp. *salamae* sv. Sakaraha PCM 2538, *S.* sp. PCM 2548, *S. enterica* subsp. *diarizonae* PCM 2511, *S. bongori* sv. Bongori PCM 2547, *S. enterica* subsp. *salamae* sv. Erlangen PCM 2533, *S. enterica* subsp. *houtenae* sv. Marina PCM 2546, *S. enterica* subsp. *enterica* sv. Sydney PCM 2551. The strains were obtained from the Polish Collection of Microorganisms (PCM), Ludwik Hirszfeld Institute of Immunology and Experimental Therapy, Polish Academy of Sciences, Wroclaw, Poland. The rest of the tested strains, shown in Table 2) had been isolated from fecal samples from children with gastroenteritis at the Lower Silesian Pediatric Center in Wroclaw during 2009-2010, and they were *S. enterica* subsp. *enterica* sv. Typhimurium (O4), *S. enterica* subsp. *enterica* sv. Enteritidis (O9), *S. enterica* subsp. *enterica* sv. Hadar (O8). Susceptibility of these serovars to 50% normal human serum was established by Sarowska et al. (2010).

Eleven strains of *Salmonella* O48 were sensitive to the bactericidal effect of human, bovine or cord serum, whereas six *Salmonella* O48 strains, and serotypes of somatic antigen groups, O4, O9, and O8 demonstrated higher resistance to the bactericidal activity of the serum. In other experiments, aimed at analyzing the mechanism of serum complement activation, serovars, which were sensitive to the bactericidal action of serum, were used. Bugla-Ploskonska et al. (2010a, 2010b, 2009b) examined serum in which AP or CP/LP pathways of C were inhibited. Authors established the following mechanisms of complement activation by *Salmonella* O48.

- CP - only the classical/lectin pathways were important in the bactericidal mechanism of complement activation,
- AP - only the alternative pathway was important in the bactericidal mechanism of complement activation,
- CP/AP - independent activation of the classical/lectin pathways and enhancing the alternative pathway in the bactericidal mechanism of complement activation,
- CL + AP - parralel activation of the classical/lectin and enhancing the alternative pathway in the antibacterial activity of complement system.

It is interesting and new information that the strains possessing the same somatic antigen group O48 present diverse susceptibility to serum and different patterns of C activation.

Sarowska and co-workers (2010) examined that *Salmonella* ESBL+ transconjugants belonging to three serovars: Enteritidis, Typhimurium, and Hadar were more sensitive to NHS than before conjugation process. It seems that the acquisition of new plasmids from *Klebsiella pneumoniae* (donor) might have unfavourable consequences for these bacteria and increased their susceptibility to serum activity. A probable explanation of this could be the remodeling of the envelope of the bacterial cells, e.g. OM composition.

It was shown, that the complex bacterial stress response may be conducted with the releasing of the outer membrane vesicles. McBroom and Kuehn (2007) demonstrated that the quantity of vesicle release correlates with the level of toxic misfolded protein accumulation in the cell envelope. Accumulation of material occurs when cells are exposured to damaging stressors such as temperature, nutrient availability, toxic agents. This process can act to selectively eliminate unwanted material. Further work is required to identify how envelope stress translates into bacterial resistance in serum. Native vesicles contain OM and periplasmic material, and they are released from the bacterial surface without loss of membrane integrity. More surprisingly, vesicles from some species contain DNA (Nikaido, 2003). These vesicles, however, have not been well characterized in most studies. For example, the reported protein composition of vesicles from *P. aeruginosa* is strikingly different from that of the OM (Kadurugamuwa and Beveridge, 1995). Vesicles were shown to be enriched in monomeric OM proteins, OmpA, OmpX, and OmpW, but contain less of the trimeric porins OmpF and OmpC (Horstman and Kuehn, 2000). Hellman et al. (2000) showed that bacterial OMPs are released into serum in complexes that also contain LPS. Release of 18-kDa OMP from *E. coli* J5 into serum was greater for bacteria in early logarithmic than in late logarithmic growth and was increased by antibiotics *in vitro* and *in vivo*. These data raise the question as to whether released OMPs, such as the 18-kDa OMP, could play a role in the pathogenesis of Gram-negative sepsis.

Strain no	Sera	Concentration of serum				OMPs (kDa)[1]
		12.5 %	25% or 30%	50%	75%	
SENSITIVE STRAINS						
S. arizonae PCM 2543	NHS	NT[2]	sensitive	sensitive	sensitive	60, 48, 45[3]
	NBS		sensitive	sensitive	sensitive	
S. arizonae PCM 2544	NHS	NT	sensitive	sensitive	sensitive	60, 31, 24, 12[3]
	NBS		sensitive	sensitive	sensitive	
S. Ngozi PCM 2514	NHS	NT	sensitive	sensitive	sensitive	58, 45, 42[3]
	NBS		sensitive	sensitive	sensitive	
S. Balboa PCM 2552	NHS	NT	sensitive	NT	sensitive	49, 46, 39[3]
	NBS		sensitive	sensitive	sensitive	
S. Hammonia PCM 2535	NHS	NT	sensitive	NT	sensitive	57[3]
	NBS		sensitive	sensitive	sensitive	
S. Hagenbeck PCM 2534	NHS	NT	sensitive	NT	sensitive	47, 31[3]
	NBS		sensitive	sensitive	sensitive	
S. Dahlem PCM 2512	NHS	NT	NT	sensitive	sensitive	50
	NCS	sensitive	sensitive	sensitive	sensitive	
	NBS	NT	sensitive	sensitive	sensitive	
S. Djakarta PCM 2513	NHS	NT	NT	sensitive	sensitive	56
	NCS	sensitive	sensitive	sensitive	sensitive	
	NBS	NT	sensitive	sensitive	sensitive	
S. Toucra PCM 2515	NHS	NT	NT	sensitive	sensitive	none[4]
	NCS	**resistant**	sensitive	sensitive	sensitive	
	NBS	NT	sensitive	sensitive	sensitive	
S. Hisingen PCM 2536	NHS	NT	NT	sensitive	sensitive	56
	NCS	**resistant**	**resistant**	sensitive	sensitive	
	NBS	NT	sensitive	sensitive	sensitive	
S. Sakaraha PCM 2538	NHS	NT	NT	sensitive	sensitive	none[4]
	NCS	**resistant**	**resistant**	sensitive	sensitive	
	NBS	NT	**resistant**	sensitive	sensitive	

RESISTANT STRAINS[5]						
S. sp. PCM 2548	NHS	NT	NT	**resistant**	**resistant**	93, 62, 30, 25, 17[3]
	NCS	NT	NT	NT	NT	
	NBS	NT	sensitive	**resistant**	**resistant**	
S. diarizonae PCM 2511	NHS	NT	NT	sensitive	sensitive	194, 84, 66, 8
	NCS	**resistant**	**resistant**	**resistant**	**resistant**	
	NBS	NT	sensitive	sensitive	sensitive	
S. Bongori PCM 2547	NHS	sensitive	sensitive	sensitive	sensitive	183, 99
	NCS	**resistant**	**resistant**	**resistant**	**resistant**	
	NBS	NT	sensitive	sensitive	sensitive	
S. Erlangen PCM 2533	NHS	sensitive	sensitive	sensitive	sensitive	69, 54, 8
	NCS	**resistant**	**resistant**	**resistant**	**resistant**	
	NBS	NT	**resistant**	sensitive	sensitive	
S. Marina PCM 2546	NHS	NT	NT	NT	**resistant**	41
	NCS	**resistant**	**resistant**	**resistant**	**resistant**	
	NBS	NT	**resistant**	**resistant**	**resistant**	
S. Sydney PCM 2551	NHS	**resistant**	sensitive	sensitive	sensitive	74
	NCS	**resistant**	**resistant**	**resistant**	**resistant**	
	NBS	NT	**resistant**	**resistant**	**resistant**	
S. Typhimurium	NHS			**resistant**	NT	82, 66, 65, 51, 41, 27, 25, 17
	NCS	NT	NT	NT	NT	
	NBS			NT	NT	
S. Enteritidis	NHS			**resistant**	NT	79, 66, 65, 53, 41, 29, 27, 17
	NCS	NT	NT	NT	NT	
	NBS			NT	NT	
S. Hadar	NHS			**resistant**	NT	82, 66, 65, 51, 41, 27, 25, 17
	NCS	NT	NT	NT	NT	
	NBS			NT	NT	

References: Bugla-Ploskonska et al. (2011, 2010a, 2010b, 2009b, 2009c); Futoma et al. (2005); Sarowska et al. (2010)

NHS - normal human serum; NCS - normal cord serum; NBS - normal bovine serum

[1] OMPs characteristic for only serum- sensitive strains (not present in serum-resistant strains) or for only serum-resistant strains (not present in serum-sensitive strains)

[2] NT - not tested

[3] data presented only in this paper

[4] there are any individual OMPs in this strain when compare to others

[5] strains were regarded as resistant when their survival was above 100% in the highest concentrations of serum

Table 2. The susceptibility of *Salmonella* strains to NHS, NCS, and NBS put together with OMPs

3.1 The role of sialylated lipopolysaccharide

Bacteria have evolved mechanisms for evading recognition by the immune system. Sialylation of LPS or LOS mediates serum resistance of *N. gonorrhoeae* (Ram et al., 1998). Sialic acids are important constituents of glycoconjugates in animal tissues, which regulate innate immunity. Covering bacterial surfaces with sialylated oligosaccharides mimic those of the host (molecular mimicry). Incorporation of NeuAc into the surface components of the cell envelope of some pathogenic bacteria inhibits the direct activation of the alternative complement pathway (Rautemaa and Meri, 1999). Activation of AP is regulated by an interaction between C3b and factor H. It is known that NeuAc can enhance the binding of factor H to C3b on the cell surface, which blocks the amplification of the AP of C activation. fH is a critical regulator of the C system, and acts a a cofactor for factor I-mediated cleavage of C3b. fH also inactivates AP convertase by dissociating Bb from the C3bBb complex (Pangburn et al., 1977). Interestingly, the positive effect of LPS sialylation on fH binding requires the presence of gonococcal porin PorB, suggesting that sialylation may cause a conformational change in the LPS that unmasks novel sites in PorB (Severi et al., 2007).

Smooth strains of *S.* Typhimurium (nonsialylated) were usually resistant to the action of serum, whereas strains of the Ra chemotype by sera of some piglets were killed (Dlabac, 1968). It was shown that the LPS O-antigen (O-Ag) plays an important role in resistance to complement-mediated serum killing in several Gram-negative bacteria (Bengoechea et al., 2004, Grossman et al., 1987, Joiner, 1988). It was shown that LPS O-antigen and the outer core of *Y. enterocolitica* do not contribute directly to complement resistance. Instead, the major *Y. enterocolitica* serum resistance determinants include OMPs such as YadA and Ail (Kirjavainen et al., 2008).

It was reported that the amount of O-Ag and its chain length distribution are important factors in protecting bacteria from serum complement. Bravo et al. (2008) demonstrated that increased amounts of length distribution produced by *S.* Typhi grown to stationary phase confered higher levels of bacterial resistance to human serum. They suggest that O-Ag is more important for survival of *S.* Typhi in serum than the Vi antigen, and that non-typhoidal serovars are more resistant than serovar Typhi to human serum.

3.2 The role of OMPs

The sensitivity of bacteria to the bactericidal activity of serum depends on the structure and organization of their outer membrane. About 50% of OM consists of proteins, so their role in the pathogenicity of Gram-negative bacteria cannot be dismissed (Koebnik et al., 2000). The resistance of bacteria to serum's lytic activity may be one of the virulence factors essential in the development of sepsis. Changes in OMPs' expression can result in Gram-negative bacteria developing resistance to the bactericidal activity of serum (Bugla and Doroszkiewicz, 2006; Weiser and Gotschlich, 1991; White et al., 2005; Attia et al., 2005; Nishio et al., 2005). Studies have shown that porins from several bacteria stimulate cells to produce and secrete cytokines (Galdiero et al., 1993). Whole bacterial cells, which express on their surface LPS and porins both use CD14 when interact with leukocydes. Galdiero and others (2001) showed that CD14 and CD11a/18 are involved in cytokine responses to LPS, but only CD11a/18 is involved in those of porins. Their previous studies (Galdiero et al., 1990) showed that S. Typhimurium porins inhibit phagocytosis by activating the adenylate cyclase system.

Some OMPs amplify the sensitivity of bacteria (Zollinger et al., 1987, Merino et al., 1998, Alberti et al., 1993) to serum. Binding of OmpK36 of the serum sensitive strain *K. pneumoniae* to C1q leads to activation of the complement classical pathway and the subsequent deposition of C components C3b and C5b-9 on the porin (Alberti et al., 1996). *Y. enterocolitica* serum resistance is dependent of the presence of proteins YadA and Ail, which bind C4b-binding protein, an inhibitor of both the classical and lectin pathways of C (Kirjavainen et al., 2008). Another example of the serum resistance phenotype of bacteria is *Actinobacillus actinomycetemcomitans* expressing surface protein Omp100, which traps factor H, an inhibitor for C3 (Asakawa et al., 2003). Futoma-Koloch et al. (2006) investigated the serial passage of *Proteus mirabilis* O18 in 90% bovine serum what contributed to over-expression of some classes of OMPs. It was also found a large heterogeneity of the OMPs' profile among *Salmonella spp.* after their passage in serum (Skwara et al., 2011). Studies of Kroll and co-authors (1983) have shown that treating *E. coli* cells with sera also generates changes in their OMPs composition.

Many years ago, some authors (Joiner et al., 1982; Taylor, 1983) suggested that the nature of bacterial resistance to the action of sera is quite complex. Galdiero et al. (1984) showed that the C system could be activated by porins isolated from *S.* Typhimurium. Chaffer et al. (1999) showed that *E. coli* O2 isolates that possess 35 kDa OmpA are higly resistant to the bactericidal effect of serum. Others (Cirillo et al., 1996) pointed out that Rck (17-19 kDa) protein in *S.* Typhimurium is associated with high-level serum resistance. This OMP probably inhibits lysis of the bacterial cell that occurs with the MAC complex. *S.* Choleraesuis' resistance to serum may be enhanced by the presence of the outer membrane protein PagC (17 kDa) (Nishio et al., 2005). Rck is a member of a family of OMP including PagC of *S.* Typhimurium (Gunn et al., 1995) and Ail of *Y. enterocolitica* (Miller et al., 1990). Site-directed mutagenesis and "domain-swapping" experiments done with Rck show that loop 3 is required for serum resistance and invasion in *E. coli* (Cirillo et al., 1996).

Bugla-Ploskonska and co-workers (2011) confirmed that certain OMPs are characteristic of the serum-resistant and serum-sensitive phenotypes of *Salmonella* O48 to the bactericidal action of cord serum (see Table 2.). But the SDS-PAGE (sodium dodecyl sulphate-polyacrylamide gel electrophoresis) analysis of the OMPs isolated from: *S.* Hisingen PCM 2536, *S.* Dahlem PCM 2512, *S.* Djakarta PCM 2513, *S.* Toucra PCM 2515, *S.* Sakaraha PCM 2538, *S. diarizonae* PCM 2511, *S.* Bongori PCM 2547, *S.* Erlangen PCM 2533, *S.* Marina PCM 2546, and *S.* Sydney PCM 2551, showed no correlation between numbers of colored stripes within the same path and the susceptibility of the tested strains to cord serum. The strain, which was most sensitive to the lytic activity of cord serum S. Dahlem PCM 2515 had 32 OMPs with distinct molecular weights, while serum-resistant S. Marina PCM 2546 had only 20 OMPs.

When comparing the results of Bugla-Ploskonska et al. (2011) (data not shown in Fig. 1.), Sarowska et al. (2010) (Fig. 1.A) and Futoma-Koloch et al. (data published in this paper) (Fig. 1.B) one may note different electrophoretic band patterns for OMPs of tested strains of *Salmonella*. The patterns of OMPs (Fig. 1.) are similar to those reported in the literature, and allow the identification of the major proteins, including the 36- to 41-kDa proteins known as porins (Kamio and Nikaido, 1977). These proteins, which were common in *S.* Typhimurium, *S.* Enteritidis, and *S.* Hadar strains, are 66-, 65-, 41-, 27-, and 17-kDa. These results are similar to that obtained for *S.* Typhi by Ortiz et al. (1989), which had 17-, 28-, and 36- to 41-kDa proteins. While studying the composition of OM of *S.* Typhimurium, Smit and Nikaido (1978) observed that these bacteria contain three porins of 34-, 35-, and 36-kDa.

As show in Fig 1., the tested strains share the same OMP peptide band located at 35 kDa, the region containing the OmpA. This protein has been shown to contribute to the increased resistance of *E. coli* to the bactericidal effect of serum by classical pathway activation. All the serum-resistant strains *S.* sp. PCM 2548 (Fig. 1.B, line 2), *S. diarizonae* PCM 2511, *S.* Bongori

PCM 2547, *S.* Erlangen PCM 2533, *S.* Marina PCM 2546, *S.* Sydney PCM 2551 (Bugla-Ploskonska et al., 2011), *S.* Enteritidis, *S.* Typhimurium, and *S.* Hadar (Sarowska et al., 2010) (Fig. 1.A, lines 3, 5, 7) possess additional proteins, not present in the strains, which were susceptible to serum. This suggests, some OMPs are characteristic of sensitive strains (group 1), as well as associated with resistant strains (group 2):

- Group 1, consisting of eleven serovars **sensitive** to the bactericidal action of serum (see Table 2.). The OMPs characteristic of this group of bacteria were not detected in the outer membranes of the strains resistant to the bactericidal action of serum: 60-, 58-, 57-, 56-, 50-, 49-, 48-, 47-, 46-, 45-, 42-, 39-, 31-, 24-, 12-kDa;
- Group 2, consisting of nine serovars **resistant** to the bactericidal action of serum (see Table 2.) The OMPs characteristic of this group of bacteria were not detected in the outer membranes of the strains sensitive to the bactericidal action of serum: 194-, 183-, 99-, 93-, 84-, 82-, 79-, 74-, 69-, 66-, 65-, 62-, 54-, 53-, 51-, 41-, 30-, 29-, 27-, 25-, 17-, 8-kDa.

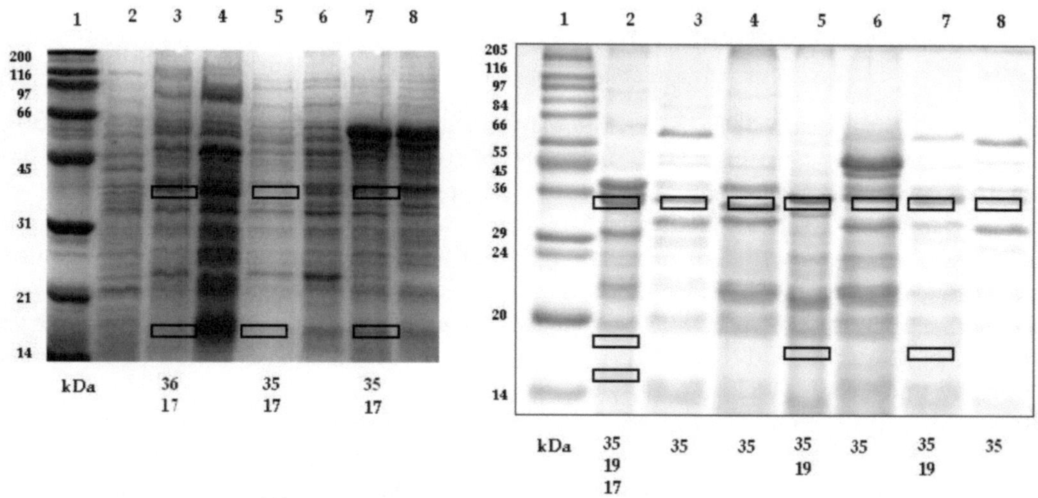

(A) (B)

Fig. 1. The SDS-PAGE OMPs isolated with Zwittergent 3-14®[1]

The results presented by Sarowska et al. (2010) show that the ESBL conjugative plasmid donor strain *K. pneumoniae*, and recipient strains (*S.* Enteritidis, *S.* Typhimurium and *S.* Hadar) were resistant to the bactericidal action of NHS, whereas the three *Salmonella* transconjugants identified as ESBL producers (*S.* Enteritidis ESBL^{+}, *S.* Typhimurium ESBL^{+}, and *S.* Hadar ESBL^{+}) demonstrated sensitivity to serum. SDS-PAGE analysis of the OMPs of *Salmonella* transconjugants revealed that the parental strains (Fig. 1.A, lines: 3-*S.* Enteritidis; 5-*S.* Typhimurium, 7-*S.* Hadar) and transconjugants (Fig. 1.A, lines 4, 6, 8) exhibited slightly

[1] Lane 1 (A, B): Molecular Weight Standards (Sigma); (A) 2: *K. pneumoniae*; 3: *S.* Enteritidis; 4: *S.* Enteritidis ESBL^{+}; 5: *S.* Typhimurium; 6: *S.* Typhimurium ESBL^{+}; Lane 7: *S.* Hadar; Lane 8: *S.* Hadar ESBL^{+} (Sarowska et al., 2010); with permission of Editor-In-Chief of *Advances in Clinical and Experimental Medicine* (B) 2: *S.* sp. PCM 2548; 3: *S.* Balboa PCM 2552; 4: *S. arizonae* PCM 2543; 5: *S. arizonae* PCM 2544; 6: *S.* Ngozi PCM 2514; 7: *S.* Hammonia PCM 2535; 8: *S.* Hagenbeck PCM 2534 (data shown only in this paper).

different outer-membrane banding patterns. These changes included the presence or absence of particular OMPs. New OMPs (absent before conjugation) with molecular masses of 25-kDa and 44-kDa were observed in *S.* Enteritidis ESBL$^+$ isolate, and 43-kDa in *S.* Typhimurium ESBL$^+$ strain. The acquisition of ESBL plasmids also resulted in the loss of some OMPs in the transconjugants compared with the parental strains. In the case of the *S.* Enteritidis ESBL$^+$ isolate, no bands for the 15-, 22-, 53-, 58- and 78-kDa protens were noted. For the remaining transconjugants no bands were observed for the 16-, 38-, 44-, 55-, and 82-kDa proteins (*S.* Typhimurium ESBL$^+$) and 27-, 65- and 66-kDa (*S.* Hadar ESBL$^+$)..

In our study, all the *Salmonella* strains tested, regardless of their susceptibility to serum, possessed the 35-kDa peptide band (Fig. 1.). Note that Rck of *S.* Typhimurium and *S.* Enteritidis, binds fH, which is accociated with resistance to the alternative pathway of complement (Ho et al., 2010), allowing to analyse OMPs patterns on this basis. In the studies of *Salmonella* O48 strains, it was shown that alternative pathway was important in the bactericidal mechanisms of C activation, in spite of the fact that some strains had 17- or 19-kDa proteins, as can be seen in Fig. 1. It seems that any identified agent masks the inhibitory properties of 17-19-kDa proteins in *Salmonella* O48 against the AP pathway.

Bugla-Ploskonska et al. (2009a, 2011), Futoma-Koloch et al. (2009), and Sarowska et al. (2010) used a method of isolating OMPs from bacteria during exponential growth using the Zwittergent Z 3-14® detergent (Calbiochem-Behring), primarily used for enrichment of proteins from cell lysates. Sulfobetaine 3-14 has a strongly basic quaternary ammonium ion and acidic sulfonate with equivalent strength and its zwitterionic character is maintained over a wide range of pH. This method was adapted for *Salmonella* strains using methods developed for isolating of OMPs of *Branhamella catarrhalis* (presently named *Moraxella catarrhalis*) (Murphy and Bartos, 1989, Faden et al., 1992), and *Haemophilus influenzae* (Murphy and Bartos, 1988). There were two modifications introduced into Murphy and Bartos's original method. The first one was that the bacteria were cultured overnight at 37°C for 18 h within liquid Brain Heart Infusion medium (not on solidified medium, similar as in bactericidal assay (YP broth)), secondly, OMPs in a buffer Z, were kept overnight at 4°C, before they were centrifuged at 8700 rpm at 4°C for 10 min. It's important to emphasize that culturing bacteria in liquid or solidified medium may influence the molecular pattern of the surface antigens. Harvesting bacteria from plates provides large numbers of cells without the need for centrifugation. In this manner, the cells are relatively free from components of the growth medium, which could interfere with subsequent procedures. Zwitterionic detergents like non-ionic detergents do not possess a net charge; they lack conductivity and electrophoretic mobility, and do not bind to ion exchange resins. Like ionic detergents, they are also suited for breaking protein-protein interactions (Srirama, 2001).

Hundreds of articles have been published with the words "*Salmonella* OMP" or "*Salmonella* porin". Of note is the review by Nikaido (2003), who has been working in that field during 30 years of his scientific carrier. He exhaustively described the molecular basis of bacterial OM permeability, taking into concideration i.a. protein channels, and LPS. Since the OMPs are surface-exposed antigens, they provide attractive targets for the development of vaccines, thus various techniques have been developed for their characterization. OMPs isolated with Zwittergent Z 3-14® can be also separated with two-dimensional electrophoresis (2-DE). Preliminary studies by Futoma-Koloch et al. (2009), Bugla-Ploskonska et al. (2009a) have reported that using the zwitterionic detergent Zwittergent Z 3-14® is suitable to isolate OMPs from *S. arizonae, S.* Dahlem, and other Gram-negative rods such as *E. coli* O56. Samples of these peptides may then be separated by 2-DE in a capillary tube system (Futoma-Koloch et al., 2009) (Fig. 2.). It was also shown that the use of the same detergent to isolate OMPs from *E. coli* O56 enables their separation by 2-DE using pH 3-10 immobilized pH gradient IPG strips (Bugla-Ploskonska et al., 2009a). Detection of hydrophobic OMPs in 2-D gels is associated with certain limitations (Fountoulakis, 2005). The poor solubility of hydrophobic OMP accounts for their absence from the 2D gel map, but the addition of zwitterionic detergents can improve protein solubilization (Shaw and Riederer, 2006).

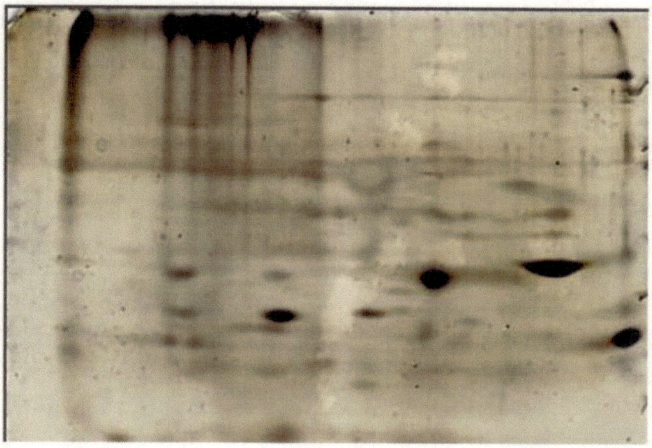

Fig. 2. 2-DE profile of OMPs isolated with Zwittergent Z 3-14®: *S. arizonae* PCM 2543 (Futoma-Koloch et al. 2009)[2]

2-DE was carried out with the Mini-PROTEAN® 3 System (Bio-Rad) and Protean IEF cell and Mini-Protean Tetra Cell (BioRad) respectively (Fig. 2.). Spots of OMPs of *S. arizonae* PCM 2543 were visualized by silver staining. Some modifications were introduced into to the original method described by O'Farrell in 1975 (O'Farrell, 1975) in order to improve the resolution of OMPs isolated with Zwittergent 3-14®. It was necessary to reduce the molar concentration of urea and replace Bio-Lyte 5/7 ampholyte with ddH_2O in three reagents: the first-dimension sample buffer, the first-dimension sample overlay buffer, and the first-dimension gel monomer solution. Tricine was used instead of glycine in the electrophoresis buffer (second dimension). The tube gels were pre-electrophoresed (electrode preparation) by running at 200 V for 10 min, 300 V for 15 min, and 400 V for 15 min (power supply adaptor - Apelex PS 900S TX) then appropriate prepared samples were loaded on the top surfaces of the gels in capillary tubes and separated by IEF on pH 3.0-10.0 at 300 V for 16 h, 400 V for 2 h, and 800 V for 1 h (Apelex PS 900S TX). Three tube gels per sample were run. After the IEF (isoelectring focusing) run was completed, gels were electrophoresed according to Laemmli (1970) for 2 h (20 mA/gel) and stained with a Silver Stain Plus™ kit (Bio-Rad). Fig. 2. contains a total of 35 spots. The major proteins were found in the acidic

[2] With permission of Editor-In-Chief of *Polish Journal of Microbiology*

regions of the gels. This procedure was described in details in paper autorship Futoma-Koloch et al. (2009).

The next issue for consideration concerns various methods developed for isolation, separation and identification of OMPs. The power of 2-DE in the OMPs analysis was demonstrated by Hamid and Jain (2008), who confirmed that OMPs provide promising targets for the development of a candidate vaccine against typhoid. 2-DE methodology in conjunction with the Western Blot has a potential for the rapid development of specific, safe, and highly efficacious vaccines against salmonellosis in human and livestock. Non-detergent sulphobetaines were also used by Blisnick and co-workers (1998) to enhance the recovery of membrane proteins and active proteases from erythrocytes infected by *Plasmodium falciparum*, a parasite. Protein extracts of parasites obtained with NDSB195 (non-detergent sulfobetaine) were separated by IEF, as well as by SDS-PAGE. Proteins were then identified with western blotting using specific antibodies. *S.* Typhimurium served as a model for isolating OMPs by the method of Foulaki et al. (1989). From the urea extract a 55-kDa protein was isolated by ion-exchange chromatography and gel filtration free of LPS. All steps in the isolation of this protein were carried out without detergents.

Huang et al. (2004) presented a newly developed method combining sucrose density centrifugation and aqueous two-phase partitioning for the isolation of pure OM from *Synechocystis* sp. The purity of the membrane fractions was verified by immunoblot analysis using Ab against specific membrane marker proteins. They have examined the protein composition by 2-DE followed by matrix-assisted laser desorption/ionization time–of-flight (MALDI-TOF) analysis. Using a combination of two nonionic detergents (CHAPS and ASB-14), proteins were solubilized and resolved within a range of pH 4.0-7.0. The studies of Ortiz et al. (1989) were undertaken to assess the ability of the OMPs of *S.* Typhi to induce a humoral immune response in human with typhoid fever. OMPs in this case were isolated with the nonionic detergent, Triton X-100. Proteins were contaminated with approximately 4% LPS. SDS-PAGE patterns showed protein bands with molecular size ranges from 17 to 70 kDa. The major group of proteins corresponded to the OmpA. Isibasi et al. (1988) isolated OMPs from *S.* Typhi also with Triton X-100, as described by Schnaitman (1971). Seleim and others (2002) performed preparation of the *Salmonella* OMPs with 2% sarkosyl in 10 mM HEPES buffer. Chooneea et al. (2010) attempted to characterize the surface proteome of *S.* Typhimurium using lipid-based protein immobilization technology in the form of LPI™ FlowCell. No detergents were required and no sample clean up was needed prior to downstream analysis. The proteins were then characterized by liquid chromatography – tandem mass spectrometry (LC-MS/MS). In these studies 54 OMPs were identified.

Proteomic analysis of the *E. coli* OM performed by Molloy and co-workers (2000) included isolation of cell membranes by carbonate extraction according to the method of Fujiki and co-workers (1982). Bolla et al. (2000) developed a method for purification of the major outer membrane protein (MOMP) of *Campylobacter*, involving outer-membrane preparation followed by specific detergent extraction and chromatography. In that study, to identify poorly expressed porin proteins, they analysed a large amount of outer membrane detergent extract by ion-exchange chromatography. This method allowed them to identify and characterize a novel porin protein Omp50 of *C. jejuni*. Extraction of the porin from the membrane was carried out in six steps. Two extractions with 0.1% sodium lauryl sarcosinate in Tris buffer to solubilize the inner membrane were followed by four successive extractions with n-octyl- polyoxyethylene (octyl-POE; Bachem AG-Switzerland) in 20 mM NaPi (pH 7.6), leading to the specific recovery of the outer membrane porin associated with octyl-POE micelles. In turn, OMPs of *Brucella* spp. were extracted with Triton X-114 (Tibor et al., 1999), and confirmed to be lipoproteins.

The preparations of OMPs in the soluble fraction in buffer Z (in a method with Zwittergent Z-14®) were assayed for the enzymatic activity of succinic dehydrogenase, a marker for the cytoplasmic membranes, according to Rockwood et al. (1987). To make certain that the extracts of proteins were free of membrane fraction contaminations, Futoma-Koloch and others (data shown only in this paper) employed transmission electron microscopy (TEM) for imaging OMPs isolated from *S. arizonae* PCM 2544.

For electron microscopy investigation:

a. The isolated material was negatively contrasted with 2 % uranyl acetate in a conventional procedure (Fig. 3.A);
b. For thin-sections isolated material was fixed in 1% osmium tetroxide, dehydrated in graded ethanol and embedded in Epon 812. Ultrathinsections were cut with a Reychert Ultracut E ultramicrotome and stained with lead citrate (Fig. 3.B).

The specimens were examined in Tesla BS 540 electron microscope. The proteins appeared bright against the dark background. Scale markers correspond to 500 nm. Note, that membrane contarrdinants are not present. If they were, they would be visible as white linear trails of phospholipid bilayers. Proteins or peptides released from the membranes tend to aggregate to assume globular or filamentous clusters of the diameter from 40 nm to about 200 nm.

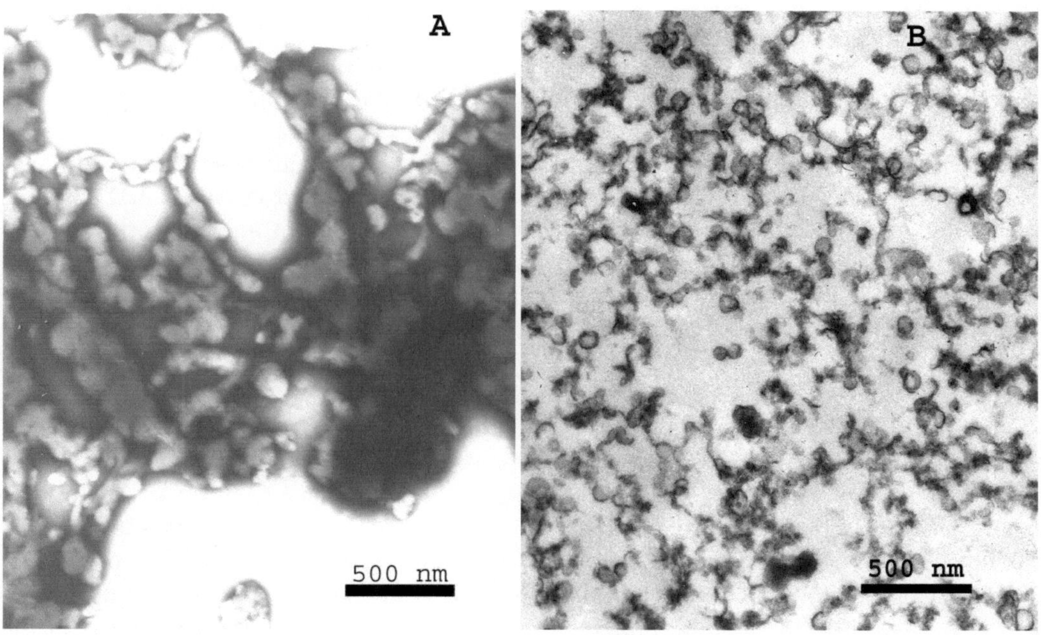

Fig. 3. Transmission electron micrographs of isolated OMPs released with Zwittergent 3-14® from *S. arizonae* PCM 2544, bar=500nm, 25 000x

4. *Salmonella*'s OMPs as potential vaccines

Another aspect of studying OMPs of Gram-negative bacteria is the potential for finding molecular candidates for vaccines. Vaccination is an effective tool for the prevention of *Salmonella* infections (Mastroeni et al., 2011). The currently available vaccines against salmonellosis can be divided into three major classes: whole-cell killed vaccines, subunit vaccines, and live attenuated vaccines. Subunit vaccines such as the ones based on the Vi polysaccharides are safe, immunogenic, and are currently licenced for human use. Other subunit vaccines such as those based on detoxified LPS, cell extracts, porins, O-polysaccharides, and O-conjugates have been tested in experimental models (Mastroeni and Menager, 2003). Recognition and neutralization of OMPs by the immune system is of great importance. When porins are used as immunogens they can ablate bacteremia and provide equivalent protection against salmonellosis. Available vaccines containing either acetone or heat-killed *S.* Typhi are of limited value, because they confer short-lived protection and they produce unacceptable side effects, due mainly to the presence of endotoxin, which prevents their use in children. At the moment there are also several vaccines prepared from Vi antigen.

The trimeric porins show stability to temperature and denaturants, and are also resistant to proteolysis. These properties make them good candidates for industrial applications towards the development of oral vaccines (Galdiero et al., 1990). Data delivered by Salazar-Gonzales et al. (2004) showed that *S.* Typhi porins-based candidate vaccine is safe and immunogenic and healthy. They observed that side effects after vaccination were mild and transient. Ortiz et al. (1989) established that sera from patients with typhiod fever contained M antibodies, which reacted with a protein of 28-kDa. Singh and others (1995) were interested in OmpC and OmpD porins from *S.* Typhimurium because of their potential role in diagnostic assays, in antibiotic resistance, and as immunogens for vaccination.

In animal models, it was shown that mouse monoclonal antibodies were raised against recombinant *S.* Typhi 36-kDa porin monomer (Kissel et al., 1994). Hamid and Jain (Hamid and Jain, 2008) investigated OMPs of *S.* Typhimurium as potential vaccine candidates for conferring protection against typhoid. They showed that OMP with an apparent molecular mass of 49-kDa were highly immunogenic, evoke humoral and cell-mediated immune responses and confer 100% protection to immunized rats. Seleim and co-workers (2002) compared patterns of OMPs bands in SDS-electrophoretic analysis, and found common protein bands in the range from 20-45 kDa in four serovars of *Salmonella* (Typhimurium, Dublin, Enteritidis, and Anatum) collected from calves' fecal samples. The OMPs of serovars Dublin and Enteritidis reacted similar in the Western Blot method with the antisera collected from infected calves. Two protein bands were characteristic, one at, 14.4- and the other at 24-kDa. The authors conclude that *Salmonella* OMPs can be employed as effective vaccine candidates. Vaccination could confer active immunity and reduce the expenses associated with treating *Salmonella*-infected calves. Studies of Maripandi and Al-Salamah (2010) were conducted on *S.* Enteritidis isolates from chicken meat samples for OMPs analysis. The immunoblotting results showed that 14.4- and 24-kDa proteins were good chicken immunogens. The authors conclude that these proteins can be used for vaccine preparation in the future. Outer membrane proteins 82- and 76-kDa are potentially involved in the attachment of *S.* Enteritidis to the intestinal mucosa. They could be used as vaccines to block or reduce *S.* Enteritidis colonization in chickens (Fadl et al., 2002). Ochoa-Reparaz et al.

(2004) state that the immunogenicity of *S.* Enteritidis porins in infected birds may serve as components of an effective subcellular vaccine for poultry salmonellosis.

VonSpecht and co-workers (1996) tested the ability of the recombinant OprI of *P. aeruginosa* to serve as a protective vaccine against this Gram-negative pathogen. Oral immunization of mice with recombinat OprI expressing *S.* Dublin, induced s-IgA antibodies in the gut mucosa against OprI. Recombinant *Lactobacillus casei* may also express SipC and OmpC antigens for vaccination against infections caused by *S.* Enteritidis (Kajikawa and Shizunobu, 2007).

Attenuated *Salmonella* species expressing heterologous antigens are promising candidates for the development of mucosal vaccines. This strategy is based on the ability of *Salmonella* bacteria to persist in the antigen-presenting cells (APC) during its migration to the lyphatic organs of the mucosal immune system. Oral live vaccines based on recombinant *Salmonella* strains were successfully developed to induce a specific immune response against human immunodeficiecy virus, *Helicobacter pylori, Clostridium difficile,* and human papilloma virus in mice and humans (Heinz et al., 2004).

The ability of OMPs to induce a protective immunity against infection caused by diverse Gram-negative bacteria, such as *H. influenzae* type b (Granoff and Cates, 1986), *N. meningitidis* group B (Wang, 1984), *P. aeruginosa* (Gilleland et al., 1984), *S.* Typhimurium (Kuusi et al., 1979) and *Borrelia bronchiseptica* (Montaraz et al., 1985), has been demonstrated previously. Witkowska and others (2006) showed that a 38-kDa OMP present in most *Enterobacteriaceae* species is a protein that generates immunological response in human organisms and is a good candidate for creating a vaccine against such species as *E. coli, Shigella flexneri, K. pneumoniae,* and *Proteus vulgaris.*

5. Conclusions

The phenomenon of serum resistance of bacteria has a multifactorial basis. Alteration of the Gram-negative bacterial envelope, including altered protein and LPS composition, may be considered as before general mechanism for survival within the host. Further studies are required to better understand all the molecular mechanisms of microbial surface remodeling and the process of recognizing of the outer membrane vesicles from the bacteria. The role of OMPs, LPSs, and LOSs in determining serum-sensitivity or serum-resistance in *Salmonella* is not entirely clear. It is important to determine which OMPs from *Salmonella* are immunogenic in animals as well as in humans, in order to improve subunit vaccines against salmonellosis.

6. Acknowledgements

The authors thank Prof. Gamian A. (Ludwik Hirszfeld Institute of Immunology and Experimental Therapy, Polish Academy of Sciences, Wroclaw, Poland) for the *Salmonella* O48 strains from the Polish Collection of Microorganisms. Special thanks to Dr. J. Kassner for assistance in transmission electron microscopy (TEM) visualisation. TEM was performed in the Workshop of Microscopy in the Institute of Genetics and Microbiology, University of Wroclaw, Poland. Dr. Sarowska would like to acknowledge Prof. Doroszkiewicz for a capacitance of doing OMPs analysis in the Department of Microbiology, Institute of Genetics and Microbiology, University of Wroclaw, Poland.

7. References

Alberti, S.; Marqués, G.; Hernández-Allés, S.; Rubires, X.; Tomás, J.M.; Vivanco, F. & Benedi, V.J. (1996). Interaction between complement subcomponent C1q and the *Klebsiella pneumoniae* porin OmpK36. *Infection and Immunity*. 64 (11): 4719-4725

Alberti, S.; Marquez, G.; Camprubi, S.; Merino, T.J.M.; Vivanco, F. & Benedi, V.J. (1993). C1q binding and activation of the complement classical pathway by *Klebsiella pneumoniae* outer membrane proteins. *Infection and Immunity*. 61 (3): 852–860

Asakawa, R.; Komatsuzawa, H.; Kawai, T.; Yamada, S.; Goncalves, R.B.; Izumi, S.; Fujiwara, T.; Nakano, Y.; Suzuki, N.; Uchida, Y.; Ouhara, K.; Shiba, H.; Taubman, M.A.; Kurihara, H. & Sugai, M. (2003). Outer membrane protein 100, a versatile virulence factor of *Actinobacillus actinomycetemcomitans*. *Molecular Microbiology*. 50 (4): 1125–1139

Attia, A.S.; Lafontaine, E.R.; Latimer, J.L.; Aebi, C.; Syrogiannopoulos, G.A. & Hansen, E.J. (2005). The UspA2 protein of *Moraxella catarrhalis* is directly involved in the expression of serum resistance. *Infection and Immunity*. 73 (4): 2400–2410

Bengoechea, J.A.; Najdenski, H. & Skurnik, M. (2004). Lipopolysaccharide O antigen status of *Yersinia enterocolitica* O:8 is essential for virulence and absence of O antigen affects the expression of other *Yersinia* virulence factors. *Molecular Microbiology*. 52 (2): 451–469

Bertrand, S.; Rimhanen-Finne, R.; Weill, F.X.; Rabsch, W.; Thornton, L.; Perevoscikovs, J.; Pelt, W. & & Heck, M. (2008). *Salmonella* infections associated with reptiles: the current situation in Europe. *Eurosurveillance*. 13 (4-6): 1-6

Biedzka-Sarek, M.; Jarva, H.; Hyytiäinen, H.; Meri, S. & Skurnik, M. (2008). Characterization of complement factor H binding to *Yersinia enterocolitica* serotype O:3. *Infection and Immunity*. 76 (9): 4100–4109

Blisnick, T.; Morales-Betoulle, M.E.; Vuillard, L.; Rabilloud T. & Braun Breton, C. (1998). Non-detergent sulphobetaines enhance the recovery of membrane and/or cytoskeleton-associated proteins and active proteases from erythrocytes infected by *Plasmodium falciparum*. *European Journal of Biochemistry*. 252 (3): 537–541

Bolla, J.M.; Dé, E.; Dorez, A. & Pagès, J.M. (2000). Purification, characterization and sequence analysis of Omp50, a new porin isolated from *Campylobacter jejuni*. *Biochemical Journal*. 352: 637–643

Boyle, E.C.; Bishop, J.L.; Grassl, G.A. & Finlay, B.B. (2007). *Salmonella*: from pathogenesis to therapeutics. *Journal of Bacteriology*. 189 (5): 1489-1495

Bravo, D.; Silva, C.; Carter, J.A.; Hoare, A.; Alvarez, S.A.; Blondel, C.J.; Zaldívar, M.; Valvano, M.A. & Contreras, I. (2008). Growth-phase regulation of lipopolysaccharide O-antigen chain length influences serum resistance in serovars of *Salmonella*. *Journal of Medical Microbiology*. 57: 938-946

Bronzan, R.N.; Taylor, T.E.; Mwenechanya, J.; Tembo, M.; Kayira, K.; Bwanaisa, L.; Njobvu, A.; Kondowe, W.; Chalira, C.; Walsh, A.L.; Phiri, A.; Wilson, L.K.; Molyneux, M.E. & Graham, S.M. (2007). Bacteremia in Malawian children with severe malaria: prevalence, etiology, HIV coinfection, and outcome. *Journal of Infectious Diseases*. 195 (6): 895–904

Bugla-Ploskonska, G.; Korzeniowska-Kowal, A. & Guz-Regner, K. (2011). Reptiles as a source of *Salmonella* O48-clinically important bacteria for children: the relationship between resistance to normal cord serum and outer membrane protein patterns. *Microbial Ecology*. 61 (1): 41-51

Bugla-Ploskonska, G.; Futoma-Koloch, B.; Rybka, J.; Gamian, A. & Doroszkiewicz, W. (2010a). The role of complement activity in the sensitivity of *Salmonella* O48 strains with sialic acid-containinig lipopolysaccharides to the bactericidal action of normal bovine serum. *Polish Journal of Veterinary Science.* 13 (1): 53-62

Bugla-Ploskonska, G.; Rybka, J.; Futoma-Koloch, B.; Cisowska, A.; Gamian, A. & Doroszkiewicz, W. (2010b). Sialic acid-containing lipopolysaccharides of *Salmonella* O48 strains - potential role in camouflage and susceptibility to the bactericidal action of normal human serum. *Microbial Ecology.* 59 (3): 601–613

Bugla-Ploskonska, G.; Futoma-Koloch, B.; Skwara, A. & Doroszkiewicz, W. (2009a). Use of zwitterionic type of detergent in isolation of *Escherichia coli* O56 outer membrane proteins improves their two-dimensional electrophoresis (2-DE). *Polish Journal of Microbiology.* 58 (3): 205-209

Bugla-Ploskonska, G.; Kiersnowski, A.; Futoma-Koloch, B. & Doroszkiewicz, W. (2009b). Killing of Gram-negative bacteria with normal human serum and normal bovine serum: use of lysozyme and complement protein in the death of *Salmonella* strains O48. *Microbial Ecology.* 58 (2): 276-289

Bugla-Ploskonska, G.; Kiersnowski, A.; Futoma-Koloch, B. & Doroszkiewicz, W. (2009c). Serum as an environment to live or not to live for Gram-negative bacteria: relationship between lysozyme and complement system in killing *Salmonella* O48 strain. Current Research Topisc in Applied Microbiology and Microbial Biotechnology (ed. A. Mendez-Vilas). Word Scientific Publishing, Singapore. 2009, chapter: 523-527, ISBN 13:978-981-283-754-7

Bugla-Ploskonska, G. & Doroszkiewicz, W. (2006). Bactericidal activity of normal bovine serum (NBS) directed against some *Enterobacteriaceae* with sialic acid-containing lipopolysaccharides (LPS) as a component of cell wall. *Polish Journal of Microbiology.* 55 (3): 169–174

Callaway, T.R.; Edrington, T.S.; Anderson, R.C.; Byrd, J.A. & Nisbet, D.J. (2008). Gastrointestinal microbial ecology and the safety of our food supply as related to *Salmonella. Journal of Animal Science.* 86 (E suppl): E163–E172

Centers for Disease Control and Prevention. (2009). Preliminary foodnet data on the incidence of infection with pathogens transmitted commonly through food-10 States, 2008. *MMWR Morbidity and Mortality Weekly Report.* 58 (13): 333-337

Chaffer, M.; Heller, E.D. & Schwartsburd, B. (1999). Relationship beetween resistance to complement, virulence and outer membrane protein patterns in pathogenic *Escherichia coli* O2 isolates. *Veterinary Microbiology.* 64 (4): 323–332

Chooneea, D.; Karlsson, R.; Encheva, V.; Arnold, C.; Appleton, H. & Shah H. (2010). Elucidation of the outer membrane proteome of *Salmonella enterica* serovar Typhimurium utilising a lipid-based protein immobilization technique. *BMC Microbiology,* 10: 44

Cirillo, D.M.; Heffernan, E.J.; Wu, L.; Harwood, J.; Fierer, J. & Guiney, D.G. (1996). Identification of a domain in Rck, a product of the *Salmonella typhimurium* virulence plasmid, required for both serum resistance and cell invasion. *Infection and Immunity.* 64 (6): 2019–2023

Cisowska, A.; Bugla-Ploskonska, G.; Tichaczek-Goska, D.; Doroszkiewicz, W. & Jankowski, S. (2004). The susceptibility of *Escherichia coli* strains with sialic acid-containing lipopolysaccharides or capsules to the bactericidal action of normal human serum, pp. 41–47 in *Proc. 7th Conf. Molecular Biology in Diagnostics of Infectious Diseases and Biotechnology*. Publishing House "Wydawnictwo SGGW", Warsaw 2004

Corrente, M.; Madio, A.; Friderich, K.G.; Grecop, G.; Desario, C.; Tagliabue, S.; D'Incau, M.; Campolo, M. & Buonavoglia, C. (2004). Isolation of *Salmonella* strains from reptile faeces and comparison of different culture media. *Journal of Applied Microbiology*. 96 (4): 709-715

de Jong, B. & Ekdahl, K. (2006). The comparative burden of salmonellosis in the European Union member states, associated and candidate countries. *BMC Public Health*. 6: 4

Dlabac, V. (1968). The sensitivity of smooth and rough mutants of *Salmonella typhimurium* to bactericidal and bacteriolytic action of serum, lysozyme and to phagocytosis. *Folia Microbiologica* (Praha). 13 (5): 439-449

Doroszkiewicz, W. (1997). Mechanism of antigenic variation in *Shigella flexneri* bacilli. IV. Role of lipopolysaccharides and their components in the sensitivity of *Shigella, flexneri* lb and its Lac+ recombinant to killing action of serum. *Archivum Immunologiae et Therapiae Experimentalis*. 45 (2): 236-240

Ekman, P.; Kirveskari, J. & Granfors, K. (2000). Modification of disease outcome in *Salmonella*-infected patients by HLA–B27. *Arthritis and Rheumatism*. 43 (7): 1527–1534

Faden, H.; Hong, J. & Murphy, T. (1992). Immune response to outer membrane antigens of *Moraxella catarrhalis* in children with otitis media. *Infection and Immunity*. 60 (9): 3824-3829

Fadl, A.A.; Venkitanarayanan, K. & Khan, M.I. (2002). Identification of *Salmonella enteritidis* outer membrane proteins expressed during attachment to human intestinal epithelial cells. *Journal of Applied Microbiology*. 92 (1): 180-186

Foster, N. & Kerr, K. (2005) The snake in the grass-*Salmonella arizonae* gastroenteritidis in a reptile handler. *Acta Paediatrica*. 94 (8): 1165-1166

Foulaki, K.; Gruber, W. & Schlecht, S. (1989). Isolation and immunological characterization of a 55-kilodalton surface protein from *Salmonella typhimurium*. *Infection and Immunity*. 57 (5): 1399-1404

Fountoulakis, M. (2005). Analysis of membrane proteins by two-dimensional gels. The Proteomics Protocols Handbook. Ed. John M. Walker. Humana Press: 133-144

Fujiki, Y.; Hubbard, A.L.; Fowler, S. & Lazarow, P.B. (1982). Isolation of intracellular membranes by means of sodium carbonate treatment: application to endoplasmic reticulum. *Journal of Cell Biology*. 93 (1): 97–102

Futoma-Koloch, B.; Bugla-Ploskonska, G. & Doroszkiewicz W. (2009). Isolation of outer membrane proteins (OMP) from *Salmonella* cells using zwitterionic detergent and their separation by two-dimensional electrophoresis (2-DE). *Polish Journal of Microbiology*. 58 (4): 363-366

Futoma-Koloch, B.; Bugla-Ploskonska, G.; Doroszkiewicz, W. & Kaca, W. (2006). Survival of *Proteus mirabilis* O3 (S1959), O9 and O18 strains in normal human serum (NHS) correlates with the diversity of their outer membrane proteins (OMPs). *Polish Journal of Microbiology*. 55 (2): 153-156

Futoma, B.; Bugla-Ploskonska, G. & Doroszkiewicz, W. (2005). Bactericidal complement activity against *Salmonella enterica* strains. *Polish Journal of Environmental Studies*. 14: 101-104

Galdiero, M.; D'Isanto, M.; Vitiello, M.; Finamore. E. & Peluso, L. (2001). Porins from *Salmonella enterica* serovar Typhimurium induce TNF-alpha, IL-6 and IL-8 release by CD14-independent and CD11a/CD18-dependent mechanisms. *Microbiology.* 147: 2697- 2704

Galdiero, F.; Cipollardo de L'Ero, G.; Benedetto, N.; Galdiero, M. & Tufano, M.A. (1993). Release of cytokines induced by *Salmonella typhimurium* porins. *Infection and Immunity.* 61 (1): 155–161

Galdiero, F.; Tufano, M.A.; Galdiero, M.; Masiello, S. & De Rosa, M. (1990). Inflammatory effects of *Salmonella typhimurium* porins. *Infection and Immunity.* 58 (10): 3183- 3188

Galdiero, E.; Tufano, M.A.; Sommese, L.; Folgore, A. & Tedesco, F. (1984). Activation of complement system by porins extracted from *Salmonella typhimurium. Infection and Immunity.* 46 (2): 559-563

Giammanco, G.M.; Pignato, S.; Mammina, C.; Grimont, F.; Grimont, P.A.D.; Nastasi, A. & Giammanco, G. (2002). Persistent endemicity of *Salmonella bongori* 48:z_{35}:- in Southern Italy: Molecular characterization of human, animal and environmental isolates. *Journal of Clinical Microbiology.* 40 (9): 3502-3505

Gilleland, H.E.; Parker, M.G.; Matthews, J.M. & Berg, R.D. (1984). Use of a purified outer membrane protein F (porin) preparation of *Pseudomonas aeruginosa* as a protective vaccine in mice. *Infection and Immunity.* 44 (1): 49–54

Gondwe, E.N.; Molyneux, M.E.; Goodall, M.; Graham, S.M.; Mastroeni, P.; Drayson, M.T. & MacLennan, C.A. (2010). Importance of antibody and complement for oxidative burst and killing of invasive nontyphoidal *Salmonella* by blood cells in Africans. *Proceedings of the National Academy of Sciences USA.* 107 (7): 3070- 3075

Granfors, K.; Merilahti-Palo, R.; Luukkainen, R.; Mottonen, T.; Lahesmaa, R.; Probst, P.; Märker-Hermann, E. & Toivanen, P. (1998). Persistence of *Yersinia* antigens in peripheral blood cells from patients with *Yersinia enterocolitica* O:3 infection with or without reactive arthritis. *Arthritis and Rheumatism.* 41 (5): 855–862

Granoff, D.M,. & Cates, K.L. (1986). *Haemophilus influenzae type b* polysaccharide vaccines. *New England Journal of Medicine.* 315 (25): 499-503

Grossman, A.D.; Straus, D.B.; Walter, W.A. & Gross, C.A. (1987). Sigma 32 synthesis can regulate the synthesis of heat shock proteins in *Escherichia coli. Genes & Development.* 1 (2): 179-184

Gunn, J.S.; Alpuche-Arande, C.M.; Loomis, W.P.; Belden, W.J. & Miller S.I. (1995). Characterization of the *Salmonella typhimurium* pagC/pagD chromosomal region. *Journal of Bacteriology.* 177 (17): 5040–5047

Hamid, N. & Jain, S.K. (2008). Characterization of an outer membrane protein of *Salmonella enterica* serovar Typhimurium that confers protection against typhoid. *Clinical and Vaccine Immunology,* 15 (9): 1461-1471

Heinz, A.; Bumann, D.; Felies, M.; Gewecke, B.; Sorensen, M.; Gessner, J.E.; Freihorst, J.; von Specht, U.B. & Baumann, U. (2004). Enhanced immunogenicity in the murine airway mucosa with an attenuated *Salmonella* live vaccine expressing OprF-OprI from *Pseudomonas aeruginosa. Infection and Immunity.* 72 (11): 6546-6553

Hellman, J.; Loiselle, P.M.; Zanzot, E.M.; Allaire, J.E.; Tehan, M.M.; Boyle, L.A.; Kurnick, J.T. & Warren, H.S. (2000). Release of gram-negative outer-membrane proteins into human serum and septic rat blood and their interactions with immunoglobulin in antiserum to *Escherichia coli* J5. *Journal of Infectious Diseases.* 181 (3): 1034-1043

Ho, D.K.; Jarva, H. & Meri, S. (2010). Human complement factor H binds to outer membrane protein Rck of *Salmonella. Journal of Immunology.* 185 (3): 1763–1769

Hohmann, E.L. (2001). Nontyphoidal salmonellosis. *Clinical Infectious Diseases.* 32 (2): 263-269

Horstman, A.L.; & Kuehn, M.J. (2000). Enterotoxigenic *Escherichia coli* secretes active heat-labile enterotoxin via outer membrane vesicles. *Journal of Biological Chemistry.* 275 (17): 12489–12496

Huang, F.; Hedman, E.; Funk, C.; Kieselbach, T.; Schroder, W.P. & Norling, B. (2004). Isolation of outer membrane of *Synechocystis* sp. PCC 6803 and its proteomic characterization. *Molecular and Cellular Proteomics.* 3 (6): 586–595

Isibasi, A.; Ortiz, V.; Vargas, M; Paniagua, J.; Gonzalez, C.; Moreno, J. & Kumate, J. (1988). Protection against *Salmonella typhi* infection in mice after immunization with outer membrane proteins isolated from *Salmonella typhi* 9,12,d,Vi. *Infection and Immunity.* 56 (11): 2953-2959

Jack, D.L.; Klein, N.J. & Turner, M.W. (2001). Mannose-binding lectin: targeting the microbial world for complement attack and opsonophagocytosis. *Immunological Reviews.* 180: 86–89

Joiner, K.A. (1988). Complement evasion by bacteria and parasites. *Annual Review of Microbiology.* 42: 201-230

Joiner, K.A.; Hammer, C.H.; Brown, E.J.; Cole, R.J. & Frank, M.M. (1982). Studies on the mechanism of bacterial resistance to complement-mediated killing. I. Terminal complement components are deposited and released from *Salmonella minnesota* S218 without causing bacterial death. *Journal of Experimental Medicine.* 155 (3): 797–808

Kadurugamuwa, J.L. & Beveridge, T.J. (1995). Virulence factors are released from *Pseudomonas aeruginosa* in association with membrane vesicles during normal growth and exposure to gentamicin: a novel mechanism of enzyme secretion. *Journal of Bacteriology.* 177 (14): 3998–4008

Kajikawa A. & Shizunobu I. (2007). Construction and evaluation of recombinant lactobacilli expressing *Salmonella* antigens for vaccination. Book of Abstracts II International Conference on Environmental, Industrial, and Applied Microbiology (BioMicroWorld2007) Seville, Spain, November-December 2007

Kamio, Y. & Nikaido, H. (1977). Outer membrane of *Salmonella typhimurium.* Identification of proteins exposed on cell surface. *Biochimica et Biophysica Acta.* 464 (3): 589-601

Kedzierska, J.; Piatkowska-Jakubas, B.; Kedzierska, A.; Biesiada, G.; Brzychczy, A.; Parnicka, A.; Miekinia, B.; Kubisz, A. & Sulowicz, W. (2008). Clinical presentation of extraintestinal infections caused by non-typhoid *Salmonella* serotypes among patients at the University Hospital in Cracow during an 7-year period. *Polish Journal of Microbiology.* 57 (1): 41-47

Kirjavainen, P.K.; Laine, R.M.; Carter, D.; Hammond, J.A. & Reid, G. (2008). Expression of anti-microbial defense factors in vaginal mucosa following exposure to *Lactobacillus rhamnosus* GR-1. *International Journal of Probiotics.* 3 (106): 1555-1431

Kissel, V.; Gonzalez, C.; Astudillo, M.; Godard, A.; Wachman B. & Cabello, F.C. (1994). *Salmonella*-specific monoclonal antibodies against recombinant *Salmonella typhi* 36-kilodalton porin. *Clinical and Diagnostic Labolatory of Immunology.* 1 (2): 250–252

Koebnik, R.; Locher, K.P. & Van Gelder, P. (2000). Structure and function of bacterial outer membrane proteins: barrels in a nutshell. *Molecular Microbiology.* 37 (2): 239–253

Kroll, H.P.; Bhakdi, S. & Taylor, P.W. (1983). Membrane changes induced by exposure of *Escherichia coli* to human serum. *Infection and Immunity.* 42 (3): 1055-1066

Kuusi, N.; Nurminen, M.; Saxen, H.; Valtonen, M.; Makela, P.H. (1979). Immunization with outer major membrane proteins in experimental salmonellosis in mice. *Infection and Immunity.* 25 (3): 857-862

Kustos, I.; Kocsis, B. & Kilar F. (2007). Bacterial outer membrane protein analysis by electrophoresis and microchip technology. *Expert Review of Proteomics.* 4 (1): 91–106

Laemmli, U.K. (1970). Cleavage of structural proteins during the assembly of the head of bacteriophage T4. *Nature.* 15 (5259): 680–685

Lazinska, B.; Rokosz, A.; Rawicka-Grzelak, A. & Łuczak M. (2005). Strains of genus *Salmonella* isolated from extraintestinal infections. *Medycyna Doswiadczalna i Mikrobiologia,* 57 (3): 287–294

Locht, H.; Kihlstrom, E. & Lindstrom, F.D. (1993). Reactive arthritis after *Salmonella* among medical doctors-study of an outbreak. *Journal of Rheumatology.* 20 (5): 845–848

MacLennan, C.A.; Gondwe, E.N.; Msefula, C.L.; Kingsley, R.A.; Thomson, N.R.; White, S.A.; Goodall, M.; Pickard, D.J.; Graham, S.M.; Dougan, G.; Hart, C.A.; Molyneux, M.E.; Drayson, M.T. (2008). The neglected role of antibody in protection against bacteremia caused by nontyphoidal strains of *Salmonella* in African children. *Journal of Clinical Investigation.* 118 (4): 1553–1562

Maripandi, A. & Al-Salamah, A.A. (2010). Analysis of *Salmonella enteritidis* outer membrane proteins and lipopolysaccharide profiles with the detection of immune dominant proteins. *American Journal of Immunology.* 6: 1-6

Mastroeni, P.; Morgan, F.J.E.; McKinley, T.J.; Shawcroft, E.; Clare, S.; Maskell, D.J.; Grant, A.J. (2011). Enhanced virulence of *Salmonella* enterica serovar Typhimurium after passage through mice. *Infection and Immunity.* 79 (2): 636–643

Mastroeni, P. & Menager, N. (2003). Development of acquired immunity to *Salmonella. Journal of Medical Microbiology.* 52: 453-459

McBroom, A.J. & Kuehn, M.J. (2007). Release of outer membrane vesicles by Gram-negative bacteria is a novel envelope stress response. *Molecular Microbiology.* 63 (2): 545–558

Merino, S.; Nogueras, M.; Aquilair, A.; Rubires, X.; Alberti, S.; Benedi, V.J. & Tomas, J.M. (1998). Activation the complement classical pathway (C1q binding) by mesophilic *Aeromonas hydrophila* outer membrane protein. *Infection and Immunity.* 66 (8): 3825-3831

Mielnik, G.; Gamian, A. & Doroszkiewicz, W. (2001). Bactericidal activity of normal cord serum (NCS) against Gram-negative rods with sialic acid-containing lipopolysaccharides (LPS). *FEMS Immunology and Medical Microbiology.* 31 (3): 169–173

Miller, V.L.; Bliska, J.B. & Falkow, S. (1990). Nucleotide sequence of the *Yersinia enterocolitica ail* gene and characterization of the Ail protein product. *Journal of Bacteriology.* 172 (2): 1062-1069

Molloy, M.P.; Herbert, B.R.; Slade, M.B.; Rabilloud, T.; Nouwens, A.S.; Williams, K.L. & Gooley, A.A. (2000). Proteomic analysis of the *Escherichia coli* outer membrane. *European Journal of Biochemistry.* 267 (10): 2871-2881

Montaraz, J.; Novotny, A.P. & Ivanyi, J. (1985). Identification of a 68-kilodalton protective protein antigen from *Bordetella bronchiseptica. Infection and Immunity.* 47 (3): 744–751

Morgan, B.P. (1999). Regulation of the complement membrane attack pathway. *Critical Reviews in Immunology.* 19 (3): 173-198

Murphy, T.F. & Bartos, L.C. (1989). Surface-exposed and antigenically conserved determinants of outer membrane proteins of *Branhamella catarrhalis. Infection and Immunity.* 57 (10): 2938–2941

Murphy, T.F & Bartos L.C. (1988). Purification and analysis with monoclonal antibodies of P2, the major outer membrane protein of nontypable *Haemophilus influenzae. Infection and Immunity.* 56 (5): 1084-1089

Nakadai, A.; Kuroki, T.; Kato, Y.; Suzuki, R.; Ymai, S.; Yaginuma, C.H.; Shiotani, R.; Yamanouchi, A. & Hayashidani, H. (2005). Prevelence of *Salmonella spp.* in pet reptiles in Japan. *Journal of Veterinary Medical Science*. 67 (1): 97-101

Nikaido, H. (2003). Molecular basis of bacterial outer membrane permeability revisited. *Microbiology and Molecular Biology Reviews*. 67 (4): 593–656

Nishio, M.; Okada, N.; Miki, T.; Haneda, T. & Danbara, H. (2005). Identification of the outer-membrane protein PagC required for the serum resistance phenotype in 946 *Salmonella enterica* serovar Choleraesuis. *Microbiology*. 151: 863-873

O'Byrne, A.M. & Mahon, M. (2008). Reptile-associated salmonellosis in residents in the South East of Ireland 2005-2007. *Eurosurveillance*. 4-6: 1-2

Ochoa-Reparaz, J.; Sesma, B.; Alvarez, M.; Renedo, M.J.; Irache J.M. & Gamazo, C. (2004). Humoral immune response in hens naturally infected with *Salmonella enteritidis* against outer membrane proteins and other surface structural antigens. *Veterinary Research*. 35 (3): 291-298

O'Farrell, P.H. (1975). High resolution two-dimensional electrophoresis of proteins. *Journal of Biological Chemistry*. 250 (10): 4007-4021

Ortiz, V.; Isibasi, A.; Garcia-Ortigoza, E. & Kumate, J. (1989). Immunoblot detection of class-specific humoral immune response to outer membrane proteins isolated from *Salmonella typhi* in humans with typhoid fever. *Journal of Clinical Microbiology*. 27 (7): 1640-1645

Pangburn, M.D.; Schreiber, R.D. & Muller-Eberhard, H.J. (1977). Human complement C3b inactivator: isolation, characterization, and demonstration of an absolute requirement for the serum protein β1H for cleavage C3b and C4b in solution. *Journal of Experimental Medicine*. 146 (1): 257-270

Pramoonjago, P.; Kaneko, M.; Kinoshita, T.; Ohtsubo, E.; Takeda, J.; Hong, K.S.; Inagi, R. & Inoue, K. (1992). Role of TraT protein, an anticomplementary protein produced in *Escherichia coli* by R100 factor, in serum resistance. *Journal of Immunology*. 148 (3): 827- 836

Rabsch, W.; Tschäpe, H. & Bäumler A.J. (2001). Non-typhoidal salmonellosis: emerging problems. *Microbes and Infection*. 3 (3): 237-247

Ram, S.; Sharma, A.K.; Simpson, S.D.; Gulati, S.; Mcquillen, D.P.; Pangburn, M.K. & Rice, P.A. (1998). A novel sialic acid binding site on factor H mediates serum resistance of sialylated *Neisseria gonorrhoeae*. *Journal of Experimental Medicine*. 187 (5): 743–752

Ramu, P.; Tanskanen, R.; Holmberg, M.; Lähteenmäki, K.; Korhonen, T.K. & Meri S. (2007). The surface protease PgtE of *Salmonella enterica* affects complement activity by proteolytically cleaving C3b, C4b and C5. *FEBS Letters*. 581 (9): 1716-1720

Rautemaa, R. & Meri, S. (1999). Complement-resistance mechanisms of bacteria. *Microbes and Infection*. 1 (10): 785–794

Rockwood, D.; Wilson, M.T. & Darley-Usmar, V.M. (1987). Isolation and characteristic of intact mitochondria. In: Darley-Usmar, V.M.; Rickwood, D. & Wilson, M.T. (eds), Mitochondria: a practical approach. IRL Press, Oxford, 1–16

Rowe, B.; Hall, M.L.; Ward, L.R. & de Sa, J.D. (1980). Epidemic spread of *Salmonella hadar* in England and Wales. *British Medical Journal*. 280 (6221): 1065-1066

Salazar-Gonzalez, R.M.; Maldonado-Bernal, C.; Ramirez-Cruz, N.E.; Rios-Sarabia, N.; Beltran-Nava, J.; Castanon-Gonzalez, J.; Castillo-Torres, N.; Palma-Aguirre, J.A.; Carrera-Camargo, M.; Lopez-Macias, C. & Isibasi, A. (2004). Induction of cellular immune response and anti-*Salmonella enterica* serovar Typhi bactericidal antibodies in healthy volunteers by immunization with a vaccine candidate against typhoid fever. *Immunology Letters*. 93 (2-3): 115–122

Sarowska, J.; Bugla-Ploskonska, G.; Futoma-Koloch, B. & Drulis-Kawa Z. (2010). The sensitivity level of *Salmonella enterica* $ESBL^+$ transconjugants to normal human serum correlated with OMPs band patterns obtained by SDS-PAGE. *Advanced of Clinical and Experimental Medicine*. 19 (6): 669-677

Sarowska, J.; Drulis-Kawa, Z.; Korzekwa, K.; Lewczyk, E.; Jankowski S. & Doroszkiewicz, W. (2005). The occurrence of acute diarrhoeas induced by rotaviruses and *Salmonella* strains in children hospitalised in the Lower Silesian J. Korczak Pediatrics Centre in Wroclaw. *Advanced of Clinical and Experimental Medicine*. 14 (4): 759–763

Scallan, E.; Hoekstra, R.M.; Angulo, F.J.; Tauxe, R.V.; Widdowson, M.A., Roy, S.L.; Jones, J.L. & Griffin, P.M. (2011). Foodborne illness acquired in the United States—major pathogens. *Emerging Infectious* Diseases. 17 (1): 7–15

Schnaitman, C.A. (1971). Solubilization of the cytoplasmic membrane of *Escherichia coli* by Triton X-100. *Journal of Bacteriology*. 108 (1): 545-552

Schröter, M.; Roggentin, P.; Hofmann, J.; Speicher, A.; Laufs, R. & Mack, D. (2004). Pet snakes as a reservoir for *Salmonella enterica* subsp. *diarizonae* (Serogroup IIIb): a prospective study. *Applied and Environmental Microbiology*. 70 (1): 613-615

Seleim, R.S.; Mohamed, S.R.; Hafez, N.M. & Gobran, R.A. (2002). *Salmonella* infection in calves: virulence proteins and its immunogenic properties. *Challenges to organic farming and sustainable land use in the tropics and subtropics*, Deutcher Tropentag, Witzenhausen, October 2002

Severi, E.; Hood, D.W. & Thomas, G.H. (2007). Sialic acid utilization by bacterial pathogens. *Microbiology*. 153 (9): 2817-2822

Shaw, M.M. & Riederer B.M. (2006). Sample preparation for two-dimensional electrophoresis. Current Advancements in the Methodology. *G.I.T Laboratory Journal*. 6: 302-303.

Siggins, M.K.; Cunningham, A.F.; Marshall, J.L.; Chamberlain, J.L.; Henderson, I.R. & MacLennan, C.A. (2011). Absent bactericidal activity of mouse serum against invasive African nontyphoidal *Salmonella* results from impaired complement function but not a lack of antibody. *Journal of Immunology*. 186 (4): 2365-2371

Simonsen, J.; Teunis, P.; Van Pelt, W.; Van Duynhoven, Y.; Krogfelt, K.A.; Sadkowska-Todys, M. & Molbak, K. (2010). Usefulness of seroconversion rates for comparing infection pressures between countries. *Epidemiology and Infection*, 139 (4): 1–8

Singh, S.P.; Singh, S.R.; Williams, Y.U.; Jones, L. & Abdullah, T. (1995). Antigenic determinants of the OmpC porin from *Salmonella typhimurium*. *Infection and Immunity*. 63 (12): 4600-4605

Skwara, A.; Bugla-Ploskonska, G.; Dudek, B.; Futoma-Koloch, B.; Kedziora, A. & Doroszkiewicz, W. (2011). Different electrophoretic patterns of outer membrane proteins in *Salmonella* O48-clinically important bacteria for children after their passages in serum. *4th Congress of European Microbiologists*, Geneva, Switzerland, June 2011

Smit, J. & Nikaido, H. (1978). Outer membrane of Gram-negative bacteria. XVIII. Electron microscopic studies on porin insertion sites and growth of cell surface of *Salmonella typhimurium*. *Journal of Bacteriology*. 135 (2): 687–702

Srirama, M.B. (2001). A guide to the properties and uses of detergents in biology and biochemistry. *Calbiochem manual*.

Taylor, P.W. (1983). Bactericidal and bacteriolytic activity of serum against gram-negative bacteria. *Microbiological Reviews*. 47 (1): 46–83

Tena, D.; Gonzales-Praetorius, A. & Bisquert J. (2007). Urinary tract infection due to non-typhoidal *Salmonella*: report of 19 cases. *Journal of Infection*. 54 (3): 245-249

Thomson, G.T.D.; DeRubeis, D.A.; Hodge, M.A.; Rajanayagam, C. & Inman R.D. (1995). Post-*Salmonella* reactive arthritis: late clinical sequelae in a point source cohort. *American Journal of Medicine*. 98 (1): 13–21

Threlfall, E. (2005). *Salmonella*. [In:] *Microbiology and Microbial Infections*. Ed. Boriello S, ASM Press, Washington, 10th ed, 54: 1398–1427

Tibor, A.; Decelle, B. & Letesson, J.J. (1999). Outer membrane proteins Omp10, Omp16, Omp19 of *Brucella spp*. are lipoproteins. *Infection and Immunity*. 67 (9): 4960–4962

Vimr, E. & Lichtensteiger, C. (2002). To sialylate, or not to sialylate: that is the question. *Trends in Microbiology*. 10 (6): 254–257

VonSpecht, B.U.; Knapp, B.; Hungerer. K.D.; Lucking, C.; Schmitt, A.; Domdey, H. (1996). Outer membrane proteins of *Pseudomonas aeruginosa* as vaccine candidates. *Journal of Biotechnology*. 44 (1-3): 145-153

Wang, L.Y. & Frasch, C.E. (1984). Development of a *Neisseria meningitidis* group B serotype 2b protein vaccine and evaluation in a mouse model. *Infection and Immunity*. 46 (2): 408-414

Weiser, J.N. & Gotschlich, E.C. (1991). Outer membrane protein A (OmpA) contributes to serum resistance and pathogenicity of *Escherichia coli* K-1. *Infection and Immunity*. 59 (7): 2252–2258

White, C.D.; Leduc, I.; Olsen, B.; Jeter, C.; Harris, C. & Elkins, C. (2005). *Haemophilus ducreyi* outer membrane determinants, including DsrA, define two clonal populations. *Infection and Immunity*. 73 (4): 2387–2399

Witkowska, D.; Maslowska, E.; Staniszewska, M.; Szostko, B.; Jankowski, A. & Gamian, A. (2006). Enterobacterial 38-kDa outer membrane protein is an age-dependent molecular marker of innate immunity and immunoglobulin deficiency as results from its reactivity with IgG and IgA antibody. *FEMS Immunology and Medical Microbiology*. 48 (2): 205–214

Woodward, D.L.; Khakhira, R. & Johnson, W.M. (1997). Human salmonellosis with exotic pets. *Journal of Clinical Microbiology*. 35 (11): 2786-2790

Würzner, R. (1999). Evasion of pathogens by avoiding recognition or eradication by complement, in part via molecular mimicry. *Molecular Immunology*. 36 (4-5): 249-260

Yu D.T. (1999). Pathogenesis of reactive arthritis. *International Medicine*. 38 (2): 97–101

Zollinger, W.D.; Boslego, J.; Froholm, L.O.; Ray, J.S.; Moran, E.E. & Brandt, B.L. (1987). Human bactericidal antibody response to meningococcal outer membrane protein vaccines. *Antonie Van Leeuwenhoek*. 53 (6): 403–411

15

Virulence Characterization of *Salmonella* Typhimurium I,4,[5],12:i:-, the New Pandemic Strain

Madalena Vieira-Pinto[1], Patrícia Themudo[2], Lucas Dominguez[3], José Francisco Fernandez-Garayzabal[3,4], Ana Isabel Vela[3,4], Fernando Bernardo[5], Cristina Lobo Vilela[5] and Manuela Oliveira[5]
[1]*Departamento das Ciências Veterinárias, CECAV Laboratório de TPA & Inspecção Sanitária, Universidade de Trás-os-Montes e Alto Douro*
[2]*Laboratório Nacional de Investigação Veterinária, Lisboa*
[3]*Centro de Vigilancia Sanitaria Veterinaria (VISAVET), Universidad Complutense, Madrid*
[4]*Departamento de Sanidad Animal, Facultad de Veterinaria, Universidad Complutense, Madrid*
[5]*Centro Interdisciplinar de Investigação em Sanidade Animal, Faculdade de Medicina Veterinária da Universidade Técnica de Lisboa, Lisboa*
[1,2,5]*Portugal*
[3,4]*España*

1. Introduction

It is really impossible to estimate the volume of ink that has been spent writing about *Salmonella* since its first description in 1885, by Daniel D. Salmon. Nowadays, performing a search on this bacterial genus using web databases originates more than 17 million references. Before the web era, the dissemination of information on *Salmonella* was extremely complex or even impossible, and this is probably the reason why *Salmonella* taxonomy has been so difficult to establish during the first century after its description. The taxonomy of this bacterial genus still today remains under revision.

Sadly, *Salmonella* is the paradigm of a popular microbe by quite regrettable reason: from the most common citizen to the most qualified microbiologist, everyone has already talked about *Salmonella*. The reason for this is, surely, its incrimination on severe food poisoning outbreaks and in many cases of illness in humans and animals and mortality in humans and animals.

Epidemiological data indicate that the cases of human or animal infections by *Salmonella* are may assume a dramatic dimension. In the European Union, the number of reported human cases is approximately 150 thousand each year, with a consistent tendency to decline during the last four years. In countries where basic health care cannot be delivered, the most dangerous clinical expression of a *Salmonella* infection, Typhoid fever, affects 16 million people per year, with almost 500,000 fatal cases, as estimated by the World Health Organization (Pang et al., 1998).

In fact, not all *Salmonella* isolates identified worldwide have such devastating consequences to human or animal health. Some of the *Salmonella* seroptypes or serovars are strictly adapted to primates (*Salmonella* Typhi, *Salmonella* Paratyphi, *Salmonella* Wien) being referred to as prototrophic for man; others are strictly adapted to some animal species (*Salmonella* Gallinarum-Pullorum, *Salmonella* Abortusovis, *Salmonella* Abortusequi), being referred to as prototrophic to animals; however, the vast majority of the serotypes are zoonotic, being able to infect both animals and humans. *Salmonella* varieties differentiation is based on its antigenic mosaic, in a complex combination of somatic (O), flagelar (H) and capsular (Vi) antigens. Serotyping according to the Kauffmann-White system, established in the middle of the last century, is still recognized as the reference method for discrimination of *Salmonella* varieties. Each combination of different antigens found in a particular *Salmonella* isolate (serotype or serovar) has a specific designation, following the international nomenclature based on one hundred years of scientific contributions, which sometimes originated peculiar designations (Popoff & Le Minor, 1997; Grimont & Weill, 2007).

Salmonella is an infectious and contagious bacterium that may be transmitted to humans, warm blood animals and reptiles by contaminated drinking water, by raw foods consumption, by direct contact with previously infected humans or animals and by iatrogenic accidents.

Food, in particular raw food, is the most common pathway for *Salmonella* infection, especially by zoonotic serotypes. Since the 1950's, zoonotic *Salmonella* became dominant in human salmonellosis cases. Virulence is strictly dependent on the serotype and it also varies with individual competences of each bacterial strain and with host susceptibility. These features explain why some serotypes have a higher prevalence in a particular host. In the last decades, two serotypes of zoonotic *Salmonella* showed a clear dominant incidence: *Salmonella* Typhimurium, firstly found in bovines, pigs, pigeons and secondarily in humans, while *Salmonella* Enteritidis, more common in poultry, but firstly found in humans, with the exception of Europe (EFSA, 2010b). These two serotypes may be discriminated more deeply using epidemiological markers like phage typing, molecular genotyping or other methodologies, including profiling for antimicrobial resistance phenotypes (R-type).

Salmonella Typhimurium is a somatic group B strain with the following antigenic formula: 4,[5],12:i:1,2. It has been early recognized as a serotype with a variable antigenic structure, like the lack of the somatic antigen [5], assuming, in this case, the designation of "variety Copenhagen" (very frequent in pigeons and bovines). The antigenic structure modulation of *Salmonella* Typhimurium may be mediated by plasmids, phages or proto-phages infections or segregations.

By the end of the 1980s, some isolates of a monophasic form of *Salmonella* Typhimurium - serotype I,4,[5],12:i:- gained epidemiological relevance, being more and more frequently referred to in the literature (Machado & Bernardo, 1990). The prevalence of this monophasic serotype has grown, presently being one of the most common *Salmonella* serotypes isolated from humans in several countries (Hopkins, et al., 2010) (Table 1). Other variants have also been found: variants lacking the 1st flagellar phase or lacking both (i and 1,2); and also variants without the somatic 1 antigen. The possibility that before the 1990s the scarce reports of *Salmonella* I,4,[5],12:i:- isolation, may reflect the difficulties in serotyping it being the isolates probably designated as *Salmonella* Typhimurium. At that time it was frequent to report some *Salmonella* serotypes as "Group B" or "untypable" (Switt et al., 2009).

Years of isolation	Country	Source
1986	Portugal	Chicken carcasses
1993	Thailand	Human
1997	Spain	Human
1991	Brazil	Human
1998	United States	Human
2000	Germany	Human, food, swine, cattle, broiler
2003	Italy	Human, swine
2005	UK	Human
2006	Luxembourg	Pork, pigs

Table 1. First time reports of *Salmonella* 4,[5],12:i: isolation (Adapted from EFSA, 2010b)

2. Occurrence of *Salmonella* I,4,[5],12:i:-

Cases of human infections with serovar I,4,[5],12:i:- have been related to severe illnesess. This serovar was responsible for an outbreak in New York City in 1998, in which 70% of the cases required hospitalization, being also associated with cases of systemic infections in Thailand and in Brazil (Switt et al., 2009).

Some foodborne outbreaks due to *Salmonella* I,4,[5],12:i:- have been reported in Europe. In 2006, Luxembourg signaled two outbreaks caused by a monophasic *S.* Typhimurium DT 193, corresponding to 133 human cases, 24 hospitalizations and one death (Mossong et al., 2007). Pork meat has been incriminated in these *Salmonella* cases (Mossong et al., 2007).

In Germany, the number of *Salmonella* I,4,[5],12:i:- related with human diseases has increased since 2000 (Hauser et al., 2010). Since 2006, the same monophasic variant of the multidrug-resistant *Salmonella* DT 193 strain has been associated with sporadic cases of salmonellosis, with increasing rates of hospitalization (Trupschuch et al., 2010). In 2008, the monophasic I,4,[5],12:i:- variant correspond to up to 42% of all *S.* Typhimurium isolates responsible for human salmonellosis (Hauser et al., 2010).

In France, official data suggest a gradual increase of *Salmonella* I,4,[5],12:i:- isolation rate in humans. After 2005, the frequency of this particular serovar raised from the eleventh to the third place (AFSSA, 2009) and a further significant increase was reported in the first five months of 2010 (Bone et al., 2010). In 2008, several outbreaks of *Salmonella* I,4,[5],12:i:- infections were identified in this country, including 13 family outbreaks, three collective infections and two hospital infections (AFSSA, 2009).

In Spain, the number of *Salmonella* I,4,[5],12:i:- illness cases has consistently increased since 1997, the year of the first report. Nowadays, the monophasic *Salmonella* is at the top five among the most frequently isolated *Salmonella* serovars in Spain (de la Torre et al., 2003). The epidemiological relevance of this serotype makes it a major cause of concern in Spain since the beginning of this Century (Echeita, et al., 1999; Guerra, et al., 2000).

In the UK, human infections by *Salmonella* I,4,[5],12:i:- began to be reported in 2005, when 47 cases occurred. In 2009 151 cases occured, representing an increase of more than 30%. Almost 30 % of the *Salmonella* I,4,[5],12:i:- isolates had a R-type ASSuT. In Scotland there was also an increase in the number of reports of *Salmonella* monophasic Group B cases.

Since 2008, sporadic and diffuse outbreaks related with ready to eat food have also been described in the UK linked to a DT 191A *Salmonella* I,4,[5],12:i:- strain, which is tetracycline-resistant (Peters et al., 2010). This strain is thought to have originated from infected frozen feeder mice imported into the UK for feeding exotic pets.

In Italy, *Salmonella* I,4,[5],12:i:- is one of the most frequent serotypes related to human cases of salmonellosis (Dionisi et al., 2009). R-type ASSuT represented 75% of the monophasic isolates identified in 2008 and 2009. Almost 50 % of the monophasic isolates were identified as *Salmonella* DT193 and 13% as *Salmonella* U302.

In The Netherlands, *S.* I,4,[5],12:i:- was related to human cases for the first time in 2004. After that, the number of cases has consistently grown, being the third most prevalent serotype responsible for human salmonellosis from 2005 to 2008 (Van Pelt et al., 2009).

There also many cases reported outside Europe. In the USA, *Salmonella* I,4,[5],12:i:- frequency in human infections has consistently increased from 2002, being now ranked in the top six. During 2007, some *Salmonella* I,4,[5],12:i:- outbreaks occurred in the USA, related to frozen chicken pies consumption and also to direct contact with turtles kept as pets (CDC, 2007a, 2007b).

Some cases have also been reported in Canada (Switt et al., 2009).

Salmonella I,4,[5],12:i:- has also been reported in Brazil quite early, in the 1970s. In São Paulo State, the occurrence of the strain in human infections was reported in the 1990s. Since then, the frequency of foodborne outbreaks and of extra-intestinal infections in humans promoted by this serovar showed a consistent tendency to increase (Tavechio et al., 2009).

In Thailand, *Salmonella* I,4,[5],12:i:- has been classified among the top five *Salmonella* serovars responsible for cases of foodborne salmonellosis (Amavisit, et al., 2005; Pornruangwong et al., 2008).

Human cases of infection with this particular serotype seem to be generally linked to raw meat. According to the EFSA zoonoses reports, in 2008 *Salmonella* I,4,[5],12:i:- has been related to 3.1% of *Salmonella* isolations in pig herds; in 2009, the same serotype has been found in 1.2% of the *Salmonella* positive bovine herds, 3.2% of positive pig herds and represented 1.4% of *Salmonella* isolations in poultry meat.

A particularly relevant feature of *Salmonella* I,4,[5],12:i:- is the fact that most virulent isolates exhibit a plasmid-mediated resistance to a wide range of antimicrobial compounds. Similar to its ancestral lineage - *Salmonella* Typhimurium DT104 - the monophasic strain I,4,[5],12:i:- frequently expresses a multiple resistance to ampicillin (A), streptomycin (S), sulphonamides (Su) and tetracyclines (T). This ASSuT antimicrobial resistance pattern is chromosomally-encoded (Hopkins et al., 2010).

The progressive increase of the incidence of this serotype lead some authors to consider *Salmonella* I,4,[5],12:i:- as a possible new pandemic strain (Hopkins, et al., 2010).

Data on the number of salmonellosis cases or outbreaks occurring in livestock due to *Salmonella* I,4,[5],12:i:- is not available. This subject needs to be further studied.

3. Characterization of monophasic *Salmonella enterica* subsp. *enterica* serovar I,4,[5],12:i:-

Serotyping divides *Salmonella* subspecies into subtypes, or serovars, based on the immunologic characterization of surface structures, such as O, H and in some cases Vi-antigens, through the use of polyvalent and monovalent antisera. The full antigenic pool of *Salmonella* [I,4,5,12:i:-] indicates that the somatic O-antigens expressed are I,4,[5],12. The underlined O factor 1 (1) means that this factor is determined by phage conversion, being present only if the culture is lysogenized by the corresponding converting phage. The factor 5 between square brackets ([5]) means that the antigen may be present or absent, not having a relation with phage conversion. So, in this serovar both factors (1 and 5) can be present or absent.

Most *Salmonella* strains are biphasic and express two serologically distinct flagellar antigens. The two antigens were historically designated as phases and the expression of two different phases is mediated at molecular level by an intricate mechanism unique to *Salmonella*. The regulation of phase 1 and phase 2 antigen expressions is under the control of the recombinase Hin. This recombinase facilitates the inversion of a promoter element so that it either (i) transcribes *flj*B (which encodes the phase 2 antigen FljB) and *flj*A (which encodes a repressor of *fli*C, the gene encoding the phase 1 antigen FliC) (Aldridge et al., 2006; Yamamoto & Kutsukake, 2006) or (ii) does not transcribe either of these genes. If the orientation of this promoter does not allow the transcription of *flj*B and *flj*A, the lack of repression of *fli*C transcription leads to the expression of phase 1 flagellar antigens.

Strains expressing both flagellar types are called biphasic. In contrast, strains defined as monophasic fail to express either phase 1 or phase 2 flagellar antigens. *S.* [1,4,5,12:i:-] possess only the phase 1 of the H-antigen "i" and lacks the second phase H antigen, encoded by *flj*B, which either is not present or contains mutation(s) affecting its expression. In 2007, Zamperini et al. screened *S.* 4,[5],12:i:- isolates for phase 1 and phase 2 antigen genes, *fli*C and *flj*B, and found that 100% of the isolates were positive for *fli*C, while 11% were positive for *flj*B. Approximately 89% of these isolates contained complete or partial deletions of the phase 2 flagellin gene, *flj*B, whereas 96% possessed the upstream gene, *hin*, which encodes the DNA invertase involved in "flipping" the *flj*B promoter.

Phage typing is a method also used for *Salmonella* typing based on the lysis of isolates with a panel of bacteriophages. Since this technique does not depend on the presence of the second phase H antigen, monophasic *Salmonella* reactions are performed with the same panel of phages used for *Salmonella* serovar Typhimurium (Echeita et al., 2001; Amavisit et al., 2005; Mossong et al., 2006). Thus, all phage types that have been recognized so far within monophasic *Salmonella* have also been found in *S.* serovar Typhimurium.

For example, the multidrug-resistant *Salmonella* 4,[5],12:i:- strain detected in Spain in 1997 was lysed by the *S.* Typhimurium phage 10 (Echeita et al., 2001). Phage type U302 was also detected among *S.* 4,[5],12:i:- isolates in other countries, such as Denmark (Ethelberg et al., 2004) and Italy (Dinosi et al., 2009). This phage type has been considered closely related to DT104 (Briggs & Fratamico, 1999).

However, *S.* 4,[5],12:i:- isolates have also been classified in other phage types linked to *S.* Typhimurium. In Germany, Hauser et al. (2010) analyzed *S.* [4,[5],12:i:- isolates obtained from different sources (human, swine and pork) and classified 70% of strains as DT193 and 19% as DT120. In another study, Hopkins et al., (2011) screened a large number of *S.* 4,[5],12:i:- strains from different countries (France, The Netherlands, England and Wales, Germany, Italy, Spain and Poland), obtained from similar sources as described by Hauser et al. (2010), and were able to identify 16 different phage types. However, the most commonly identified phage types were DT193, DT120 and RDNC ("Reaction Does Not Conform"). DT193 was the most common phage type identified in England and Wales, France, Germany, Spain and the Netherlands, while DT120 predominated in Italy and Poland. In other studies, *S.* 4,[5],12:i:- DT193 strains were also isolated from human cases of infection and/or pigs in United Kingdom, Luxembourg, United States and Spain (Hampton et al., 1995; Gebreyes & Altier, 2002; de la Torre et al., 2003; Mossong et al., 2006), while monophasic DT120 strains were identified in Italy (Dionisi et al., 2009).

According to serological characterization, it is difficult to identify the origin of the monophasic strains. This strain may be a new variant of the rare serovar Lagos (4,[5],12:i:-), or a new variant of the very common serovar Typhimurium [4,5,12:i:1,2], or even a new variant of other serovars with similar antigenic pools, such as *S.* Agama [4,12:i:1,6], *S.* Farsta [4,12:i:e,n,x], *S.* Tsevie [4,12:i:e,n,z15], *S.* Cloucester [1,5,12,27:i:l,w], *S.* Tumodi [1,4,12:i:z6] or as *S.* 4,5,27:i:z35, an unnamed serotype (Switt et al., 2009). However, large scale studies suggest that *S.* 4,[5],12:i:- is genetically related to Typhimurium [4,5,12:i:1,2], and is likely to have originated from a *S.* Typhimurium ancestor (Echeita et al., 2001; Zamperini et al., 2007). Monophasic *Salmonella* could have evolved by two distinct pathways. It could represent ancestral forms which did not acquire, though evolution, a second flagellar antigen or the required switching mechanism. Alternatively, it could originate as mutants of biphasic *Salmonella*, which have lost either the switching mechanism or the ability to express the second flagellar antigen (Burnens et al., 1996).

The atypical *fljB*-negative and multidrug-resistant *S.* 4,[5],12:i:- which emerged and spread in Spain in 1997 had a unique sequence specific for *S.* Typhimurium phage types DT104 and U302 and also an IS*200* fragment located in a Typhimurium serovar-specific location. Both facts strongly suggest that these strains are monophasic variants of *S.* Typhimurium (Echeita et al., 2001).

On other hand, *S.* 4,[5],12:i:- DT193 and DT120 strains were classified as monophasic variants of *S.* Typhimurium due to the presence of a Typhimurium-specific fragment of the malic acid dehydrogenase gene (Hopkins et al., 2011). However, these strains were negative for the DT104- and U302-specific region. Houser et al. (2010) indicated that phage type DT193 and DT120 isolates of both serovars presented genetic differences and represent different Pulsed-field Gel Electrophoresis (PFGE) clusters. Such differences seem to indicate that the *S.* Typhimurium phage type DT193 lineage was not a direct ancestor of the monophasic phage type DT193. In contrast, *S.* 4,[5],12:i:- phage type DT120 strains showed a higher genetic similarity with the *S. enterica* Typhimurium phage type DT120 strains, suggesting that this biphasic subtype was the recent common ancestor of the monophasic variant.

Different mutations and deletions have been associated with the lack of phase 2 flagella expression in *S.* 4,[5],12:i:- isolates. Specifically, some Spanish *S.* 4,[5],12:i:- isolates appear to be characterized by the deletion of a large fragment, that included *fljB*, *hin*, and a DNA invertase essential for *fljB* expression (Garaizar et al., 2002). Most USA isolates characterized so far also present deletions that eliminate *fljB* but maintain *hin* (Zamperini et al., 2007; Soyer et al., 2009). These genetic differences among American and Spanish *S.* 4,[5],12:i:- isolates have also been made evident by PFGE typing (Soyer et al., 2009). Genetic data indicate that American and Spanish isolates represent different clonal groups with distinct genome deletion patterns. This is consistent with the observation that most Spanish *S.* 4,[5],12:i:- isolates are phage type U302 (Echeita et al., 2001). Moreover, PFGE and Multiple-Locus Variable Number Tandem Repeat Analysis (MLVA) techniques showed that Spanish phage type U302 strains seem to be more homogeneous than groups constituted by isolates from other countries (Soyer et al., 2009), supporting a clonal origin. Soyer et al. (2009) suggested that Spanish *Salmonella* 4,[5],12:i:- strains might have emerged from a multidrug-resistant *S.* Typhimurium strain, while American *S.* 4,[5],12:i:- strains might have emerged from a non-drug-resistant *S.* Typhimurium strain, through independent events.

Strains belonging to S. 4,[5],12:i:- that have been recently implicated in infections both in humans and farm animals have been further typed using genetic techniques. Guerra et al. (2000) studies showed a high genetic homogeneity among 16 Spanish S. 4,[5],12:i:- isolates using techniques such as ribotyping, RAPD (Random Amplified Polymorphic DNA analysis) and plasmid profiling. However, the use of PFGE techniques could originate degrees of heterogeneity that may range from moderate to high, even when applied to strains from a single country (Agasan et al., 2002; de la Torre et al., 2003; Zamperini et al., 2007; Soyer et al., 2009). For example, at least 13 different *Xba*I PFGE types were found among 32 S. 4,[5],12:i:- isolates from Georgia (Zamperini et al., 2007), 44 different *Xba*I PFGE types were detected among 148 isolates from Germany (Hauser et al., 2010) and at least 11 *Xba*I PFGE types were found among 23 Spanish S. 4,[5],12:i:- isolates (de la Torre et al., 2003). Despite their heterogeneity, S. 4,[5],12:i:- strains have been reported to be less heterogenic than *S.* Typhimurium strains (Guerra et al., 2000; Agasan et al., 2002; Soyer et al., 2009; Hauser et al., 2010).

Studies also have showed the occurence of common genetic profiles among *S.* 4,[5],12:i:- isolates obtained from different sources and countries. Zamperini et al. (2007) studies revealed the same PFGE profile among poultry and bovine *S.* 4,[5],12:i:- isolates. In 2011, Hopkins et al. compared isolates from humans, pigs and pork using PFGE and detected several prevalent genetic profiles common to these three sources (StYMXB.0131, STYMXB.0083, STYMXB.0079, STYMXB.0010, STYMXB.0022). Moreover, these profiles were detected in isolates from different countries. One PFGE profile, STYMXB.0010, was identified in isolates obtained in all the countries surveilled in the referred study. However, the authors also found some country-specific differences in the distribution of PFGE patterns. For example, nine of the 12 STYMXB.0079 strains originated from Italy, three of the five Polish strains were STYMXB.0010 and six of 10 strains from the Netherlands were STYMXB.0131. The STYMXB.0079 profile was also the predominant one among 146 human *S.* 4,[5],12:i:- isolates obtained in Italy by Dionisi et al. (2009).

Typing of monophasic strains using molecular techniques, such as PFGE, have showed that these strains differ from *S.* Lagos strains (Soyer et al., 2009). Data also showed the occurrence of some profiles common to *S.* Typhimurium. Zamperini et al. (2007) examined isolates of *S.* 4,[5],12:i:- and *S.* Typhimurium collected from animal sources that presented the same PFGE profile. In another study, Agasan et al. (2002) compared the PFGE profile of *S.* 4,[5],12:i:– strains found in humans in New York City to the profile of *S.* Typhimurium isolates, including *S.* serovar Typhimurium DTI04, and found that *S.* 4,[5],12:i:– isolates were related to some of the *S.* Typhimurium isolates examined. Amavisit et al. (2005) compared the PFGE profiles of human isolates identified as *S.* Typhimurium DTI04, Typhimurium U302 and 4,[5],12:i:–, showing that four of the *S.* 4,[5],12:i:– isolates presented the same or similar profiles as *S.* Typhimurium phage type U302.

In another study, Alcaine et al. (2006) used Multilocus Sequence Typing (MLST) to show that ST6 type comprises not only bovine and human *S.* 4,[5],12:i:– isolates but also Typhimurium isolates obtained in the United States. ST6 was unique to *S.* Typhimurium and 4,[5],12:i:–, which supports the initial findings based on characterization of Spanish isolates (de la Torre et al., 2003), that *S.* [4,5,12:i:-] may have emerged from a *S.* Typhimurium ancestor. A MLST technique based on four genes applied to American and Spanish isolates belonging to *S.* 4,[5],12:i:– and to *S.* Typhimurium classified the vast majority of isolates as ST1 (Soyer et al., 2009). Similar results were obtained with other molecular fingerprinting techniques e.g. RAPD analysis, plasmid profiling (Sala, 2002; de la Torre et al., 2003), MLST (Alcaine et al., 2006) and MLVA/Variable Number of Tandem Repeats (VNTR) typing (Laorden et al., 2009; Torpdahl et al., 2009; Hauser et al., 2010; Hopkins et al., 2011). All these studies lead to the conclusion that *S.* 4,[5],12:i:– isolates belong to a single genetic lineage or clone and seem closely related to *S.* Typhimurium (Zamperini et al., 2007; Dionisi et al., 2009; Hopkins et al., 2011).

Overall, the genomic characterization of *S.* 4,[5],12:i:– isolates suggests that this serovar is likely to gather several clones or strains that have independently emerged from *S.* Typhimurium during the last two decades, and have changed through multiple independent events involving different clonal groups (Garaizar et al., 2002; Laorden et al., 2009; Laorden et al., 2010). Although the driver for this evolution remains to be enlightened for many epidemic strains antimicrobial resistance may be implicated (Zaidi et al., 2007; Bailey et al., 2010).

4. Antimicrobial resistance traits of *Salmonella* I,4,[5],12:i:-

The characterization of zoonotic bacteria virulence factors, including the presence of antimicrobial resistance traits, is of major importance for assuring the safeguard of health in the wider concept of "one health". The dissemination of antimicrobial resistant bacteria is a well-recognized hazard for public and animal health.

Several *Salmonella* serovars are frequently related to human and animal diseases, and this genus is recognized worldwide as a major foodborne pathogen. Gastroenteritis due to *Salmonella* is usually characterized by mild to moderate self-limiting symptoms, such as diarrhea, abdominal cramps, vomiting and fever. However, some strains are responsible for severe infections, such as septicemia, osteomyelitis, pneumonia, and meningitis that occur, especially in children and in elderly and immunocompromised individuals (Folley and Lynne, 2008a).

Generally, salmonellosis cases caused by *Salmonella* I,4,[5],12:i:- strains are severe, requiring hospitalization (EFSA, 2010b). The control of severe infections requires antimicrobial therapy, generally with fluoroquinolones or ceftriaxone, administrated to children in order to avoid the cartilage damage frequently associated with fluoroquinolone therapy (Folley and Lynne, 2008a). Therefore, *Salmonella* represents a bacterial genus of special concern regarding antimicrobial resistance dissemination.

This serotypes' resistance profiles may vary, worldwide, from 100% susceptible to multidrug resistance. Although *S.* Typhimurium resistance levels have been decreasing in several European countries, the incidence of resistant *S.* Typhimurium I,4,[5],12:i:- strains seems to be escalating (Switt et al., 2009). There are only a few studies available on antimicrobial resistance traits and genes present in antimicrobial drug-resistant *Salmonella* serotype 4,[5],12:i:- isolates, which have identified some specific resistance genes and genetic mechanisms. The limited data available still hasn't allowed researchers to identify the common ancestor responsible for the emergence of 4,[5],12:i:- isolates with a multidrug resistance pattern (MDR), information essential to understand resistance evolution and dissemination (Switt et al., 2009).

Antimicrobial resistance in *Salmonella* spp. may be due to several resistance determinants that can be located either in the bacterial chromosome or in plasmids (Folley and Lynne, 2008a; Switt et al., 2009). These genetic determinants can be responsible for the expression of intrinsic resistant mechanisms, related to the production of ß -lactamases, to the modification of the antimicrobial compound by bacterial enzymes, to the variation of bacterial permeability, to the presence of efflux pumps or to the modification of target receptors (Folley and Lynne, 2008a).

Antimicrobial resistance may also result from the expression of acquired resistance mechanisms, emerging through the occurrence of point mutations in chromosomal genes or the acquisition of mobile elements such as plasmids, transposons, and genomic islands (Switt et al., 2009). The transfer of resistance determinants may occur directly from the same or different bacterial species/genera, or indirectly through the environment (Folley and Lynne 2008a; EFSA, 2010b). Intestinal microbiota from humans and animals is often exposed to antimicrobial compounds of different classes, concentrations and exposure frequencies, used for therapy, prophylaxis or methaphylaxis. This exposure may derive from food/feed products or from the environment (Martins da Costa et al., 2007). Emergence, selection and dissemination of antimicrobial resistant bacteria are still mainly attributed to the selective pressure of antibiotic misuse and abuse (Monroe & Polk, 2000; Sayah et al., 2005), so intestinal bacteria can became resistant to some antimicrobial compounds, and therefore transmit these resistant traits to *Salmonella,* which occupies the same ecological niche.

The presence of one or the combination of several of the above mentioned mechanisms may also confer a MDR profile to bacteria. These MDR profiles may comprise major antimicrobial compounds, hampering the treatment of severe *Salmonella* infections (EFSA, 2010b).

In 1997, MDR *Salmonella* 4,[5],12:i:- isolates were identified for the first time in Spain (Guerra et al., 2001). The most frequent MDR pattern is the ASSuT tetraresistance pattern, isolated from 30% of the human infection cases in the last 5 years and also from farm animals (Lucarelli et al., 2010; EFSA, 2010b). This pattern emerged in Italy during the 2000s, and has already been identified in Denmark, the United Kingdom, the United States, Spain, France, and the Czech Republic (Lucarelli et al., 2010). Genes responsible for this MDR phenotype are present in a chromosomal resistance island that usually includes the *bla*TEM, *str*A-*str*B, *sul*2 and *tet*(B) genes (Hauser et al., 2010; Lucarelli et al., 2010), having some strains additional resistances (Lucarelli et al., 2010; EFSA, 2010b).

Other multirresistant patterns identified in 4,[5],12:i:- isolates worldwide are the ACKGSuTm (showing resistance to ampicillin, chloramphenicol, kanamycin, gentamicin, sulfamethoxazole and trimethoprim) and ACKGSuTm with additional resistance to nalidixic acid patterns, found in Thailand (Switt et al., 2009); the ACSuGSTTm (showing resistance to ampicillin, chloramphenicol, sulfamethoxazole, gentamicin, streptomycin and tetracycline) and ACGSSuTSTm patterns, found in Spain (Echeita et al., 1999); the ACSSuT pattern, found in the United States (Agasan et al., 2002; Switt et al., 2009); and the ACSSpSuT pattern, found in the United Kingdom and other countries (Lucarelli et al., 2010). The isolation of multiresistant isolates was also described in Brazil (Switt et al., 2009) and Germany (Hauser et al., 2010).

The MDR phenotypes include 4,[5],12:i:- strains harboring class 1 integrons or large resistant plasmids, resistant to ampicillin, chloramphenicol, gentamicin, streptomycin, sulfamethoxazole, tetracyclines and trimethoprim. These resistance traits are mainly due to the expression of *bla*TEM-1, which codes for broad spectrum *b*-lactamases responsible for resistance to penicillin and amino-penicillins; of *bla*CTX-M-1, which codes for extended-spectrum ß-lactamases; of *cml*A1, which codes for an efflux pump responsible for chloramphenicol resistance; of *aac*(3)-IV and *aad*A2, which code for enzymes that modify gentamycin and streptomycin active sites, impairing the action of these drugs; of *aad*A1, *sul*1 and *sul*2, which code for enzymes responsible for resistance to sulfonamides; of *sul*3 and *tet*(A), which code for an efflux pump mechanism responsible for tetracycline resistance; and of *dfrA*12, which codes for an enzyme responsible for resistance to trimethoprim (Folley and Lynne, 2008a; Guerra et al., 2001; Switt et al., 2009).

It is important to refer that, despite the road book aiming at controlling antimicrobial use and abuse, antimicrobial resistance remains a worldwide problem for both human and veterinary medicine. In this context, the boundaries between human and animal health, as well as between living organisms and the environment are insubstantial. Besides data from clinical studies, resistant bacteria have been described from a variety of environmental sources, including domestic sewage, drinking water, rivers, and lakes (Sayah et al., 2005).

5. *Salmonella* virulence factors

Salmonella enterica includes many serovars that cause disease in avian and mammalian hosts (Eswarappa et al., 2008). Also, *Salmonella* sp. is one of the most frequent bacterial food-borne pathogens affecting humans. In both animal and human hosts, infections may be present in a variety of presentations, from asymptomatic colonization to inflammatory diarrhoea or typhoid fever, depending on serovar- and host-specific factors. Colonization of reservoir hosts often occurs in the absence of clinical signs; however, some *S. enterica* serovars threaten animal health due to their ability to cause acute enteritis or to translocate from the intestine to other organs, causing fever and septicaemia (Stevens, 2009). Also, while certain serovars of *S. enterica* are ubiquitary and cause disease in humans and in a variety of animals, other serovars are highly restricted to a specific host (Hensel, 2004). For example, ubiquitous serovars such as Typhimurium and Enteritidis tend to produce an acute but self-limiting enteritis in a wide range of hosts, whereas host-specific serovars are associated with severe systemic disease that may not involve diarrhoea, usually affecting healthy adults of a single species (e.g. *S.* Typhi in humans, *S.* Gallinarum in poultry) (Stevens, 2009).

Differences in virulence among *Salmonella* serovars and variations in the evolution of *Salmonella* spp. infections in several host species have been attributed to the acquisition and expression of virulence genes (Zhao, 2001). *Salmonella* spp. virulence requires the coordinated expression of complex arrays of virulence factors that allow the bacterium to evade the host's immune system. All *Salmonella* serotypes share the ability to invade the host by inducing their own uptake into the intestinal epithelial cells. In addition, *Salmonella* serotypes associated with gastroenteritis trigger an intestinal inflammatory and secretory response, whereas serotypes that cause enteric fever give raise to systemic infections through their ability to survive and replicate in mononuclear phagocytes (Ohl & Miller, 2001).

Many virulence phenotypes of *Salmonella enterica* are encoded by genes located in distinct chromosome regions, organized in 12 pathogenicity islands (Bhunia, 2008; Eswarappa et al., 2008; Saroj et al., 2008). These gene clusters, known as *Salmonella* pathogenicity islands (SPIs), are thought to be acquired by horizontal gene transfer. They present a G-C content that differs from the remaining chromosome, suggesting acquisition by horizontal transfer. While some SPIs are conserved throughout the genus, others are specific for certain serovars (Amavisit et al., 2003; Bhunia, 2008; Eswarappa et al., 2008). According to Saroj et al., (2008), pathogenicity islands can be transferred between bacteria of different genera, leading to an accumulation of different virulence mechanisms in some strains. Therefore, the occurrence of SPIs varies between serovars and strains (Hensel, 2004). Pathogenicity islands often contain multiple genes functionally related, and required for the expression of a specific virulence phenotype, which suggests that the acquisition of a pathogenicity island during evolution may in one "quantum leap" open up new host niches for the pathogen (Ohl & Miller, 2001; Eswarappa et al., 2008). According to Bhunia (2008), the virulence genes responsible for invasion, survival, and extraintestinal spread are distributed in the *Salmonella* pathogenicity islands. For instance, the virulence genes that are involved in the intestinal phase of infection are located in SPI-1 and SPI-2. Many pathogenicity islands, including SPI-1 and SPI-2, encode specialized devices for the delivery of virulence proteins into host cells, termed type III secretion systems (TTSSs) (Eswarappa et al., 2008). The remaining SPIs are required for causing systemic infections, intracellular survival, fimbrial expression, antibiotic resistance, and Mg2+ and iron uptake (Bhunia, 2008).

Besides the SPIs, some virulence factors can be encoded in virulence plasmids. Six serovars (Typhimurium, Gallinarum, Gallinarum biovar Pullorum, Enteritidis, Dublin, Choleraesuis and Abortusovis) typically harbor virulence plasmids of 60-95 kb that contain the *spv* locus, which holds some of the genes that are involved in intracellular survival and multiplication of this facultative intracellular pathogen (Tierrez & Garcia-del Portillo, 2005). The typical virulence plasmid of *S.* Typhimurium (pSLT90), is about 90-95 kb, and belongs to the FII incompatibility group.

Regarding the monophasic *S.* Typhimurium, this serotype has only recently emerged, but it comprises a wide variety of different strains (Soyer et al., 2008). For that, consistent data on virulence mechanisms are limited. Nevertheless, several studies have already shown that not only *Salmonella* serotype 4,[5],12:i:- isolates are genetically and phenotypically closely related to *Salmonella* serotype Typhimurium (Agasan et al., 2002; Amavisit et al., 2005; de la Torre et al. 2003; Delgado et al., 2006; Echeita et al., 2001; Zamperini et al., 2007) but also, virulence genes of monophasic *S.* Typhimurium and their variability are identical to those found in *S.* Typhimurium (Garaizar et al., 2002; Hauser et al., 2009; Soyer et al., 2009; Hauser et al., 2010). For example, studies developed by del Cerro et al. (2003) and Guerra et al. (2000), demonstrated that strains of monophasic *S.* Typhimurium presented an homology regarding virulence plasmid genes *spv*C, *inv*E and *inv*A invasion genes, *stn* enterotoxin genes, *sly*A cytolysin genes and genes associated with survival within macrophages (*pho*), when compared to those typically found in *S.* Typhimurium

For all these reasons, it should be noted that, presently, most of the knowledge on SPIs and other *Salmonella* virulence genes of monophasic *S.* Typhimurium is based on observations made in serovar Typhimurium. This serovar is considered a model organism for genetic studies, and a wide variety of classical and molecular tools are available for the identification and characterization of potential *Salmonella* virulence genes.

5.1. *Salmonella* Pathogenicity Islands

As above referred, there are at least twelve chromosomally-encoded *Salmonella* pathogenicity islands (SPIs) (Table 2), as follows:

- SPI-1 is a 43-kb chromosomal locus that was acquired by horizontal gene transfer from other pathogenic bacteria during evolution. It contains 31 genes with a major role in the invasion of host cells and induction of macrophage apoptosis. It also encodes components of the Type III secretion system (TTSS) designated as the Inv/Spa-Type III secretion apparatus that includes the secretion apparatus components, effectors, chaperones, and regulator (Amavisit et al., 2003; Bhunia, 2008; Eswarappa et al., 2008). The major genes present in SPI-1 are *inv*A, *inv*B, *inv*C, *inv*F, *inv*G, *hil*A, *sip*A, *sip*C, *sip*D, *spar, org*A, *sop*B, and *sop*E. *inv*ABCD genes, responsible for the expression of several invasion factors that promote bacterial attachment and invasion of M-cells, allowing them to cross the epithelial barrier which is the preferential route of *Salmonella* translocation. For example, InvA is an inner membrane protein involved in the formation of a channel through which polypeptides are exported. InvH and HilD are accessory proteins involved in *Salmonella* adhesion. InvG is an outer membrane protein of the TTSS that plays a critical role in bacterial uptake and protein secretion.

  There are two kinds of effector proteins secreted by the TTSS. One subclass consists of InvJ and SpaO, which are involved in the protein secretion through the TTSS. The other subclass modulates host cytoskeleton and induces its uptake. SipB and SipC are the major proteins, which interact with host cytoskeletal proteins to promote *Salmonella* uptake. Inv/Spa are also responsible for macrophage apoptosis. SipA is an actin-binding protein. SopB is an inositol phosphate phosphatase and SopE activates GTP-binding proteins. HilA is the central transcriptional regulator of genes located on SPI-1 (Bhunia, 2008).

- SPI-2 is a 40-kb segment that encodes for 32 genes, only present in members of *S. enterica*, and other type III secretion systems involved in systemic pathogenesis (Amavisit et al., 2003; Eswarappa et al., 2008; Bhunia, 2008). The gene products are essential for systemic infection and mediate bacterial replication, rather than survival within host macrophages (Bhunia, 2008). The majority of these genes are expressed during bacterial growth inside the host-cells. SPI-2 carries genes for Spi/Ssa and TTSS apparatus, i.e., SpiC, which inhibits the fusion between the *Salmonella*-containing phagosome and the lysosome (Bhunia, 2008).
- Type III Secretion Systems are expressed by many bacterial pathogens to deliver virulence factors to the host cell and to interfere with or subvert normal host cell

signaling pathways (Marcus et al., 2000). The TTSS structural genes (including *inv*G, *prg*H and *prg*K) encode proteins that may form a needle-like structure and are responsible for contact dependent secretion or for the delivery of virulence proteins to host cells (Zhao, 2001; Bhunia, 2008). This needle-like organelle located in the bacterial periphery has four parts: a needle, outer rings, neck, and inner rings. The needle is constituted by PrgI and a putative inner rod protein, PrgJ; the outer rings structure by InvG; the neck by PrgK; and the base by PrgH that forms the inner rings. The inner membrane components include InvC, InvA, SpaP, SpaQ, SpaR, and SpaS proteins (Bhunia, 2008). When *Salmonella* adheres to a target cell, this needle-like structure is assumed to form a channel with its base anchored in the cell wall and its tip puncturing the membrane of the host cell. Through this channel, *Salmonella* effectors proteins such as SipC, SipA, SopE/E2, and SopB, are injected into the host cell cytoplasm, promoting actin polymerization and membrane remodelling which allows the active uptake of bacteria by the host cell (Zhao, Y., 2001).

- SPI-3 is a 17-kb locus conserved between *S. enterica* serovar Typhi and Typhimurium that is also found in *S. bongori*, being variable in other serovars. SPI-3 harbors 10 genes, including the *mgt*CB operon, which is regulated by PhoPQ and is required for intra-macrophage survival and virulence and for magnesium uptake under low magnesium concentrations (Amavisit et al., 2003; Bhunia, 2008; Eswarappa et al., 2008). PhoQ is a sensor and PhoP is a transcriptional activator that expresses different genes that are required for bacterial survival inside the macrophage, as well as in various stressing environments including carbon and nitrogen starvation, low pH, low O2 levels, and the presence of defensins. In addition, PhoP regulates genes such as *spi*C and *tass*C that prevent lysosome fusion with the *Salmonella*-containing vacuole. PhoQ regulon activates *pags* genes that are essential for adaptation during the intracellular life cycle (Bhunia, 2008).

Salmonella present in the subcellular lamina propria are either engulfed by the macrophages or by the dendritic cells, which allows its extraintestinal dissemination. The survival of *Salmonella* within macrophages is generally considered to be essential for the translocation of bacteria from the gut-associated lymphoid tissue to the mesenteric lymph nodes and from there to the liver and spleen.

- SPI-4 is a 27-kb locus located next to a putative tRNA gene, containing 18 genes. It is thought to encode genes for the Type I secretion system and is suspected to be required for intramacrophage survival (Amavisit et al., 2003; Bhunia, 2008).
- SPI-5 is a 7.6-kb region and encodes six genes. It appears that SPI-5 encodes effector proteins for TTSS. SopB, which is translocated by TTSS, is an inositol phosphatase involved in triggering fluid secretion responsible for diarrhea. Thus, it is believed that SPI-5 is possibly responsible for enteric infections (Bhunia, 2008; Eswarappa et al., 2008).
- SPI-6 is a 59-kb locus present in both serovars Typhi and Typhimurium. It contains the *saf* gene cluster responsible for fimbriae development, *pag*N responsible for invasion traits, and several genes with unknown function (Bhunia, 2008).

In many studies, bacterial motility was found to be essential for adherence or invasion. In many systems, flagella provide the driving force that enable the bacteria to penetrate the host mucus layer and reach the host cell surface more rapidly (Zhao, 2001). *Salmonella* expresses different types of fimbriae that promote adhesion to M-cells and colonization of intestinal epithelial cells. Type I fimbriae (Fim) binds to α-d-mannose receptor in the host cell; long polar fimbriae (Lpf) bind to cells located in the Peyer's patch; and plasmid-encoded fimbriae (Pef) and curli, thin aggregative fimbriae, aid in bacterial adhesion to intestinal epithelial cells. Curli helps bacteria to autoaggregate, which enhances survival in the presence of stomach acid or biocides (Bhunia, 2008).

- SPI-7 or Major Pathogenicity Island (MPI) is a 133-kb locus specific for serovar Typhi, Dublin, and Paratyphi. Its genes encode for Vi antigen, a capsular polysaccharide that illicits high fever in typhoid fever infections. SPI-7 also carries the *pil* gene cluster responsible for type IV pili synthesis and the gene that encodes for the SopE effector protein of TTSS (Bhunia, 2008).
- SPI-8 is a 6.8-kb locus that appears to be specific for serovar Typhi. It carries genes for putative bacteriocin biosynthesis but its functional traits have not been fully investigated (Bhunia, 2008).
- SPI-9 is a locus of approximately 16-kb that carries genes for type I secretion system and a large putative RTX (repeat in toxin)-like toxin (Bhunia, 2008). SPI-9 is present in S. Typhi, and also as a pseudogene in S. Typhimurium (EFSA, 2010)
- SPI-10 is a 32.8-kb locus found in serovars Typhi and Enteritidis. It contains genes that encode for Sef fimbriae (Bhunia, 2008).
- *Salmonella* Genomic Island 1 is a 43-kDa locus that contains genes responsible for antimicrobial resistance. It was identified in S. Typhimurium DT104, Paratyphi and Agona, which are resistant to multiple antibiotics. The DT104 strain has been implicated in outbreaks worldwide. It includes genes responsible for five antimicrobial resistance phenotypes (ampicillin, chloramphenicol, streptomycin, sulphonamides, and tetracycline) that are clustered in a multidrug resistance region and are composed of two integrons (Bhunia, 2008).
- High Pathogenicity Island (HPI) contains genes responsible for siderophore biosynthesis, required for iron uptake. The HPI is found in *S. enterica* (Bhunia, 2008).

Islands	Salmonella serovars	Length Kb)	Functions
SPI - 1	*S. enterica* and *S. bongori*	43	TTSS, invasion of host cells
SPI - 2	*S. enterica*	40	TTSS, systemic infection
SPI - 3	*S. enterica* and *S. bongori*	17	Mg2+ uptake, macrophage survival
SPI - 4	*S. enterica* and *S. bongori*	27	Macrophage survival
SPI - 5	*S. enterica* and *S. bongori*	7.6	Enteropathogeniticity
SPI - 6	*S. enterica* subsp. *enterica*	59	Fimbriae
SPI - 7	S. Typhi, S. Dublin, S. Paratphy	133	Vi antigen
SPI - 8	S. Typhi,	6.8	Unknown; putative bacteriocin biosynthesis
SPI - 9	S. Typhy	16.3	Type I secretion system and RTX - like toxin
SPI - 10	S. Typhi, S. Enteritidis	32.8	Sef fimbriae
SGI - 1	S. Typhimurium (DT104), S. Partyphi, S. Agona	43	Antibiotic resistance genes
HPI	*S. enterica* subsp. IIIa, IIIb, IV	?	High affinity iron uptake

Table 2. Main properties and functions of *Salmonella* pathogenicity islands (SPI) (Adapted from Hensel, 2004 and Bhunia, 2008)

Presently, there are over 30 *Salmonella* specific genes that have been used as targets for PCR (Polymerase Chain Reaction) to detect and characterize *Salmonella*. These include *inv*A gene sequences that are highly conserved among all *Salmonella* serotypes, other gene sequences also present throughout the genus, and fimbriae protein-encoding genes and antibiotic resistance genes (Table 3).

Gene Description	Description
invA	Triggers internalization required for invasion of deep tissue cells
InvE/A	Invase proteins
phoP/Q	Intramacrophage survival and enhanced bile resistance
stnB	*Salmonella* enterotoxin gene
irob	Iron regulation
slyA	Salmolysin
hin/H2	Flagellar phase variation
afgA	Thin aggregative fimbriae
fimC	Pathogen related fimbrae gene of *S. enterica*
sefA	Major subunit fimbrial protein of serotype Enterica strains
pefA	Fimbrial virulence gene of *S.* Typhimurium
spvA	Virulence plasmid region
spvB	Virulence plasmid region
spvC	Virulence plasmid region that interacts with the host immune system and is responsible for an increased growth rate in host cells
rep-FIIA	Plasmid incompatibility group
sprC	Virulence gene
sipB-sipC	Junction of virulence genes *sip*B–*sip*C
himA	Encodes a binding protein
his	*Salmonella* genus specific histidine transport operon
prot6e	Virulence plasmid region specific for *S.* Enteritidis
ST M3357	Regulatory protein whose start codon sequence determines the DT phenotype exhibiting enhanced virulence

Table 3. Genes Used for the PCR Identification of *Salmonella* spp. (Adapted from Levin, 2010)

6. Conclusions

Salmonella spp. is one of the major foodborne pathogen responsible for outbreaks worldwide (EECDC, EFSA, 2009; Switt et al., 2009), being estimated to be the main pathogen responsible for foodborne mortality in the United States (Mead et al., 1999). This bacterial genus includes 2,500 identified serotypes, distributed between 2 species: *Salmonella* enterica and *Salmonella* bongori (Foley and Lynne, 2008a). The emergence of new pathogenic strains and serotypes has been described (EFSA, 2010b; Hauser et al., 2010). Due to their increased virulence, these strains can rapidly spread among production animals and humans, representing a major public health issue (EFSA, 2010b; Hauser et al., 2010). In the mid-1990s the emergence of *Salmonella enterica* subsp. *enterica* serotype I,4,[5],12:i:-, a monophasic variant of *Salmonella* Typhimurium, has been reported in Europe (Foley et al., 2008b; Hauser et al., 2010; Switt et al., 2009). Nowadays it seems to be one of the major serotypes responsible for human salmonellosis cases worldwide (EECDC, EFSA, 2009; Switt et al., 2009). It has also been isolated from several animal species, such as poultry, cattle, swine, and turtles, and also from food products, such as poultry and pork products.

In 2010, the European Food Safety Authority (EFSA) Panel on Biological Hazards (BIOHAZ) published a Scientific Opinion alerting for the increasing number of outbreaks in the European Union member states promoted by "*Salmonella* Typhimurium-like" strains. The Panel has recommended that these strains should be further typed and characterized, particularly in terms of antimicrobial resistance (EFSA, 2010b).

Studies aiming at fully characterizing the monophasic variants of *Salmonella* Typhimurium-like strains (4,[5],12:i:–) isolated from different sources, such as food products, animals and the environment, in terms of molecular typing, antimicrobial resistance, virulence traits and immune response modulation, are extremely relevant. Data provided by such studies will have repercussions in preventive and therapeutic strategies, both in human and veterinary medicine.

7. Acknowledgements

This work was supported by CIISA ("Centro de Investigação Interdisciplinar em Sanidade Animal") from the Faculty of Veterinary Medicine, Lisbon. Manuela Oliveira is a FCT ("Fundação para a Ciência e a Tecnologia") funded scientist from the program "Ciência 2007".

8. References

AFSSA (2009). Opinion of the French Food Safety Agency concerning two draft amendments to Orders for controlling salmonellae in the *Gallus gallus* species. 2009-SA-0182, pp-22.

Agasan, A., Kornblum, J., Williams, G., Pratt, C.C., Fleckenstein, P., Wong, M., Ramon, A. (2002). Profile of *Salmonella enterica* subsp. *enterica* (subspecies I) serotype 4,5,12:i:- strains causing food-borne infections in New York City. *Journal of Clinical Microbiology,* 40, 6, (Jun 2002), pp. 1924-1929, ISSN 0095-1137.

Alcaine, S.D., Soyer, Y., Warnick, L.D., Su, W.L., Sukhnanand, S., Richards, J, Fortes, E.D., McDonough, P., Root, T.P., Dumas, N.B., Grohn, Y., Wiedmann. M. (2006). Multilocus sequence typing supports the hypothesis that cow- and human-associated *Salmonella* isolates represent distinct and overlapping populations. *Applied and Environmental Microbiology,* 72, 12, (Dec 2006), pp. 7575-7585, ISSN 0099-2240.

Aldridge, P.D., Wu, C., Gnerer, J., Karlinsey, J.E., Hughes, K.T., Sachs, M.S. (2006). Regulatory protein that inhibits both synthesis and use of the target protein controls flagellar phase variation in *Salmonella enterica. Proceedings of the National Academy of Sciences of The United States of America,* 103, 30, (Jul 2006), pp. 11340–11345, ISSN 0027-8424.

Amavisit, P., Lightfoot, D., Browning, G.F., Markham, P.F. (2003). Variation between pathogenic serovars within *Salmonella* Pathogenicity Islands. *Journal of Bacteriology,* 185, 12, (Jun 2003), pp. 3624–3635, ISSN 0021-9193.

Amavisit, P., Boonyawiwat ,W., Bangtrakulnont, A. (2005). Characterization of *Salmonella* enteric serovar typhimurium and monophasic *Salmonella* serovar I,4,[5],12 : i : - isolates in Thailand. *Journal of Clinical Microbiology*, 43, 6, (Jun 2005), pp. 2736-2740, ISSN 0095-1137.

Antunes, P., Mourão, J., Freitas, A., Peixe, L. (2010). Population structure of multidrug-resistant nontyphoidal *Salmonella enterica* isolates from Portugal. *Clinical Microbiology and Infection*, 16, S371-372, ISSN 1469-0691.

Bailey, A.M., Ivens, A., Kingsley, R., Cottell, J.L., Wain, J., Piddock, L.J. (2010). RamA, a member of the AraC/XylS family, influences both virulence and efflux in *Salmonella enterica* serovar Typhimurium. *Journal of Bacteriology*, 192, 6, (Mar 2010), pp. 1607-1616, ISSN 0021-9193.

Barone, D.L., Dal Vecchio, A., Pellissier, N., Viganò, A., Romani, C., Pontello, M. (2008). Emergence of *Salmonella* Typhimurium monophasic serovar: determinants of antimicrobial resistance in porcine and human strains. *Annali di igiene: medicina preventive e di comunità*, 20, 3, (May-Jun 2008), pp. 199-209, ISSN 11209135.

Bhunia, A.K. (2008). *Salmonella enterica. Foodborne Microbial Pathogens: Mechanisms and Pathogenesis*. Springer, pp 201-216, ISBN: 038774536X, USA.

Bone, A., Noel, H., Le Hello, S., Pihier, N., Danan, C., Raguenaud, M.E., Salah, S., Bellali, H., Vaillant, V., Weill, F.X., Jourdan-da Silva, N. (2010). Nationwide outbreak of *Salmonella enterica* serotype 4,12:i:- infections in France, linked to dried pork sausage. Euro Surveillance, 15, 24, (Mar-May 2010), pp. 1-3.

Briggs, C.E., Fratamico, P. (1999). Molecular characterization of an antibiotic resistance gene cluster of *Salmonella* typhimurium DT104. *Antimicrobial Agents and Chemotherapy*, 43, 4, (Apr 1999), pp. 846-849, ISSN 0305-7453.

Burnens, A., Stanley, J., Sechter, I., Nicolet, J. (1996). Evolutionary origin of a monophasic *Salmonella* serovar, 9,12:l,v:-, revealed by IS200 profiles and restriction fragment polymorphisms of the fljB gene. *Journal of Clinical Microbiology*, 34, 7, (Jul 1996), pp. 1641–1645, ISSN 0095-1137.

Carattoli, A., Tosini, F., Visca, P. (1998). Multidrug-resistant *Salmonella enterica* serotype Typhimurium infections. *The New England Journal of Medicine*. 339, (Sep 1998), pp. 921-922.

CDC. (2007a). Investigation of Outbreak of Human Infections Caused by *Salmonella* I 4,[5],12:i:-. In: *Centers for Disease Control and Prevention*. 15 July 2011. Available from: <http://www.cdc.gov/Salmonella/4512eyeminus.html>.

CDC (2007b). Turtle-Associated Salmonellosis in Humans - United States, 2006-2007. *Morbidity and Mortality Weekly Report*, 56, pp. 649-652.

CDC (2008). *Salmonella* Surveillance: Annual Summary, 2006. *US Department of Health and Human Services*. CDC, Atlanta, Georgia, USA.

de la Torre, E., Zapata, D., Tello, M., Mejia, W., Frias, N., Pena, F.J.G., Mateu, E.M., Torre, E. (2003). Several *Salmonella enterica* subsp *enterica* serotype 4,5,12:i: - Phage types isolated from swine originate from serotype typhimurium DT U302. *Journal of Clinical Microbiology*, 41, 6, (Jun 2003), pp. 2395-2400, ISSN 0095-1137.

del Cerro A., Soto S. M., Mendoza M. C. (2003). Virulence and antimicrobial-resistance gene profiles determined by PCR-based procedures for *Salmonella* isolated from samples of animal origin. *Food Microbiology*, 20, 24, (Aug 2003), pp. 431-438, ISSN 0740-0020.

Delgado R.N., Munoz Bellido J.L., García García M.I., Ibanez Perez R., Munoz Criado S., Serrano Heranz R., Saenz Gonzalez M.C., García Rodríguez J.A. (2006). Molecular epidemiology of drug-resistant *Salmonella* Typhimurium in Spain. *Revista Espanola de Quimioterapia*. 19, 2, (Jun 2006), pp. 152–160, ISSN 0214-3429.

Dionisi, A.M., Graziani, C., Lucarelli, C., Filetici, E., Villa, L., Owczarek, S., Caprioli, A., Luzzi, I. (2009). Molecular Characterization of Multidrug-Resistant Strains of *Salmonella enterica* Serotype Typhimurium and Monophasic Variant (S. 4,[5], 12:i:-) Isolated from Human Infections in Italy. *Foodborne Pathogens and Disease*, 6, 6, (Jul-Aug 2009), pp. 711-717, ISSN 1535-3141.

Echeita, M.A., Díez, R., Usera, M.A. (1999). Distribución de serotipos de *Salmonella spp.* aislados en España durante un periodo de 4 años (1993–1996), 1999. Enfermedades infecciosas y microbiologia clinica. 17, 1, pp. 9–14.

Echeita, M.A., Aladueña, A., Cruchaga, S., Usera, M.A. (1999). Emergence and Spread of an Atypical *Salmonella enterica* subsp. *enterica* Serotype 4,5,12:i:– Strain in Spain. *Journal of Clinical Microbiology*. 37, 10, (Oct 1999), pp. 3425.

Echeita, M.A., Herrera, S., Usera, M.A. (2001). Atypical, fljB-negative *Salmonella enterica* subsp *enterica* strain of serovar 4,5,12:i: appears to be a monophasic variant of serovar typhimurium. *Journal of Clinical Microbiology*, 39, 8, (Aug 2001), pp. 2981-2983, ISSN 0095-1137.

EFSA (2009). Analysis of the baseline survey on the prevalence of *Salmonella* in holdings with breeding pigs, in the EU, 2008, Part A: *Salmonella* prevalence estimates. *EFSA Journal*, 7, 12, (Dec 2008), pp. 1-93.

EFSA (2010a). Trends and Sources of Zoonoses and Zoonotic Agents and Food-borne Outbreaks in the European Union in 2008. *EFSA Journal*, 8, 1, (Jan 2010), pp. 1-48.

EFSA Panel on Biological Hazards (BIOHAZ). (2010b). Scientific Opinion on monitoring and assessment of the public health risk of "*Salmonella* Typhimurium-like" strains. *EFSA Journal*. 8, 10, (Oct 2010), pp. 1-48.

EFSA (2011). EU summary report on trends and sources of zoonoses and zoonotic agents and food-borne outbreaks 2009. *EFSA Journal*. 9, 3, (Mar 2011), pp.1-2.

EECDC; EFSA - Panel on Biological Hazards (BIOHAZ); CVMP-EMA; SCENIHR. (2009). Joint Opinion on antimicrobial resistance (AMR) focused on zoonotic infections. *EFSA Journal*. 7, 11, (Nov 2009), pp. 1-78.

Eswarappa, S.M., Janice, J., Nagarajan, A.G., Balasundaram, S.V., Karnam, G. (2008) Differentially Evolved Genes of *Salmonella* Pathogenicity Islands: Insights into the Mechanism of Host Specificity in *Salmonella*. *PLoS ONE*, 3, 12, (Dec 2008), pp. e3829, ISSN 1932-6203.

Ethelberg, S., Lisby, M., Torpdahl, M., Sorensen, G., Neimann, J., Rasmussen, P., Bang, S., Stamer, U., Hansson, H.B., Nygard, K., Baggesen, D.L., Nielsen, E.M., Molbak, K., Helms, M. (2004). Prolonged restaurant-associated outbreak of multidrug-resistant *Salmonella* Typhimurium among patients from several European countries. *Clinical Microbiology and Infection*, 10, 10, (Oct 2004), pp. 904–910, ISSN 1198-743X.

Foley, S.L., Lynne, A.M. (2008a). Food animal-associated *Salmonella* challenges: Pathogenicity and antimicrobial resistance. *Journal of Animal Science*, 86, 14, (Apr 2008), pp. E173–E187, ISSN 0021-8812.

Foley, S.L., Lynne, A.M., Nayak, R. (2008b). *Salmonella* challenges: Prevalence in swine and poultry and potential pathogenicity of such isolates. *Journal of Animal Science*, 86, 14, (Apr 2008), pp. E149-E162, ISSN 0021-8812.

Friedrich, A., Dorn, C., Schroeter, A., Szabo, I., Jaber, M., Berendonk, G., Brom, M., Ledwolorz, J., Helmuth, R. (2010). [Report on *Salmonella* isolates in livestock, food and feed, received at the German national reference laboratory for Salmonella during 2004-2008]. *Berliner und Münchener tierärztliche Wochenschrift*, 123, 7-8, (Jul-Aug 2010), pp. 265-277, ISSN 0005-9366.

Garaizar, J., Porwollik, S., Echeita, A., Rementeria, A., Herrera, S., Wong, R.M.Y., Frye, J., Usera, M.A., McClelland, M. (2002). DNA microarray-based typing of an atypical monophasic *Salmonella* enterica serovar. *Journal of Clinical Microbiology*, 40, 6, (Jun 2002), pp. 2074-2078, ISSN 0095-1137.

Garaizar, J., Porwollik, S., Echeita, A., Rementeria, A., Herrera, S., Wong, R. M.Y., Frye, J., Usera, M.A., McClelland, M M. (2003). DNA microarray-based typing of atypical monophasic *Salmonella* serovar (4,5,12:i:-) strains emergent in Spain. *Infection, Genetics and Evolution*, 2, pp. 286-287, ISSN 1567- 1348.

Gebreyes, W.A., Altier, C. (2002). Molecular characterization of multidrug-resistant *Salmonella enterica* subsp. *enterica* serovar Typhimurium isolates from swine. *Journal of Clinical Microbiology*, 40, 8, (Aug 2002), pp. 2813–2822, ISSN 0095-1137.

Grimont, P.A.D., Weill, F-X. (2007). *Antigenic formulae of the* Salmonella *serovars* (9th edition). WHO Collaborating Centre for Reference and Research on *Salmonella*. Institute Pasteur, Paris, France

Guerra, B., Laconcha, I., Soto, S.M., Gonzalez-Hevia, M.A., Mendoza, M.C. (2000). Molecular characterisation of emergent multiresistant *Salmonella enterica* serotype [4,5,12:i:-] organisms causing human salmonellosis. *FEMS Microbiology Letters*, 190, 2, (Sep 2000), pp. 341-347, ISSN 0378-1097.

Guerra, B., Soto, S.M., Arguelles, J.M., Mendoza, M.C. (2001). Multidrug resistance is mediated by large plasmids carrying a class 1 integron in the emergent *Salmonella* enterica serotype [4,5,12 : i :-]. *Antimicrobial Agents and Chemotherapy*, 45, 4, (Apr 2001), pp. 1305-1308, ISSN 0066-4804.´

Hampton, M.D., Threlfall, E.J., Frost, J.A., Ward, L.R., Rowe, B. (1995). *Salmonella* typhimurium DT 193: differentiation of an epidemic phage type by antibiogram, plasmid profile, plasmid fingerprint and *Salmonella* plasmid virulence (spv) gene probe. *Journal of Applied Bacteriology*, 78, 4 (Apr 1995), pp. 402-408, ISSN 0370-1778.

Hauser, E., Huhn, S., Junker, E., Jaber, M., Schroeter, A., Helmuth, R., Rabsch, W., Winterhoff, N., Malorny, B. (2009). Characterisation of a phenotypic monophasic variant belonging to *Salmonella enterica* subsp *enterica* serovar Typhimurium from wild birds and its possible transmission to cats and humans. *Berliner und Münchener tierärztliche Wochenschrift*, 122, 5-6, (May-Jun 2009), pp. 169-177, ISSN 0005-9366.

Hauser, E., Tietze, E., Helmuth, R., Junker, E., Blank, K., Prager, R., Rabsch, W., Appel, B., Fruth, A., Malorny. B. (2010a). Pork contaminated with *Salmonella enterica* serovar 4,[5],12:i:-, an emerging health risk for humans. *Applied and Environmental Microbiology*, 76, 14, (Jul 2010), pp. 4601-4610, ISSN 0099-2240.

Helaine, S., Thompson, J.A., Watson, K.G., Liu, M., Boyle, C., Holden, D.W. (2010). Dynamics of intracellular bacterial replication at the single cell level. *Proceedings of the National Academy of Sciences of the United States of America*, 107, (Feb 2010), pp. 3746- 3751, ISSN 0027-8424.

Hoelzer, K., Soyer, Y., Rodriguez-Rivera, L.D., Cummings, K.J., McDonough, P.L., Schoonmaker-Bopp, D.J., Root, T.P., Dumas, N.B., Warnick, L.D., Grohn, Y.T., Wiedmann, M., Baker, K.N., Besser, T.E., Hancock, D.D., Davis, M.A. (2010). The prevalence of multidrug resistance is higher among bovine than human *Salmonella enterica* serotype Newport, Typhimurium, and 4,5,12:i:- isolates in the United States but differs by serotype and geographic region. *Applied and Environmental Microbiology*, 76, 17, (Sep 2010), pp. 5947-5959, ISSN 0099-2240.

Hopkins, K.L., Kirchner, M., Guerra, B., Granier, S.A., Lucarelli, C., Porrero, M.C., Jakubczak, A., Threlfall, E.J., Mevius, D.J. (2010). Multiresistant *Salmonella enterica* serovar 4,[5],12:i:- in Europe: a new pandemic strain?. Eurosurveillance, 15, 22, (Jun 2010), pp. 1-9.

Hopkins, K.L., Nair, S., Kirchner, M., Guerra, B., Granier, S., Lucarelli, C., Porrero, C., Jakubczak, A., Threlfall, E.J., Mevius, D. (2010). Genetic variation in emerging multidrug-resistant *Salmonella enterica* 4,[5],12:i:- from seven European countries. *Proceedings of the 110th General Meeting of the American Society for Microbiology*, ISBN 1555816231, San Diego, CA, May 2010.

Ibarra, J.A., Steele-Mortimer, O. (2009). *Salmonella*--the ultimate insider. *Salmonella* virulence factors that modulate intracellular survival. *Cell Microbiology*, 11, 11, pp. 1579-1586, ISSN: 1462-5822

Kirk, M.D., Veitch, M.G., Hall, G.V. (2010). Gastroenteritis and food-borne disease in elderly people living in long-term care. *Clinical Infectious Diseases*, 50, 3 (Feb 2010), pp. 397-404, ISSN 1058-4838.

Laorden, L., Bikandi, J., Herrera-Leon, S., Sanchez, A., Echeita, A., Rementeria, A., Garaizar. J. (2009). Characterisation and evolutionary study of *Salmonella enterica* [4,5,12:i:-] using PFGE, MLVA, PCR and sequencing techniques. *Proceedings of the 3rd ASM Conference on Salmonella: Biology, Pathogenesis and Prevention*, ISBN 9781555815448, Aix-en-Provence, France, October 2009.

Laorden, L., Herrera-León, S., Sanchez, A., Bikandi, J., Rementeria, A., Echeita, A., Garaizar, J. (2010). Six types of deletions detected in monophasic *Salmonella enterica* 4,[5],12:i:- strains. *Proceedings of the 9th International Meeting on Molecular Epidemiological Markers*, Wernigerode, Germany, September 2010.

Levin, R.E. (2010). *Salmonella. Rapid Detection and Characterization of Foodborne Pathogens by Molecular techniques*, CRC Press, Taylor & Francis Group, ISBN 10 1420092421, Amherst, USA, pp. 79-138.

Lucarelli, C., Dionisi, A.M., Torpdahl, M., Villa, L., Graziani, C., Hopkins, K., Threlfall, J., Caprioli, A., Luzzi, I. (2010). Evidence for a second genomic island conferring multidrug resistance in a clonal group of strains of *Salmonella enterica* serovar Typhimurium and its monophasic variant circulating in Italy, Denmark, and the United Kingdom. *Journal of Clinical Microbiology*, 48, 6, (Jun 2010), pp. 2103-2109, ISSN: 0095-1137.

Machado, J., Bernardo, F. (1990). Prevalence of *Salmonella* in chicken carcasses in Portugal. *Journal of Applied Bacteriology*, 69, 4, (Oct 1990), pp. 477-480, ISSN 1364-5072.

Marcus, S.L., Brumell, J.H., Pfeifer, C.G., Finlay, B.B. (2000). *Salmonella* pathogenicity islands: big virulence in small packages. *Microbes and Infection*, 2, 2, (Feb 2000), pp. 145–156, ISSN 1286-4579.

Martins da Costa, P., Oliveira, M., Bica, A., Vaz-Pires, P., Bernardo, F. (2007). Antimicrobial resistance in *Enterococcus* spp. and *Escherichia coli* isolated from poultry feed and feed ingredients. *Veterinary Microbiology,* 120, 1-2, (Feb 2007), pp. 122–131, ISSN 0378-1135.

Mead, P.S., Slutsker, L., Dietz, V., McCaig, L.F., Bresee, J.S., Shapiro, C., Griffin, P.M., Tauxe, R.V. (1999). Food-Related Illness and Death in the United States. *Emerging Infectious Diseases*, 5, 5, (Oct 1999), pp. 607-625, ISSN 1080-6059.

Monroe, S., Polk, R. (2000). Antimicrobial use and bacterial resistance. *Current Opinion in Microbiology*, 3, 5, (Oct 2000), pp. 496–501, ISSN 1369- 5274.

Mossong, J., Marques, P., Ragimbeau, C., Huberty-Krau, P., Losch, S., Meyer, G., Moris, G., Strottner, C., Rabsch, W. Schneider, F. (2007). Outbreaks of monophasic *Salmonella enterica* serovar 4,[5],12:i:- in Luxembourg, 2006. *Eurosurveillance*, 12, 6, (Jun 2007), pp. 156-158, ISSN 1560-7917.

Pang, T., Levine, M.M., Ivanoff, B., Wain, J., Finlay, B.B. (1998). Typhoid fever—important issues still remain. *Trends in Microbiology*, 6, 4, (April 1998), pp. 131–133, ISSN 0966-842X.

Peters, T., Hopkins, K.L., Lane, C., Nair, S., Wain, J., de Pinna, E. (2010). Emergence and characterization of *Salmonella enterica* serovar Typhimurium phage type DT191a. *Journal of Clinical Microbiology*, 48, 9, (Sep 2010), pp. 3375- 3377, ISSN 0095-1137.

Popoff, M.Y., Le Minor, L. (1997). *Antigenic formulas of the Salmonella serovars* (7th edition). WHO Collaborating Centre for Reference and Research on *Salmonella,* Institut Pasteur, Paris, France.

Pornruangwong, S., Sriyapai, T., Pulsrikarn, C., Sawanpanyalert, P., Boonmar, S., Bangtrakulnonth, A. (2008). The epidemiological relationship between *Salmonella enterica* serovar typhimurium *and Salmonella enterica* serovar 4,[5],12:1:- isolates from humans and swine in Thailand. *Southeast Asian Journal of Tropical Medicine and Public Health,* 39, 2, pp. 288-296, ISSN 0125-1562.

Sala, A. (2002). Tracing the origin of monophasic serovar *S. enterica* I 4, 5,12: I:-: Genetic similarity with *S. enterica* typhimurium. *Medicina (Ribeirao Preto),* 35, 1, 510-511, ISSN 2176-7262.

Saroj, S.D., Shashidhar, R., Karani, M., Bandekar, J.R. (2008). Distribution of *Salmonella* pathogenicity island (SPI)-8 and SPI-10 among different serotypes of *Salmonella.* Journal of Medical Microbiology, 57, 4, (Apr 2008), pp. 424-427, ISSN 0022-2615.

Sayah, R.S., Kaneene, J.B., Johnson, Y., Miller, R. (2005). Patterns of antimicrobial resistance observed in *Escherichia coli* isolates obtained from domestic- and wild animal fecal samples, human septage, and surface water. *Applied and Environmental Microbiology,* 71, 3, (Mar 2005), pp. 1394–1404, ISSN 0099-2240.

Soyer, Y., Switt, A.M., Davis, M.A., Maurer, J., McDonough, P.L., Schoonmaker-Bopp, D.J., Dumas, N.B., Root, T., Warnick, L.D., Grohn, Y.T., Wiedmann, M. (2009). *Salmonella* enterica serotype 4,5,12:i:-, an emerging *Salmonella* serotype that represents multiple distinct clones. *Journal of Clinical Microbiology,* 47, 11, (Nov 2009), pp. 3546-3556, ISSN 0095-1137.

Stevens, M.P., Humphrey, T.J., Maskell, D.J. (2009). Molecular insights into farm animal and zoonotic *Salmonella* infections. *Philosophical Transations of the Royal Society B,* 364, 1530, (Sep 2009), pp. 2709–2723, ISSN 0962-8436.

Switt, A.I.M., Soyer, Y., Warnick, L.D., Wiedmann, M. (2009). Emergence, distribution and molecular and phenotypic characteristics of *Salmonella enterica* serotype 4,5,12:i:-. *Foodborne Pathogens and Disease,* 6, 4, (May 2009), pp. 407–415, ISSN 1535-3141.

Tavechio, A.T., Fernandes, S.A., Ghilardi, A.C.R., Soule, G., Ahmed, R., Melles, C.E.A. (2009). Tracing lineage by phenotypic and genotypic markers in *Salmonella enterica* subsp *enterica* serovar I,4,[5],12:i:- and *Salmonella* Typhimurium isolated in state of Sao Paulo, Brazil. *Memórias Do Instituto Oswaldo Cruz,* 104, 7, (Nov 2009), pp. 1042-1046, ISSN 0074-0276.

Téllez, S., Briones, V., González, S., García-Pena, F.J., Altimira, A., Vela, A.I., Blanco, M.M., Ballesteros, C., Fernández-Garayzábal, J.F., Goyache, J. (2002). *Salmonella* septicaemia in a beauty snake (*Elaphe taeniura taeniura*): a case report. *The Veterinary Record,* 151, 1, (Jul 2002), pp. 28-29, ISSN 0042-4900.

Tierrez A., Garcia-del Portillo F. (2005). New concepts in *Salmonella* virulence: the importance of reducing the intracellular growth rate in the host. *Cellular Microbiology,* 7, 7, (Jul 2005), pp. 901-909, ISSN 1462-5822.

Torpdahl, M., Litrup, E., Nielsen, E.M. (2009). Caracterisation and prevalence of *Salmonella* 4,5,12:i:- in Denmark, the monophasic variant of *Salmonella* Typhimurium. *Proceedings of the 3rd ASM Conference on Salmonella: Biology, Pathogenesis and Prevention,* ISBN 9781555815448, Aix-en-Provence, France, October 2009.

Trupschuch, S., Gomez J.A.L., Ediberidze, I., Flieger, A., Rabsch, W. (2010). Characterisation of multidrug-resistant *Salmonella Typhimurium* 4,[5],12:i:- DT193 strains carrying a novel genomic island adjacent to the thrW tRNA locus. *International Journal of Medical Microbiology,* 300, 5, pp. 279-288, ISSN 1438-4221.

Van Pelt, W., Schimmer, B., Stenvers, O.F.J., Langelaar M.F.M. (2009). *Staat van zoönosen 2007-2008.* National Institute for Public Health and the Environment, pp. 64.

Vieira-Pinto, M., Temudo, P., Martins, C. (2005). Occurrence of *Salmonella* in the ileum, ileocolic lymph nodes, tonsils, mandibular lymph nodes and carcasses of pigs slaughtered for consumption. *Journal of Veterinary Medicine Serie B,* 52, 10, pp. 476-481, ISSN 0931-1793.

Yamamoto, S., Kutsukake, K. (2006). *fljA*-mediated posttranscriptional control of phase 1 flagellin expression in flagellar phase variation of *Salmonella enterica* serovar Typhimurium. *Journal of Bacteriology,* 188, 3, (Feb 2006), pp. 958–967, ISSN 0021-9193.

Zaidi, M.B., Leon, V., Canche, C., Perez, C., Zhao, S., Huber, S.K., Abbott, J., Blickenstaff, K., McDermott, P.F. (2007). Rapid and widespread dissemination of multidrug-resistant blaCMY-2 *Salmonella* Typhimurium in Mexico. *Journal of Antimicrobial Chemotherapy,* 60, (May 2007), pp. 398-401, ISSN 0305-7453.

Zamperini, K., Soni, V., Waltman, D., Sanchez, S., Theriault, E.C., Bray, J., Maurer, J.J. (2007). Molecular Characterization Reveals *Salmonella* enterica Serovar 4,[5],12:i:2-from Poultry Is a Variant Typhimurium Serovar. *Avian Diseases,* 51, 4, (Dec 2007), 958-964, ISSN 0005-2086.

Zhao, Y. (2001). *Virulence factors of Salmonella enterica serovar Enteritidis*. PhD Thesis. Faculty of Veterinary Medicine, Utrecht University, Utrech, The Netherlands, pp. 96.

16

Salmonella: Invasion, Evasion & Persistence

Belal Chami and Shisan Bao
The University of Sydney, Bosch Institute
Australia

1. Introduction

The gastrointestinal tract, home to a large flora of commensal bacteria, performs the essential role of degradation and absorption of food via gastrointestinal epithelia. The semi-permeability of the epithelial barrier allows for food-derived nutrients to pass through and enter the bloodstream, while simultaneously acting as a physical and chemical barricade towards microbes. Despite this, many bacteria have evolved the means to elude the gastrointestinal tract and migrate to underlying host tissue, causing disease. These disease-causing bacteria are largely thought to obtain their virulence through horizontal gene transfer, which has enabled the bacterium to overcome the epithelial barrier and disguise itself from the intestinal immune system (Flannagan et al., 2009).

Salmonella species are facultative, gram-negative intracellular bacteria harbouring over 2000 serovars; however, only a handful is associated with disease in humans. While *Salmonella* remains the leading cause of bacterial gastroenteritis, it is also one the most extensively studied and well characterised bacterial species. Worldwide, *Salmonella* is thought to cause ~1.3 billion cases of human disease, including diarrhoea and typhoid fever (McGhie et al., 2009). Moreover, 3-5% of patients with typhoid fever develop persistent infection of the gallbladder which acts as a crucial reservoir to the human-specific *Salmonella enteric serotype* typhi (S. Typhi). The recent development of the streptomycin pre-treated murine model of *Salmonella* enterica serovar typhimurium (S. Typhimurium) has become the pinnacle in gaining critical insight into the pathogenesis of diseases caused by *Salmonella*. More specifically, it has enabled scientists to investigate molecular mechanisms of invasion, evasion, intracellular survival and persistence of *Salmonella* in host tissue.

In this chapter, we aim to decipher the pathogenesis of *Salmonell*a by breaking down and exploring the effects of various virulence factors in *Salmonella*. The knowledge of the molecular basis of host-pathogen interactions will bring help bridge the gap between molecular events and clinical presentations of Salmonellosis.

2. Internalization of Salmonella

2.1 M cells

Membraneous epithelilal (M) cells are sparsely distributed, specialized cells characterized by an irregular microvilli apical surface and a basolateral cytoplasmic invagination (or an intraepithelial pocket) which can harbour lymphocytes or macrophages. M cells are not randomly distributed; rather they reside in the specialised follicle-associated epithelium (FAE) overlying lymphoid aggregates such as Peyer's patches. The molecular features of the apical surface of M cells promote adherence, uptake and sampling of inert particles and microbes within the lumen, which are transferred to the underlying lymphoid tissue where immunological responses are initiated (Kraehenbuhl & Neutra, 2000). In most cases, only antigens that adhere to the surface of M cells induce strong immunological responses. However, several types of bacteria and viruses are known to exploit M cells by selectively adhering to the apical surface, internalising themselves and evading mucosal immune responses (Neutra et al., 1996; Sansonetti & Phalipon, 1999). Numerous studies have shown both S. Typhi (Kohbata et al., 1986; Pascopella et al., 1995) and S. Typhimurium (Clark et al., 1994; Jones et al., 1994) preferentially target and invade mouse M cells and that S. Typhimurium also invades M cells in calf ileal loops (Frost et al., 1997). Despite these reports, there is a lack of direct evidence that human M cells are a major site of *Salmonella* invasion, although it is widely speculated that sites of *Salmonella* evasion in humans parallel mice and calf studies. Supporting this is the presence of ulcerations corresponding to the position of Peyer's patches in human typhoid (Owen, 1994).

Studies of S. Typhimurium invasion in murine and calf M cells have revealed active processes of internalization. Membrane ruffles are a crucial determinate of salmonella invasion, as demonstrated in cultured epithelial cell lines (Galan & Collmer, 1999). The membrane 'ruffler' formation results from extensive rearrangement of M cell apical membranes due to the redistribution of polymerised actin to form membrane protrusions (Clark et al., 1994; Frost et al., 1997; Jones et al., 1994). This process is triggered by a active process in which the ultimate result is engulfment of *Salmonella*. It should be noted that not all bacterial uptake by M cells involves specialised adaptive processes. Some of the bacteria entry, such as in the case of *Salmonella*, is performed in a passive fashion by taking advantage of the M cell sampling and uptaking abilities. Although M cells appear to play a major role in salmonella internalization and evasion, this highly adaptive pathogen is able to exploit other routes that all amount to the pathogenesis of *Salmonella*.

2.2 Macrophages

Professional antigen presenting cells, such as macrophages are endlessly sampling luminal contents, phagocytising potential pathogens and presenting antigens to adaptive immune cells, in a process of maintaining host protection against potentially harmful microbes. Phagocytic uptake of gram-negative bacteria (such as *Salmonella*) is a complex mechanism which involves various receptors and interactions. Of particular importance are Pattern-recognition receptors that recognise pathogen-associated molecular patterns that include lipopolysaccharides and flagellin. Macrophages are thought to readily recognise and engulf *Salmonella* in a independent fashion, thus offering an alternative independent point of entry.

2.3 Enterocytes

Enterocytes are simple columnar epithelial cells found in the intestine which offer the first line of defence against microbes in the lumen. Despite employing a vast array of protective features, many microbes including *Salmonella* have evolved strategies to secure their survival in host cells by manipulating cellular structures, as observed in M cells. Therefore, *Salmonella* also invades enterocytes by employing membrane ruffles.

2.4 Dendritic cells (DC)

DCs are a heterogeneous group of cells that are categorized primarily by their resident tissue. They are best known for their ability to capture and present antigens and have been heavily implicated in host immune responses and self-tolerance. *Salmonella* appears to possess the ability to cross the gut epithelial via DCs. It has been proposed that *Salmonella* from the intestinal lumen is absorbed via dendritic projections that pass between adjacent intestinal epithelial cells without disturbing the epithelial barrier integrity (Rescigno et al., 2001). This is through the utilization of fimbriae which selectively adheres *Salmonella* to dendritic projections, allowing *Salmonella* to invade DCs, thereby utilizing DCs as an additional entry point, as demonstrated in a recent study (Guo et al., 2007).

3. Virulence genes

The presence of virulence determinants in S. Typhimurium, and the somewhat related pathogenic *E.coli,* are thought to be acquired by lateral gene transfer (Boyd & Brussow, 2002; Schmidt & Hensel, 2004). Pathogenicity islands (PAI) describe chromosomal regions that contain virulence genes which are otherwise absent in non-pathogenic or closely related strains species (Hacker et al., 1990; Lavigne & Blanc-Potard, 2008). They are typically inserted adjacent to tRNA genes and their overall base composition differs markedly from the native bacterial chromosome, thereby implying they are acquired from a foreign source (Daigle, 2008). According to Schmidt and Hensel, 2004., five major PAI's have been identified in S. Typhimurium, which are referred to as *Salmonella* pathogenicity islands (SPI) (Schmidt & Hensel, 2004). The human-specific S. Typhi contains a chromosomal region of virulence, SPI-7, not present in S. Typhimurium which causes unique clinical presentations in patients affected, such as typhoid fever.

3.1 SPI-1

T3SS-1, encoded by SPI-1, is required for SPI-1-dependant internalisation of non-pathogenic cells, such as M cells and epithelial cells, and mediates the translocation of effector proteins into eukaryotic cells (Ehrbar et al., 2002; Lostroh & Lee, 2001; Mills et al., 1995). At least 15 effectors can be translocated by T3SS-1, most of which are encoded on the SPI-1, such as SptP, SipA, SipB and AvrA (McGhie et al., 2009). Until recently, T3SS-1 effectors were thought only important for the internalization of *Salmonella;* however recent of studies have revealed that many effectors of T3SS-1 have important roles in post-invasion processes that are discussed later in this chapter.

3.2 SPI-2

T3SS-2, encoded by SPI-2, is required for intracellular replication and immune evasion (Ochman et al., 1996; Shea et al., 1996; Waterman & Holden, 2003). Known effectors of T3SS-2, encoded on SPI-2, include SpiC, SseF, SseG, whereas SifA, SifB, PipB, PipB2, SseI, SseJ, SseL, SspH2, GogB are other effectors of T3SS-2 which are encoded on a different loci (Lavigne & Blanc-Potard, 2008). To date, the effectors of T3SS-2 remain less understood than effectors of T3SS-1, although it is widely established that T3SS-2 is required for survival within host cells (Hensel et al., 1998). Several studies have also highlighted the importance of SPI-2 in systemic infection, while noting its contribution in intestinal disease and inflammation (Bispham et al., 2001; Coburn et al., 2005; Coombes et al., 2005; Hapfelmeier et al., 2005). T3SS-2 evasion processes are discussed in greater detail later in this chapter.

3.3 SPI-3

SPI-3 encodes virulence factors that are important in intestinal colonization and intracellular survival. MgtC is an inner membrane protein, common to several intracellular pathogens, required for intramacrophage survival (Alix & Blanc-Potard, 2007; Blanc-Potard & Groisman, 1997). SPI-2 also encodes MisL, a type V secretion system (T5SS) (Blanc-Potard et al., 1999; Henderson et al., 2004). Although not much is known about MisL, a recent study of S. Typhimurium demonstrates that MisL is important for intestinal colonization by promoting S. Typhimurium binding to fibronectin (Dorsey et al., 2005).

3.4 SPI-4

SPI-4 encodes a type I secretion system (T1SS) and also a substrate of T1SS, SiiE, a large (600kDa) surface-associated non-fimbrial adhensin that contributes to invasion and adhension to eukaryotic cells (Gerlach et al., 2007). Although encoded by SPI-4, SiiE is also coregulated by SPI-1. Little is known about the precise function of SPI-4, however a study in both calf and mouse models have revealed a role of SiiE in colonization and intestinal inflammation (Morgan et al., 2007).

3.5 SPI-5

Many additional effectors of T3SS-1, including SopA, SopB, SopD, SopE, SopE2, Ssph1 and Slrp, are not encoded on SPI-1; rather they are encoded by other horizontally acquired elements, such as on SPI-5 (Lavigne & Blanc-Potard, 2008; Wood et al., 1998). Some of these effectors, namely SopB and SopE/SopE2 induce dramatic rearrangement of the actin cytoskeleton in host cells, which results in large membrane ruffles and subsequent internalization of *Salmonella* (McGhie et al., 2009).

3.6 SPI-7

SPI-7 is a large 134 kb segment that encodes the Vi capsular polysaccharide antigen, Type IV pili and SopE (Hornick et al., 1970). The *viaB* locus is a 14Kb region within SPI-7 that prevents host recognition of *Salmonella* by TLR4 and TLR5 (Raffatellu et al., 2005). The locus contains genes that synthesize, regulate and export the Vi capsular antigen. The presence of the Vi antigen contributes greatly to the virulence in *S. Typi*, which is required for intracellular survival in phagocytes and has been implicated in system dissemination by virtue of its role in serum resistance (Hirose et al., 1997; Looney & Steigbigel, 1986). It should be noted that SPI-7 is expressed in S. Typhi and is absent in S. Typhimurium.

3.7 Fimbriae & biofilm

Four different types of fimbriae are known to be expressed by *Salmonella* that include type 1 fimbriae, plasma-encoded fimbriae, long polar fimbriae and thin aggregrative fimbriae (curli), all of which seem to have specificities for different cell types (Darwin & Miller, 1999). A recent study has shown fimbriae, namely type 1 fimbrial adhesion FimH, mediates *Salmonella* uptake into murine DCs in a T3SS-independent fashion (Guo et al., 2007). It is thought that 13 fimbrial loci exist in *Salmonella*, which are thought to aid the internalization process through biofilm formation, attachment to host cells and colonization (Humphries et al., 2001). Conversely, an earlier study has demonstrated a more invasive behavior of an S. Typhi mutant strain carrying a deletion of the *fim* genes (encoding type 1 fimbriae) compared to its wild-type strain (Miyake et al., 1998). It is thought that in the absence of type 1 fimbrial adhesions, various interactions between bacterial surface proteins and host cells may become more enhanced and result in a higher degree of invasion. BapA, a large cell-surface protein is also required for biofilm formation and subsequent evasion and colonization, similar to FimH (Latasa et al., 2005). BapA is secreted through T1SS (BapBCD) and its expression is orchestrated with genes encoding other fimbriae, suggesting important interplay in overall biofilm formation. The significance of the biofilm stems from the extreme environmental conditions the bacteria are subjected to, and their successful survival lies in their ability to grow in surface-attached biofilms protected by an extracellular matrix (Costerton et al., 1995; Davey & O'Toole G, 2000). The formation of biofilms, particularly in the gall bladder, contributes greatly to pathogenesis of chronically infected S. Typhi individuals.

3.8 Flagella

The role of flagella in *Salmonellosis* remains controversial due, in part, to seemingly conflicting studies and poorly understood intracellular mechanisms. For example, the evasiveness of *Salmonella* is increased via flagellar-based motility, despite the fact several studies have demonstrated that flagellin monomers are potent inducers of innate immunity (Franchi et al., 2006; Miao et al., 2006; Schmitt et al., 2001). Conversely, it has been well demonstrated that flagellin interacts with T3SS-1 from *Salmonella*-infected macrophages and is translocated into the cytosol resulting in activation of the inflammasome and subsequent cell death via caspase-1 pathway (discussed later in the chapter) (Miao et al., 2007; Ren et al., 2006; Sun et al., 2007).

4. Evasion of salmonella

4.1 The *Salmonella*-containing vacuole (SCV)

Following internalization, *Salmonella* becomes engrossed within a vacuole in which it is able to survive and replicate intracellularly. These vacuoles, termed *Salmonella*-containing vacuole (SCV) are characterised by the transformation of cell markers as the vacuole matures, displaying late endosome and lysosome markers, particularly lysosomes glycoprotein markers (Steele-Mortimer et al., 1999). Concurrent to marker transformation post-invasion, SCVs migrate from the periphery plasma membrane to a juxtanuclear position at the microtubule-organising centre (Deiwick et al., 2006; Salcedo & Holden, 2003). In some cell types, the onset of intracellular replication are marked by the presence of *Salmonella*-induced filaments (Sifs) which are branched membrane tubules expelling from the SCV (Drecktrah et al., 2008). Within the SCV, various processes occur, such as *Salmonella* transformation and immune modulation, which are imperative for survival, replication and dissemination of *Salmonella*. Following internalisation of *Salmonella* and translocation of SPI, SPI-effectors are localized to different cellular compartments, such as the Golgi apparatus and lysosomes (Freeman et al., 2003; Haraga & Miller, 2003; Knodler et al., 2003; Salcedo & Holden, 2003). The differential localisation pattern indicates the ability of SPI-effectors and thereby *Salmonella* to manipulate various aspects of host cell function.

4.2 Maturation and trafficking of SCV

Initially, when SCV form, they are characterized by early endocytic markers, such as transferrin receptor (TfnR), early endosomal antigen 1 (EEA1) and several Rab GTPases, such as Rab4/5 & 11. In an effort to curb or delay lysosomal fusion, SCV deviates from the endocytic pathway, thereby reducing the likelihood of lysis of *Salmonella*. (Steele-Mortimer, 2008). Maturing SCVs are characterised by replacement of earlier endocytic markers by later markers including Rab7, vacuolar ATPase (v-ATPase) and lysosomal membrane glycoproteins (1pgs), such as LAMP-1 (Steele-Mortimer, 2008).

Several studies have implicated the effectors of T3SS-1, namely SopE and SopB in the maturation of SCV and replication of *Salmonella* within. SopE and SopB are required for the recruitment of Rab5 within the SCV, which binds the phosphatidylinositol 3-kinase (PI(3)P) Vps34 required for LAMP-1 recruitment (Mallo et al., 2008; Mukherjee et al., 2001; Steele-Mortimer, 2008). Vps34 also acts via PI(3)P on the SCV membrane, which enables recruitment of EEA1(Mallo et al., 2008). SopB acts by inhibiting the degradation of epidermal growth factor receptor (EGFR) by lysosomes (Dukes et al., 2006). In a recent study, SopB has been attributed to the disappearance of late endosomal markers by recruiting sorting nexin-1 (SNX-1) which is speculated to down-regulate mannose 6-phosphate receptor from maturing SCV (Bujny et al., 2008). Collectively, the current data pins a role for SopB in diverting SCV trafficking from the endosomal maturation pathway. In addition to this, SopB has also been demonstrated to indirectly increase intracellular *Salmonella* replication, via activation of Akt, which in turn deactivates Rab14 GAP, AS160 (Layton & Galyov, 2007). The activated Rab14 increases intracellular *Salmonella* replication most likely by delaying SCV-lysosomal fusion (Kuijl et al., 2007). On the same note, SpiC, an effector of T3SS-2 is thought to prevent fusion of macrophage-late lysosomes with SCV (Steele-Mortimer, 2008).

SseJ, another effector of T3SS-2 on the SPI-2, is localised to the SCVs and SIFs. A study in SseJ null mutant mice has revealed that SseJ is required for full virulence of *Salmonella* (Ruiz-Albert et al., 2002). More specifically, an *in vitro* study has revealed deacylase activity of SseJ, while portraying its role in esterification of cholesterol, which is enriched in SCV (Brumell et al., 2001; Catron et al., 2002; Garner et al., 2002; Ohlson et al., 2005). It is thought the esterification of cholesterol could disrupt cell-signalling platforms or inhibit molecular interactions of complexes on the SCV, ultimately interfering with vesicular trafficking (Ohlson et al., 2005).

SopA, an effector of SPI-1, promotes bacterial escape from the SCV in HeLa cells (Diao et al., 2008). It is one of several effectors that is structurally and functionally similar to HECT E3 ubiquitin ligases and is thought to have a role in disrupting SCV membrane integrity (Steele-Mortimer, 2008; Zhang et al., 2006).

4.3 Sif biogenesis

As mentioned previously, maturing SCVs migrate from the peripheral towards the perinuclear region of the host cell, strategically positioning themselves adjacent to the Golgi apparatus. This seems to be important for promoting bacterial replication and survival, and, as a recent study suggests, the close proximity of SCV to the Golgi apparatus may enable interception of endocytic and exocyclic transport vesicles to stockpile nutrients and/or membrane materials (Ramsden et al., 2007). In line with this, exocytic transport vesicles are able to be averted from their normal path under the influence of SifA, SseG and SseF towards the SCV (Kuhle et al., 2006).

In epithelial cells, SseG and SseF are required for the maintenance of SCV at the perinuclear region, while also appearing to be important for intracellular replication (Deiwick et al., 2006). SseG and Ssef are thought to either form 'tethers' from the SCV to the Golgi apparatus or manipulate dynein activity in an attempt to 'glue' the SCV to the microtubule-organising centre (MTOC) (Kuhle & Hensel, 2002; Ramsden et al., 2007; Salcedo & Holden, 2003). SopB is also required for the retention of the SCV within the perinuclear region by mediating the phosphorylation of actin-associated motor myosin II light chain (MLC) (Wasylnka et al., 2008).

Once the SCV has positioned itself near the perinuclear region of the host cell, replication is initiated and is characterised by LAMP-rich specialised tubulovesicular structures called *Salmonella*-induced filaments (Sifs) that project from the SCV. The fusion of late endosome with the SCV is thought to induce Sif formation, however the precise role of Sifs remains elusive (McGhie et al., 2009; Steele-Mortimer, 2008). SifA is essential for the formation and maintenance of Sifs, by which SifA and two other T3SS-2 effectors, PibB2 and SseJ, cooperate to induce and drive extensions of Sif tubules from the juxtanuclear SCV towards the periphery of the host cell (Brumell et al., 2002; Henry et al., 2006; Knodler & Steele-Mortimer, 2005). SifA is localised to the SCV by the TS33-1 effector SipA, where it forms a functional complex with the host protein SKIP (SifA and kinesin-interacting protein) (Brawn et al., 2007). SKIP has been shown to bind to the PibB2-induced microtubule-based motor kinesin-1 that drives Sif extensions (Boucrot et al., 2005; Brawn et al., 2007; Henry et al., 2006). SKIP also directly interacts with various GTPases such as rab9 which is implicated in lysosome positioning and function, potentially displacing it from this complex (Barbero et al., 2002; Ganley et al., 2004; Jackson et al., 2008). In addition to this, SifA is also able to bind to rab7, uncoupling it from RILP and recruiting RhoA, another GTPase that promotes membrane tubulation when activated in the presence of SKIP and SseJ (Harrison et al., 2004; Lossi et al., 2008; Ohlson et al., 2008; Ramsden et al., 2007). Moreover, SseF and SseG are believed to augment Sif formation via modulation of aggregated endosomal compartments. In studies of *Salmonella* mutants lacking SseF and and SseG, SCVs induced fewer Sifs compared to wild type bacteria (Ramsden et al., 2007).

Salmonella within the SCV have evolved mechanisms that allow it to escape the ubiquitination process by employing three T3SS-2 effectors that interfere with host ubiquitin pathways (Quezada et al., 2009). SseL is a deubiquitinase that acts via modulation of NF-KB, although the downstream effects are unclear (Coombes et al., 2007; Le Negrate et al., 2008; Rytkonen et al., 2007). SspH1 and SspH2 are both members of the ubiquitin E3 ligases family. More research is required to clearly define a role for these two effectors. Nevertheless a study has identified that SspH1 can ubiquitinate ubiquitin (Rohde et al., 2007).

5. Surviving intracellularly

Salmonella has successfully evolved several strategies to manipulate and supress cellular immune responses. SptP GAP and tyrosine phosphatase activities play critical roles in reversing MAPK activation while AvrA acetyltransferase activity towards MAPK kinases inhibits Jnk activation (Jones et al., 2008; Lin et al., 2003; Murli et al., 2001). Moreover, SpvC has been shown to directly inhibit Erk, Jnk and p38 MAPKs via its phosphothreonine lyase activity (Li et al., 2007; Mazurkiewicz et al., 2008).

The deubiquitinase activity of SPI-2 effector, SseL, is able to suppress NFκB activation by impairing IκBα ubiquitination and degradation (Le Negrate et al., 2008). This is thought to be an additional measure by which *Salmonella* is able to target transcription factors downstream from MAPK pathways to ensure immune suppression. AvrA also has a reportedly redundant role to SseL deubiquitinase activity and thereby acts in a similar manner (Ye et al., 2007). Furthermore, SspH1 inhibits NFkB-dependant gene expression, although the precise mechanisms are unclear (Rohde et al., 2007). The production of reactive host species by many host cells is imperative for killing intracellular pathogens. This is essentially through the employment of NADPH oxidase (NOX2) activity found in lysosomes. *Salmonella* is able to evade this activity by utilizing SodCl, a superoxide dismutase, which protects itself from the reactive oxygen species.

Metal availability in host eukaryotic cells is required for full virulence of *Salmonella*. Of many trace elements reportedly utilised by *Salmonella*, iron appears most important. Iron is a cofactor for various fundamental enzymes and metabolic processes in *Salmonella*, which must compete with the host cell to obtain this ion (Schaible & Kaufmann, 2004). Epidemiological evidence from patients with β-thalassaemia has demonstrated an increased susceptibility of *Salmonella* infection (Wanachiwanawin, 2000). Similarly, *Salmonella* virulence was exacerbated in laboratory conditions replicating iron overload (Sawatzki et al., 1983). Further evidence of increased virulence of *Salmonella* in iron favouring conditions stems from the attenuated intracellular growth of mutant S. Typhi whose iron uptake abilities are impaired (Furman et al., 1994).

In light of the importance of iron in *Salmonella* virulence, it is not surprising that *Salmonella* has evolved strategies in acquiring various metals for intracellular survival. The iron availability in eukaryotic hosts is limited due to activity of transferrin and natural resistance-associated macrophage protein one (Nramp1) (Nairz et al., 2009). Additionally, during bouts of inflammation, the antimicrobial protein lipocalin-2 further inhibits bacterial iron acquisition, creating an environment highly unfavourable for *Salmonella* and other intracellular bacteria (Raffatellu et al., 2009). *Salmonella* therefore employs two siderophores, enterobactin and salmonchelin, when acquiring iron in highly competitive conditions (Muller et al., 2009). Salmonechelin, a glucoslyated derivative of enterobactin, is thought to resist or inhibit lipocalin-2 function (Raffatellu et al., 2009). Furthermore, SCVs in macrophages contain enough iron to affect activity of metal-responsive promoters, independently of Nramp1 (Taylor et al., 2009).

Magnesium is also significant for intracellular survival of *Salmonella* and is delivered by three distinct systems for uptake: CorA, MgtA and MgtB (Blanc-Potard & Groisman, 1997). Zinc and potassium are also implicated in intracellular survival of *Salmonella*. In low zinc conditions, ZnuABC Zn^{2+} uptake system demonstrates its importance intracellularly, while further studies with ZnuABC mutants have supported the importance of zinc acquisition for virulence of *Salmonella* (Ammendola et al., 2007). Finally, the Trk complex system functions as a low-affinity K^+ transporter and resist host antimicrobial peptides(Parra-Lopez et al., 1994).

6. Effector modulation of host immunity

Many SPI effectors can induce symptoms that are the hallmark feature of salmonellosis, such as acute intestinal inflammation and diarrhoea, through activation of immune cells and release of cytokines. During *Salmonella* invasion, transcription factors AP-1 and NFκB are activated via stimulation of Cdc42 by SPI-1 effectors SopE/SopE2 and SopB. More specifically, Erk, Jnk and p38 mitogen-activated protein kinase (MAPK) are unregulated in a Raf1-dependant fashion that ultimately result in transcription of AP-1 and NFκB to release proinflammatory cytokines such as IL-8, recruiting polymorphonuclear leukocytes (PMNs) (Layton & Galyov, 2007; Patel & Galan, 2006, 2005). Concomitantly, SipA triggers the Arf6- and phospholipase D signalling cascade, releasing PMN chemoattractant hepoxillin A3 apically via protein kinase Cα (Layton & Galyov, 2007; Wall et al., 2007). As a result, PMN chemoattractant hepoxillin A3 promotes transmigration of PMN across the epithelium into the intestinal lumen. The actions of SopB, SopE, SopE2 and SipA are likely to disturb the integrity in the epithelial barrier and result further in PMN transmigration whilst promoting fluid flux, thereby contributing to diarrhoea (Boyle et al., 2006). SopB is also known to play a role in the induction of diarrhoea due to its inositol phosphatase activity, producing Ins(1,4,5,6)P_4, which promotes cellular chloride ion secetion and fluid flux (Layton & Galyov, 2007). Contrary to this, the SPI-1 effector, AvrA,, has been shown to have countering effects on ion secretion by stabilising cell permeability and tight junctions in intestinal epithelial cells (Liao et al., 2008). This action is believed to have a strategic advantage to bacterial survival since disruption of the epithelial lining also increases the inflammatory response. Therefore AvrA may help *Salmonella* survive in the host during by dampening intestinal inflammation.

7. Cell death

'From death comes life' A proverb that seems to rings true during *Salmonella* infection of host cells. The relationship between *Salmonella* invasion and cell death has been long implicated; however the once simplistic model has now evolved to include many different mechanisms in which *Salmonella* prompts cell death.

In many ways the epithelium provides a barrier, both physical and chemical, that demarcates two environments whilst selectively allowing particles to migrate to their new world. The internalization of *Salmonella* alone, mostly by epithelial lining cells, does not guarantee access to the underlying tissue. Rather, the phenomenon of cell death is thought to create the perfect opportunity for *Salmonella* to reach and infect Peyer's patches and disseminate to systemic tissues in the host. Internalized *Salmonella* in cultured epithelial cells is able to exploit and induce apoptosis *in vitro* after 8-12 hours, in a manner that is characteristic of apoptosis, such as activation of apoptotic caspase-3 and caspase-8 (Kim et al., 1998; Paesold et al., 2002; Zeng et al., 2006). Apoptosis is best defined as an active, controlled, genetically regulated and ATP-requiring process that results in cell death in the face of aging or damaged cells (Danial & Korsmeyer, 2004; Kerr et al., 1972). The bacterial invasion and synthesis of bacterial proteins from SPI-2 T3SS-II and *spv* genes are required for intracellular proliferation and induction of apoptosis (Paesold et al., 2002). Additionally, following bacterial invasion, host cellular production of inflammatory mediators, such as TNF-α and nitric oxide, are all thought to contribute to epithelial cell apoptosis. It should be noted that apoptosis of *Salmonella*-infested epithelial cells is a relatively delayed event, which is thought to favour intracellular reproduction, increasing the overall niche of intracellular *Salmonella* (Kim et al., 1998).

A relatively newly defined form of apoptosis utilized by *Salmonella* and other intracellular residing bacteria is termed pyroptosis. Its unique mechanism, features and inflammatory outcome distinguishes it from our current understanding of apoptosis (Fink & Cookson, 2007; Hersh et al., 1999). Pyroptosis is caspase-1 dependant which is activated in the inflammasome during *Salmonella* infection. This differs from apoptosis in that caspase-3 and not caspase-1 is central to cell death (Brennan & Cookson, 2000; Jesenberger et al., 2000). Additionally, Caspase-3 is not activated in pyroptosis, nor is caspase-6 and caspase-8. Furthermore, the characteristic mitochondrial release of cytochrome *c* in apoptosis does not occur during pyroptosis (Jesenberger et al., 2000). Finally, the unique inflammatory outcome of pyroptosis stems from caspase-1 ability to release proinflammatory cytokines IL-1β and IL-18 by cleaving their precursor molecules (Fantuzzi & Dinarello, 1999).

The SPI-1 effector, SipB has been heavily implicated in host cell death of following *Salmonella* internalization of macrophages, as supported by a study which showed reduced apoptosis following infection of SPI-1 mutant *Salmonella* (Monack et al., 2004). SipB is able to bind and activate caspase-1, triggering rapid pyroptosis. Flagellin is also demonstrated to be necessary in caspase-1-mediated, SPI-1-dependent pyroptosis, as observed in flagellin void *Salmonella* mutants (Franchi et al., 2006; Miao et al., 2006). It should be noted that pyroptosis is not limited in macrophages, as caspase-1-dependant death has also been observed in *Salmonella*-infected DCs (van der Velden et al., 2003). Another described pyroptosis in *Salmonella* infected macrophages, dubbed 'Delayed SPI-2-dependant caspase-1-mediated pyroptosis, is thought to be important during the systemic phase of infection, as SPI-1 effectors and flagellin are both repressed during this stage (Cummings et al., 2005; Fink & Cookson, 2007; Schlumberger & Hardt, 2006). Delayed macrophage death also requires expression of the *spvB* gene, as mutations in this gene prevent induction of delayed macrophage death (Browne et al., 2002; Libby et al., 2000). Despite this, *Spv* genes may not directly affect cytotoxicity as Spv mutants show attenuated intracellular replication and therefore may indirectly affect cytotoxicity through intracellular proliferation of *Salmonella* (Fink & Cookson, 2007). Delayed macrophage pyroptosis may heavily contribute to virulence of *Salmonella*, as dissemination is largely through *Salmonella*-infected macrophages (Fields et al., 1986). Therefore, delaying cell death and the subsequent release of *Salmonella* will allow the bacterium to disseminate further virtually undetected. Finally, an extremely late event of apoptosis in *Salmonella*-infected macrophages has been observed in caspase-1-deficient macrophages, which is caspase-1-indepedant (Hernandez et al., 2003; Jesenberger et al., 2000). SPI-1 and more notably, sipB, are shown to be required for this caspase-1-indepenant apoptosis in macrophages (Hernandez et al., 2003; Jesenberger et al., 2000). This process acts via the release of mitochondrial cytochrome *c* and activation of caspase-2, caspase-3, caspase-6 and caspase-8, resulting in apoptosis (Jesenberger et al., 2000). More research is required to clarify the role of caspase-1-independent apoptosis in the physiological setting of Salmonellosis.

The many failsafe's of *Salmonella* mediated cell death has caused greater debate on the effects in the virulence of *Salmonella*. In light of the fact that pyroptosis produces an inflammatory outcome, one may speculate that this pathway may have important implications in host protection. Contrarily, epithelial cell death via apoptosis is believed to enhance bacterial migration and dissemination as this would likely result in a breach of the epithelial barrier and thereby allow more *Salmonella* to pass into underlying tissue. Further research in *Salmonella* mediated cell death may help clarify this seemly paradoxical event.

8. Serum resistance

Serum resistance and subsequent typhoid fever is a characteristic phenomenon observed in cases of S. Typhi infection. Unlike S. Typhimurium, S. Typhi is host specific and it does not persist in animals and thus is inherently difficult to study *in vivo* conditions. As a result, volunteer studies have been essential in establishing the pathogenesis of typhoid fever. Following mucosa invasion of S. Typhimurium, host pattern recognition receptors recognise various pathogen-associated molecular patterns (PAMPs) that are unique to bacteria. Such receptors include Toll-like receptor 4 (TLR-4) which recognises lipopolysaccharide (LPS) and TLR-5 that is exclusively expressed on the basolateral surface of epithelial cells which recognises and binds flagellin (Gewirtz et al., 2001; Hayashi et al., 2001; Poltorak et al., 1998). Activation of TLR signalling induces expression of various proinflammatory cytokines such as TNF-α and chemokine IL-8, recruiting neutrophils to the intestinal mucosa. These inflammatory markers are essential to the containment and clearance of *Salmonella* infection in the mucosa (Raffatellu et al., 2006). Contrasting this, S. Typhi invasion of the intestinal mucosa does not initiate effective immune response, nor triggers the neutrophil influx that is characteristic of S. Typhimurium. This is due to the expression of the Vi capsular antigen on the SPI-7 that is absent in S. Typhimurium. The expression of the Vi capsular antigen in S. Typhi is thought to down-regulate the TLR-mediated host response in the intestinal mucosa, ultimately allowing bacteria to escape the immune defence line and disseminate to the liver, bone marrow and gall bladder (Tsolis et al., 2008). In human colonic epithelial cell lines, capsulated S. Typhi reduces IL-8 production, while in a similar study, noncapsulated S. Typhi triggers more IL-8 and TNF-alpha production (Hirose et al., 1997; Raffatellu et al., 2005; Sharma & Qadri, 2004). Capsulated S. Typhi interferes with TLR5 and TLR4/MD2/CD14 stimulation by flagella and LPS, respectively (Miyake et al., 1998). In this view, the Vi capsular antigen appears to deafen the immune system by simply reducing immunological stimulation and subsequent response. An earlier study has revealed an approximate 10,000-fold decrease in the virulence of non-capsulated S. Typhi in an intraperitoneal mouse model of infection (Hone et al., 1988). Similarly, a volunteer study has demonstrated a significant increase in disease activity amongst those infected with capsulated S. Typhi (Hornick et al., 1970). Finally, vaccination with the Vi antigen has confirmed protection during human infection with capsulated S. Typhi (Klugman et al., 1987).

Numerous theories by which the Vi capsular antigen inhibits inflammation have been proposed, two of which are most widely accepted. Primarily, Vi capsular antigen may physically mask PAMPs, thereby interfering with TLR stimulation (Raffatellu et al., 2006). This is supported by studies which found that the Vi antigen blocks the agglutination of S. Typhi with anti-LPS serum (Felix, 1934). Vi antigen also inhibits type 1 fimbriae mediated agglutination in *Saccharomyces cerevisiae*, collectively insinuating that the capsule physically masks surface structures (Miyake et al., 1998). Secondly, it has been suggested that the Vi antigen may attenuate downstream signalling related to IL-8 production (Qadri, 1997; Sharma & Qadri, 2004). Despite its early discovery, many questions regarding Vi capsular antigen mechanisms remain unanswered. This is due to the limitations of directly studying the Vi capsular antigen *in vivo* in laboratory condition. Vi antigen expression is markedly reduced, if not obliterated, when transferred to the laboratory. This characteristic loss of the Vi capsular antigen is ascribed to the genetic instability of the SPI-7, which frequently is lost in the laboratory passage (Bueno et al., 2004).

S. Typhi blood isolates from infected patients suggests that Vi antigen expression is invariable (Robbins & Robbins, 1984). However, S. Typhi isolates in human stool samples revealed a lack of Vi capsular antigen expression, compared to blood samples in the same patients (James Craigie, 1936). Moreover, recent *in vitro* studies have suggested that S. Typhi downregulates the expression of the Vi capsular antigen in the intestinal lumen as a result of the inherent high osmolarity of the region (Pickard et al., 1994). Concurrently, flagella expression is unregulated, while T3SS-1 genes are expressed (Arricau et al., 1998). These studies have revealed the transient nature of Vi expression during various stages of S. Typhi infection. The environmental shift between the high osmolarity of the intestinal lumen and low osmolarity inside the host tissue appears to promote expression of the Vi capsular antigen, while simultaneously repressing mobility and invasiveness. Upon invasion into the underlying epithelium, S. Typhi encounters low osmolarity within its new environment, thus triggering two component regulatory systems RcsBC and OmpR EnvZ. Both components activate Vi antigen expression while the expression of flagella and T3SS-1 genes are reduced (Arricau et al., 1998; Pickard et al., 1994; Virlogeux et al., 1996). The effects of Vi antigen expression on S. Typhi virulence are demonstrated in recent *in vitro* studies in which capsulated S. Typhi is resistant to phagocytosis (Looney & Steigbigel, 1986). These findings perplex the role virulent T3SS-1 effectors in intracellular survival of macrophages.

9. Typhoid fever or septic shock?

Unlike S. Typhi, S. Typhimurium and other non-typhoidal *Salmonella* serotypes generally do not elicit typhoid fever due to the absence of the SPI-7 and therefore Vi capsular antigen. In immunocompetent individuals, non-typhoidal *Salmonella* serotypes prompt a strong immune response, marked by neutrophil influx and inflammatory diarrhoea which help contain the infection in the intestinal mucosa. Conversely, immunocompromised patients infected with non-typhoidal *Salmonella* serotypes develop fulminant bacteraemia, a clinical presentation markedly different to that of typhoid fever (Tsolis et al., 2008). The failed containment of non-typhoidal *Salmonella* to the intestinal mucous leads to bacterial dissemination to the blood stream, prompting an aggressive immune response towards bacteria associated LPS. LPS, a known inducer of endotoxic shock, binds the TLR4-MD-2-CD14 receptor complex inducing an excessive inflammatory response marked by release of TNF-α, IFN-γ and IL-1β (Hoebe et al., 2004). Endotoxic shock is characterised by a decrease in hypotension and microvascular thrombosis as the result of fibrin deposition in capillaries (Waage et al., 1991). LPS is thought to contribute to septic shock and mortality in patients with non-typhoidal *Salmonella*, in part due to the rapid production of TLR4-dependant TNF-α in macrophages (Engelberts et al., 1991; Wilson et al., 2008). The synergic induction of nitric oxide synthase, by TNF-α, IFN-γ and IL-1β, increases production of nitric oxide which is a powerful vasodilator contributing to hypotension (Petros et al., 1991). In addition to this, TNF-α increases tissue-factor expression on monocytes, resulting in cleavage of serum fibrinogen to fibrin (Carlsen et al., 1988). Deposits of fibrin in microvasculature lead to intravascular coagulopathy, which can cause organ failure (Waage et al., 1991). Contrary to the robust immunological response to non-typhoidal *Salmonella* serotypes, S. Typhi induces only a weak immune response. This is paralleled in the clinical setting as coagulatory abnormalities are not apparent in patients with typhoid fever (Butler et al., 1978). Furthermore, serum cytokine levels in patients with typhoid fever were relatively lower when compared to patients with gram-negative septic shock (Raffatellu et al., 2006). The impaired identification and host response towards S. Typhi is attributed to its ability to conceal two important molecular signatures, LPS and flagellin. As mentioned previously, the Vi capsular antigen is thought to mask the physical structure of LPS, thereby evading TLR4 recognition and subsequent response. Additionally, *viaB* locus in SPI-7 is also able to attenuate TLR5 signalling, albeit via a different mechanism. TviA, a regulatory protein encoded by the *viaB*, suppresses the transcription of locus *flhC* and *flhD*, both of which encode the master regulator of flagella expression (Winter et al., 2008). As a result, the transcription of the flagellin gene *fliC* is reduced and therefore flagellin is downregulated. This unique mechanism allows S. Typhi to evade TLR5 recognition of flagellin.

10. Persistence

The vast majority of patients with acute typhoid fever recover following adequate treatment; however 3-5% of cases develop a chronic infection in the gall bladder (Levine et al., 1982; Merselis et al., 1964). In light of the fact that S. Typhi is a human restrictive pathogen, these chronically affected individuals form crucial reservoirs for future spread via the faecal and urinal oral route (Bhan et al., 2005; Khatri et al., 2009). Furthermore, chronically affected individuals are almost always asymptomic, making identification of possible carriers a difficult task (Shpargel et al., 1985; Sinnott & Teall, 1987).

Epidemiological studies have revealed a strong association between chronic carriers of S. Typhi and gallstones (Schioler et al., 1983). Moreover, 90% of chronically affected individuals have gallstones (Karaki & Matsubara, 1984). Alongside S. Typhi, many other bacterium have been implicated in the development of gallstones and later cholecystitis, an inflammation and obstruction of the gallbladder (Capoor et al., 2008; Swidsinski & Lee, 2001). Despite much research, it remains unclear whether S. Typhi and other bacterium directly cause cholecystitis, or rather colonise previously damaged gall bladders (Cohen et al., 1987; Vaishnavi et al., 2005; Vogelsang & Boe, 1948).

Being the site of bile storage, the gall bladder possesses a harsh environment and therefore can only be inhabited by organisms resistant to the bile (van Velkinburgh & Gunn, 1999) (Thanassi et al., 1997). S. Typhi is known to form biofilms in abiotic and biotic surfaces and it is therefore not surprising that S. Typhi forms biofilms in the gall bladder (Ledeboer & Jones, 2005). Interestingly, however, formation of *Salmonella* biofilms on gallstones is dependent on the presence of bile (Prouty et al., 2002). Bile is known to interact and manipulate gene expression in *Salmonella* biofilms, such as downregulating SPI-1 genes and mobility genes (Crawford et al., 2010; Prouty & Gunn, 2000). Despite this, the effects are believed to be minimal and may not dramatically affect the abilitiy of *Salmonella's* to invade via effectors of SPI-1 or migrate via flagella. As S. Typhi is a human-restricted pathogen, utilising laboratory models such as S. Typhimurium does not truly mimic the pathogenesis of typhoid fever as S. Typhimurium induces a characteristic neutrophil response that is otherwise absent in S. Typhi. Therefore, much of our current understanding of S. Typhi resistance in gall bladders stems from *in vitro* biofilm models, such as tube biofilm assays (TBA)(Gonzalez-Escobedo et al., 2011). Earlier studies have established the essential role of biofilm formation on gallstones removed from patients chronically infected with S. Typhi (Prouty et al., 2002). More recently, TBAs have revealed the bile-dependant enhancement of S. Typhi biofilms and specific binding to cholesterol-coated surfaces, such as in some cases of gallstones (Crawford et al., 2008). Furthermore, TBA's have also confirmed that the flagellin subunit *fliCI* is necessary for initial binding to cholesterol-coated surfaces. In addition to this, outer-membrance protein C (OmpC) also affects binding of S. Typhi biofilms to cholesterol (Crawford et al., 2010). Following the initial attachment phase, formation of microcolonies typically precedes the development to mature biofilm. During these two latter stages, extracellular polymeric substances (EPS) help biofilm structural development and cell-cell interaction (Costerton et al., 1999). In S. Typhi infected gallbladders, EPS is primarily composed of cellulose, colanic acid, Vi capsular antigen, curli fimbriae, O antigen capsule and biofilm associated proteins (Gibson et al., 2006; Gonzalez-Escobedo et al., 2011; Jonas et al., 2007; Ledeboer & Jones, 2005). Although the role of some elements in the EPS remain minor, other elements such as cellulose, colonic acid and O antigen capsule are crucial for S. Typhi persistence and biofilm development (Crawford et al., 2008; Prouty & Gunn, 2003; Prouty et al., 2002).

Biofilm development is an important component of bacterial survival and persistence. In order to decipher the complex interaction between S. Typhi biofilm and gallbladder further research is required. Humanised moue models are currently in development and may provide useful data by allowing S. Typhi to be studied directly in biofilm formation and gallbladder persistence (Song et al., 2010).

11. Conclusion

In the last two decades, incredible progress has been made in our understanding of the very complex host-*Salmonella* interactions. Furthermore, current therapeutic developments reflect our current knowledge of molecular events during Salmonellosis. Despite this, existing animal models used to decipher *Salmonella* and host interactions have severe limitations and implications in the clinical scenario. For example, the scarcity of data on S. Typhi, due to no suitable animal models available, has limited our understanding and therefore therapeutic development in human typhoid. Although the recently developed streptomycin pre-treated murine model has greatly enhanced our understanding of S. Typhimurium, we must caution ourselves in over interpreting data as S. Typhimurium mouse model does not always reflect the human disease. Until laboratory based *in vivo* models of S. Typhi are established, scientists must rely on a combination of existing models to help increase our understanding of the infectious processes.

12. References

Alix, E. & A. B. Blanc-Potard (2007). MgtC: a key player in intramacrophage survival. *Trends Microbiol,* Vol.15, No.6, (Jun), pp. 252-256, 0966-842X.

Ammendola, S., P. Pasquali, et al. (2007). High-affinity Zn2+ uptake system ZnuABC is required for bacterial zinc homeostasis in intracellular environments and contributes to the virulence of *Salmonella* enterica. *Infect Immun,* Vol.75, No.12, (Dec), pp. 5867-5876, 0019-9567

Arricau, N., D. Hermant, et al. (1998). The RcsB-RcsC regulatory system of *Salmonella* typhi differentially modulates the expression of invasion proteins, flagellin and Vi antigen in response to osmolarity. *Mol Microbiol,* Vol.29, No.3, (Aug), pp. 835-850, 0950-382X

Barbero, P., L. Bittova, et al. (2002). Visualization of Rab9-mediated vesicle transport from endosomes to the trans-Golgi in living cells. *J Cell Biol,* Vol.156, No.3, (Feb 4), pp. 511-518, 0021-9525.

Bhan, M. K., R. Bahl, et al. (2005). Typhoid and paratyphoid fever. *Lancet,* Vol.366, No.9487, (Aug 27-Sep 2), pp. 749-762, 0140-6736

Bispham, J., B. N. Tripathi, et al. (2001). *Salmonella* pathogenicity island 2 influences both systemic salmonellosis and *Salmonella*-induced enteritis in calves. *Infect Immun,* Vol.69, No.1, (Jan), pp. 367-377, 0019-9567.

Blanc-Potard, A. B. & E. A. Groisman (1997). The *Salmonella* selC locus contains a pathogenicity island mediating intramacrophage survival. *EMBO J,* Vol.16, No.17, (Sep 1), pp. 5376-5385, 0261-4189

Blanc-Potard, A. B., F. Solomon, et al. (1999). The SPI-3 pathogenicity island of *Salmonella* enterica. *J Bacteriol,* Vol.181, No.3, (Feb), pp. 998-1004, 0021-9193.

Boucrot, E., T. Henry, et al. (2005). The intracellular fate of *Salmonella* depends on the recruitment of kinesin. *Science,* Vol.308, No.5725, (May 20), pp. 1174-1178, 0036-8075

Boyd, E. F. & H. Brussow (2002). Common themes among bacteriophage-encoded virulence factors and diversity among the bacteriophages involved. *Trends Microbiol,* Vol.10, No.11, (Nov), pp. 521-529, 0966-842X.

Boyle, E. C., N. F. Brown, et al. (2006). Salmonella enterica serovar typhimurium effectors SopB, SopE, SopE2 and SipA disrupt tight junction structure and function. *Cell Microbiol,* Vol.8, No.12, (Dec), pp. 1946-1957, 1462-5814.

Brawn, L. C., R. D. Hayward, et al. (2007). Salmonella SPI1 effector SipA persists after entry and cooperates with a SPI2 effector to regulate phagosome maturation and intracellular replication. *Cell Host Microbe,* Vol.1, No.1, (Mar 15), pp. 63-75, 1931-3128

Brennan, M. A. & B. T. Cookson (2000). Salmonella induces macrophage death by caspase-1-dependent necrosis. *Mol Microbiol,* Vol.38, No.1, (Oct), pp. 31-40, 0950-382X.

Browne, S. H., M. L. Lesnick, et al. (2002). Genetic requirements for salmonella-induced cytopathology in human monocyte-derived macrophages. *Infect Immun,* Vol.70, No.12, (Dec), pp. 7126-7135, 0019-9567

Brumell, J. H., P. Tang, et al. (2001). Characterization of Salmonella-induced filaments (Sifs) reveals a delayed interaction between Salmonella-containing vacuoles and late endocytic compartments. *Traffic,* Vol.2, No.9, (Sep), pp. 643-653, 1398-9219

Brumell, J. H., P. Tang, et al. (2002). Disruption of the Salmonella-containing vacuole leads to increased replication of Salmonella enterica serovar typhimurium in the cytosol of epithelial cells. *Infect Immun,* Vol.70, No.6, (Jun), pp. 3264-3270, 0019-9567

Bueno, S. M., C. A. Santiviago, et al. (2004). Precise excision of the large pathogenicity island, SPI7, in Salmonella enterica serovar typhi. *J Bacteriol,* Vol.186, No.10, (May), pp. 3202-3213, 0021-9193

Bujny, M. V., P. A. Ewels, et al. (2008). Sorting nexin-1 defines an early phase of Salmonella-containing vacuole-remodeling during Salmonella infection. *J Cell Sci,* Vol.121, No.Pt 12, (Jun 15), pp. 2027-2036, 0021-9533.

Butler, T., W. R. Bell, et al. (1978). Typhoid fever. Studies of blood coagulation, bacteremia, and endotoxemia. *Arch Intern Med,* Vol.138, No.3, (Mar), pp. 407-410, 0003-9926.

Capoor, M. R., D. Nair, et al. (2008). Microflora of bile aspirates in patients with acute cholecystitis with or without cholelithiasis: a tropical experience. *Braz J Infect Dis,* Vol.12, No.3, (Jun), pp. 222-225, 1413-8670

Carlsen, E., A. Flatmark, et al. (1988). Cytokine-induced procoagulant activity in monocytes and endothelial cells. Further enhancement by cyclosporine. *Transplantation,* Vol.46, No.4, (Oct), pp. 575-580, 0041-1337

Catron, D. M., M. D. Sylvester, et al. (2002). The Salmonella-containing vacuole is a major site of intracellular cholesterol accumulation and recruits the GPI-anchored protein CD55. *Cell Microbiol,* Vol.4, No.6, (Jun), pp. 315-328, 1462-5814

Clark, M. A., M. A. Jepson, et al. (1994). Preferential interaction of Salmonella typhimurium with mouse Peyer's patch M cells. *Res Microbiol,* Vol.145, No.7, (Sep), pp. 543-552, 0923-2508

Coburn, B., Y. Li, et al. (2005). Salmonella enterica serovar typhimurium pathogenicity island 2 is necessary for complete virulence in a mouse model of infectious enterocolitis. *Infect Immun,* Vol.73, No.6, (Jun), pp. 3219-3227, 0019-9567

Cohen, J. I., J. A. Bartlett, et al. (1987). Extra-intestinal manifestations of salmonella infections. *Medicine (Baltimore),* Vol.66, No.5, (Sep), pp. 349-388, 0025-7974

Coombes, B. K., B. A. Coburn, et al. (2005). Analysis of the contribution of Salmonella pathogenicity islands 1 and 2 to enteric disease progression using a novel bovine ileal loop model and a murine model of infectious enterocolitis. *Infect Immun,* Vol.73, No.11, (Nov), pp. 7161-7169, 0019-9567

Coombes, B. K., M. J. Lowden, et al. (2007). SseL is a salmonella-specific translocated effector integrated into the SsrB-controlled salmonella pathogenicity island 2 type III secretion system. *Infect Immun,* Vol.75, No.2, (Feb), pp. 574-580, 0019-9567

Costerton, J. W., Z. Lewandowski, et al. (1995). Microbial biofilms. *Annu Rev Microbiol,* Vol.49, pp. 711-745, 0066-4227.

Costerton, J. W., P. S. Stewart, et al. (1999). Bacterial biofilms: a common cause of persistent infections. *Science,* Vol.284, No.5418, (May 21), pp. 1318-1322, 0036-8075

Crawford, R. W., D. L. Gibson, et al. (2008). Identification of a bile-induced exopolysaccharide required for Salmonella biofilm formation on gallstone surfaces. *Infect Immun,* Vol.76, No.11, (Nov), pp. 5341-5349, 0019-9567.

Crawford, R. W., K. E. Reeve, et al. (2010). Flagellated but not hyperfimbriated Salmonella enterica serovar typhimurium attaches to and forms biofilms on cholesterol-coated surfaces. *J Bacteriol,* Vol.192, No.12, (Jun), pp. 2981-2990, 0021-9193.

Cummings, L. A., S. L. Barrett, et al. (2005). FliC-specific CD4+ T cell responses are restricted by bacterial regulation of antigen expression. *J Immunol,* Vol.174, No.12, (Jun 15), pp. 7929-7938, 0022-1767.

Daigle, F. (2008). typhi genes expressed during infection or involved in pathogenesis. *J Infect Dev Ctries,* Vol.2, No.6, pp. 431-437, 1972-2680 (Electronic) 1972-2680 (Linking).

Danial, N. N. & S. J. Korsmeyer (2004). Cell death: critical control points. *Cell,* Vol.116, No.2, (Jan 23), pp. 205-219, 0092-8674

Darwin, K. H. & V. L. Miller (1999). Molecular basis of the interaction of Salmonella with the intestinal mucosa. *Clin Microbiol Rev,* Vol.12, No.3, (Jul), pp. 405-428, 0893-8512.

Davey, M. E. & A. O'Toole G (2000). Microbial biofilms: from ecology to molecular genetics. *Microbiol Mol Biol Rev,* Vol.64, No.4, (Dec), pp. 847-867, 1092-2172

Deiwick, J., S. P. Salcedo, et al. (2006). The translocated Salmonella effector proteins SseF and SseG interact and are required to establish an intracellular replication niche. *Infect Immun,* Vol.74, No.12, (Dec), pp. 6965-6972, 0019-9567

Diao, J., Y. Zhang, et al. (2008). Crystal structure of SopA, a Salmonella effector protein mimicking a eukaryotic ubiquitin ligase. *Nat Struct Mol Biol,* Vol.15, No.1, (Jan), pp. 65-70, 1545-9985

Dorsey, C. W., M. C. Laarakker, et al. (2005). Salmonella enterica serotype typhimurium MisL is an intestinal colonization factor that binds fibronectin. *Mol Microbiol,* Vol.57, No.1, (Jul), pp. 196-211, 0950-382X.

Drecktrah, D., S. Levine-Wilkinson, et al. (2008). Dynamic behavior of Salmonella-induced membrane tubules in epithelial cells. *Traffic,* Vol.9, No.12, (Dec), pp. 2117-2129, 1398-9219.

Dukes, J. D., H. Lee, et al. (2006). The secreted Salmonella dublin phosphoinositide phosphatase, SopB, localizes to PtdIns(3)P-containing endosomes and perturbs normal endosome to lysosome trafficking. *Biochem J,* Vol.395, No.2, (Apr 15), pp. 239-247, 0264-6021

Ehrbar, K., S. Mirold, et al. (2002). Characterization of effector proteins translocated via the SPI1 type III secretion system of Salmonella typhimurium. *Int J Med Microbiol,* Vol.291, No.6-7, (Feb), pp. 479-485, 1438-4221

Engelberts, I., E. J. von Asmuth, et al. (1991). The interrelation between TNF, IL-6, and PAF secretion induced by LPS in an in vivo and in vitro murine model. *Lymphokine Cytokine Res,* Vol.10, No.1-2, (Apr), pp. 127-131, 1056-5477.

Fantuzzi, G. & C. A. Dinarello (1999). Interleukin-18 and interleukin-1 beta: two cytokine substrates for ICE (caspase-1). *J Clin Immunol,* Vol.19, No.1, (Jan), pp. 1-11, 0271-9142.

Felix, A., and R. M. Pitt (1934). A new antigen of B. typhosus. *The Lancet,* Vol.224, No. 57, (28 July 1934), pp. 186 - 191.

Fields, P. I., R. V. Swanson, et al. (1986). Mutants of Salmonella typhimurium that cannot survive within the macrophage are avirulent. *Proc Natl Acad Sci U S A,* Vol.83, No.14, (Jul), pp. 5189-5193, 0027-8424

Fink, S. L. & B. T. Cookson (2007). Pyroptosis and host cell death responses during Salmonella infection. *Cell Microbiol,* Vol.9, No.11, (Nov), pp. 2562-2570, 1462-5814

Flannagan, R. S., G. Cosio, et al. (2009). Antimicrobial mechanisms of phagocytes and bacterial evasion strategies. *Nat Rev Microbiol,* Vol.7, No.5, (May), pp. 355-366, 1740-1526

Franchi, L., A. Amer, et al. (2006). Cytosolic flagellin requires Ipaf for activation of caspase-1 and interleukin 1beta in salmonella-infected macrophages. *Nat Immunol,* Vol.7, No.6, (Jun), pp. 576-582, 1529-2908.

Freeman, J. A., M. E. Ohl, et al. (2003). The Salmonella enterica serovar typhimurium translocated effectors SseJ and SifB are targeted to the Salmonella-containing vacuole. *Infect Immun,* Vol.71, No.1, (Jan), pp. 418-427, 0019-9567

Frost, A. J., A. P. Bland, et al. (1997). The early dynamic response of the calf ileal epithelium to Salmonella typhimurium. *Vet Pathol,* Vol.34, No.5, (Sep), pp. 369-386, 0300-9858.

Furman, M., A. Fica, et al. (1994). Salmonella typhi iron uptake mutants are attenuated in mice. *Infect Immun,* Vol.62, No.9, (Sep), pp. 4091-4094, 0019-9567

Galan, J. E. & A. Collmer (1999). Type III secretion machines: bacterial devices for protein delivery into host cells. *Science,* Vol.284, No.5418, (May 21), pp. 1322-1328, 0036-8075.

Ganley, I. G., K. Carroll, et al. (2004). Rab9 GTPase regulates late endosome size and requires effector interaction for its stability. *Mol Biol Cell,* Vol.15, No.12, (Dec), pp. 5420-5430, 1059-1524.

Garner, M. J., R. D. Hayward, et al. (2002). The Salmonella pathogenicity island 1 secretion system directs cellular cholesterol redistribution during mammalian cell entry and intracellular trafficking. *Cell Microbiol,* Vol.4, No.3, (Mar), pp. 153-165, 1462-5814

Gerlach, R. G., D. Jackel, et al. (2007). Salmonella Pathogenicity Island 4 encodes a giant non-fimbrial adhesin and the cognate type 1 secretion system. *Cell Microbiol,* Vol.9, No.7, (Jul), pp. 1834-1850, 1462-5814

Gewirtz, A. T., T. A. Navas, et al. (2001). Cutting edge: bacterial flagellin activates basolaterally expressed TLR5 to induce epithelial proinflammatory gene expression. *J Immunol,* Vol.167, No.4, (Aug 15), pp. 1882-1885, 0022-1767

Gibson, D. L., A. P. White, et al. (2006). Salmonella produces an O-antigen capsule regulated by AgfD and important for environmental persistence. *J Bacteriol,* Vol.188, No.22, (Nov), pp. 7722-7730, 0021-9193.

Gonzalez-Escobedo, G., J. M. Marshall, et al. (2011). Chronic and acute infection of the gall bladder by Salmonella typhi: understanding the carrier state. *Nat Rev Microbiol,* Vol.9, No.1, (Jan), pp. 9-14, 1740-1526

Guo, A., M. A. Lasaro, et al. (2007). Adhesin-dependent binding and uptake of Salmonella enterica serovar typhimurium by dendritic cells. *Microbiology,* Vol.153, No.Pt 4, (Apr), pp. 1059-1069, 1350-0872

Hacker, J., L. Bender, et al. (1990). Deletions of chromosomal regions coding for fimbriae and hemolysins occur in vitro and in vivo in various extraintestinal Escherichia coli isolates. *Microb Pathog,* Vol.8, No.3, (Mar), pp. 213-225, 0882-4010

Hapfelmeier, S., B. Stecher, et al. (2005). The Salmonella pathogenicity island (SPI)-2 and SPI-1 type III secretion systems allow Salmonella serovar typhimurium to trigger colitis via MyD88-dependent and MyD88-independent mechanisms. *J Immunol,* Vol.174, No.3, (Feb 1), pp. 1675-1685, 0022-1767

Haraga, A. & S. I. Miller (2003). A Salmonella enterica serovar typhimurium translocated leucine-rich repeat effector protein inhibits NF-kappa B-dependent gene expression. *Infect Immun,* Vol.71, No.7, (Jul), pp. 4052-4058, 0019-9567.

Harrison, R. E., J. H. Brumell, et al. (2004). Salmonella impairs RILP recruitment to Rab7 during maturation of invasion vacuoles. *Mol Biol Cell,* Vol.15, No.7, (Jul), pp. 3146-3154, 1059-1524.

Hayashi, F., K. D. Smith, et al. (2001). The innate immune response to bacterial flagellin is mediated by Toll-like receptor 5. *Nature,* Vol.410, No.6832, (Apr 26), pp. 1099-1103, 0028-0836.

Henderson, I. R., F. Navarro-Garcia, et al. (2004). Type V protein secretion pathway: the autotransporter story. *Microbiol Mol Biol Rev,* Vol.68, No.4, (Dec), pp. 692-744, 1092-2172

Henry, T., C. Couillault, et al. (2006). The Salmonella effector protein PipB2 is a linker for kinesin-1. *Proc Natl Acad Sci U S A,* Vol.103, No.36, (Sep 5), pp. 13497-13502, 0027-8424

Hensel, M., J. E. Shea, et al. (1998). Genes encoding putative effector proteins of the type III secretion system of Salmonella pathogenicity island 2 are required for bacterial virulence and proliferation in macrophages. *Mol Microbiol,* Vol.30, No.1, (Oct), pp. 163-174, 0950-382X

Hernandez, L. D., M. Pypaert, et al. (2003). A Salmonella protein causes macrophage cell death by inducing autophagy. *J Cell Biol,* Vol.163, No.5, (Dec 8), pp. 1123-1131, 0021-9525

Hersh, D., D. M. Monack, et al. (1999). The Salmonella invasin SipB induces macrophage apoptosis by binding to caspase-1. *Proc Natl Acad Sci U S A,* Vol.96, No.5, (Mar 2), pp. 2396-2401, 0027-8424

Hirose, K., T. Ezaki, et al. (1997). Survival of Vi-capsulated and Vi-deleted Salmonella typhi strains in cultured macrophage expressing different levels of CD14 antigen. *FEMS Microbiol Lett,* Vol.147, No.2, (Feb 15), pp. 259-265, 0378-1097.

Hoebe, K., E. Janssen, et al. (2004). The interface between innate and adaptive immunity. *Nat Immunol,* Vol.5, No.10, (Oct), pp. 971-974, 1529-2908

Hone, D. M., S. R. Attridge, et al. (1988). A galE via (Vi antigen-negative) mutant of Salmonella typhi Ty2 retains virulence in humans. *Infect Immun,* Vol.56, No.5, (May), pp. 1326-1333, 0019-9567

Hornick, R. B., S. E. Greisman, et al. (1970). Typhoid fever: pathogenesis and immunologic control. *N Engl J Med,* Vol.283, No.13, (Sep 24), pp. 686-691, 0028-4793

Humphries, A. D., S. M. Townsend, et al. (2001). Role of fimbriae as antigens and intestinal colonization factors of Salmonella serovars. *FEMS Microbiol Lett,* Vol.201, No.2, (Jul 24), pp. 121-125, 0378-1097

Jackson, L. K., P. Nawabi, et al. (2008). The Salmonella virulence protein SifA is a G protein antagonist. *Proc Natl Acad Sci U S A,* Vol.105, No.37, (Sep 16), pp. 14141-14146, 0027-8424.

James Craigie, K. F. B. (1936). The identification of the V and W forms of B. typhosus and the occurrence of the V form in cases of typhoid fever and carriers. *The Journal of Pathology and Bacteriology,* Vol.43, No.2, pp. 249-260.

Jesenberger, V., K. J. Procyk, et al. (2000). Salmonella-induced caspase-2 activation in macrophages: a novel mechanism in pathogen-mediated apoptosis. *J Exp Med,* Vol.192, No.7, (Oct 2), pp. 1035-1046, 0022-1007.

Jonas, K., H. Tomenius, et al. (2007). Roles of curli, cellulose and BapA in Salmonella biofilm morphology studied by atomic force microscopy. *BMC Microbiol,* Vol.7, pp. 70, 1471-2180

Jones, B. D., N. Ghori, et al. (1994). Salmonella typhimurium initiates murine infection by penetrating and destroying the specialized epithelial M cells of the Peyer's patches. *J Exp Med,* Vol.180, No.1, (Jul 1), pp. 15-23, 0022-1007.

Jones, R. M., H. Wu, et al. (2008). Salmonella AvrA Coordinates Suppression of Host Immune and Apoptotic Defenses via JNK Pathway Blockade. *Cell Host Microbe,* Vol.3, No.4, (Apr 17), pp. 233-244, 1931-3128

Karaki, K. & Y. Matsubara (1984). [Surgical treatment of chronic biliary typhoid and paratyphoid carriers]. *Nihon Shokakibyo Gakkai Zasshi,* Vol.81, No.12, (Dec), pp. 2978-2985, 0446-6586

Kerr, J. F., A. H. Wyllie, et al. (1972). Apoptosis: a basic biological phenomenon with wide-ranging implications in tissue kinetics. *Br J Cancer,* Vol.26, No.4, (Aug), pp. 239-257, 0007-0920.

Khatri, N. S., P. Maskey, et al. (2009). Gallbladder carriage of Salmonella paratyphi A may be an important factor in the increasing incidence of this infection in South Asia. *Ann Intern Med,* Vol.150, No.8, (Apr 21), pp. 567-568, 0003-4819.

Kim, J. M., L. Eckmann, et al. (1998). Apoptosis of human intestinal epithelial cells after bacterial invasion. *J Clin Invest,* Vol.102, No.10, (Nov 15), pp. 1815-1823, 0021-9738

Klugman, K. P., I. T. Gilbertson, et al. (1987). Protective activity of Vi capsular polysaccharide vaccine against typhoid fever. *Lancet,* Vol.2, No.8569, (Nov 21), pp. 1165-1169, 0140-6736

Knodler, L. A. & O. Steele-Mortimer (2005). The Salmonella effector PipB2 affects late endosome/lysosome distribution to mediate Sif extension. *Mol Biol Cell,* Vol.16, No.9, (Sep), pp. 4108-4123, 1059-1524.

Knodler, L. A., B. A. Vallance, et al. (2003). Salmonella type III effectors PipB and PipB2 are targeted to detergent-resistant microdomains on internal host cell membranes. *Mol Microbiol,* Vol.49, No.3, (Aug), pp. 685-704, 0950-382X.

Kohbata, S., H. Yokoyama, et al. (1986). Cytopathogenic effect of Salmonella typhi GIFU 10007 on M cells of murine ileal Peyer's patches in ligated ileal loops: an ultrastructural study. *Microbiol Immunol,* Vol.30, No.12, pp. 1225-1237, 0385-5600.

Kraehenbuhl, J. P. & M. R. Neutra (2000). Epithelial M cells: differentiation and function. *Annu Rev Cell Dev Biol,* Vol.16, pp. 301-332, 1081-0706

Kuhle, V., G. L. Abrahams, et al. (2006). Intracellular Salmonella enterica redirect exocytic transport processes in a Salmonella pathogenicity island 2-dependent manner. *Traffic,* Vol.7, No.6, (Jun), pp. 716-730, 1398-9219

Kuhle, V. & M. Hensel (2002). SseF and SseG are translocated effectors of the type III secretion system of Salmonella pathogenicity island 2 that modulate aggregation of endosomal compartments. *Cell Microbiol,* Vol.4, No.12, (Dec), pp. 813-824, 1462-5814

Kuijl, C., N. D. Savage, et al. (2007). Intracellular bacterial growth is controlled by a kinase network around PKB/AKT1. *Nature,* Vol.450, No.7170, (Nov 29), pp. 725-730, 0028-0836.

Latasa, C., A. Roux, et al. (2005). BapA, a large secreted protein required for biofilm formation and host colonization of Salmonella enterica serovar Enteritidis. *Mol Microbiol,* Vol.58, No.5, (Dec), pp. 1322-1339, 0950-382X.

Lavigne, J. P. & A. B. Blanc-Potard (2008). Molecular evolution of Salmonella enterica serovar typhimurium and pathogenic Escherichia coli: from pathogenesis to therapeutics. *Infect Genet Evol,* Vol.8, No.2, (Mar), pp. 217-226, 1567-1348.

Layton, A. N. & E. E. Galyov (2007). Salmonella-induced enteritis: molecular pathogenesis and therapeutic implications. *Expert Rev Mol Med,* Vol.9, No.18, pp. 1-17, 1462-3994.

Le Negrate, G., B. Faustin, et al. (2008). Salmonella secreted factor L deubiquitinase of Salmonella typhimurium inhibits NF-kappaB, suppresses IkappaBalpha ubiquitination and modulates innate immune responses. *J Immunol,* Vol.180, No.7, (Apr 1), pp. 5045-5056, 0022-1767

Ledeboer, N. A. & B. D. Jones (2005). Exopolysaccharide sugars contribute to biofilm formation by Salmonella enterica serovar typhimurium on HEp-2 cells and chicken intestinal epithelium. *J Bacteriol,* Vol.187, No.9, (May), pp. 3214-3226, 0021-9193.

Levine, M. M., R. E. Black, et al. (1982). Precise estimation of the numbers of chronic carriers of Salmonella typhi in Santiago, Chile, an endemic area. *J Infect Dis,* Vol.146, No.6, (Dec), pp. 724-726, 0022-1899.

Li, H., H. Xu, et al. (2007). The phosphothreonine lyase activity of a bacterial type III effector family. *Science,* Vol.315, No.5814, (Feb 16), pp. 1000-1003, 0036-8075.

Liao, A. P., E. O. Petrof, et al. (2008). Salmonella type III effector AvrA stabilizes cell tight junctions to inhibit inflammation in intestinal epithelial cells. *PLoS One,* Vol.3, No.6, pp. e2369, 1932-6203

Libby, S. J., M. Lesnick, et al. (2000). The Salmonella virulence plasmid spv genes are required for cytopathology in human monocyte-derived macrophages. *Cell Microbiol,* Vol.2, No.1, (Feb), pp. 49-58, 1462-5814.

Lin, S. L., T. X. Le, et al. (2003). SptP, a Salmonella typhimurium type III-secreted protein, inhibits the mitogen-activated protein kinase pathway by inhibiting Raf activation. *Cell Microbiol,* Vol.5, No.4, (Apr), pp. 267-275, 1462-5814

Looney, R. J. & R. T. Steigbigel (1986). Role of the Vi antigen of Salmonella typhi in resistance to host defense in vitro. *J Lab Clin Med,* Vol.108, No.5, (Nov), pp. 506-516, 0022-2143

Lossi, N. S., N. Rolhion, et al. (2008). The Salmonella SPI-2 effector SseJ exhibits eukaryotic activator-dependent phospholipase A and glycerophospholipid : cholesterol acyltransferase activity. *Microbiology,* Vol.154, No.Pt 9, (Sep), pp. 2680-2688, 1350-0872.

Lostroh, C. P. & C. A. Lee (2001). The Salmonella pathogenicity island-1 type III secretion system. *Microbes Infect,* Vol.3, No.14-15, (Nov-Dec), pp. 1281-1291, 1286-4579

Mallo, G. V., M. Espina, et al. (2008). SopB promotes phosphatidylinositol 3-phosphate formation on Salmonella vacuoles by recruiting Rab5 and Vps34. *J Cell Biol,* Vol.182, No.4, (Aug 25), pp. 741-752, 0021-9525

Mazurkiewicz, P., J. Thomas, et al. (2008). SpvC is a Salmonella effector with phosphothreonine lyase activity on host mitogen-activated protein kinases. *Mol Microbiol,* Vol.67, No.6, (Mar), pp. 1371-1383, 0950-382X

McGhie, E. J., L. C. Brawn, et al. (2009). Salmonella takes control: effector-driven manipulation of the host. *Curr Opin Microbiol,* Vol.12, No.1, (Feb), pp. 117-124, 1369-5274

Merselis, J. G., Jr., D. Kaye, et al. (1964). Quantitative Bacteriology of the Typhoid Carrier State. *Am J Trop Med Hyg,* Vol.13, (May), pp. 425-429, 0002-9637

Miao, E. A., C. M. Alpuche-Aranda, et al. (2006). Cytoplasmic flagellin activates caspase-1 and secretion of interleukin 1beta via Ipaf. *Nat Immunol,* Vol.7, No.6, (Jun), pp. 569-575, 1529-2908.

Miao, E. A., E. Andersen-Nissen, et al. (2007). TLR5 and Ipaf: dual sensors of bacterial flagellin in the innate immune system. *Semin Immunopathol,* Vol.29, No.3, (Sep), pp. 275-288, 1863-2297.

Mills, D. M., V. Bajaj, et al. (1995). A 40 kb chromosomal fragment encoding Salmonella typhimurium invasion genes is absent from the corresponding region of the Escherichia coli K-12 chromosome. *Mol Microbiol,* Vol.15, No.4, (Feb), pp. 749-759, 0950-382X

Miyake, M., L. Zhao, et al. (1998). Vi-deficient and nonfimbriated mutants of Salmonella typhi agglutinate human blood type antigens and are hyperinvasive. *FEMS Microbiol Lett,* Vol.161, No.1, (Apr 1), pp. 75-82, 0378-1097.

Monack, D. M., D. M. Bouley, et al. (2004). Salmonella typhimurium persists within macrophages in the mesenteric lymph nodes of chronically infected Nramp1+/+ mice and can be reactivated by IFNgamma neutralization. *J Exp Med,* Vol.199, No.2, (Jan 19), pp. 231-241, 0022-1007

Morgan, E., Bowen, A.J, et al (2007). SiiE is secreted by the Salmonella enterica serovar Typhimurium pathogenicity island 4-encoded secretion system and contributes to intestinal colonization in cattle. *Infect Immun.* Vol. 75 No. 3, (Mar), pp.1524-33. 0019-9567

Mukherjee, K., S. Parashuraman, et al. (2001). SopE acts as an Rab5-specific nucleotide exchange factor and recruits non-prenylated Rab5 on Salmonella-containing phagosomes to promote fusion with early endosomes. *J Biol Chem,* Vol.276, No.26, (Jun 29), pp. 23607-23615, 0021-9258

Muller, S. I., M. Valdebenito, et al. (2009). Salmochelin, the long-overlooked catecholate siderophore of Salmonella. *Biometals,* Vol.22, No.4, (Aug), pp. 691-695, 0966-0844.

Murli, S., R. O. Watson, et al. (2001). Role of tyrosine kinases and the tyrosine phosphatase SptP in the interaction of Salmonella with host cells. *Cell Microbiol,* Vol.3, No.12, (Dec), pp. 795-810, 1462-5814

Nairz, M., G. Fritsche, et al. (2009). Slc11a1 limits intracellular growth of Salmonella enterica sv. typhimurium by promoting macrophage immune effector functions and impairing bacterial iron acquisition. *Cell Microbiol,* Vol.11, No.9, (Sep), pp. 1365-1381, 1462-5814

Neutra, M. R., A. Frey, et al. (1996). Epithelial M cells: gateways for mucosal infection and immunization. *Cell,* Vol.86, No.3, (Aug 9), pp. 345-348, 0092-8674

Ochman, H., F. C. Soncini, et al. (1996). Identification of a pathogenicity island required for Salmonella survival in host cells. *Proc Natl Acad Sci U S A,* Vol.93, No.15, (Jul 23), pp. 7800-7804, 0027-8424

Ohlson, M. B., K. Fluhr, et al. (2005). SseJ deacylase activity by Salmonella enterica serovar typhimurium promotes virulence in mice. *Infect Immun,* Vol.73, No.10, (Oct), pp. 6249-6259, 0019-9567.

Ohlson, M. B., Z. Huang, et al. (2008). Structure and function of Salmonella SifA indicate that its interactions with SKIP, SseJ, and RhoA family GTPases induce endosomal tubulation. *Cell Host Microbe,* Vol.4, No.5, (Nov 13), pp. 434-446, 1931-3128

Owen, R. L. (1994). M cells--entryways of opportunity for enteropathogens. *J Exp Med,* Vol.180, No.1, (Jul 1), pp. 7-9, 0022-1007

Paesold, G., D. G. Guiney, et al. (2002). Genes in the Salmonella pathogenicity island 2 and the Salmonella virulence plasmid are essential for Salmonella-induced apoptosis in intestinal epithelial cells. *Cell Microbiol,* Vol.4, No.11, (Nov), pp. 771-781, 1462-5814

Parra-Lopez, C., R. Lin, et al. (1994). A Salmonella protein that is required for resistance to antimicrobial peptides and transport of potassium. *EMBO J,* Vol.13, No.17, (Sep 1), pp. 3964-3972, 0261-4189

Pascopella, L., B. Raupach, et al. (1995). Host restriction phenotypes of Salmonella typhi and Salmonella gallinarum. *Infect Immun,* Vol.63, No.11, (Nov), pp. 4329-4335, 0019-9567

Patel, J. C. & J. E. Galan (2005). Manipulation of the host actin cytoskeleton by Salmonella--all in the name of entry. *Curr Opin Microbiol,* Vol.8, No.1, (Feb), pp. 10-15, 1369-5274.

Patel, J. C. & J. E. Galan (2006). Differential activation and function of Rho GTPases during Salmonella-host cell interactions. *J Cell Biol,* Vol.175, No.3, (Nov 6), pp. 453-463, 0021-9525.

Petros, A., D. Bennett, et al. (1991). Effect of nitric oxide synthase inhibitors on hypotension in patients with septic shock. *Lancet,* Vol.338, No.8782-8783, (Dec 21-28), pp. 1557-1558, 0140-6736

Pickard, D., J. Li, et al. (1994). Characterization of defined ompR mutants of Salmonella typhi: ompR is involved in the regulation of Vi polysaccharide expression. *Infect Immun,* Vol.62, No.9, (Sep), pp. 3984-3993, 0019-9567

Poltorak, A., X. He, et al. (1998). Defective LPS signaling in C3H/HeJ and C57BL/10ScCr mice: mutations in Tlr4 gene. *Science,* Vol.282, No.5396, (Dec 11), pp. 2085-2088, 0036-8075

Prouty, A. M. & J. S. Gunn (2000). Salmonella enterica serovar typhimurium invasion is repressed in the presence of bile. *Infect Immun,* Vol.68, No.12, (Dec), pp. 6763-6769, 0019-9567

Prouty, A. M. & J. S. Gunn (2003). Comparative analysis of Salmonella enterica serovar typhimurium biofilm formation on gallstones and on glass. *Infect Immun,* Vol.71, No.12, (Dec), pp. 7154-7158, 0019-9567.

Prouty, A. M., W. H. Schwesinger, et al. (2002). Biofilm formation and interaction with the surfaces of gallstones by Salmonella spp. *Infect Immun,* Vol.70, No.5, (May), pp. 2640-2649, 0019-9567.

Qadri, A. (1997). Identification of specific recognition molecules on murine mononuclear phagocytes and B lymphocytes for Vi capsular polysaccharide: modulation of MHC class II expression on stimulation with the polysaccharide. *Immunology,* Vol.92, No.1, (Sep), pp. 146-152, 0019-2805.

Quezada, C. M., S. W. Hicks, et al. (2009). A family of Salmonella virulence factors functions as a distinct class of autoregulated E3 ubiquitin ligases. *Proc Natl Acad Sci U S A,* Vol.106, No.12, (Mar 24), pp. 4864-4869, 0027-8424.

Raffatellu, M., D. Chessa, et al. (2005). The Vi capsular antigen of Salmonella enterica serotype typhi reduces Toll-like receptor-dependent interleukin-8 expression in the intestinal mucosa. *Infect Immun,* Vol.73, No.6, (Jun), pp. 3367-3374, 0019-9567.

Raffatellu, M., D. Chessa, et al. (2006). Capsule-mediated immune evasion: a new hypothesis explaining aspects of typhoid fever pathogenesis. *Infect Immun,* Vol.74, No.1, (Jan), pp. 19-27, 0019-9567

Raffatellu, M., M. D. George, et al. (2009). Lipocalin-2 resistance confers an advantage to Salmonella enterica serotype typhimurium for growth and survival in the inflamed intestine. *Cell Host Microbe,* Vol.5, No.5, (May 8), pp. 476-486, 1931-3128

Ramsden, A. E., D. W. Holden, et al. (2007). Membrane dynamics and spatial distribution of Salmonella-containing vacuoles. *Trends Microbiol,* Vol.15, No.11, (Nov), pp. 516-524, 0966-842X.

Ren, T., D. S. Zamboni, et al. (2006). Flagellin-deficient Legionella mutants evade caspase-1- and Naip5-mediated macrophage immunity. *PLoS Pathog,* Vol.2, No.3, (Mar), pp. e18, 1553-7366

Rescigno, M., G. Rotta, et al. (2001). Dendritic cells shuttle microbes across gut epithelial monolayers. *Immunobiology,* Vol.204, No.5, (Dec), pp. 572-581, 0171-2985

Robbins, J. D. & J. B. Robbins (1984). Reexamination of the protective role of the capsular polysaccharide (Vi antigen) of Salmonella typhi. *J Infect Dis,* Vol.150, No.3, (Sep), pp. 436-449, 0022-1899.

Rohde, J. R., A. Breitkreutz, et al. (2007). Type III secretion effectors of the IpaH family are E3 ubiquitin ligases. *Cell Host Microbe,* Vol.1, No.1, (Mar 15), pp. 77-83, 1931-3128.

Ruiz-Albert, J., X. J. Yu, et al. (2002). Complementary activities of SseJ and SifA regulate dynamics of the Salmonella typhimurium vacuolar membrane. *Mol Microbiol,* Vol.44, No.3, (May), pp. 645-661, 0950-382X

Rytkonen, A., J. Poh, et al. (2007). SseL, a Salmonella deubiquitinase required for macrophage killing and virulence. *Proc Natl Acad Sci U S A,* Vol.104, No.9, (Feb 27), pp. 3502-3507, 0027-8424

Salcedo, S. P. & D. W. Holden (2003). SseG, a virulence protein that targets Salmonella to the Golgi network. *EMBO J,* Vol.22, No.19, (Oct 1), pp. 5003-5014, 0261-4189

Sansonetti, P. J. & A. Phalipon (1999). M cells as ports of entry for enteroinvasive pathogens: mechanisms of interaction, consequences for the disease process. *Semin Immunol,* Vol.11, No.3, (Jun), pp. 193-203, 1044-5323

Sawatzki, G., F. A. Hoffmann, et al. (1983). Acute iron overload in mice: pathogenesis of Salmonella typhimurium infection. *Infect Immun,* Vol.39, No.2, (Feb), pp. 659-665, 0019-9567.

Schaible, U. E. & S. H. Kaufmann (2004). Iron and microbial infection. *Nat Rev Microbiol,* Vol.2, No.12, (Dec), pp. 946-953, 1740-1526

Schioler, H., E. D. Christiansen, et al. (1983). Biliary calculi in chronic Salmonella carriers and healthy controls: a controlled study. *Scand J Infect Dis,* Vol.15, No.1, pp. 17-19, 0036-5548.

Schlumberger, M. C. & W. D. Hardt (2006). Salmonella type III secretion effectors: pulling the host cell's strings. *Curr Opin Microbiol,* Vol.9, No.1, (Feb), pp. 46-54, 1369-5274.

Schmidt, H. & M. Hensel (2004). Pathogenicity islands in bacterial pathogenesis. *Clin Microbiol Rev,* Vol.17, No.1, (Jan), pp. 14-56, 0893-8512.

Schmitt, C. K., J. S. Ikeda, et al. (2001). Absence of all components of the flagellar export and synthesis machinery differentially alters virulence of Salmonella enterica serovar typhimurium in models of typhoid fever, survival in macrophages, tissue culture invasiveness, and calf enterocolitis. *Infect Immun,* Vol.69, No.9, (Sep), pp. 5619-5625, 0019-9567.

Sharma, A. & A. Qadri (2004). Vi polysaccharide of Salmonella typhi targets the prohibitin family of molecules in intestinal epithelial cells and suppresses early inflammatory responses. *Proc Natl Acad Sci U S A,* Vol.101, No.50, (Dec 14), pp. 17492-17497, 0027-8424.

Shea, J. E., M. Hensel, et al. (1996). Identification of a virulence locus encoding a second type III secretion system in Salmonella typhimurium. *Proc Natl Acad Sci U S A,* Vol.93, No.6, (Mar 19), pp. 2593-2597, 0027-8424

Shpargel, J. S., R. S. Berardi, et al. (1985). Salmonella typhi carrier state 52 years after illness with typhoid fever: a case study. *Am J Infect Control,* Vol.13, No.3, (Jun), pp. 122-123, 0196-6553

Sinnott, C. R. & A. J. Teall (1987). Persistent gallbladder carriage of Salmonella typhi. *Lancet,* Vol.1, No.8539, (Apr 25), pp. 976, 0140-6736

Song, J., T. Willinger, et al. (2010). A mouse model for the human pathogen Salmonella typhi. *Cell Host Microbe,* Vol.8, No.4, (Oct 21), pp. 369-376, 1931-3128

Steele-Mortimer, O. (2008). The Salmonella-containing vacuole: moving with the times. *Curr Opin Microbiol,* Vol.11, No.1, (Feb), pp. 38-45, 1369-5274

Steele-Mortimer, O., S. Meresse, et al. (1999). Biogenesis of Salmonella typhimurium-containing vacuoles in epithelial cells involves interactions with the early endocytic pathway. *Cell Microbiol,* Vol.1, No.1, (Jul), pp. 33-49, 1462-5814

Sun, Y. H., H. G. Rolan, et al. (2007). Injection of flagellin into the host cell cytosol by Salmonella enterica serotype typhimurium. *J Biol Chem,* Vol.282, No.47, (Nov 23), pp. 33897-33901, 0021-9258.

Swidsinski, A. & S. P. Lee (2001). The role of bacteria in gallstone pathogenesis. *Front Biosci,* Vol.6, (Oct 1), pp. E93-103, 1093-4715

Taylor, C. M., D. Osman, et al. (2009). Differential expression from two iron-responsive promoters in Salmonella enterica serovar typhimurium reveals the presence of iron in macrophage-phagosomes. *Microb Pathog,* Vol.46, No.2, (Feb), pp. 114-118, 0882-4010

Thanassi, D. G., L. W. Cheng, et al. (1997). Active efflux of bile salts by Escherichia coli. *J Bacteriol,* Vol.179, No.8, (Apr), pp. 2512-2518, 0021-9193.

Tsolis, R. M., G. M. Young, et al. (2008). From bench to bedside: stealth of enteroinvasive pathogens. *Nat Rev Microbiol,* Vol.6, No.12, (Dec), pp. 883-892, 1740-1526

Vaishnavi, C., S. Singh, et al. (2005). Prevalence of Salmonella enterica serovar typhi in bile and stool of patients with biliary diseases and those requiring biliary drainage for other purposes. *Jpn J Infect Dis,* Vol.58, No.6, (Dec), pp. 363-365, 1344-6304.

van der Velden, A. W., M. Velasquez, et al. (2003). Salmonella rapidly kill dendritic cells via a caspase-1-dependent mechanism. *J Immunol,* Vol.171, No.12, (Dec 15), pp. 6742-6749, 0022-1767

van Velkinburgh, J. C. & J. S. Gunn (1999). PhoP-PhoQ-regulated loci are required for enhanced bile resistance in Salmonella spp. *Infect Immun,* Vol.67, No.4, (Apr), pp. 1614-1622, 0019-9567

Virlogeux, I., H. Waxin, et al. (1996). Characterization of the rcsA and rcsB genes from Salmonella typhi: rcsB through tviA is involved in regulation of Vi antigen synthesis. *J Bacteriol,* Vol.178, No.6, (Mar), pp. 1691-1698, 0021-9193.

Vogelsang, T. M. & J. Boe (1948). Temporary and chronic carriers of Salmonella typhi and Salmonella paratyphi B. *J Hyg (Lond),* Vol.46, No.3, (Sep), pp. 252-261, 0022-1724

Waage, A., P. Brandtzaeg, et al. (1991). Current understanding of the pathogenesis of gram-negative shock. *Infect Dis Clin North Am,* Vol.5, No.4, (Dec), pp. 781-791, 0891-5520

Wall, D. M., W. J. Nadeau, et al. (2007). Identification of the Salmonella enterica serotype typhimurium SipA domain responsible for inducing neutrophil recruitment across the intestinal epithelium. *Cell Microbiol,* Vol.9, No.9, (Sep), pp. 2299-2313, 1462-5814

Wanachiwanawin, W. (2000). Infections in E-beta thalassemia. *J Pediatr Hematol Oncol,* Vol.22, No.6, (Nov-Dec), pp. 581-587, 1077-4114

Wasylnka, J. A., M. A. Bakowski, et al. (2008). Role for myosin II in regulating positioning of Salmonella-containing vacuoles and intracellular replication. *Infect Immun,* Vol.76, No.6, (Jun), pp. 2722-2735, 0019-9567

Waterman, S. R. & D. W. Holden (2003). Functions and effectors of the Salmonella pathogenicity island 2 type III secretion system. *Cell Microbiol,* Vol.5, No.8, (Aug), pp. 501-511, 1462-5814.

Wilson, R. P., M. Raffatellu, et al. (2008). The Vi-capsule prevents Toll-like receptor 4 recognition of Salmonella. *Cell Microbiol,* Vol.10, No.4, (Apr), pp. 876-890, 1462-5814

Winter, S. E., M. Raffatellu, et al. (2008). The Salmonella enterica serotype typhi regulator TviA reduces interleukin-8 production in intestinal epithelial cells by repressing flagellin secretion. *Cell Microbiol,* Vol.10, No.1, (Jan), pp. 247-261, 1462-5814.

Wood, M. W., M. A. Jones, et al. (1998). Identification of a pathogenicity island required for Salmonella enteropathogenicity. *Mol Microbiol,* Vol.29, No.3, (Aug), pp. 883-891, 0950-382X

Ye, Z., E. O. Petrof, et al. (2007). Salmonella effector AvrA regulation of colonic epithelial cell inflammation by deubiquitination. *Am J Pathol,* Vol.171, No.3, (Sep), pp. 882-892, 0002-9440

Zeng, H., H. Wu, et al. (2006). Flagellin/TLR5 responses in epithelia reveal intertwined activation of inflammatory and apoptotic pathways. *Am J Physiol Gastrointest Liver Physiol,* Vol.290, No.1, (Jan), pp. G96-G108, 0193-1857.

Zhang, Y., W. M. Higashide, et al. (2006). The inflammation-associated Salmonella SopA is a HECT-like E3 ubiquitin ligase. *Mol Microbiol,* Vol.62, No.3, (Nov), pp. 786-793, 0950-382X

The Different Strategies Used by *Salmonella* to Invade Host Cells

Rosselin Manon, Abed Nadia, Namdari Fatémeh,
Virlogeux-Payant Isabelle, Velge Philippe and Wiedemann Agnès
INRA Centre de Tours, UR1282 Infectiologie Animale et Santé Publique, Nouzilly
IFR 136, Agents Transmissibles et Infectiologie, Nouzilly
France

1. Introduction

Salmonella enterica are members of a Gram-negative enteropathogenic bacteria family, which are able to infect a great diversity of hosts, including human. According to serotypes and hosts, *Salmonella enterica* cause a wide range of food- and water-borne diseases ranging from self-limiting gastroenteritis to systemic typhoid fever. Moreover, no other known bacterial pathogens belonging to a single species show such a remarkable variation in their host specificity. Ubiquitous serotypes such as Typhimurium and Enteritidis tend to produce acute but self-limiting enteritis in a wide range of hosts, whereas host-specific serotypes are associated with severe systemic disease in healthy outbred adults of a single species that may not involve diarrhoea (e.g. Gallinarum in poultry). Host-restricted serotypes are primarily associated with systemic disease in one host (e.g. Dublin in cattle, Choleraesuis in pigs), but may cause disease in a limited number of other species (Velge *et al.*, 2005).

For all these serotypes, the intestinal barrier crossing constitutes a crucial step for infection establishment. As shown in Figure 1, *Salmonella* can induce their own entry into enterocytes, but M cells and CD18-expressing phagocytes also facilitate their translocation through the intestinal epithelium (Watson & Holden, 2010). During gastroenteritis pathology, host colonization is restricted to the intestinal tract. However, *Salmonella* also have the ability to disseminate to extra-intestinal sites at least via CD18-expressing phagocytes, leading to deep organ colonization (Vazquez-Torres *et al.*, 1999).

Bacterial pathogens have developed two different mechanisms to invade non-phagocytic host cells by hijacking physiological cellular processes. Bacteria, such as *Listeria monocytogenes* and *Yersinia pseudotuberculosis* express surface proteins that interact with receptor on the host cell plasma membrane. This interaction promotes an activation of host cell signaling pathways, leading to actin remodelling. This process is referred to as a Zipper mechanism and is characterized by the induction of little protrusive activity and thin membrane extensions (Figure 2A and C) (Cossart & Sansonetti, 2004). Other bacteria, such as *Shigella flexneri*, do not require a receptor but trigger internalization from "inside" via the action of pathogen-effector proteins delivered by specialized protein secretion systems (Schroeder & Hilbi, 2008). Translocated effector proteins effectively allow the bacteria to "hijack" many essential intracellular processes and induce a massive reorganization of the host actin cytoskeleton, resulting in intense membrane ruffling and internalization of the bacteria. This invasion process is referred to as a Trigger mechanism (Figure 2B and D) (Cossart & Sansonetti, 2004).

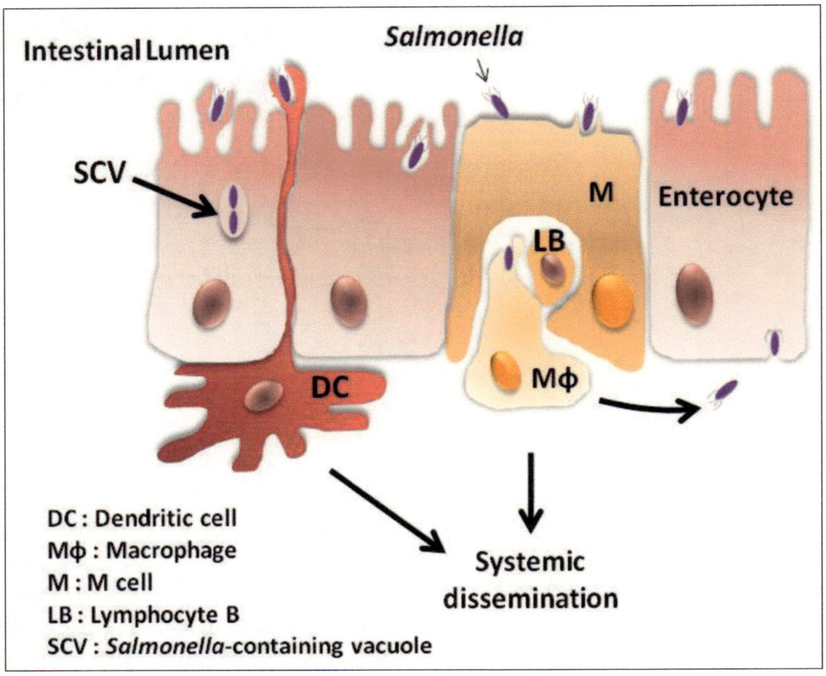

Fig. 1. Intestinal barrier crossing by *Salmonella enterica* through M cells, enterocytes or following a luminal capture by CD18+ phagocytes such as dendritic cells.

The reorganization of actin cytoskeleton at the entry site is a crucial step for Trigger and Zipper bacterial internalization. In eukaryotic cells, actin exists as a globular monomer (G-actin) which can assemble to form a filamentous structure (F-actin). In physiological conditions, actin polymerization requires different steps. First, nucleation of actin which consists in regrouping three actin monomers, is stimulated by cellular factors such as the Arp2/3 complex (Mullins *et al.*, 1998). Once nucleated, the addition of ATP-actin-monomers at the barbed extremity of the filaments allows actin elongation (Pollard *et al.*, 2000). The three-dimensional structure of actin filaments is ensured by capping proteins and other actin-binding proteins such as actinin, gelsolin, and villin that enable bundling of filaments (Bretscher, 1991; Hartwig & Kwiatkowski, 1991). Actin dynamics regulation is closely associated with small Rho guanosine triphosphatase protein (RhoGTPase) activity. RhoGTPases cycle between an inactive guanine di-phosphate (GDP)-bound form and an active guanine tri-phosphate (GTP)-bound form. The switch between inactive and active state is regulated by guanine exchange factors (GEF) which catalyze the exchange of GDP with GTP and GTPase activating proteins (GAP) which hydrolyze GTP into GDP to switch off their active state. When bound to GTP, Rho GTPases target and activate downstream effectors such as proteins from the Wiscott-Aldrich Syndrome protein (WASP) / N-WASP Family, leading to nucleator activation and actin reorganization. All these steps are required during bacterial internalization.

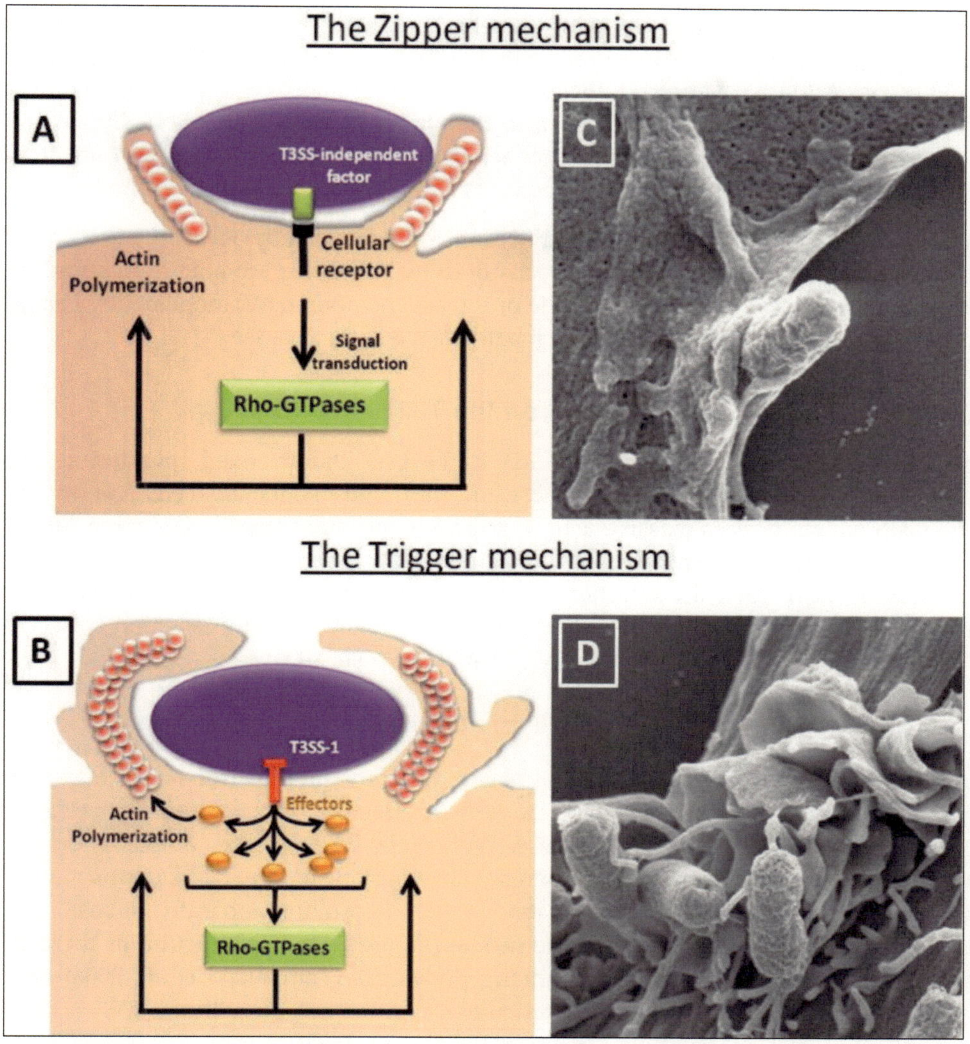

Fig. 2. Models of Zipper and Trigger invasion mechanisms. (A) The Zipper process is initiated by an interaction between a host cell receptor and a bacterial surface protein which allows the activation of RhoGTPases and actin polymerization at the entry site. (B) In contrast, during the Trigger mechanism, RhoGTPases are targeted by bacterial effectors which are directly translocated into host cell via a type-three secretion system, leading to actin polymerization and internalization. Electron scanning microscopy pictures show (C) *S.* Enteritidis invading fibroblasts via a Zipper process which is characterized by weak membrane rearrangements and (D) via a Trigger process which is characterized by intense membrane rearrangements.

The study of host cell invasion by *Salmonella* has been initiated in 1967 by Takeuchi (Takeuchi, 1967). For decades, it was described in the literature that *Salmonella* can enter cells only via a "Trigger" mechanism mediated by a type-three secretion system (T3SS-1) encoded by the *Salmonella* pathogenicity island-1 (SPI-1) (Ibarra & Steele-Mortimer, 2009). Recent data have showed that cell invasion could occur despite the absence of the T3SS-1

(Aiastui *et al.*, 2010; Radtke *et al.*, 2010; Rosselin *et al.*, 2011), indicating that the dominant paradigm postulating that a functional SPI-1/T3SS is absolutely required for cell entry, should be reconsidered. Moreover, the characterization of one T3SS-1-independent invasion pathway revealed that *Salmonella* have also the ability to enter cells via a Zipper process mediated by the Rck invasin (Rosselin *et al.*, 2011). Consequently *Salmonella* are the first bacteria found to be able to invade cells both via a Zipper and a Trigger mechanism.

Here, our current understanding of the different strategies used by *Salmonella* to invade host cells will be summarized and we will focus on how *Salmonella* are able to manipulate the host actin cytoskeleton, leading to discrete or intense membrane rearrangements. The gap of our knowledge about these different entry pathways will be discussed.

2. Invasion mechanism dependent on the T3SS-1

The Type-Three Secretion System (T3SS-1) is the best characterized invasion system of *Salmonella*. It allows bacterial internalization into non-phagocytic cells via a Trigger mechanism which induces massive actin rearrangements and intense membrane ruffling at the entry site (Cossart & Sansonetti, 2004). Under environmental conditions that enable the expression of the T3SS-1, the secretion apparatus is assembled at the bacterial surface and effectors are translocated into the eukaryotic cytosol following an interaction between the bacteria and the host cell (Garner *et al.*, 2002; Hayward *et al.*, 2005).

2.1 T3SS-1 structure

T3SSs are supramolecular complexes that play a major role in the virulence of many Gram-negative pathogens by injecting bacterial protein effectors directly into host cells in an energy-dependent (ATP) manner (Galan & Wolf-Watz, 2006). These complexes cross both inner and outer membranes of bacteria and are able to create a pore in eukaryotic membrane upon contact with a host cell. They are made of an exportation apparatus, a basal body, a needle and a translocon at the tip of the needle (Figure 3A). The structure of these T3SSs shows a high degree of conservation among pathogens (Tampakaki *et al.*, 2004) and the *Salmonella* T3SS-1 apparatus shares in particular a high homology with the T3SS of *Shigella*, also involved in host cell invasion (Groisman & Ochman, 1993).

The basal body of the T3SS anchors the complex into the bacterial inner and outer membranes (Figure 3A). It is composed of PrgH, PrgK and InvG proteins which assemble into an inner ring (PrgH and PrgK) and an outer ring (InvG) (Schraidt & Marlovits, 2011). Anchored to the basal body via its transmembrane part, the needle protrudes from the outer membrane as a long filament of 50 nm length and is composed of the single PrgI protein (Kimbrough & Miller, 2000). At the extremity of the needle, a complex of three proteins (SipB, SipC, SipD), known as the translocon, is able to form a pore in the eukaryotic target cell, allowing the secretion of effector proteins (Mattei *et al.*, 2011). SipB, SipC and SipD proteins (also referred to Ssp proteins) share homology with other translocon proteins such as IpaB, IpaC and IpaD proteins of *Shigella* (Hueck, 1998). SipD has a hydrophilic domain and interacts directly with the PrgI needle protein (Rathinavelan *et al.*, 2011) while the two other proteins of the translocon (SipB and SipC) have a hydrophobic domain and are therefore directly involved in the pore formation (Hayward *et al.*, 2000; Miki *et al.*, 2004). Particularly, it has been shown that the interaction of SipB with cellular cholesterol is necessary for effector translocation (Hayward *et al.*, 2005). Finally, the translocation of T3SS-1 effector proteins requires an exportation apparatus located at the inner membrane level and made of highly conserved proteins among T3SSs (SpaP, SpaQ, SpaR, SpaS, InvA, InvC and OrgB). The unfolded effectors in association with their chaperone are targeted to the exportation apparatus and the ATPase InvC produces the energy necessary to the transport of these proteins through the needle (Akeda & Galan, 2004). The appropriate hierarchy in the secretion process is established by a cytoplasmic sorting platform composed of SpaO, OrgA and OrgB (Lara-Tejero *et al.*, 2011). This platform sequentially loads the secreted proteins by interacting with their chaperones to ensure a specific order of secretion and optimize host cell invasion.

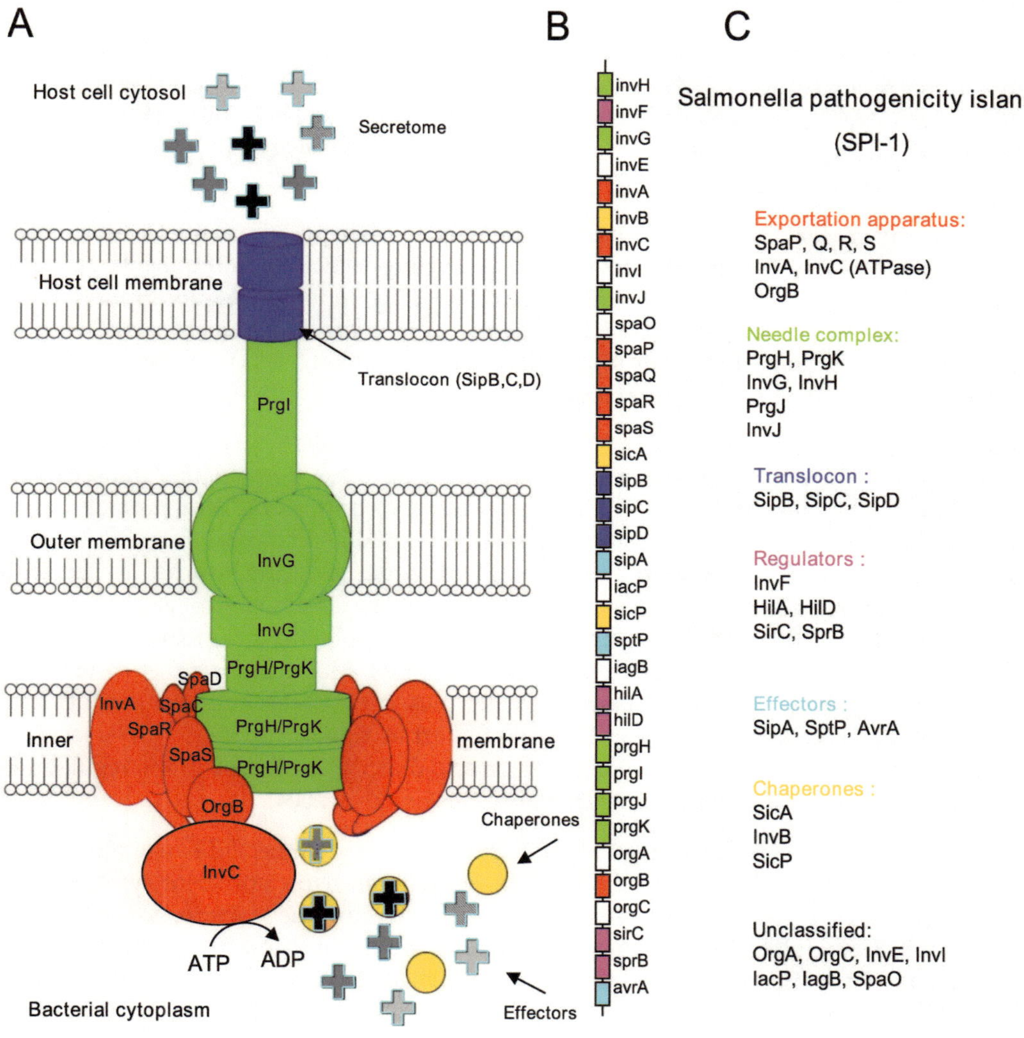

Adapted from Kimbrough and Miller, 2002.
A. Localization of the T3SS-1 structure proteins. **B.** Schematic representation of SPI-1 island encoding the T3SS-1 proteins. **C.** Functional classification of SPI-1-encoded proteins.

Fig. 3. Structure and organization of *Salmonella* T3SS-1.

2.2 Regulation of T3SS-1 expression

During *Salmonella* infection, a crucial step is the crossing of the intestinal barrier. The host environment encountered by the bacteria, and more particularly the small intestine environment, plays a major role in the invasion as it controls expression of the secretion apparatus. Coordination of T3SS-1 expression genes, almost all located on the *Salmonella* Pathogenicity Island 1 (SPI-1) is complex and well-timed. In response to different environmental stimuli, a sophisticated regulatory network controlling the expression of SPI-1 has been established (Figure 4). Our purpose here is not to set up the thorough state-of-the-art on all the regulators involved in *Salmonella* invasion, but to give a general overview of this system (for a review, see (Ellermeier & Slauch, 2007)).

SPI-1 contains 39 genes encoding structural T3SS-1 proteins (*inv/spa* and *prg* operon), translocon proteins (SipB, C, D), some effectors (SipA, SptP and AvrA), some chaperones (SicA, InvB, SicP) and finally four transcriptional regulators (HilA, hilC, HilD and InvF) (Figure 3B and C). Other genes encoding secreted effectors (*sopA, sopB, sopD, sopE, sopE2, slrP, sspH1, sspH2*) are located elsewhere on the chromosome.

HilA is central for SPI-1 transcriptional regulation. This protein activates directly the transcription of *prg, inv/spa* and *sip* operons, encoding structural components and some secreted effectors of T3SS-1 respectively. In addition, HilA induces the transcription of *invF*, encoding a transcriptional activator and targeting, among others, *sip* operon, *sopE* and *sopB* genes (Darwin & Miller, 1999). The sequential expression of HilA and InvF regulators allows a hierarchical regulation of invasion genes.

Then, a second crucial level of SPI-1 transcriptional regulation takes place through the regulation of HilA *via* a feed-forward loop, involving three homologous transcriptional regulators: HilC, HilD and RtsA. Each of them binds directly to the *hilA* promoter and is able to activate its own expression. In fact, HilC, HilD and probably RtsA, act as derepressors of *hilA* transcription by counteracting the silencing exerted by nucleoid-structuring proteins such as H-NS or Hha (Akbar *et al.*, 2003; Queiroz *et al.*, 2011). The reason why HilC, HilD and RtsA play such an important role in T3SS-1 expression through *hilA* regulation is that they are at the integration point of a lot of signals that control SPI-1 expression (Figure 4). In this regulatory circuit, it is currently admitted that HilD has a predominant role whereas HilC and RtsA simply act as signal amplifiers. However, it has also been shown that these three regulators are also directly implicated in the regulation of others invasion genes (Akbar *et al.*, 2003; Ellermeier & Slauch, 2004).

Moreover, besides these direct regulators, a great number of other *hilA* regulators, acting mainly through HilD, have been identified. Among them, two-component systems play a major role. They sense environmental conditions and allow the transmission of different signals which modulate T3SS-1 genes expression. Some are able to activate indirectly HilA expression such as BarA/SirA and OmpR/EnvZ, whereas others such as PhoP/PhoQ and PhoB/PhoR repress it. In fact, HilA expression can also be inhibited. HilE has been identified as a negative regulator of *hilA* transcription preventing HilD activity (Fahlen *et al.*, 2000; Baxter *et al.*, 2003). It has been suggested that the two-component systems PhoP/PhoQ and PhoB/PhoR act through HilE to regulate SPI-1 (Baxter & Jones, 2005).

As stated above, environmental signals play a major role in *Salmonella* invasion. Low oxygen tension, high osmolarity, high iron concentration, neutral pH are conditions found in the ileum, known to be the preferential invasion site of *Salmonella*. Thus, as expected in these conditions, invasion genes are activated through *hilA* expression. In contrast, when *Salmonella* are located at unfavorable sites for invasion in the host organism, the presence of signals such as bile, secreted into the proximal small intestine or cationic peptides, known to exist in macrophages, inhibits T3SS-1 expression (Figure 4).

Although much has already been identified about the regulation of SPI-1, recently, it became more evident that mechanisms regulating this system are more complex than previously thought.

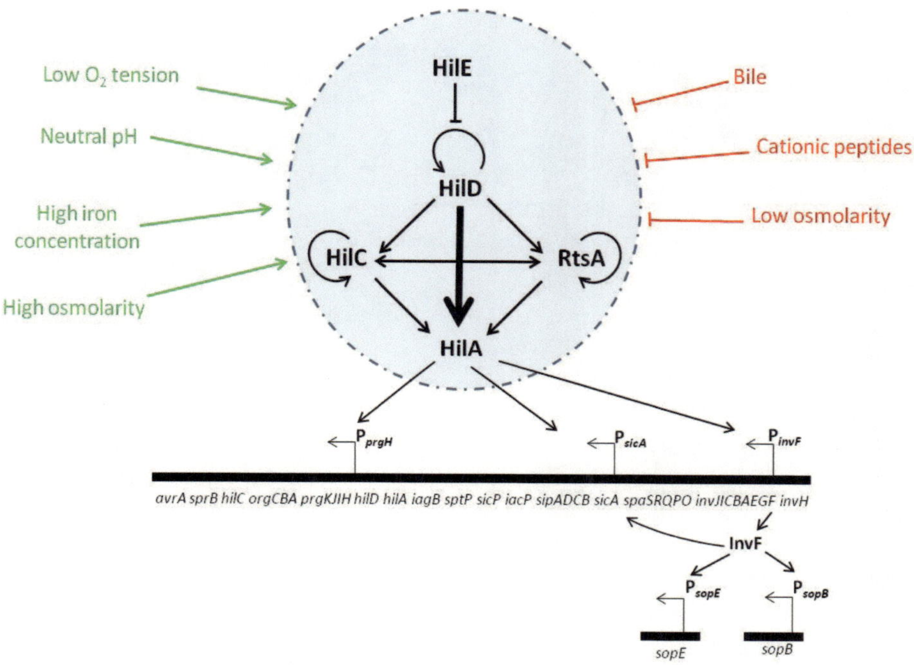

Fig. 4. Environmental and transcriptional regulation of SPI-1 encoded genes. HilA is the major regulator of SPI-1 and is itself regulated by other regulators such as HilC, HilD, RtsA and HilE. When *Salmonella* reach the small intestine, a low O_2 tension, a neutral pH, a high iron concentration and a high osmolarity activate SPI-1 expression. In contrast, the presence of bile or cationic peptides represses its expression.

2.3 Subversion of the cellular machinery during T3SS-1-dependent entry

Among the effectors that are translocated into host cell by the T3SS-1, six are essential to cell invasion (SipA, SipC, SopB, SopD, SopE, SopE2) while the other effectors contribute to a variety of post-invasion processes such as host cell survival and modulation of the inflammatory response (Patel & Galan, 2005). To trigger internalization into cells, effectors manipulate actin cytoskeleton either directly or indirectly. They also manipulate the delivery of vesicles to the site of bacterial entry to provide additional membrane and allow the extension and ruffling of the plasma membrane necessary to promote invasion. In later steps, membrane fission occurs to induce the sealing of the future *Salmonella*-containing vacuole (SCV) and actin filaments are depolymerized, enabling the host cell to recover its normal shape (Figure 5).

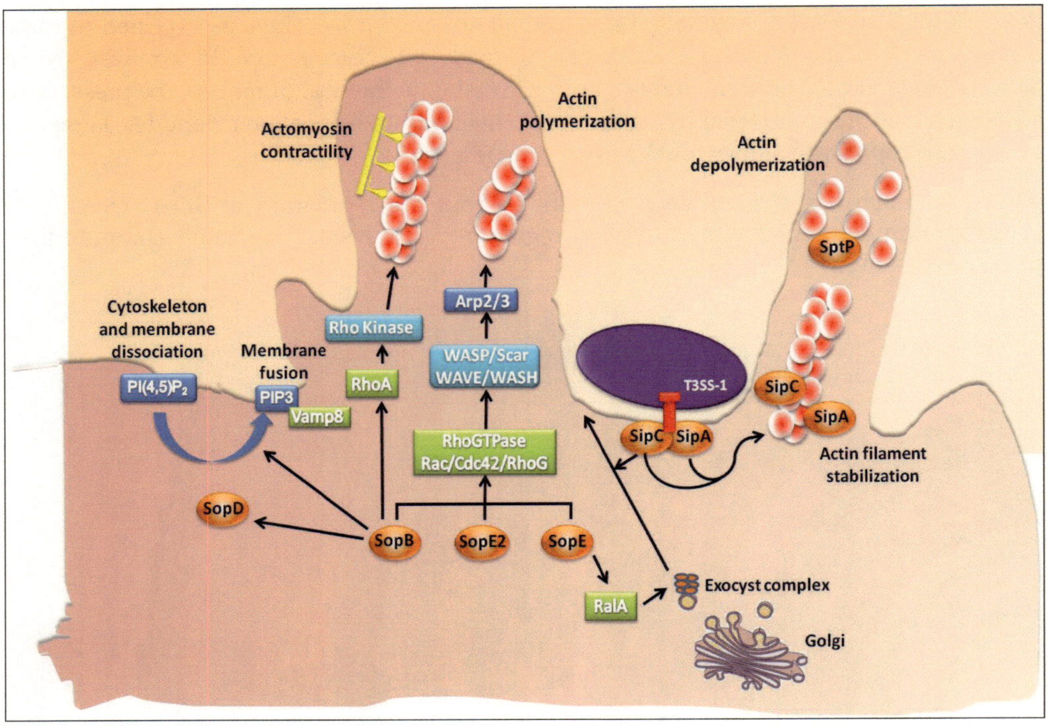

Fig. 5. Intracellular activities of the T3SS-1 effectors: SipA and SipC bind actin directly whereas SopE, SopE2 and SopB stimulate RhoGTPase activity. SipC and SopE also act in cooperation to recruit exocytic vesicles at the entry site. SopB plays diverse roles during invasion: it promotes actomyosin contractility and changes phosphoinositide concentrations to facilitate the dissociation between actin cytoskeleton and membrane at the entry site. SopB also probably triggers the delivery of vesicles to the bacterial entry site in a VAMP-8 dependent way and activate SopD which seems to contribute to the sealing and the formation of the SCV. The last effector SptP turns off the activity of RhoGTPases to allow the host cell to regain its initial shape.

2.3.1 Actin manipulation

Actin polymerization is an essential process induced by T3SS-1 effectors during entry. Some effectors stimulate actin rearrangements indirectly and two effectors, SipA and SipC, manipulate actin directly. SipA and SipC are localized at the eukaryotic plasma membrane during entry (Scherer *et al.*, 2000) but they are also translocated into the host cell cytoplasm (Hueck *et al.*, 1995; Kaniga *et al.*, 1995).

SipC, as part of the translocon, is required for T3SS-1 effector translocation and involved in actin nucleation and bundling. Due to its various functions, a 95% decrease in invasion is observed when *sipC* is deleted (Chang *et al.*, 2005). The C-terminal region of SipC (amino-acids A321-A409) encodes the effector translocation activity (Chang *et al.*, 2005) and its central region (amino-acids N201–S220) binds to actin and induces a rapid nucleation and elongation of actin filaments. More precisely the regions containing the amino acids from H221–M260 and L381–A409 bind to and bundle actin filaments *in vitro* (Myeni & Zhou,

2010). The bundling activity of SipC is essential for internalization as a *sipC* mutant lacking bundling activity is impaired in cell invasion. SipC dimerization / multimerization seems to be required for nucleation and a *sipC* mutant deficient for multimerization and actin nucleation failed to cause severe colitis in a mouse model (Chang *et al.*, 2007).

As SipC, SipA binds directly to actin (amino acids P446-R685) and modulates cytoskeleton dynamics in different ways (Galkin *et al.*, 2002; Higashide *et al.*, 2002). A *Salmonella* Typhimurium *sipA* mutant exhibits a 60-80% decrease in invasion compared to the wild-type strain (Perrett & Jepson, 2009), which can be correlated to the fact that SipA is a multifunctional effector. First, Zhou *et al.* (1999b) have observed that SipA reduces the critical concentration of G-actin in the cytosol required for polymerization. In addition, to facilitate polymerization, SipA also stabilizes actin filaments by displacing ADF / cofilin factor which stimulates actin depolymerization and by protecting F-actin from gelsolin severing (McGhie *et al.*, 2004). Moreover, SipA enhances actin cross-linking both by interacting with T-Plastin, a cellular bundling protein, and by enhancing SipC activity (Zhou *et al.*, 1999a; McGhie *et al.*, 2001). Interestingly, Perrett and Jepson have demonstrated that a *sipA* deletion induces a decrease in host cell invasion but without affecting the frequency of membrane ruffle formation (Perrett & Jepson, 2009). By visualizing the membrane ruffles in the absence of SipA, they have observed that SipA is required to ensure the spatial localization of actin rearrangement beneath invading *Salmonella* for efficient uptake of bacteria.

In contrast to SipA and SipC, SopB, SopE and SopE2 exert their activity into host cells by inducing actin polymerization in an indirect way. They activate RhoGTPases which are key cellular effectors that regulate actin cytoskeleton remodeling (Patel & Galan, 2005).

During *Salmonella* T3SS-1 dependent invasion, SopE and SopE2 effectors mimic GEF activity to activate RhoGTPases. Their activation induces actin polymerization by stimulating downstream cellular proteins such as N-WASP, WAVE and WASH which activate the Arp2/3 nucleator complex (Buchwald *et al.*, 2002; Schlumberger *et al.*, 2003). SopE specifically targets the Rho GTPases Rac and Cdc42 *in vitro* whereas SopE2 only activates Cdc42 (Friebel *et al.*, 2001). The role of Rac in *Salmonella* T3SS-1-dependent entry is well characterized but the role of Cdc42 is controversial. Criss *et al.* (2001) have demonstrated by using dominant negative forms and by pull-down assays that, in contrast to non-polarized cells, Cdc42 is not required and not activated during invasion of MCDK polarized epithelial cells. In the same way, Patel and Galan have observed that the depletion of Cdc42 by RNA interference (RNAi) in COS-2 and Henle-407 had no effect on membrane ruffling and efficient uptake (Patel & Galan, 2006). In contrast, a recent genome-scale RNAi screening in HeLA cells indicated that Cdc42 depletion induced a 70% decrease in invasion, suggesting that it is required for the T3SS-1-dependent invasion process (Misselwitz *et al.*, 2011). All together, it is difficult to conclude about the involvement of Cdc42 during T3SS-1-dependent entry.

Salmonella mutant strains lacking both *sopE* and *sopE2* are still able to invade cells in a SopB dependent way (Zhou *et al.*, 2001). SopB is an inositol phosphatase which shares homology with eukaryotic phopho-inositol (PI) phosphatases (Norris *et al.*, 1998). Like SopE and SopE2, SopB targets a GTPase from the Rho family, RhoG, but in an indirect manner since SopB activates the GEF protein that allows RhoG activation (Patel & Galan, 2006). Once activated, RhoG induces actin polymerization at the entry site presumably by stimulating the Arp2/3 complex (Patel & Galan, 2006). A *sopB* deletion in *S.* Typhimurium induces a 50% decrease in invasion. But when *sopB* deletion is coupled with a *sopE* deletion, *Salmonella* uptake is drastically impaired (Zhou *et al.*, 2001), demonstrating that all the T3SS-1 effectors work in concert to trigger entry.

Recently, SopB was also shown to manipulate actomyosin contractility to mediate invasion. SopB recruits myosin II by activating RhoA and its Rho kinase downstream effector. In contrast to the process leading to actin polymerization during *Salmonella* entry, myosin II recruitment at the entry site is independent on Arp2/3 nucleator activity (Hanisch *et al.*, 2011).

In addition, different cellular proteins are involved during the T3SS-1 dependent entry of *Salmonella* without the identification of the bacterial effector responsible of this effect. This includes the focal adhesion kinase FAK, the Abelson tyrosine kinase Abl, and Shank3 (Shi & Casanova, 2006; Huett *et al.*, 2009; Ly & Casanova, 2009). During *Salmonella* uptake, FAK acts as a scaffolding protein, but not as a protein tyrosine kinase and its interaction with p130Cas is involved in actin reorganization and membrane ruffle formation (Shi & Casanova, 2006). But how *Salmonella* can nucleate assembly of focal adhesion-like complexes is still unclear and further research is needed to determine if this mechanism involves secreted bacterial effector proteins, other transmembrane host proteins, or both. Another scaffolding protein Shank3 also seems to regulate actin rearrangement during entry but the mechanisms leading to its recruitment and its activation have to be elucidated (Huett *et al.*, 2009). As the experiments were performed using HeLa cells which are highly permissive to the T3SS-1-dependent entry and with bacterial culture conditions that allow T3SS-1 expression, it is more probable that the *Salmonella* entry process inducing Shank3 recruitment is dependent on the T3SS-1. However, a T3SS-1-independent invasion process could also be involved because no mutant deficient for T3SS-1 expression was used as a control to analyze the involvement of Shank3.

Abelson tyrosine kinase Abl is also involved during *Salmonella* invasion as well as its effectors Abi1, a member of the WAVE2 complex, and CrkII (Ly & Casanova, 2009). Abi1 could thus enhance actin polymerization at the entry site but the role of CrkII during the invasion process remains poorly characterized.

2.3.2 Subversion of exocytosis machinery and membrane fusion during entry

Recent data indicate that membrane fusion is a major process involved during entry, suggesting that membrane ruffling requires the addition of intracellular membrane. A study focusing on the subversion of the host exocyst complex during *Salmonella* entry has showed cooperation between SipC and SopE (Nichols & Casanova, 2010). The exocyst is an octomeric complex (Sec3, Sec5, Sec6, Sec8, Sec10, Sec15, Exo70, Exo84) involved in vesicular trafficking which directs post-Golgi vesicules at specific site on the plasma membrane prior to their fusion. Nichols and Casanova have demonstrated that the mature exocyst complex is recruited at the entry site through an interaction between its subunit Exo70 and SipC. A depletion of exo70 or Sec5, another component of the exocyst complex, impairs *S.* Typhimurium invasion. Moreover, they have shown that SopE activates the Ras-related protein RalA, a small GTPase required for exocyst complex assembly (Nichols

& Casanova, 2010). It appears that SopE and SipC effectors manipulate the host exocyst to bring new membrane at the entry site in order to allow the formation of membrane ruffles and internalization.

SopB is also involved in this membrane fusion process through its inositol phosphatase activity. Dai *et al.* (2007) have shown that SopB-generated PI3P at the entry site leads to the recruitment of VAMP8, a host V-SNARE protein that mediates fusion between early and late endosomes. Moreover, depletion of VAMP8 by RNAi induces a decrease in invasion rate of a wild-type *S.* Typhimurium strain which is equivalent to that obtained with a *sopB* mutant. Thus, it seems that SopB promotes invasion by manipulating eukaryotic vesicular trafficking probably to induce fusion of intracellular vesicles to the cell membrane at the entry site.

How these events of vesicle-membrane fusion interact with actin cytoskeleton rearrangements to trigger entry has not been investigated yet. These different processes may synergize to induce internalization since actin dynamics is closely related to the metabolism of phosphoinosides (Honda *et al.*, 1999; Sechi & Wehland, 2000). However, VAMP8 which seems to be a marker of membrane fusion involved during *S.* Typhimurium invasion does not co-localize with F-actin during entry (Dai *et al.*, 2007). In addition, it could be interesting to better characterize the role of the cellular factor IQGAP1 which is required for *Salmonella* uptake and acts following an interaction with actin and the RhoGTPases Rac1 and Cdc42 (Brown *et al.*, 2007). Indeed, IQGAP1 is known to regulate actin architecture and interestingly, it also seems to act as a regulator of exocytosis by interacting with Exo70 (Rittmeyer *et al.*, 2008). IQGAP1 could thus be one of the missing links between actin rearrangement and membrane fusion during *Salmonella* entry. Further studies could overcome this issue.

2.3.3 Phagosome closure and restoration of the host cell normal shape

As described above, inositol phosphatase activity of SopB drives to changes in cellular phosphoinosite concentrations at the bacteria/cell contact. In addition to generate PI3P at the entry site, translocation of SopB into host cells also induces $PI(4,5)P_2$ hydrolysis, which leads to an almost complete absence of $PI(4,5)P_2$ at the membrane invagination regions (Terebiznik *et al.*, 2002). By reducing the local concentration of $PI(4,5)P_2$, SopB destabilizes cytoskeleton-plasma membrane interactions, thus reducing the rigidity of the membrane and promoting invasion by facilitating the fission and the sealing of the future *Salmonella*-containing vacuole. In addition to SopB, SopD also contributes to membrane fission. Boonyom *et al.* have demonstrated that a *sopD* deletion, like the *sopB* mutant, leads to a decrease in membrane fission during invasion and that SopD is recruited at the bacterial invasion site dependently on the phosphatase activity of SopB (Bakowski *et al.*, 2007). Thus, SopD seems to cooperate with SopB and contribute to *Salmonella* uptake by facilitating membrane fission at the entry site leading to the formation of the SCV (Bakowski *et al.*, 2007).

Following the formation of intense membrane ruffling and internalization, the eukaryotic cell regains its normal shape, inducing the closure of the vacuole of endocytosis containing the bacteria. The restoration of actin cytoskeleton is promoted by the effector SptP, a tyrosine phosphatase which inactivates the RhoGTPases Rac-1 and Cdc42 by stimulating their intrinsic GTPase activity (Fu & Galan, 1998; Fu & Galan, 1999). The N- terminal region of SptP interacts with Rac-1 and Cdc42 and a structural study of SptP indicates that this effector mimics the activity of host cell GAPs factors (Stebbins & Galan, 2000). Interestingly, SptP is regulated by two different mechanisms in order to delay its activity in host cell compared to that of SopE or SipA. A microscopy analysis revealed that SipA is injected earlier than SptP in the host cytoplasm, which would imply that SipA has a higher affinity for the exportation apparatus of the T3SS-1 than SptP (Winnen *et al.*, 2008). Moreover, SptP degradation by the host cell proteasome occurs later than SopE degradation (Kubori & Galan, 2003).

2.4 T3SS-1 contribution to *Salmonella* pathogenesis

The T3SS-1 is the main invasion factor of *Salmonella in vitro*. Nevertheless, its contribution to pathogenesis depends on the model used. *In vivo* studies with *S.* Dublin and *S.* Typhimurium serotypes have demonstrated that the T3SS-1 is essential for intestinal colonization and is required to induce enterocolitis in bovine, rabbit and murine models (Wallis & Galyov, 2000). In contrast, recent studies demonstrate that different serotypes of *Salmonella* lacking T3SS-1 still have the ability to invade *in vitro* cells of diverse origins and can be pathogenic in different *in vivo* infection models (Aiastui *et al.*, 2010; Rosselin *et al.*, 2011). In addition, it was shown that the T3SS-1 is not required for *Salmonella* internalization into a 3-Dimensional intestinal epithelium (Radtke *et al.*, 2010). Moreover, a SPI-1 mutant of *S.* Gallinarum exhibits a reduced invasiveness into avian cells but is fully virulent in adult chicken (Jones *et al.*, 2001). In *S.* Enteritidis and *S.* Typhimurium, the T3SS-1 is not essential during systemic infection of one week-old chicken or BalB/c mouse nor during the intestinal colonization of rabbit ileal loops (Coombes *et al.*, 2005; Jones *et al.*, 2007; Karasova *et al.*, 2010). Moreover, *S.* Senftenberg strains lacking SPI-1 are isolated from human clinical cases, suggesting that the T3SS-1 is dispensable by this serotype for the establishment of infection in humans (Hu *et al.*, 2008).

Taken together, these results indicate that T3SS-1- independent invasion mechanisms also play an important role in *Salmonella* infection and pathogenesis.

3. Invasion mechanisms independent of the T3SS-1

A *Salmonella* mutant, unable to express its T3SS-1 is still able to invade numerous cell lines and cell types and is shown to induce both intense and local membrane rearrangements (Rosselin et al., 2011). However, to date, little is known about the entry factors mediating these T3SS-1 independent invasion mechanisms. Here, we describe and sum up the state-of-art regarding these new invasion systems. Rck, PagN and HlyE are the three invasins identified as involved in *Salmonella* uptake. Moreover, Rosselin *et al.* (2011) have described that others unknown invasion factors exist although they are still not identified.

3.1 The Rck invasin

Among invasins that play a role in *Salmonella* invasion in a T3SS-1-independent way, Rck is clearly the best characterized. Rck is an 17kDa outer membrane protein (OMP) encoded by the large virulence plasmid of *S.* Enteritidis and *S.* Typhimurium (Heffernan *et al.*, 1992; Rotger & Casadesus, 1999). In addition to its ability to induce adhesion to and invasion of eukaryotic cells, Rck confers a high resistance level to complement killing by preventing the formation of the membrane attack complex (Heffernan *et al.*, 1992; Cirillo *et al.*, 1996; Rosselin *et al.*, 2010).

3.1.1 Rck structure

Rck is a member of an outer membrane protein family named "Ail/Lom family". This family consists of five members (Rck, Ail, Lom, OmpX and PagC) which are predicted to have eight transmembrane beta-sheets and four cell surface-exposed loops. Even if these proteins present a similar conformation, they have different functions. Rck and Ail (encoded by a chromosomal gene of *Yersinia Enterocolitica*) share the ability to promote serum resistance and epithelial cell invasion. These proteins do not exhibit homologous regions that could be related to these two identical roles. In Ail, the cell invasion property is associated with loop2 whereas loop3 and more precisely the region from the amino acids G113 to V159 was shown to be the minimal region of Rck required and sufficient for cell adhesion and invasion (Miller *et al.*, 2001; Rosselin *et al.*, 2010).

Another member of this family involved in virulence is PagC which is encoded by a *phoP*-regulated gene on the *Salmonella* chromosome and plays a role in intracellular macrophage survival in *Salmonella* (Miller *et al.*, 1989; Gunn *et al.*, 1995). Others members of this family are OmpX of *Enterobacter cloacae* (Mecsas *et al.*, 1995) and Lom, a protein expressed by bacteriophage λ from lysogenic *E. coli* (Reeve & Shaw, 1979) but none of them have known virulence-associated phenotype.

3.1.2 Rck regulation

A genetic screening performed in *S.* Typhimurium to identify genes regulated by SdiA (*s*uppressor of *d*ivision *i*nhibition), a transcriptional regulator of quorum sensing, has suggested that *rck* belongs to a putative operon called the "*rck* operon" whose expression is activated by SdiA in an Acyl Homoserine Lactone (AHLs)-dependent manner (Figure 6) (Ahmer *et al.*, 1998; Michael *et al.*, 2001).

The *rck* operon contains 6 open reading frames: *pefI*, *srgD*, *srgA*, *srgB*, *rck* and *srgC* (Figure 6). Two genes in this operon, *pefI* (*p*lasmid *e*ncoded *f*imbriae) and *srgA* (*s*diA-*r*egulated *g*ene), affect the expression and function of the *pef* operon located upstream of the *rck* operon and involved in the biosynthesis of the Pef fimbriae. *pefI* encodes a transcriptional regulator of the *pef* operon, and SrgA is a DsbA paralog that efficiently oxidizes the disulfide bond of PefA, the major structural subunit of the Pef fimbriae (Bouwman *et al.*, 2003). These fimbriae are involved in biofilm formation, adhesion to murine small intestine and fluid accumulation in the infant mouse (Baumler *et al.*, 1996; Ledeboer *et al.*, 2006). Also localized on the *rck* operon, *srgD* encodes a putative transcriptional regulator. Recently, it has been shown that SrgD acts in cooperation with PefI to induce a synergistic negative regulation of flagellar genes expression (Wozniak *et al.*, 2009; Wallar *et al.*, 2011). The remaining genes on the *rck* operon have unknown functions and encode a putative outer membrane protein, SrgB, and a putative transcriptional regulator, SrgC.

Another locus regulated by SdiA-AHLs has been identified during screening. This chromosomal locus encodes a single gene named *srgE* (STM1554) (Ahmer *et al.*, 1998). No function for SrgE is described but a computational approach has suggested that SrgE is secreted by the T3SS-1 (Samudrala *et al.*, 2009) (Figure 6).

As *E. coli* and *Klebsiella*, *Salmonella* lack an AHL synthase and thus do not produce AHLs. However, SdiA can detect and bind AHLs produced by others bacterial species (Michael *et al.*, 2001). SdiA is a LuxR homologue and has two functional domains. The C-terminal region contains a predicted helix-turn-helix motif implicated in DNA binding and a N-terminal domain called "autoinducer domain" that interacts with AHLs. By NMR analysis, Yao *et al.* (2007) have shown that a direct interaction between SdiA and AHLs is required for SdiA folding and function.

Temperature also affects *rck* operon expression. At temperature below 30°C, the transcription of *rck* operon is repressed, while *srgE* is repressed only at temperature below 22°C (Smith & Ahmer, 2003)(Figure 6). As SdiA expression is not temperature regulated, another level of *rck* operon regulation remains to be identified.

In addition, a transcriptomic study has shown that Hha and its paralogue YdgH could be involved in the regulation of the *rck* operon (Vivero *et al.*, 2008).

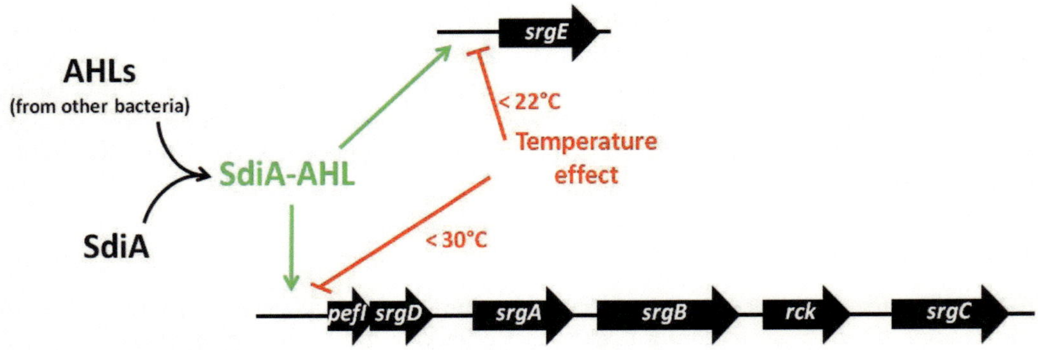

Fig. 6. Regulation of *rck* operon expression. When bound to AHLs, SdiA activates the expression of *rck* operon and *srgE*. Under temperatures that are lower than 30°C or 22°C, the expression of *rck* operon and *srgE* is inhibited, respectively.

3.1.3 Rck-mediated entry mechanism

When a *rck* mutant is grown under swarming conditions known to induce SdiA expression, a 2-3 fold decrease in epithelial cell invasion has been observed compared to the wild-type strain (Rosselin *et al.*, 2010). Moreover, in standard culture conditions, Rck overexpression leads to an increase in invasion.

By using both an initially non-invasive *E. coli* strain overexpressing Rck and latex beads coated with the minimal region of Rck inducing invasion (G113-V159), it was demonstrated that Rck alone is able to induce entry by a receptor-mediated process. This mechanism promotes local actin remodelling and weak and closely adherent membrane extensions (Rosselin *et al.*, 2010). *Salmonella* can thus enter cells through two distinct mechanisms: the Trigger mechanism mediated by its T3SS-1 apparatus and a Zipper mechanism induced by Rck. A model of this Zipper entry process is shown in figure 7. Following an interaction between Rck and its unknown cellular receptor, it was shown by using specific drugs and a dominant negative form that the class I PI3-kinase made of the p85-p110 heterodimer is required for Rck mediated entry. Moreover, Rck induces an increase in the interactions between p85 and phosphotyrosine residues, leading to the class I PI3-Kinase activation. Pharmacological approaches or Akt knockout cells also demonstrate that Akt is necessary to Rck-mediated internalization. Probably by binding to PI(3,4,5)P_3, Akt is recruited at the entry site and activated in a PI3-Kinase dependent way (Mijouin *et al.*, 2012).

The GTPase Rho is not involved during the Rck entry process but the use of dominant negatives demonstrates that Rac1 and Cdc42 are required (Rosselin *et al.*, 2010). Moreover, Rac1 is recruited at the entry site and Rck induces an increase in the level of active Rac1, demonstrating that it activates this GTPase (Rosselin *et al.*, 2010; Mijouin *et al.*, 2012). Rac1 activation occurs downstream on the PI-3kinase activity. Finally, overexpression of inhibitory constructs has shown that actin polymerization is dependent on the Arp2/3 nucleator complex during Rck-mediated entry (Rosselin *et al.*, 2010).

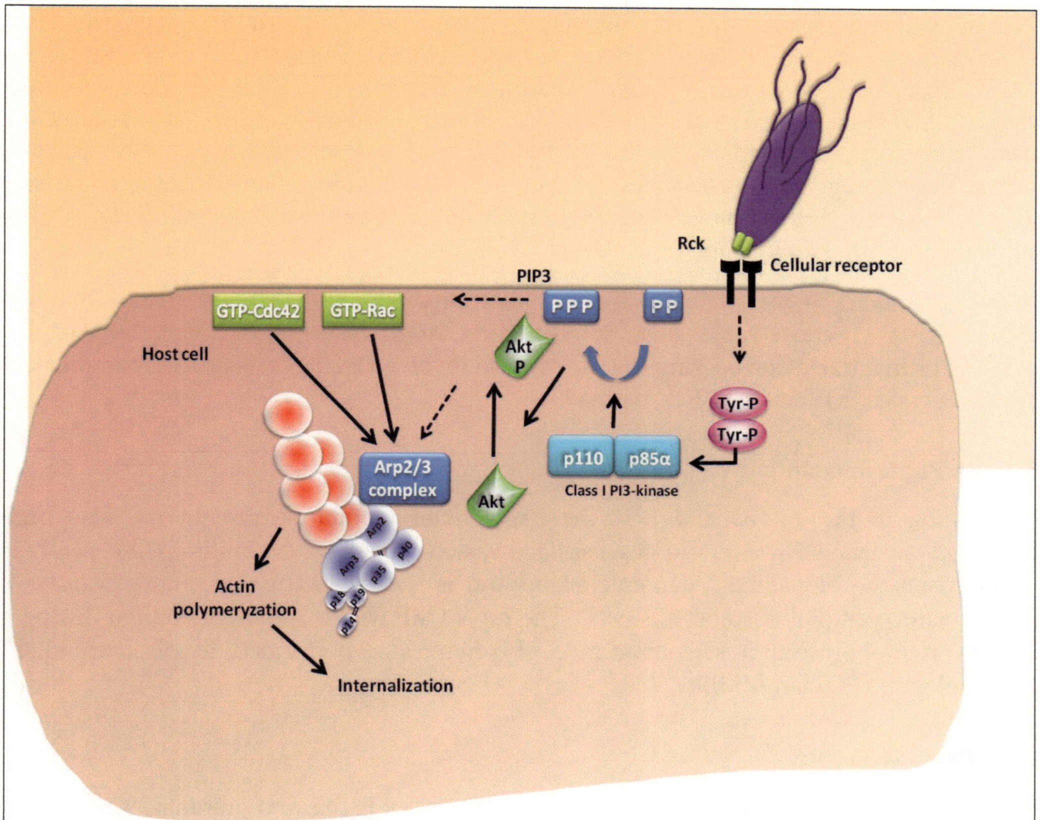

Fig. 7. Model of the cellular signaling pathway induces by Rck and leading to invasion. This Zipper entry process involves different cellular proteins: Class I PI3-Kinase, Akt, Rac and Cdc42, the Arp2/3 complex and actin. Dotted arrows: possible signalling events and/or interactions.

3.1.4 Rck contribution to *Salmonella* pathogenesis

The role of Rck in *Salmonella* invasion is clearly demonstrated *in vitro*, but its role in *Salmonella* pathogenesis is poorly understood. Indeed, *in vivo* conditions allowing *rck* expression are unclear. The fact that Rck is regulated by SdiA, a quorum sensing regulator suggests an intestinal role of this invasin (Ahmer *et al.*, 1998). However, the mechanisms leading to SdiA activation and *rck* expression are not well characterized. SdiA activation has been investigated in different hosts including rabbit, guinea pig, cow, turtle, mouse, pig and chicken but no activated-SdiA has been detected in the gastro-intestinal tract of these animals, except for turtles which were found to be co-infected with AHLs-producing *Aeromonas hydrophila* (Smith *et al.*, 2008). Another work has demonstrated that SdiA is activated in mice previously infected with *Yersinia enterocolitica,* which is able to synthesize AHLs (Dyszel *et al.*, 2010). However, in these conditions, SdiA activation does not confer a fitness advantage for *Salmonella* intestinal colonization in comparison to a *sdiA* mutant (Dyszel *et al.*, 2010). These results suggest that even if SdiA activation is achieved when AHL-producing strains colonize the gastrointestinal tract, it is not always sufficient to induce the expression of its regulon including *rck.* To assess the role of SdiA and its regulon during intestinal infection, Dyszel *et al.* (2010) have constructed a *Salmonella* strain able to produce AHLs. After co-infection of mice with the AHL-producing *Salmonella* strain and a *sdiA* mutant, it was shown that the constant activation of SdiA confers a selective advantage to *Salmonella.* Moreover, a loss of this selective advantage was observed when all individual SdiA-regulated genes were deleted, including *rck,* suggesting a role during intestinal colonization. Nevertheless, an *in vivo* model allowing a physiological activation of SdiA would be needed to assess the contribution of Rck to intestinal infection.

In addition, as *rck* is also regulated by an unidentified SdiA-independent system (Smith *et al.*, 2008), it is conceivable that Rck invasion mechanism is not restricted to the gastrointestinal tract. Considering that Rck is also involved in the resistance to complement killing, a systemic function of Rck is possible.

3.2 The PagN invasin

In addition to the T3SS-1 and Rck, the PagN outer membrane protein has also been identified as being involved in *Salmonella* invasion (Lambert & Smith, 2008). *pagN,* is localized on the centisome 7 genomic island and is widely distributed among *Salmonella enterica* serotypes (Folkesson *et al.*, 1999). The *pagN* ORF was originally identified during a Tn*phoA* random-insertion screening in *S.* Typhimurium performed to discover PhoP-activated genes (Belden & Miller, 1994).

3.2.1 PagN structure

PagN shares similarity to both the Tia and Hek invasins of *E. coli,* and presents 39% and 42% identity in amino acids with these two invasins, respectively. Tia and Hek are predicted to have eight transmembrane regions, four long exposed extracellular loops and three short periplasmic turns (Mammarappallil & Elsinghorst, 2000; Fagan *et al.*, 2008). Thus, PagN probably adopts a similar conformation as that of Hek and Tia.

3.2.2 PagN regulation

The *pagN* (*phoP*-activated gene) gene is *phoP*-regulated. The PhoP/PhoQ system is a two-component transcriptional regulatory system which modulates transcription of a multitude of virulence genes in *Salmonella.* This regulatory system is composed of the PhoQ sensor kinase (located at the membrane) and the PhoP response regulator. In response to specific stimuli such as acidified macrophage phagosome environment or low Mg^{2+} concentration, PhoQ is auto-phosphorylated and transfers its phosphates to the cytoplasmic DNA-binding protein PhoP, regulating specific genes.

3.2.3 PagN-mediated entry mechanism

Lambert & Smith (2008) have demonstrated that *pagN* deletion in *S.* Typhimurium leads to a 3-fold decrease in invasion of enterocytes without altering cell adhesion. At the cellular level, the PagN-mediated entry process is poorly characterized. It was only shown that actin polymerization is required during invasion (Lambert & Smith, 2008) and that PagN is able to interact with extracellular heparin proteoglycans (Lambert & Smith, 2009). However, proteoglycans cannot transduce a signaling cascade so it is probable that they act as co-receptors for invasion and not as the receptor itself. Moreover, although an interaction between PagN and heparin has been suggested, no clear heparin-binding motif was detected. Moreover, all PagN loops are required for invasion in epithelial cells (Lambert & Smith, 2009).

3.2.4 PagN contribution to *Salmonella* pathogenesis

PagN is required for survival in BALB/c mice (Heithoff *et al.*, 1999) and a *pagN* mutant is less competitive to colonize the spleen of mice compared to its parental strain (Conner *et al.*, 1998). However, the role of PagN in *Salmonella* pathogenesis is still unclear. *pagN* is activated by PhoP and thus maximally expressed intracellularly, a condition in which the SPI-1 island encoding the T3SS-1 is downregulated (Conner *et al.*, 1998; Heithoff *et al.*, 1999; Eriksson *et al.*, 2003). Lambert & Smith (2008) thus postulate that bacteria which exit epithelial cells or macrophages have an optimal level of PagN expression, but have a low T3SS-1 expression and this might facilitate subsequent interactions with mammalian cells that the pathogen encounters after host cell destruction.

3.3 The HlyE invasin

The *hlyE* gene is localized on the *Salmonella* pathogenicity island SPI-18 and is expressed by serotypes associated with systemic infection in humans including *S.* Typhi and *S.* Paratyphi A (Fuentes *et al.*, 2008). The *hlyE* sequence shares more than 90% identity with that of *Escherichia coli* HlyE (ClyA) hemolysin.The HlyE protein is able to lyse epithelial cells when exported from bacterial cell via outer membrane vesicule release (Wai *et al.*, 2003). Recently, Fuentes *et al.* (2008) have demonstratred that HlyE contributes to epithelial cell invasion of *S.* Typhi. However, the cellular events leading to HlyE-mediated invasion have not been characterized.

In vivo studies have shown that HlyE contributes to colonization of mouse deep organs (Fuentes *et al.*, 2008). However, how HlyE participates in establishment of systemic infection of *Salmonella* is not well understood.

3.4 Non-identified invasion factors

Several studies have revealed that invasion systems in *S.* Typhimurium and *S.* Enteritidis are not restricted to the T3SS-1, Rck and PagN. Indeed, a strain which does not express *rck*, *pagN* and the T3SS-1 is still able to significantly invade fibroblasts, epithelial and endothelial cells (Rosselin *et al.*, 2011). Results obtained by Aiastui *et al.* (2010) and van Sorge *et al.* (2011) have reinforced the idea that non-identified invasion factors are involved during entry into these cell types since *Salmonella* strains that cannot express the

T3SS-1 still enter into epithelial cells, endothelial cells and fibroblasts in a significant way. Moreover, invasion analyses of a 3-D intestinal epithelium by *S.* Typhimurium have also highlighted the fact that *Salmonella* possess non-characterized invasion factors (Radtke *et al.*, 2010).

Actin network remodeling and membrane rearrangements induced by these unknown factors have been visualized by confocal and electron microscopy as well as both Zipper-like and Trigger-like membrane alterations (Rosselin *et al.*, 2011). Identification of these factors is required to confirm these observations. It suggests that *Salmonella* express non-identified invasins able to mediate a Zipper process and factor(s) other than the T3SS-1 that induce Trigger-like invasion process(es). Type IV or type VI secretion systems are good candidates to induce Trigger-like cellular structures as they are able to translocate proteins directly into the host cell cytosol and as they are major virulence determinants involved in the pathogenesis of diverse Gram-negative bacteria (Oliveira *et al.*, 2006; Filloux *et al.*, 2008; Blondel *et al.*, 2010).

These observations thus open new avenues for identification of new invasion factors.

4. Conclusions and perspectives

Until recently, it was accepted that *Salmonella* enter cells only via its T3SS-1, which mediates a Trigger entry process. The T3SS-1-dependent invasion system has been widely described in the literature both at the bacterial and the cellular molecular levels. Moreover, the requirement of the T3SS-1 during intestinal and systemic infections has been demonstrated in some animals (Wallis & Galyov, 2000). However, an increasing number of reports describe that different serotypes of *Salmonella* can induce host infection without a functional T3SS-1 (Penheiter *et al.*, 1997; Jones *et al.*, 2001; Karasova *et al.*, 2010). This has been demonstrated with T3SS-1 mutants but also with clinical *Salmonella* strains (Hu *et al.*, 2008). However, the majority of *Salmonella* invasion system studies have focused on the T3SS-1 and we have little information concerning the T3SS-1-independent entry processes. Several invasins including PagN, Rck and HlyE have been recently identified in *Salmonella* and different investigations have provided evidences for other non-identified invasion factors (Aiastui *et al.*, 2010; Radtke *et al.*, 2010; Rosselin *et al.*, 2011; van Sorge *et al.*, 2011). In addition, the vast majority of this information has been obtained in a mouse model and with *S.* Typhimurium and much less data are available for other serotypes especially those adapted to pigs, cattle or poultry which represent major reservoirs of *Salmonella*. *Salmonella enterica* contain, over 2,500 diverse serotypes that have different host ranges, and cause diseases with severity ranging from subclinical colonization to serious systemic disease. Because the essential feature of the pathogenicity of *Salmonella* is its interaction with host cells, the identification of new entry routes could, in part, explain their different host ranges and disease symptoms.

The finding that *Salmonella* serotypes use different cell receptors and cell routes for host infection shows that the contribution of *Salmonella* genes to pathogenesis may be more complex than previously thought. These findings are changing our classical view of *Salmonella* pathogenicity. This new paradigm will modify the understanding of the mechanisms that lead to the different *Salmonella*-induced diseases and could allow us to revisit the host specificity bases.

5. References

Ahmer, B. M., van Reeuwijk, J., Timmers, C. D., Valentine, P. J. & Heffron, F. (1998). *Salmonella* typhimurium encodes an SdiA homolog, a putative quorum sensor of the LuxR family, that regulates genes on the virulence plasmid. *J Bacteriol*. Vol. 180, No. 5, pp. 1185-93.

Aiastui, A., Pucciarelli, M. G. & Garcia-del Portillo, F. (2010). *Salmonella* enterica serovar typhimurium invades fibroblasts by multiple routes differing from the entry into epithelial cells. *Infect Immun*. Vol. 78, No. 6, pp. 2700-13.

Akbar, S., Schechter, L. M., Lostroh, C. P. & Lee, C. A. (2003). AraC/XylS family members, HilD and HilC, directly activate virulence gene expression independently of HilA in *Salmonella* typhimurium. *Mol Microbiol*. Vol. 47, No. 3, pp. 715-28.

Akeda, Y. & Galan, J. E. (2004). Genetic analysis of the *Salmonella* enterica type III secretion-associated ATPase InvC defines discrete functional domains. *J Bacteriol*. Vol. 186, No. 8, pp. 2402-12.

Bakowski, M. A., Cirulis, J. T., Brown, N. F., Finlay, B. B. & Brumell, J. H. (2007). SopD acts cooperatively with SopB during *Salmonella* enterica serovar Typhimurium invasion. *Cell Microbiol*. Vol. 9, No. 12, pp. 2839-55.

Baumler, A. J., Tsolis, R. M., Bowe, F. A., Kusters, J. G., Hoffmann, S. & Heffron, F. (1996). The pef fimbrial operon of *Salmonella* typhimurium mediates adhesion to murine small intestine and is necessary for fluid accumulation in the infant mouse. *Infect Immun*. Vol. 64, No. 1, pp. 61-8.

Baxter, M. A., Fahlen, T. F., Wilson, R. L. & Jones, B. D. (2003). HilE interacts with HilD and negatively regulates hilA transcription and expression of the *Salmonella* enterica serovar Typhimurium invasive phenotype. *Infect Immun*. Vol. 71, No. 3, pp. 1295-305.

Baxter, M. A. & Jones, B. D. (2005). The fimYZ genes regulate *Salmonella* enterica Serovar Typhimurium invasion in addition to type 1 fimbrial expression and bacterial motility. *Infect Immun*. Vol. 73, No. 3, pp. 1377-85.

Belden, W. J. & Miller, S. I. (1994). Further characterization of the PhoP regulon: identification of new PhoP-activated virulence loci. *Infect Immun*. Vol. 62, No. 11, pp. 5095-101.

Blondel, C. J., Yang, H. J., Castro, B., Chiang, S., Toro, C. S., Zaldivar, M., Contreras, I., Andrews-Polymenis, H. L. & Santiviago, C. A. (2010). Contribution of the type VI secretion system encoded in SPI-19 to chicken colonization by *Salmonella* enterica serotypes Gallinarum and Enteritidis. *PLoS One*. Vol. 5, No. 7, pp. e11724.

Boonyom, R., Karavolos, M.H., Bulmer, D.M. & Khan, C.M. (2010). */Salmonella/* pathogenicity island 1 (SPI-1) type III secretion of SopD involves N- and C-terminal signals and direct binding to the InvC ATPase. Microbiology. vol.156, No.6, pp 1805-14.

Bouwman, C. W., Kohli, M., Killoran, A., Touchie, G. A., Kadner, R. J. & Martin, N. L. (2003). Characterization of SrgA, a *Salmonella* enterica serovar Typhimurium virulence plasmid-encoded paralogue of the disulfide oxidoreductase DsbA, essential for biogenesis of plasmid-encoded fimbriae. *J Bacteriol*. Vol. 185, No. 3, pp. 991-1000.

Bretscher, M. S. (1991). Lipid flow in locomoting cells. *Science*. Vol. 251, No. 4991, pp. 317-8.

Brown, M. D., Bry, L., Li, Z. & Sacks, D. B. (2007). IQGAP1 regulates *Salmonella* invasion through interactions with actin, Rac1, and Cdc42. *J Biol Chem*. Vol. 282, No. 41, pp. 30265-72.

Buchwald, G., Friebel, A., Galan, J. E., Hardt, W. D., Wittinghofer, A. & Scheffzek, K. (2002). Structural basis for the reversible activation of a Rho protein by the bacterial toxin SopE. *EMBO J*. Vol. 21, No. 13, pp. 3286-95.

Chang, J., Chen, J. & Zhou, D. (2005). Delineation and characterization of the actin nucleation and effector translocation activities of *Salmonella* SipC. *Mol Microbiol*. Vol. 55, No. 5, pp. 1379-89.

Chang, J., Myeni, S. K., Lin, T. L., Wu, C. C., Staiger, C. J. & Zhou, D. (2007). SipC multimerization promotes actin nucleation and contributes to *Salmonella*-induced inflammation. *Mol Microbiol*. Vol. 66, No. 6, pp. 1548-56.

Cirillo, D. M., Heffernan, E. J., Wu, L., Harwood, J., Fierer, J. & Guiney, D. G. (1996). Identification of a domain in Rck, a product of the *Salmonella* typhimurium virulence plasmid, required for both serum resistance and cell invasion. *Infect Immun*. Vol. 64, No. 6, pp. 2019-23.

Conner, C. P., Heithoff, D. M. & Mahan, M. J. (1998). In vivo gene expression: contributions to infection, virulence, and pathogenesis. *Curr Top Microbiol Immunol*. Vol. 225, No., pp. 1-12.

Coombes, B. K., Wickham, M. E., Lowden, M. J., Brown, N. F. & Finlay, B. B. (2005). Negative regulation of *Salmonella* pathogenicity island 2 is required for contextual control of virulence during typhoid. *Proc Natl Acad Sci U S A*. Vol. 102, No. 48, pp. 17460-5.

Cossart, P. & Sansonetti, P. J. (2004). Bacterial invasion: the paradigms of enteroinvasive pathogens. *Science*. Vol. 304, No. 5668, pp. 242-8.

Criss, A. K., Ahlgren, D. M., Jou, T. S., McCormick, B. A. & Casanova, J. E. (2001). The GTPase Rac1 selectively regulates *Salmonella* invasion at the apical plasma membrane of polarized epithelial cells. *J Cell Sci*. Vol. 114, No. Pt 7, pp. 1331-41.

Dai, S., Zhang, Y., Weimbs, T., Yaffe, M. B. & Zhou, D. (2007). Bacteria-generated PtdIns(3)P recruits VAMP8 to facilitate phagocytosis. *Traffic*. Vol. 8, No. 10, pp. 1365-74.

Darwin, K. H. & Miller, V. L. (1999). InvF is required for expression of genes encoding proteins secreted by the SPI1 type III secretion apparatus in *Salmonella* typhimurium. *J Bacteriol*. Vol. 181, No. 16, pp. 4949-54.

Dyszel, J. L., Smith, J. N., Lucas, D. E., Soares, J. A., Swearingen, M. C., Vross, M. A., Young, G. M. & Ahmer, B. M. (2010). *Salmonella* enterica serovar Typhimurium can detect acyl homoserine lactone production by Yersinia enterocolitica in mice. *J Bacteriol*. Vol. 192, No. 1, pp. 29-37.

Ellermeier, C. D. & Slauch, J. M. (2004). RtsA coordinately regulates DsbA and the *Salmonella* pathogenicity island 1 type III secretion system. *J Bacteriol*. Vol. 186, No. 1, pp. 68-79.

Ellermeier, J. R. & Slauch, J. M. (2007). Adaptation to the host environment: regulation of the SPI1 type III secretion system in *Salmonella* enterica serovar Typhimurium. *Curr Opin Microbiol*. Vol. 10, No. 1, pp. 24-9.

Eriksson, S., Lucchini, S., Thompson, A., Rhen, M. & Hinton, J. C. (2003). Unravelling the biology of macrophage infection by gene expression profiling of intracellular *Salmonella* enterica. *Mol Microbiol*. Vol. 47, No. 1, pp. 103-18.

Fagan, R. P., Lambert, M. A. & Smith, S. G. (2008). The hek outer membrane protein of Escherichia coli strain RS218 binds to proteoglycan and utilizes a single extracellular loop for adherence, invasion, and autoaggregation. *Infect Immun*. Vol. 76, No. 3, pp. 1135-42.

Fahlen, T. F., Mathur, N. & Jones, B. D. (2000). Identification and characterization of mutants with increased expression of hilA, the invasion gene transcriptional activator of *Salmonella* typhimurium. *FEMS Immunol Med Microbiol*. Vol. 28, No. 1, pp. 25-35.

Filloux, A., Hachani, A. & Bleves, S. (2008). The bacterial type VI secretion machine: yet another player for protein transport across membranes. *Microbiology*. Vol. 154, No. Pt 6, pp. 1570-83.

Folkesson, A., Advani, A., Sukupolvi, S., Pfeifer, J. D., Normark, S. & Lofdahl, S. (1999). Multiple insertions of fimbrial operons correlate with the evolution of *Salmonella* serovars responsible for human disease. *Mol Microbiol*. Vol. 33, No. 3, pp. 612-22.

Friebel, A., Ilchmann, H., Aepfelbacher, M., Ehrbar, K., Machleidt, W. & Hardt, W. D. (2001). SopE and SopE2 from *Salmonella* typhimurium activate different sets of RhoGTPases of the host cell. *J Biol Chem*. Vol. 276, No. 36, pp. 34035-40.

Fu, Y. & Galan, J. E. (1998). The *Salmonella* typhimurium tyrosine phosphatase SptP is translocated into host cells and disrupts the actin cytoskeleton. *Mol Microbiol*. Vol. 27, No. 2, pp. 359-68.

Fu, Y. & Galan, J. E. (1999). A *Salmonella* protein antagonizes Rac-1 and Cdc42 to mediate host-cell recovery after bacterial invasion. *Nature*. Vol. 401, No. 6750, pp. 293-7.

Fuentes, J. A., Villagra, N., Castillo-Ruiz, M. & Mora, G. C. (2008). The *Salmonella* Typhi hlyE gene plays a role in invasion of cultured epithelial cells and its functional transfer to S. Typhimurium promotes deep organ infection in mice. *Res Microbiol*. Vol. 159, No. 4, pp. 279-87.

Galan, J. E. & Wolf-Watz, H. (2006). Protein delivery into eukaryotic cells by type III secretion machines. *Nature*. Vol. 444, No. 7119, pp. 567-73.

Galkin, V. E., Orlova, A., VanLoock, M. S., Zhou, D., Galan, J. E. & Egelman, E. H. (2002). The bacterial protein SipA polymerizes G-actin and mimics muscle nebulin. *Nat Struct Biol*. Vol. 9, No. 7, pp. 518-21.

Garner, M. J., Hayward, R. D. & Koronakis, V. (2002). The *Salmonella* pathogenicity island 1 secretion system directs cellular cholesterol redistribution during mammalian cell entry and intracellular trafficking. *Cell Microbiol*. Vol. 4, No. 3, pp. 153-65.

Groisman, E. A. & Ochman, H. (1993). Cognate gene clusters govern invasion of host epithelial cells by *Salmonella* typhimurium and Shigella flexneri. *EMBO J*. Vol. 12, No. 10, pp. 3779-87.

Gunn, J. S., Alpuche-Aranda, C. M., Loomis, W. P., Belden, W. J. & Miller, S. I. (1995). Characterization of the *Salmonella* typhimurium pagC/pagD chromosomal region. *J Bacteriol*. Vol. 177, No. 17, pp. 5040-7.

Hanisch, J., Kolm, R., Wozniczka, M., Bumann, D., Rottner, K. & Stradal, T. E. (2011). Activation of a RhoA/myosin II-dependent but Arp2/3 complex-independent pathway facilitates *Salmonella* invasion. *Cell Host Microbe*. Vol. 9, No. 4, pp. 273-85.

Hartwig, J. H. & Kwiatkowski, D. J. (1991). Actin-binding proteins. *Curr Opin Cell Biol*. Vol. 3, No. 1, pp. 87-97.

Hayward, R. D., Cain, R. J., McGhie, E. J., Phillips, N., Garner, M. J. & Koronakis, V. (2005). Cholesterol binding by the bacterial type III translocon is essential for virulence effector delivery into mammalian cells. *Mol Microbiol*. Vol. 56, No. 3, pp. 590-603.

Hayward, R. D., McGhie, E. J. & Koronakis, V. (2000). Membrane fusion activity of purified SipB, a *Salmonella* surface protein essential for mammalian cell invasion. *Mol Microbiol*. Vol. 37, No. 4, pp. 727-39.

Heffernan, E. J., Harwood, J., Fierer, J. & Guiney, D. (1992). The *Salmonella* typhimurium virulence plasmid complement resistance gene rck is homologous to a family of virulence-related outer membrane protein genes, including pagC and ail. *J Bacteriol*. Vol. 174, No. 1, pp. 84-91.

Heithoff, D. M., Conner, C. P., Hentschel, U., Govantes, F., Hanna, P. C. & Mahan, M. J. (1999). Coordinate intracellular expression of *Salmonella* genes induced during infection. *J Bacteriol.* Vol. 181, No. 3, pp. 799-807.

Higashide, W., Dai, S., Hombs, V. P. & Zhou, D. (2002). Involvement of SipA in modulating actin dynamics during *Salmonella* invasion into cultured epithelial cells. *Cell Microbiol.* Vol. 4, No. 6, pp. 357-65.

Honda, A., Nogami, M., Yokozeki, T., Yamazaki, M., Nakamura, H., Watanabe, H., Kawamoto, K., Nakayama, K., Morris, A. J., Frohman, M. A. & Kanaho, Y. (1999). Phosphatidylinositol 4-phosphate 5-kinase alpha is a downstream effector of the small G protein ARF6 in membrane ruffle formation. *Cell.* Vol. 99, No. 5, pp. 521-32.

Hu, Q., Coburn, B., Deng, W., Li, Y., Shi, X., Lan, Q., Wang, B., Coombes, B. K. & Finlay, B. B. (2008). *Salmonella* enterica serovar Senftenberg human clinical isolates lacking SPI-1. *J Clin Microbiol.* Vol. 46, No. 4, pp. 1330-6.

Hueck, C. J. (1998). Type III protein secretion systems in bacterial pathogens of animals and plants. *Microbiol Mol Biol Rev.* Vol. 62, No. 2, pp. 379-433.

Hueck, C. J., Hantman, M. J., Bajaj, V., Johnston, C., Lee, C. A. & Miller, S. I. (1995). *Salmonella* typhimurium secreted invasion determinants are homologous to Shigella Ipa proteins. *Mol Microbiol.* Vol. 18, No. 3, pp. 479-90.

Huett, A., Leong, J. M., Podolsky, D. K. & Xavier, R. J. (2009). The cytoskeletal scaffold Shank3 is recruited to pathogen-induced actin rearrangements. *Exp Cell Res.* Vol. 315, No. 12, pp. 2001-11.

Ibarra, J. A. & Steele-Mortimer, O. (2009). *Salmonella*--the ultimate insider. *Salmonella* virulence factors that modulate intracellular survival. *Cell Microbiol.* Vol. 11, No. 11, pp. 1579-86.

Jones, M. A., Hulme, S. D., Barrow, P. A. & Wigley, P. (2007). The *Salmonella* pathogenicity island 1 and *Salmonella* pathogenicity island 2 type III secretion systems play a major role in pathogenesis of systemic disease and gastrointestinal tract colonization of *Salmonella* enterica serovar Typhimurium in the chicken. *Avian Pathol.* Vol. 36, No. 3, pp. 199-203.

Jones, M. A., Wigley, P., Page, K. L., Hulme, S. D. & Barrow, P. A. (2001). *Salmonella* enterica serovar Gallinarum requires the *Salmonella* pathogenicity island 2 type III secretion system but not the *Salmonella* pathogenicity island 1 type III secretion system for virulence in chickens. *Infect Immun.* Vol. 69, No. 9, pp. 5471-6.

Kaniga, K., Trollinger, D. & Galan, J. E. (1995). Identification of two targets of the type III protein secretion system encoded by the inv and spa loci of *Salmonella* typhimurium that have homology to the Shigella IpaD and IpaA proteins. *J Bacteriol.* Vol. 177, No. 24, pp. 7078-85.

Karasova, D., Sebkova, A., Havlickova, H., Sisak, F., Volf, J., Faldyna, M., Ondrackova, P., Kummer, V. & Rychlik, I. (2010). Influence of 5 major *Salmonella* pathogenicity islands on NK cell depletion in mice infected with *Salmonella* enterica serovar Enteritidis. *BMC Microbiol.* Vol. 10, No., pp. 75.

Kimbrough, T. G. & Miller, S. I. (2000). Contribution of *Salmonella* typhimurium type III secretion components to needle complex formation. *Proc Natl Acad Sci U S A.* Vol. 97, No. 20, pp. 11008-13.

Kimbrough, T. G. & Miller, S. I. (2002). Assembly of the type III secretion needle complex of *Salmonella* typhimurium. *Microbes Infect.* Vol. 4, No. 1, pp. 75-82.

Kubori, T. & Galan, J. E. (2003). Temporal regulation of *Salmonella* virulence effector function by proteasome-dependent protein degradation. *Cell.* Vol. 115, No. 3, pp. 333-42.

Lambert, M. A. & Smith, S. G. (2008). The PagN protein of *Salmonella* enterica serovar Typhimurium is an adhesin and invasin. *BMC Microbiol*. Vol. 8, No., pp. 142.

Lambert, M. A. & Smith, S. G. (2009). The PagN protein mediates invasion via interaction with proteoglycan. *FEMS Microbiol Lett*. Vol. 297, No. 2, pp. 209-16.

Lara-Tejero, M., Kato, J., Wagner, S., Liu, X. & Galan, J. E. (2011). A sorting platform determines the order of protein secretion in bacterial type III systems. *Science*. Vol. 331, No. 6021, pp. 1188-91.

Ledeboer, N. A., Frye, J. G., McClelland, M. & Jones, B. D. (2006). *Salmonella* enterica serovar Typhimurium requires the Lpf, Pef, and Tafi fimbriae for biofilm formation on HEp-2 tissue culture cells and chicken intestinal epithelium. *Infect Immun*. Vol. 74, No. 6, pp. 3156-69.

Ly, K. T. & Casanova, J. E. (2009). Abelson tyrosine kinase facilitates *Salmonella* enterica serovar Typhimurium entry into epithelial cells. *Infect Immun*. Vol. 77, No. 1, pp. 60-9.

Mammarappallil, J. G. & Elsinghorst, E. A. (2000). Epithelial cell adherence mediated by the enterotoxigenic Escherichia coli tia protein. *Infect Immun*. Vol. 68, No. 12, pp. 6595-601.

Mattei, P. J., Faudry, E., Job, V., Izore, T., Attree, I. & Dessen, A. (2011). Membrane targeting and pore formation by the type III secretion system translocon. *FEBS J*. Vol. 278, No. 3, pp. 414-26.

McGhie, E. J., Hayward, R. D. & Koronakis, V. (2001). Cooperation between actin-binding proteins of invasive *Salmonella*: SipA potentiates SipC nucleation and bundling of actin. *EMBO J*. Vol. 20, No. 9, pp. 2131-9.

McGhie, E. J., Hayward, R. D. & Koronakis, V. (2004). Control of actin turnover by a *Salmonella* invasion protein. *Mol Cell*. Vol. 13, No. 4, pp. 497-510.

Mecsas, J., Welch, R., Erickson, J. W. & Gross, C. A. (1995). Identification and characterization of an outer membrane protein, OmpX, in Escherichia coli that is homologous to a family of outer membrane proteins including Ail of Yersinia enterocolitica. *J Bacteriol*. Vol. 177, No. 3, pp. 799-804.

Michael, B., Smith, J. N., Swift, S., Heffron, F. & Ahmer, B. M. (2001). SdiA of *Salmonella* enterica is a LuxR homolog that detects mixed microbial communities. *J Bacteriol*. Vol. 183, No. 19, pp. 5733-42.

Mijouin, L., Rosselin, M., Bottreau, E., Pizarro-Cerda, J., Cossart, P., Velge, P. & Wiedemann A (2012). /*Salmonella*/ Enteritidis Rck-mediated invasion requires activation of Rac1 dependent of Class I PI 3-kinases-Akt signalling pathway. /FASEB J./ vol.26, No.4, pp 1569-81.

Miki, T., Okada, N., Shimada, Y. & Danbara, H. (2004). Characterization of *Salmonella* pathogenicity island 1 type III secretion-dependent hemolytic activity in *Salmonella* enterica serovar Typhimurium. *Microb Pathog*. Vol. 37, No. 2, pp. 65-72.

Miller, S. I., Kukral, A. M. & Mekalanos, J. J. (1989). A two-component regulatory system (phoP phoQ) controls *Salmonella* typhimurium virulence. *Proc Natl Acad Sci U S A*. Vol. 86, No. 13, pp. 5054-8.

Miller, V. L., Beer, K. B., Heusipp, G., Young, B. M. & Wachtel, M. R. (2001). Identification of regions of Ail required for the invasion and serum resistance phenotypes. *Mol Microbiol*. Vol. 41, No. 5, pp. 1053-62.

Misselwitz, B., Dilling, S., Vonaesch, P., Sacher, R., Snijder, B., Schlumberger, M., Rout, S., Stark, M., von Mering, C., Pelkmans, L. & Hardt, W. D. (2011). RNAi screen of *Salmonella* invasion shows role of COPI in membrane targeting of cholesterol and Cdc42. *Mol Syst Biol*. Vol. 7, No., pp. 474.

Mullins, R. D., Heuser, J. A. & Pollard, T. D. (1998). The interaction of Arp2/3 complex with actin: nucleation, high affinity pointed end capping, and formation of branching networks of filaments. *Proc Natl Acad Sci U S A*. Vol. 95, No. 11, pp. 6181-6.

Myeni, S. K. & Zhou, D. (2010). The C terminus of SipC binds and bundles F-actin to promote *Salmonella* invasion. *J Biol Chem*. Vol. 285, No. 18, pp. 13357-63.

Nichols, C. D. & Casanova, J. E. (2010). *Salmonella*-directed recruitment of new membrane to invasion foci via the host exocyst complex. *Curr Biol*. Vol. 20, No. 14, pp. 1316-20.

Norris, F. A., Wilson, M. P., Wallis, T. S., Galyov, E. E. & Majerus, P. W. (1998). SopB, a protein required for virulence of *Salmonella* dublin, is an inositol phosphate phosphatase. *Proc Natl Acad Sci U S A*. Vol. 95, No. 24, pp. 14057-9.

Oliveira, M. J., Costa, A. C., Costa, A. M., Henriques, L., Suriano, G., Atherton, J. C., Machado, J. C., Carneiro, F., Seruca, R., Mareel, M., Leroy, A. & Figueiredo, C. (2006). Helicobacter pylori induces gastric epithelial cell invasion in a c-Met and type IV secretion system-dependent manner. *J Biol Chem*. Vol. 281, No. 46, pp. 34888-96.

Patel, J. C. & Galan, J. E. (2005). Manipulation of the host actin cytoskeleton by *Salmonella*--all in the name of entry. *Curr Opin Microbiol*. Vol. 8, No. 1, pp. 10-5.

Patel, J. C. & Galan, J. E. (2006). Differential activation and function of Rho GTPases during *Salmonella*-host cell interactions. *J Cell Biol*. Vol. 175, No. 3, pp. 453-63.

Penheiter, K. L., Mathur, N., Giles, D., Fahlen, T. & Jones, B. D. (1997). Non-invasive *Salmonella* typhimurium mutants are avirulent because of an inability to enter and destroy M cells of ileal Peyer's patches. *Mol Microbiol*. Vol. 24, No. 4, pp. 697-709.

Perrett, C. A. & Jepson, M. A. (2009). Regulation of *Salmonella*-induced membrane ruffling by SipA differs in strains lacking other effectors. *Cell Microbiol*. Vol. 11, No. 3, pp. 475-87.

Pollard, T. D., Blanchoin, L. & Mullins, R. D. (2000). Molecular mechanisms controlling actin filament dynamics in nonmuscle cells. *Annu Rev Biophys Biomol Struct*. Vol. 29, No., pp. 545-76.

Queiroz, M. H., Madrid, C., Paytubi, S., Balsalobre, C. & Juarez, A. (2011). Integration Host Factor alleviates H-NS silencing of the *Salmonella* enterica serovar Typhimurium master regulator of SPI1, hilA. *Microbiology*. Vol. No.

Radtke, A. L., Wilson, J. W., Sarker, S. & Nickerson, C. A. (2010). Analysis of interactions of *Salmonella* type three secretion mutants with 3-D intestinal epithelial cells. *PLoS One*. Vol. 5, No. 12, pp. e15750.

Rathinavelan, T., Tang, C. & De Guzman, R. N. (2011). Characterization of the interaction between the *Salmonella* type III secretion system tip protein SipD and the needle protein PrgI by paramagnetic relaxation enhancement. *J Biol Chem*. Vol. 286, No. 6, pp. 4922-30.

Reeve, J. N. & Shaw, J. E. (1979). Lambda encodes an outer membrane protein: the lom gene. *Mol Gen Genet*. Vol. 172, No. 3, pp. 243-8.

Rittmeyer, E. N., Daniel, S., Hsu, S. C. & Osman, M. A. (2008). A dual role for IQGAP1 in regulating exocytosis. *J Cell Sci*. Vol. 121, No. Pt 3, pp. 391-403.

Rosselin, M., Abed, N., Virlogeux-Payant, I., Bottreau, E., Sizaret, P. Y., Velge, P. & Wiedemann, A. (2011). Heterogeneity of type III secretion system (T3SS)-1-independent entry mechanisms used by *Salmonella* Enteritidis to invade different cell types. *Microbiology*. Vol. 157, No. Pt 3, pp. 839-47.

Rosselin, M., Virlogeux-Payant, I., Roy, C., Bottreau, E., Sizaret, P. Y., Mijouin, L., Germon, P., Caron, E., Velge, P. & Wiedemann, A. (2010). Rck of *Salmonella* enterica, subspecies enterica serovar enteritidis, mediates zipper-like internalization. *Cell Res*. Vol. 20, No. 6, pp. 647-64.

Rotger, R. & Casadesus, J. (1999). The virulence plasmids of *Salmonella. Int Microbiol.* Vol. 2, No. 3, pp. 177-84.

Samudrala, R., Heffron, F. & McDermott, J. E. (2009). Accurate prediction of secreted substrates and identification of a conserved putative secretion signal for type III secretion systems. *PLoS Pathog*. Vol. 5, No. 4, pp. e1000375.

Scherer, C. A., Cooper, E. & Miller, S. I. (2000). The *Salmonella* type III secretion translocon protein SspC is inserted into the epithelial cell plasma membrane upon infection. *Mol Microbiol*. Vol. 37, No. 5, pp. 1133-45.

Schlumberger, M. C., Friebel, A., Buchwald, G., Scheffzek, K., Wittinghofer, A. & Hardt, W. D. (2003). Amino acids of the bacterial toxin SopE involved in G nucleotide exchange on Cdc42. *J Biol Chem*. Vol. 278, No. 29, pp. 27149-59.

Schraidt, O. & Marlovits, T. C. (2011). Three-dimensional model of *Salmonella*'s needle complex at subnanometer resolution. *Science*. Vol. 331, No. 6021, pp. 1192-5.

Schroeder, G. N. & Hilbi, H. (2008). Molecular pathogenesis of Shigella spp.: controlling host cell signaling, invasion, and death by type III secretion. *Clin Microbiol Rev*. Vol. 21, No. 1, pp. 134-56.

Sechi, A. S. & Wehland, J. (2000). The actin cytoskeleton and plasma membrane connection: PtdIns(4,5)P(2) influences cytoskeletal protein activity at the plasma membrane. *J Cell Sci*. Vol. 113 Pt 21, No., pp. 3685-95.

Shi, J. & Casanova, J. E. (2006). Invasion of host cells by *Salmonella* typhimurium requires focal adhesion kinase and p130Cas. *Mol Biol Cell*. Vol. 17, No. 11, pp. 4698-708.

Smith, J. N. & Ahmer, B. M. (2003). Detection of other microbial species by *Salmonella*: expression of the SdiA regulon. *J Bacteriol*. Vol. 185, No. 4, pp. 1357-66.

Smith, J. N., Dyszel, J. L., Soares, J. A., Ellermeier, C. D., Altier, C., Lawhon, S. D., Adams, L. G., Konjufca, V., Curtiss, R., 3rd, Slauch, J. M. & Ahmer, B. M. (2008). SdiA, an N-acylhomoserine lactone receptor, becomes active during the transit of *Salmonella* enterica through the gastrointestinal tract of turtles. *PLoS One*. Vol. 3, No. 7, pp. e2826.

Stebbins, C. E. & Galan, J. E. (2000). Modulation of host signaling by a bacterial mimic: structure of the *Salmonella* effector SptP bound to Rac1. *Mol Cell*. Vol. 6, No. 6, pp. 1449-60.

Takeuchi, A. (1967). Electron microscope studies of experimental *Salmonella* infection. I. Penetration into the intestinal epithelium by *Salmonella* typhimurium. *Am J Pathol*. Vol. 50, No. 1, pp. 109-36.

Tampakaki, A. P., Fadouloglou, V. E., Gazi, A. D., Panopoulos, N. J. & Kokkinidis, M. (2004). Conserved features of type III secretion. *Cell Microbiol*. Vol. 6, No. 9, pp. 805-16.

Terebiznik, M. R., Vieira, O. V., Marcus, S. L., Slade, A., Yip, C. M., Trimble, W. S., Meyer, T., Finlay, B. B. & Grinstein, S. (2002). Elimination of host cell PtdIns(4,5)P(2) by bacterial SigD promotes membrane fission during invasion by *Salmonella. Nat Cell Biol*. Vol. 4, No. 10, pp. 766-73.

van Sorge, A. J., Termote, J. U., de Vries, M. J., Boonstra, F. N., Stellingwerf, C. & Schalij-Delfos, N. E. (2011). The incidence of visual impairment due to retinopathy of prematurity (ROP) and concomitant disabilities in the Netherlands: a 30 year overview. *Br J Ophthalmol*. Vol. 95, No. 7, pp. 937-41.

Vazquez-Torres, A., Jones-Carson, J., Baumler, A. J., Falkow, S., Valdivia, R., Brown, W., Le, M., Berggren, R., Parks, W. T. & Fang, F. C. (1999). Extraintestinal dissemination of *Salmonella* by CD18-expressing phagocytes. *Nature*. Vol. 401, No. 6755, pp. 804-8.

Velge, P., Cloeckaert, A. & Barrow, P. (2005). Emergence of *Salmonella* epidemics: the problems related to *Salmonella* enterica serotype Enteritidis and multiple antibiotic resistance in other major serotypes. *Vet Res*. Vol. 36, No. 3, pp. 267-88.

Vivero, A., Banos, R. C., Mariscotti, J. F., Oliveros, J. C., Garcia-del Portillo, F., Juarez, A. & Madrid, C. (2008). Modulation of horizontally acquired genes by the Hha-YdgT proteins in *Salmonella* enterica serovar Typhimurium. *J Bacteriol*. Vol. 190, No. 3, pp. 1152-6.

Wai, S. N., Lindmark, B., Soderblom, T., Takade, A., Westermark, M., Oscarsson, J., Jass, J., Richter-Dahlfors, A., Mizunoe, Y. & Uhlin, B. E. (2003). Vesicle-mediated export and assembly of pore-forming oligomers of the enterobacterial ClyA cytotoxin. *Cell*. Vol. 115, No. 1, pp. 25-35.

Wallar, L. E., Bysice, A. M. & Coombes, B. K. (2011). The non-motile phenotype of *Salmonella* hha ydgT mutants is mediated through PefI-SrgD. *BMC Microbiol*. Vol. 11, No., pp. 141.

Wallis, T. S. & Galyov, E. E. (2000). Molecular basis of *Salmonella*-induced enteritis. *Mol Microbiol*. Vol. 36, No. 5, pp. 997-1005.

Watson, K. G. & Holden, D. W. (2010). Dynamics of growth and dissemination of *Salmonella* in vivo. *Cell Microbiol*. Vol. 12, No. 10, pp. 1389-97.

Winnen, B., Schlumberger, M. C., Sturm, A., Schupbach, K., Siebenmann, S., Jenny, P. & Hardt, W. D. (2008). Hierarchical effector protein transport by the *Salmonella* Typhimurium SPI-1 type III secretion system. *PLoS One*. Vol. 3, No. 5, pp. e2178.

Wozniak, C. E., Lee, C. & Hughes, K. T. (2009). T-POP array identifies EcnR and PefI-SrgD as novel regulators of flagellar gene expression. *J Bacteriol*. Vol. 191, No. 5, pp. 1498-508.

Yao, Y., Dickerson, T. J., Hixon, M. S. & Dyson, H. J. (2007). NMR detection of adventitious xylose binding to the quorum-sensing protein SdiA of Escherichia coli. *Bioorg Med Chem Lett*. Vol. 17, No. 22, pp. 6202-5.

Zhou, D., Chen, L. M., Hernandez, L., Shears, S. B. & Galan, J. E. (2001). A *Salmonella* inositol polyphosphatase acts in conjunction with other bacterial effectors to promote host cell actin cytoskeleton rearrangements and bacterial internalization. *Mol Microbiol*. Vol. 39, No. 2, pp. 248-59.

Zhou, D., Mooseker, M. S. & Galan, J. E. (1999a). An invasion-associated *Salmonella* protein modulates the actin-bundling activity of plastin. *Proc Natl Acad Sci U S A*. Vol. 96, No. 18, pp. 10176-81.

Zhou, D., Mooseker, M. S. & Galan, J. E. (1999b). Role of the *S*. typhimurium actin-binding protein SipA in bacterial internalization. *Science*. Vol. 283, No. 5410, pp. 2092-5.

18

A Tale of 6 Sigmas: How Changing Partners Allows *Salmonella* to Thrive in the Best of Times and Survive the Worst of Times

R. Margaret Wallen and Michael H. Perlin
University of Louisville
USA

1. Introduction

Salmonella enterica are rod-shaped, facultative anaerobic, Gram-negative members of the Enterobacteriacae family (Dougan et al., 2011). Most people have heard of the bacteria and generally associate it with food-borne illness. Despite general public knowledge of the health risks associated with and precautions taken to prevent its spread, *Salmonella* continues to cause many problems. One approach toward curbing this spread and reducing the negative impact of *S. enterica* could be genetic analysis, with an ultimate goal of understanding why the bacteria are able to survive attempts to destroy them.

It has been suggested that the *Salmonella* genus diverged from *Escherichia coli* somewhere between 100 and 150 million years ago (Dougan et al., 2011). While there is evoluntionary distance between the two genera, much of the genetic information has been conserved, and as a result, the study of one organism has provided insight into the study of the other. *Salmonella* spp. are generally considered to be pathogenic and can have both warm- and cold-blooded hosts (Dougan et al., 2011). More recent evolution has occurred within the *Salmonella* genus itself. *Salmonella enterica* has evolved into many different subspecies and serovars that manifest in dramatically different ways across a variety of hosts despite sharing 95% of the same genetic information (McDermott et al., 2011). From a medical perspective, *Salmonella* genetics are particularly important. Although a single-celled organism, due to its long evolutionary history with humans and other organisms, these bacteria has developed several sophisticated mechanisms to survive the immune systems of its hosts and evade sanitation efforts to kill it. Understanding how this survival at the most fundamental of levels, it may be possible to more specifically combat the bacteria.

Salmonella typically reach their hosts through the consumption of contaminated food or water. Once inside its host, the bacteria must persist through various levels of pH, temperature, osmolarity, and nutrient availability (Ohl & Miller, 2001). The pathogen must also face various attempts by the host's immune system to eliminate it. Each different environment and each assault on the bacteria's integrity must be addressed by the organism in order to survive. The ability of the organism to thrive in a multitude of environments and persist to establish infection in its host is governed by the expression of different genes.

While there are a multitude of regulatory pathways within *Salmonella* that can influence gene expression, one of the most fundamental comes from the usage of alternate sigma factors by the cell's RNA polymerase, as is the case for most prokaryotes. Sigma factors facilitate differential gene expression by reversibly binding to the RNA polymerase core enzyme and providing specificity for certain promoter regions. The various sigma factors have different affinities for particular promoters as well as for the core enzyme itself. Similar to other cellular proteins, sigma factors are regulated at a variety of levels. Transcription in *Salmonella,* as in all prokaryotes, requires a sigma factor, and ultimately all gene expression is affected by sigma factors and their activity.

Sigma factors were originally discovered as protein factors that stimulate RNA synthesis from DNA using DNA-dependent RNA polymerase (Burgess & Travers, 1969). These proteins all share four regions of similarity indicative of a common function (Kutasake et al., 1994). For the group of closely related sigma factors, special regions within the protein recognize specific regions of the DNA as promoters versus non-promoter regions of DNA (Dombroski et al., 1992). These DNA regions include conserved sequences centered around the -35 and -10 positions with respect to the transcription initiation site. By truncating the sigma protein at various locations, researchers were able to determine that four conserved regions of the sigma factors were responsible for locating different areas of the promoter region. For example, region 4 of the sigma factor is found to recognize the consensus sequence around -35, while regions 2 and 3 recognize the -10 consensus sequence (Dombroski et al., 1992). Region 1 of the sigma factor, the amino terminus of the protein, blocks regions 2, 3, and 4 from interacting with the DNA (Dombroski et al., 1993). Binding of the sigma factor to the core enzyme blocks region 1 and allows interaction of the other three regions with the DNA (Dombroski et al., 1992). In this way, the sigma factor cannot interact with DNA without being bound by RNA polymerase. While it was understood that a sigma factor was necessary to facilitate transcription, their power to regulate gene expression was not fully understood.

2. Early virulence-related genetic studies

As with most pathogenic microorganisms, early genetic research focused on the disease-causing properties of *Salmonella.* Preliminary studies involving virulence properties of *Samonella* revealed that in the absence of a functional copy of several genes, the bacteria was unable to survive to cause infection inside its host. Further studies of each of these genes revealed that while all of the genes were required for optimal virulence, the gene expression was not under the same regulatory control. Baumler and his colleagues examined nearly 30 mutant strains of *Salmonella* Typhimurium that had shown attenuated ability to infect and survive inside mouse macrophages (Baumler et al., 1994). Baumler concluded that these genes all made contributions to the virulence properties of *Salmonella.*

Some of the particular genes that Baumler concluded were disrupted in the attenuated strains were *purD, prc, fliD,* and *nagA* (Baumler et al., 1994). Other researchers have examined the transcriptional control of these genes to understand why they are so essential to the virulence capabilities of *Salmonella.*

As many sigma factors are closely related, there is a high degree of homology between their structures and therefore promoter affinities. However, as few as one or two base pair change can dramatically change which sigma factor recognizes the promoter (Römling et al., 1998). The *purD* gene encodes 5′-phosphoribosylglycinamide synthetase, which is involved in purine nucleotide synthesis (Aiba & Mizobuchi, 1989). While these genes have easily identifiable -10 consensus sequences, none appear to have the -35 region similar to those typically recognized by the primary sigma factor (Kilstrup et al., 1998). Potentially, the ambiguity of the promoter region shows the ability to be used by multiple sigma factors.

A second gene, *prc*, encodes a protease that in closely related organisms has been found to play a role in response to cell wall stress (Wood et al., 2006). In these organisms, *prc* is preceded by a consensus sequence for a sigma factor showing a great deal of similarity to the sigma factor in *E. coli* and *Salmonella* that responds to a variety of global stresses, including damage to the cellular envelope (Wood et al., 2006).

The *fliD* gene encodes part of the flagella filament, needed for the motility of the bacteria (Kutsukake et al., 1994). This gene is proceeded by a consensus sequence that can only be used by the flagella-specific sigma factor (Kutsukake et al., 1994) and is part of a highly temporally and spatially regulated pathway that ensures flagella are expressed readily in times that motility is necessary and repressed when the bacteria have not formed the appropriate primary structures for the flagellar.

The *nagA* gene product is N-acetylglucosamine-6-phosphate deacetylase in *E. coli* and has the same function in *Salmonella* Typhimurium (Baumler et al., 1994). This gene was found to have consensus sequence in the -10 region requiring the activation of a magnesium sensitive regulator in the presence of the housekeeping sigma (Minagawa et al., 2003). Based only on the extracellular availability of magnesium, the primary sigma factor is responsible for the transcription of the gene, provided a secondary regulatory system is activated.

With the genes that Baumler examined, in combination with other research indicating that each of these types of genes was under different regulatory control by particular sigma factors, a pattern began to emerge. Genes responsible for the organism's response to particular threats to its integrity were under the transcriptional direction of particular sigma factors. The importance of sigma factors as transcriptional regulators is further revealed by their stability over time (Sutton et al., 2000) and the high degree of homology between closely related species (Guiney et al., 1995).

3. A tale of six sigmas

To date, six different sigma factors have been discovered to be encoded within the *Salmonella* genome that are responsible for transcription from a variety of promoters in response to different phases of the organism's life as well as environmental conditions. Acting together in a complex, as an interconnected web of gene regulation, they enable *Salmonella* to withstand and thrive inside infected hosts.

Sigma factors were characterized as proteins before their function as essential elements of the holoenzyme became clear. As such, each sigma factor is known by a variety of names. Designations with *rpo* or Rpo are used across species and refer to the particular stress to which the sigma factor responds. A more contemporary convention is to use a lower case Greek sigma with the molecular weight of the sigma factor as a superscript. In this text, all molecular weights refer to those found in *Salmonella* and *E. coli.*

Most of these proteins, σ^{70}, σ^{E}, σ^{H}, σ^{S}, and σ^{F}, belong to the same family of sigma factors, potentially all derived from some ancestral form or ancestral regulatory process. The other sigma factor, σ^{N}, belongs to a different family, although it is the only modern day example found, and may belong to a more ancient regulatory system that has become obsolete with current patterns of growth and reproduction for bacteria like *Salmonella*. While the housekeeping sigma was found to facilitate most gene expression during exponential growth, each of the other sigma factors was found to help the organism address different environmental stresses. Each sigma factor recognizes a different consensus sequence within the promoter region. The relative affinities of multiple sigma factors for the same promoter region determine which recognizes it more often at a specific intracellular concentration.

3.1 σ^{N} – Nitrogen regulation

σ^{N} seems to be more evolutionarily distant from the other alternate sigma factors and it may be the remnants of a more ancient regulatory system. In fact, the processes governed by σ^{N} may not be essential or may be under transcriptional control of another sigma factor (Morett & Segovia, 1993). These processes include nitrogen fixation, dicarboxylic acid transport, and hydrogen oxidation (Morett & Segovia, 1993). Down-regulating expression from RpoN-dependent genes provides increased resistance to killing by host cationic antimicrobial peptides (Barchiesi et al., 2009), indicating that some of these processes may even be detrimental to the organism in certain conditions. In some related species σ^{N} is related to pathogenicity, but that does not appear to be in *Salmonella* (Studholme, 2002).

The differences between σ^{N} and the rest of the sigma factors are profound. There is almost no sequence similarity between the *rpoN* gene and genes for other known sigma factors, also suggesting a different origin (Morett & Segovia, 1993). σ^{N} promoters are unique in that they have conserved consensus sequences centered at -24 and -12 nucleotides from the transcription start site, as opposed to -35 and -10 (Barrios et al., 1999). A highly conserved RpoN-Box is involved in the recognition of the -24 and -12 DNA sequences (Barrios et al., 1999). The distance between the -24 and -12 elements is more stringent than the analogous distance between the -35 and -10 elements for the σ^{70} family of sigma factors, indicating a highly controlled regulation (Barrios et al., 1999). Moreover, the sequences at the -24 and -12 elements have highly conserved GG and GC regions respectively, also suggesting a high level of regulatory control (Barrios et al., 1999).

While the σ^{N} protein is very different from other alternate sigma factors, the interaction between the sigma factor and template DNA is also distinct. The σ^{70} family of sigma factors do not form stable closed complexes and transcription will start spontaneously (Barrios et al., 1999). Unlike other sigma factors, the σ^{N} and core enzyme form a stable closed complex. In this way, σ^{N} binding to the core enzyme actually blocks transcription because the open complex must be activated (Buck & Cannon, 1992). The binding of the RNA polymerase holoenzyme with σ^{N} as the sigma factor cannot induce DNA melting alone, similar to the RNA polymerase II system in eukaryotes (Buck et al., 2000). σ^{N} may bind to DNA first rather than binding to the core enzyme first (Buck et al., 2000). This is supported by the fact that σ^{N} binds to a different location on the core enzyme than σ^{70} and in doing so may be able to assist in DNA melting once activated (Buck et al., 2000).

Because it forms a stable closed complex, the RNA polymerase with σ^N as the sigma factor requires enhancer proteins for activation. Each enhancer protein is under the regulation of its own signal transduction pathway, allowing response to various environmental conditions (Buck et al., 2000). All the enhancer proteins have hidden ATPase activity that allows for the DNA melting necessary to initiate transcription (Buck et al., 2000).

3.2 The housekeeping sigma σ^{70}

The other five sigma factors appear to be evolutionarily related, developing from the original or primary sigma factor. RpoD or σ^{70} is the housekeeping sigma factor and is responsible for the transcription of most of the genes in bacterial cells growing exponentially (Ishihama, 1993). When *rpoD* was found in the genome for *E. coli*, it was determined that the gene sequence had a high degree of homology between other *rpoD* genes from closely related species (Scaife et al., 1979). Further genomic analysis determined that *rpoD* is found in a transcript with the 30S ribosomal protein S21 and DNA primase (Burton et al., 1983). This operon was the first discovered operon containing proteins involved in transcription, translation, and replication (Burton et al., 1983). Eσ^{70} (the holoenzyme containing the core enzyme associated with σ^{70}) does not form a stable closed complex and transcription begins spontaneously (Barrios et al., 1999), requiring no enhancer proteins. Moreover, the σ^{70} concentration found inside a cell undergoing exponential growth is less than the concentration of core enzymes, indicating the level of the sigma factor present may regulate the level of transcription (Burton et al., 1983).

3.3 σ^E – Response to extracytoplasmic stress

When the bacteria face stressors, other sigma factors are involved in the expression of genes necessary to survive the stress, such as σ^E, σ^{24}, or RpoE which results in transcription of genes to combat envelop stress (Kenyon et al., 2005). RpoE is constitutively expressed in the bacteria, held inactive by interaction with various binding proteins. The *rpoE* gene seems to be the most highly conserved of alternate sigma factors across several species, as are the genes under its transcriptional control.

RpoE must be able to respond to a signal coming from outside of the cell, while the protein itself resides inside the bacterium. It appears that a transmembrane protein, RseA, interacts with RseB on the periplasmic side and with σ^E on the cytoplasmic side. An area of the DegS protein on the periplasmic side recognizes unfolded proteins resulting in proteolysis of the periplasmic side of RseA. Cleaved RseA is a target for RseP, which then cleaves the transmembrane portion of RseA, releasing the RseA/ σ^E complex from the membrane and the unstable cytoplasmic portion of RseA is quickly degraded by cytoplasmic proteases (Muller et al., 2009). RseB also interacts on the periplasmic side with both DegS and RseP to control the activity of these proteases in the absence of a stress response (Muller et al., 2009). The strength of the signal is directly proportional to the number of misfolded outer membrane proteins.

While response to envelop stress is typically the signal necessary to release RpoE from RseA, acid stress may also result in the same response. It was found that mutants deficient in RpoE activity showed increased susceptibility to acid and reduced ability to survive inside macrophages. The RseP domain was required for this response to the acid shock, but its proteolytic activity was not dependent on DegS (Muller et al., 2009). It is proposed that the acidic milieu affects the interaction between RseB and RseP, which normally keeps RseP inactive, so that RseP is released to act on RseA, discontinuing negative control over σ^E (Muller et al., 2009). Both DegS and RseP have cytoplasmic and periplasmic domains, and the acid response appears to be independent of the envelope stress response. Again, the response strength is contingent upon the acidity of conditions and the length of exposure.

Once σ^E is released to interact with RNA polymerase, not all σ^E - dependent genes are transcribed equally. Within the approximately 60 promoters examined that required σ^E for transcription, there were few very strong promoters (showing high affinity) but many relatively weak promoters. The strong promoters were conserved across both *E. coli* and *S. enterica*, and were typically involved in maintaining porin homeostasis (Mutalik et al., 2009). Varying strength of promoters allow quick and efficient adaptation to different environments by being able to transcribe different genes in response to various signals (Mutalik et al., 2009). If the stress signal is strong, the cellular concentration of σ^E will increase to transcribe at high rates from weak promoters.

In order to prevent wasted energy and further damage to the cell, the activation of σ^E also results in the down-regulation of *omp* (outer membrane protein) mRNA (Papenfort et al., 2006). The cell also prevents these nascent mRNAs from producing misfolded proteins while avoiding destruction by the exocytoplasmic stress. Two small non-coding RNAs, RybB and MicA, not under the control of RpoE, collectively expedite the destruction of *omp* mRNAs. Under normal conditions, the cellular machinery making OMPs is still not perfect and some misfolded proteins are generated. In this case, the same two sRNAs are involved in the response to fix the problem by inducing the σ^E response, but at a much lower level than would be found in bacteria responding to prolonged stress (Papenfort et al., 2006). As such, the two sRNAs are most likely under the transcriptional control of the housekeeping sigma factor and their increased activity helps to induce σ^E activity.

As far as specific genes governed by σ^E, the parts of the σ^E regulon that are highly conserved across species are involved in making the cell wall and outer membrane of Gram-negative bacteria (Rhodius et al., 2006). The variable portion may be involved in the alternative lifestyles that the studied species utilize. A genome-wide search was done for σ^E-dependent genes in several species including *E. coli* and *Salmonella* Typhimurium, determining that several genes were at the core of the σ^E regulon. Some genes were involved in making lipoproteins, such as *yfiO*, *yeaY*, and *yraP*. Others were involved in outer membrane protein synthesis and modification, like *yeaT*, *skp*, *fkpA*, and *degP*. And still others were involved in cell envelope structure, such as *plsB*, *bacA*, *ahpF*, and *ygiM*. Interestingly, both *rpoE* and *rpoH* were both under regulatory control of σ^E, indicating that σ^E promotes its own transcription and the transcription of other sigma factors (Rhodius et al., 2006). By autoregulation, σ^E can create a multi-fold increase in gene product from its regulon. All of the genes found to be under the control of σ^E are related to making proteins for cellular structure.

3.4 σ^H – Response to heat shock

One of the genes under the transcriptional control of RpoE is another sigma factor, RpoH or σ^{32} (Rhodius et al., 2006). This sigma factor has been found to be involved in the transcription of genes that help *Salmonella* withstand high temperatures, potentially as a result of fever response within the host. Whereas σ^E appears to mediate the response to misfolded outer membrane proteins, σ^H is involved with proteins within the cytoplasm that are misfolded (Bang et al., 2005). Concomitant with increased heat exposure, cell wall and membrane proteins begin to misfold and denature. As the concentration of σ^E increases in response to the misfolded proteins, σ^H also accumulates to respond to a sustained stressor. This is supported by the finding that *rpoH* expression is directly proportional to σ^E activity at temperatures above 42°C (Testerman et al., 2002), a temperature at which protein denaturing begins with the cell.

RpoH governs the transcription of genes such as those encoding proteases that allow for the removal of misfolded proteins within the cytoplasm. For example, an operon composed of *opdA* and *yhiQ* was found to be immediately proceeded by a consensus sequence for the RpoH promoter (Conlin & Miller, 2000). While the function of these two proteins has not been directly studied in the heat shock response, OpdA is metalloprotease oligopeptidase A that would be helpful in degrading misfolded proteins.

Some researchers have also hypothesized that σ^H is related to RNA thermometers, which are other regulatory means for activating and utilizing heat shock genes. RNA thermometers are areas of 5′-untranslated region that fold and complementary pair in such a way as to block the Shine-Dalgarno (SD) sequence of downstream genes (Waldminghaus et al., 2007). When heated to high enough temperatures, these areas unpair to allow the ribosome access to the SD sequence. A previously undescribed RNA thermometer was found within the 5′-UTR of the *agsA* gene in *S. enterica*. This gene is known to be involved in response to heat shock, and has a promoter region that is a consensus sequence for RpoH. Within the *agsA* mRNA appear to be RNA thermometer sequences (Waldminghaus et al., 2007).

In *E. coli,* the *rpoH* mRNA itself contains RNA thermometers. In this species, the cellular level of the RpoH is controlled by complementary base pairing in its mRNA. Unlike other RNA thermometers, the SD sequence is not blocked but the start codon is inaccessible to the ribosome and two halves of the ribosome-binding site pair at low temperatures (Waldminghaus et al., 2007). A similar mechanism is likely at play in *Salmonella*.

While responding to heat shock is vitally important for survival of the bacteria, the most important function of σ^H is to mediate σ^E regulation of σ^S through *hfq* gene expression. In *E. coli,* the promoter sequence found upstream of the *hfq* gene was found to be σ^H -dependent. The same promoter was found in *S.* Typhimurium (Bang et al., 2005). In conditions with scarce nutrients, σ^E appears to upregulate σ^S through the increase of σ^H (Bang et al., 2005).

The product of the *hfq* gene, HF-I, is important for translation of RpoS. This small protein is heat stable and binds to RNA to facilitate translation (Brown & Elliot, 1996) by associating with the ribosome (Brown & Elliot, 1997). Several possible mechanisms for the manner in which the protein encoded by *hfq* regulated σ^S translation have been suggested, including preventing the interaction of some sort of antisense mRNA or by being directly involved in the transcription of *rpoS* (Cunning & Elliot, 1999). Most evidence supports the assertion that the function of HF-I is as an RNA chaperone, after it was demonstrated to bring the mRNA and ribosome in correct association for translation (Sittka et al., 2007).

3.5 σ^S – Stationary phase growth, response to stress, and response to starvation

The role of this sigma factor, also called σ^{38}, is slightly more difficult to define than that of RpoE or RpoH. However, it is clear that the function of RpoS is essential. The conserved sequence of *rpoS* across multiple species and within the same species found in different geographical areas speaks to its importance. When *rpoS* genes are characterized in clinical isolates, the mutations found are not clonal but rather novel, implying that there is some selection against mutants. Even when strains demonstrated different abilities to survive certain stresses like exposure to hydrogen peroxide, it did not appear to be related to different *rpoS* genes (Robbe-Saule et al., 2007).

The number and types of genes that seem to be under transcriptional control of σ^S have a variety of functions and respond to a wide variety of lifestyle requirements and threats to survival. The only known constant about the genes transcriptionally governed by RpoS is their dependence on growth phase (Ibanez-Ruiz et al., 2000). Previously, work has determined that during logarithmic growth, any activity from σ^S promoters is repressed by cyclic-AMP receptor activity (Fang et al., 1996). Stationary phase growth is characterized by a lack of cellular multiplication and decreasing cell density. The transition from exponential growth to stationary phase growth is the result of the concentration of a regulatory protein (Hirsch & Elliot, 2005). The concentration of Fis (factor for inversion stimulation), a DNA binding protein, is high during exponential growth and low in stationary phase. Fis binds to a region of DNA upstream of the promoter for *rpoS* and with decreasing concentration, allows the switch to stationary phase (Hirsch & Elliot, 2005).

A genome-wide search has been done for genes under the transcriptional control of RpoS. The project found that, like RpoE, the σ^S regulon includes promoters of various strengths. Despite the assumed similarities between the *E. coli* and *S.* Typhimurium genome, there were several genes within the *Salmonella* genome that were not homologous with any genes of *E. coli*. Several genes of unknown function were found under the control of σ^S, as was *ogt*, which encodes the enzyme O^6-methylguanine DNA methyltransferase (Ibanez-Ruiz et al., 2000). This enzyme is responsible for repairing DNA damaged by alkylation (Fang et al., 1992).

σ^S also seems to play a role in a wide variety of other functions that ensure the survival of the bacteria, such as protection from acid shock and nutrient depletion. Decreased pH unfolds the secondary structure stem and loops of the *rpoS* mRNA, allowing availability for translation (Audia & Foster, 2003). Constitutive degradation of the sigma factor coupled with no more being made results in the system reset after the acid threat has passed (Audia & Foster, 2003). RpoS also seems to be involved in survival of the bacteria in starvation conditions. σ^S has been found to act as both a positive regulator for *stiA* and *stiC* and a negative regulator for *stiB*. These three genes are part of the multiple-nutrient starvation-induced loci. σ^S was required for phosphate, carbon, and nitrogen starvation survival through induction of *stiA* and *stiC*. σ^S also acted as a negative regulator of *stiB* during phosphate and carbon starvation induced stationary growth (O'Neal et al., 1994).

3.6 σ^F – Flagellar formation and chemotaxis

Flagellar assembly was originally assumed to be under the control of σ^{70}, because it seemed essential to survival. However, examining promoters of known flagellar genes found no consensus sequences for σ^{70} (Helmann & Chamberlin, 1987). Instead, researchers found promoter sequences in *Salmonella* known to be used by alternative sigma factors in closely related species (Helmann & Chamberlin, 1987). σ^F, more commonly called FliA, or σ^{28}, has the most specific function of all the alternate sigma factors. FliA is involved in the transcription of genes related to the formation of flagella, specifically the formation of the flagellar filament (Ohnishi et al., 1990). Operons of flagellar assembly are proceeded by one of three classes of promoters, class 1, 2, or 3 (Bonifield & Hughes, 2003, Karlinsey et al., 2000, Karlinsey et al., 2006) which allow for a temporal regulation of gene expression. From these operons, more than 50 genes are transcribed to allow complete flagellar assembly and function (Kutsukake et al., 1994).

There is only one class 1 operon which encodes the *flhD* and *flhC* genes (Karlinsey et al., 2000). Class 1 is the master operon, with FlhD and FlhC acting as a global regulator of flagellar assembly (Karlinsey et al., 2006). FlhD and FlhC form a heterotetrameric complex that is a positive transcriptional activator of class 2 promoters through σ^{70}, by interacting with the α subunit of the core enzyme (Bonifield & Hughes, 2003, Liu et al., 1995, Liu & Matsumura, 1994). Class 2 operons include genes for the assembly of the hook and basal body complex (HBB), σ^F, and FlgM (Bonifield & Hughes, 2003). The basal body, containing the motor, penetrates the cell membrane and includes the hook element on the extracellular side of the cell (Brown & Hughes, 1995). The filament protrudes from the hook into the extracellular matrix and turns to provide motility.

The third class of flagellar operons requires σ^{28} or FliA for transcription (Bonifield & Hughes, 2003). Proteins generated from these operons are for the flagellar filament, the generation of motor force, and chemotaxis (Karlinsey et al., 2006). FlgM, which is also transcribed from class 2 operons along with FliA, acts as an anti-sigma factor, keeping FliA inactive until the completion of the HBB. The C-terminal portion of FliA has a binding site for FlgM (Kutsukake et al., 1994). FlgM prevents RNA polymerase core enzyme from interacting with FliA to transcribe class 3 flagellar operons (Chadsey et al., 1998). The FlgM protein is able to assess the completion of the HBB because the protein itself is an exported substrate (Hughes et al., 1993). Decreasing concentrations of FlgM release FliA to interact with the RNA polymerase core enzyme and transcribe class 3 operons (Hughes et al., 1993). The relative concentration of FliA to FlgM determines the number of flagella that a single cell will have (Kutsukake & Iino, 1994). Additionally, the FlhD/FlhC complex may assist FliA in association with the RNA polymerase (Kutsukake & Iino, 1994). FlhD is involved in assessing nutrient state (Chilcott & Hughes, 2000), which may be requisite for bacterial motility.

The intracellular concentration of FliA and FlgM is governed by other regulatory mechanisms as well. The genes from both of these proteins can be transcribed from either class 2 or class 3 promoters (Wozniak et al., 2010). In this way, FliA can positively and negatively regulate its own intracellular concentration dependent upon the concentration of FlgM within the cell (Ikebe et al., 1999). Mutants lacking FlgM overproduce flagella via overexpression from class 3 operons (Yokoseki et al., 1996).

4. Changing partners

The presence of alternate sigma factors has been well studied, but how do the alternate sigma factors displace the housekeeping sigma or each other to govern gene transcription? Most of the answer points to concentration dependence; that is, the concentration of a particular sigma factor changes in response to different environmental conditions. For example, RpoE, as discussed above, is expressed constitutively but held inactive by various other proteins until an extracellular signal is received. This signal activates a series of proteolytic activities that gradually increases the intracellular concentration of RpoE. Once RpoE is released, it is free to interact with the core enzyme. RpoE is positively autoregulated and as genes are transcribed from RpoE-response promoters, the intracellular concentration increases exponentially so that the intracellular concentration of RpoE can outcompete other sigma factors for binding access to the core enzyme. RpoE, in turn, allows for transcription of *rpoH*, which summarily mediates *rpoS* expression, increasing the intracellular level of all three alternative sigma factors. Fine tuning of these concentrations allows for precise control of gene expression. If a finite amount of RNA polymerase is available, increasing the presence of one sigma factor can repress expression of genes requiring a different sigma factor (Farewell et al., 1998).

Growth phase also appears to play a role in the intracellular concentration of certain sigma factors. During exponential growth, intracellular concentrations of σ^{70} remain relatively constant and σ^S is basically absent (Jishage & Ishihama, 1995). During stationary phase growth, the intracellular concentration of σ^S increases to nearly 30% of σ^{70} concentration (Jishage & Ishihama, 1995). Moreover, the concentration of the core enzyme decreases during stationary phase growth (Jishage & Ishihama, 1995), meaning that a 30% increase in concentration is more than a 30% increase in competitive advantage. RpoS activity is repressed by the products of *uspA* and *uspB*, which are both under the transcriptional control of σ^{70} (Farewell et al., 1998). During exponential growth, σ^S is highly unstable (Jishage & Ishihama, 1995). In stationary phase growth, σ^S is released and free to interact with RNA polymerase core enzyme. Researchers have hypothesized that there may be a σ^{70} anti-sigma factor under transcriptional control of σ^S or that a change in the cytoplasm may favor σ^S - mediated transcription (Farewell et al., 1998). Most genes expressed during exponential growth are not expressed during stationary phase growth, so σ^{70} proteins need to be rendered inactive (Jishage & Ishihama, 1995). Interestingly, the intracellular levels of σ^S reach those of σ^{70} during osmotic shock (Jishage & Ishihama, 1995), indicating that the change in concentration of a sigma factor can be a gradual or dramatic.

Environmental conditions can also play a role in the stability of the proteins, which can affect transcriptional efficiency. For example, RpoH, the heat shock sigma factor, is highly unstable at low temperatures; but, above 42°C intracellular concentrations will transiently increase (Jishage & Ishihama, 1995). Higher temperatures may provide increased efficiency of σ^H - mediated transcription or they may stabilize the protein itself so that it is able to interact with the core enzyme (Jishage & Ishihama, 1995).

5. *Salmonella* as pathogenic bacteria

In determining how alternate sigma factors are able to promote survival and spread of *Salmonella*, it is important to understand how *Salmonella* lives. *Salmonella* typically enters its host through the oral route. If sufficient numbers are ingested, some organisms will survive the low pH conditions of the stomach to reach the small intestine (Dougan et al., 2011). Sometimes the bacterial infection is halted here. For a systemic infection to occur, the bacteria must invade the gut epithelium (Hansen-Wester & Hensen, 2001). *Salmonella* preferentially invade epithelial cells in the distal ileum of the small intestine by adhering to and then injecting effector proteins into the host cell that facilitates bacterial entrance into membrane bound vesicles (Bueno et al., 2010). The small intestine provides an environment of near-neutral pH and high osmolarity, condusive to invasion not found in the large intestine (Lawhon et al., 2002).

Within the small intestines, *Salmonella* specifically invades Peyer's patches through M cells. Peyer's patches are specialized lymphoid tissues that are designed to sample intestinal antigens and lead to immune responses (Slauch et al., 1997). *Salmonella* exclusively enter M cells found within the follicle-associated epithelium of Peyer's patches (Jones & Falkow, 1994). M cells are epithelial cells responsible for the uptake of luminal antigens (Slauch et al., 1997) and can engulf large particles, making them ideal for target by *Salmonella* (Jones & Falkow, 1994). When one bacterium makes entry into the host epithelial cell, it recruits other pathogens to its location (Francis et al., 1992).

6. Islands of pathogenicity

An estimated 5-10% of genes within the *Salmonella* genome can be considered virulence genes (Slauch et al., 1997). These genes have been found arranged in clusters within the *Salmonella* chromosome, the so called *Salmonella* Pathogenicity Islands (SPIs). It has been theorized that these gene clusters were acquired by horizontal transfer based on their higher G-C content compared with other parts of the *Salmonella* chromosome (Slauch et al., 1997) and because similar regions are not found in closely related commensal species such as *E. coli* (Galán, 1996). There are at least five known SPIs, but SPI-1 and SPI-2 seem to the most important in the initial phases of infection. Both SPI-1 and SPI-2 encode type III secretion systems (TTSS) (Shea et al., 1996). Additionally, genes within the SPIs encode effector proteins and regulatory proteins (Hansen-Wester & Hensen, 2001). These secretion systems allow the insertion of effector proteins into the extracellular environment and inside the host cell.

SPI-1 appears to contain genes involved in bacterial uptake by the host cell, while SPI-2 genes are involved in survival inside cells (Lara-Tejero & Galán, 2009). However, there is some evidence indicating that SPI-1 may also be important for bacterial life inside the vacuole and for their survival and replication intracellularly (Steele-Mortimer et al., 2002). Secreted proteins from genes transcribed from SPI-1 leads to actin cytoskeleton rearrangement of the host cell that facilitates bacterial entrance into membrane bound vesicles (Chen et al., 1996). Once inside the cell, a variety of functions can be hijacked to serve the bacteria's purpose, including cytoskeleton arrangement, vesicular trafficking, cell cycle progression, and programmed cell death (Lara-Tejero & Galán, 2009). These effector proteins activate GTP-binding proteins such as Cdc42, Rac-1, and Rho, which coordinate intracellular activities in the host cell (Chen et al., 1996). Effector proteins also down-regulate actin rearrangement (Fu & Galán, 1999) to reverse the actin rearrangement.

Transcription of all SPI-1 operons is activated by a regulatory loop beginning with HilA (Matsui et al., 2008). Through other regulator proteins like HilC, HilD, and InvF, expression of invasion genes is modulated with HilA as the central player (Lucas et al., 2000). Interestingly, the rising concentration of acetate in the distal intestine activates the expression of HilA, bypassing normal positive regulators (Lawhon et al., 2002).

While SPI-1 may play a role in the procession of the infection past the initial invasion of epithelial cells, SPI-2 is vital for the migration of the bacteria to other parts of the host (Löber et al., 2006). SPI-2 was the second pathogenicity island discovered and is required for virulence after the bacteria has entered into the epithelial cells (Shea et al., 1996). This claim is further supported by evidence that mutants without SPI-2 genes could enter Peyer's patches but were unable to spread to mesenteric lymph nodes (Cirillo et al., 1998). Not all members of the SPI-2 pathogenicity island are equally vital for the ability of the pathogen to establish systemic infection. Mutants with various genes knocked out show a varying level of attenuation (Cirillo et al., 1998, Hensel et al., 1998). However, the genes within the SPI-2 are responsible for avoiding destruction by lysosomes within dendritic cells and macrophages (Tobar et al., 2006). Expression of SPI-2 genes seems to be induced by the slightly acidic conditions inside the initial vacuole formed when the bacteria are initially internalized by the host cell (Löber et al., 2006).

6.1 Regulation of *Salmonella pathogenicity islands* by sigma factors

Regulatory control of SPIs can be exerted by sigma factors without sigma factors being directly involved in the transcription of these genes. SPI-1 genes are typically transcribed using σ^{70}. σ^{H} mediates SPI-1 expression by regulating activators of SPI-1. Systems mediated by RpoH negatively regulate HilD post-translationally and HilA transcriptionally (Matsui et al., 2008). HilD is responsible for activating HilA transcription, and HilA in turn activates all the genes within SPI-1. σ^{H} directs the production of Lon protease which specifically degrades HilD (Matsui et al., 2008). By modulating the activation of σ^{H}, the bacterial cell can control SPI-1 expression, restricting expression to specific regions within the host cell (Matsui et al., 2008). The cell can repress invasion genes long enough to replicate, escape, and invade a new macrophage before cell death (Matsui et al., 2008).

Promoters for SPI-2 genes all have consensus sequences for σ^{70} (Osborne & Coombes, 2009). However, upstream of some SPI-2 genes seem to be consensus sequences for σ^{E} recognition (Osborne & Coombes, 2009). It is postulated that these σ^{E} binding sites may serve a couple of different purposes. The σ^{E} - recognized promoters may allow the bacteria to express TTSS in response to host factors that compromise bacterial cellular integrity (Osborne & Coombes, 2009). Alternatively, σ^{E} may fine-tune the expression of SPI-2 genes through σ^{70} (Osborne & Coombes, 2009) by preferentially overexpressing certain genes while all others are expressed at basal levels by σ^{70}.

Stationary phase *Salmonella* are unable to cause actin rearrangement in the host epithelial cell that is necessary for entry (Francis et al., 1992). Invasion factors are either not functional or not expressed in stationary phase bacteria (Francis et al., 1992). As growth phase has been demonstrated to change intracellular concentrations of different sigma factors and virulence genes do not appear to be under the transcriptional control of σ^{S}, it stands to reason that these bacteria would not be able to invade; invasion genes would be inactive since the activity of the necessary sigma factor is repressed.

6.2 Other genetic sources of virulence

Virulence genes may be found outside of *Salmonella* pathogenicity islands. These genes are similarly essential to survival and also are responsive to changes in sigma factor availability. While the genetic location of the Spv regulon varies among *Salmonella* species from chromosomal to plasmid-encoded, all species carry the regulon and it functions to increase intracellular growth in host cells once the bacteria have spread outside of the small intestine (Guiney et al., 1995). σ^{S} mutants are unable to efficiently express the Spv regulon. Expression of one of the members of the Spv regulon, *spvB*, decreased by 86% when σ^{S} was knocked out (Fang et al., 1992). The lethal dosage in mice for a strain without a functional *rpoS* gene was 1000 fold greater than the wild type (Fang et al., 1992).

The dependence of Spv regulon expression on growth phase also indicates a dependence on σ^S for transcription. However, it seems to be nutrient availability, not cell density, that is most important in mediating Spv regulon expression (Guiney et al., 1995). σ^S associated with RNA polymerase results in expression of genes that are essential to help the bacteria survive nutrient depleted conditions, such as those found in deeper tissues beyond the small intestine (Guiney et al., 1995).

σ^S increases expression of *spv* virulence genes by interacting with SpvR, a repressor protein for the virulence plasmid (Kowarz et al., 1994). Competition for RNA polymerase between σ^S and σ^{70} led to less efficient transcription of *spvR* from its promoter as σ^S has a greater affinity for RNA polymerase than σ^{70} but a lower affinity for the promoter for *spvR* (Kowarz et al., 1994). σ^S affinity for RNA polymerase is enhanced by its interaction with the Crl protein, giving it the ability to displace σ^{70} as the preferred promoter (Robbe-Saule et al., 2007). The presence of SpvR regulates its own transcription (Kowarz et al., 1994) so the lack of efficient transcription leads to decreasing cellular levels and derepression of *spv* plasmid virulence genes. σ^S ensures that enough SpvR is present to activate transcription from the *spvA* promoter, the first gene in the regulon (Guiney et al., 1995).

7. Sigma factors and surviving the best of times and the worst of times

While *Salmonella* Pathogenicity Islands allow the bacteria to invade host cells, the pathogen must then survive the hostile environment found inside. While differential gene expression from various sigma factors ensures the appropriate expression of SPIs to gain access to the intracellular milieu of the host, the use of alternate sigma factors also permits survival.

7.1 A sigma factor cascade for survival in phagocytic cells

Ferric Fang describes a cascade of transcriptional and translational events that involve sigma factors associating with the core enzyme to transcribe genes for each other and those necessary to respond to a variety of assaults in the intracellular environment (Fang, 2005). The first step in the cascade is activation of σ^E, which is constitutively expressed through σ^{70} promoters, but held inactive by a pair of negative regulators, RseA and RseB (De Las Peñas et al., 1997). RseA interacts with σ^E in such a way as to block the binding site for RNA polymerase (Muller et al., 2009). When an extracytoplasmic stress is perceived, σ^E is released by RseA and freed to bind to RNA polymerase. Interaction of σ^E with the core enzyme allows for transcription from other promoters. These promoters include those before the σ^E regulon of genes but also before the *rpoH* gene, which encodes the alternative sigma factor, σ^H. σ^H provides specificity for RNA polymerase to transcribe genes in the σ^H regulon, which respond to cytoplasmic stress. Additionally, σ^H allows transcription of *hfq*. The Hfq protein interacts with the *rpoS* mRNA to facilitate its translation. The σ^S then allows transcription of genes under its transcriptional control, which allow for a starvation response (Fang, 2005). This overall cascade allows for coordinated response by the pathogen. To ensure that sigma factors help transcribe genes needed to respond to stress only as long as it exists, there must be some mechanism of turnover (Fang, 2005). In this way, the use of an interconnected web of sigma factors allows *Salmonella* to gain access to various cell types and then survive to be able to spread to other areas of the host.

This cascade's vital importance to survival, in particular within macrophages, is illustrated by the increased levels of σ^S inside the macrophage following infection. Some aspect of being inside a macrophage results in increased transcription of the *rpoS* gene. While levels of the housekeeping sigma σ^{70} decreased, levels of σ^{S} increased about 10-fold a few hours after infection (Khan et al., 1998). Conditions inside the macrophage induce the stress response and restrict nutrient availability, which induces the sigma cascade of gene expression to help the bacteria survive, although not necessarily to increase/induce virulence.

7.2 Sigma factors coordinate gene expression

Rarely is gene expression controlled in a strictly linear manner. That is, multiple sigma factors may work together to fine tune an expression of a group of genes to provide the bacteria with high probability of survival. The cascade of sigma factors used to allow survival inside phagocytic cells (described above) is just one example. There are many other instances of sigma factors working simultaneously.

One way to determine if one sigma factor plays a role in the efficient transcription by the other is to knock out one of them and see how the function of gene products mediated by the other are affected. In this way, investigators determined a relation between RpoE and FliA. Mutants without *rpoE* showed defective or limited mobility (Du et al., 2011). In these mutants, expression from class 1 flagellar promoters remained unaffected while some class 2 and most class 3 promoters showed decreased activity as compared to wild type (Du et al., 2011). It was concluded that RpoE may promote expression from class 3 promoters by mediating expression of FliA during osmotic stress, such as the hyperosmotic conditions found in the small intestine (Du et al., 2011).

RpoH and RpoN also appear to be related based on their ability to control the same genes as well as their dependence on one another. Expression of some heat shock operons appear to be under the control of RpoN in certain conditions, as expression from σ^{H} operons is down-regulated in mutants with an *rpoN* knockout (Studholme, 2002). In this way, RpoN may be responsible for fine tuning some gene expression during heat shock response. The expression of topoisomerases also appears to be governed by both σ^{N} and σ^{H} (Studholme, 2002), which may also indicate an interdependence of the activities of the two sigma factors.

Insufficient expression of one sigma factor can be compensated for by over-expression of other sigma factors. For example, researchers expected that because RpoS was vital to survival within macrophages, this sigma factor would be important for expressing virulence genes inside these phagocytic cells. However, within macrophages while RpoS only moderately increased following infection, RpoH and RpoE showed dramatic increases in intracellular concentration (Eriksson et al., 2003). While RpoS is typically associated with virulence inside phagocytic cells, it may be possible for other sigma factors to express other genes in response to a different environmental stimulus while still ultimately resulting in virulence. Research has also demonstrated that RpoN can compensate for insufficient RpoS in the formation of certain lipopolysaccharides (Bittner et al., 2004).

7.3 Survival outside of a host

While *Salmonella* is an important enteric pathogen to study because it infects many hosts and can be transmitted from species to species, it also is able to survive for long periods of time outside a host. Because of this characteristic, it has been an important target of sanitation processes to eliminate possible sources of transmission.

One mean of *Salmonella* transmission to human hosts is through food products, such as poultry. The same mechanisms of alternate sigma factor used to survive acid challenges in the mammalian gut are also utilized in surviving the fowl gastrointestinal tract and can lead to transmission of the pathogen (Dunkley et al., 2008).

Other studies specific to food handling procedures and alternate sigma factors have determined that RpoS, for example, is essential to *Salmonella*'s ability to withstand normal sanitation procedures common in the food service industry and that early induction of RpoS can cause the cells to enter stationary growth phase prematurely, negating the protective nature of stationary growth on the pathogen's ability to survive (Komitopoulou et al., 2004). Other studies have demonstrated that certain food handling processes, such as washing in various antimicrobial agents, can induce RpoS to protect the bacteria from destruction (Dodd & Aldsworth, 2002). Significant drops in temperature have also been found to activate transcription from σ^S dependent promoters rather than from the σ^{70} promoters from which genes are normally transcribed (Rajkumari & Gowrishankar, 2001).

Multiple alternate sigma factors contribute to survival through food processing. For example, σ^S and σ^E were both found to be important in surviving refrigeration and changes in osmotic pressure. Depending on the nature of the stress, either σ^S or σ^E may be more important and their relative concentrations dictate the response (McMeechan et al., 2007).

8. Transcriptional and translational regulation of sigma factors

Because sigma factors are capable of effecting dramatic changes in cellular protein composition and energy use, their actions must be closely guarded to ensure that the pathogen is responding to the stress without exhausting cellular resources.

8.1 Regulation of sigma factors

Some alternate sigma factors are constitutively expressed but held inactive until they are needed by regulatory proteins that change conformation or leave the cell in response to a particular signal. RpoE is held inactive until an extracellular signal of extracytoplasmic stress is received and FliA is held inactive by FlgM until the FlgM is exported out of the cell by the completed hook and basal body structure. Some regulation of sigma factors is accomplished by the optimal conditions under which they can influence gene expression. *rpoH* cannot be translated below a certain temperature because at lower temperatures the mRNA folds back on itself blocking the start codon. And RpoS shows increased efficiency during stationary phase growth and is almost nonexistent during exponential growth.

Because much of the efficiency of sigma factors to influence transcription is itself influenced by their relative concentrations within the cells, many mechanisms to regulate them change the available concentration of these proteins. Different proteases target specific sigma factors and depending on the relative concentration of these proteases, the relative availability of the sigma factors can be adjusted.

RpoS is needed to transcribe the most genes and is therefore the most highly regulated. Several novel pathways of regulation have been discovered. DksA is required for efficient translation of *rpoS* but not as an RNA chaperone (Webb et al., 1999). Another protein, RstA, decreases the expression of RpoS controlled genes and appears to decrease cellular levels of

RpoS independently of proteolytic activity (Cabeza et al., 2007). Translation of the *rpoS* mRNA is elevated in the presence of appropriate carbon sources, indicating a growth rate dependent control of sigma factor availability (Cunning & Elliot, 1999). In response to increased glucose levels, StpA prevents overactivation of σ^S indirectly enhancing its turnover (Lucchini et al., 2009). Some small mRNAs such as DsrA and RprA, are highly conserved as are their antisense elements within the *rpoS* mRNA, but they only have small effects on RpoS availability (Jones et al., 2006). DsrA interaction with *rpoS* mRNA disrupts the stem and loop base pairing of *rpoS* mRNA to allow high levels of translation (Majdalani et al., 2001). The same study discovered another small RNA, RprA, that interacts in a similar way to positively regulate RpoS translation (Majdalani et al., 2001).

8.2 Sigma factors and other regulatory mechanisms

Differential gene expression through alternate sigma factors is far from the only regulatory mechanism found in *Salmonella*. When these other regulatory systems respond to environmental stimuli, alternate sigma factors influence gene expression related to these systems as well. Two important regulators that intersect differential gene expression with sigma factors are the PhoP/PhoQ regulatory system and the Fis global regulator.

The PhoP/PhoQ regulatory system influences the expression of many genes and is functionally a sensor of extracellular magnesium concentration. It has been hypothesized to have evolved differently in closely related species like *E. coli* and *Salmonella* as a result of different lifestyles (Monsieurs et al., 2005). The relation between the PhoP/PhoQ regulatory system and σ^S appears to be essential. Even in cells with functional copies of *rpoS,* mutants lacking PhoP cannot form functional phagosomes within phagocytic cells (Alpuche-Aranda et al., 1994). Mutants with a double knockout of the RpoS and PhoP/PhoQ show decreased virulence and decreased invasion of host cells (Lee et al., 2007). It has even been suggested that because of their inability to cause lasting infections, these double knockouts should be used to make a *Salmonella* vaccine (Lee et al., 2007).

PhoP controls the level of available RpoS by controlling proteins, which enable its degradation by ClpXP. PhoP acts as a transcriptional activator for *iraP*, which encodes a protein that interacts with RssB. RssB facilitates ClpXP degradation of σ^S (Tu et al., 2006). By blocking RssB activity, the level of σ^S accumulates during PhoP/PhoQ activation, which includes low levels of magnesium as found inside macrophages. This is very different than the type of regulation seen in the commensal *E. coli* (Tu et al., 2006), indicating that while there is some similarity in the genes expressed between the two, the regulation of the alternative sigma pathways is not the same. Interestingly, RpoE seems to be involved in the regulation of PhoP/PhoQ activity through Hfq, the same RNA chaperone through which it mediates RpoS expression (Coornaert et al., 2010).

Fis (factor for inversion stimulation) is a global transcription regulator and facilitates site-specific DNA recombination (Mallik et al., 2004). The intracellular concentrations of Fis are high during exponential growth and low in late exponential and stationary phase growth (Walker et al., 2004). The *fis* promoter itself is of some interest as to how these concentration differences are maintained. The σ^{70} dependent and growth-phase dependent regulation from this promoter is achieved through a weak -35 sequence, a second RNA polymerase binding site, and the relative concentration of nucleotides within the cell (Walker et al., 1999). The *fis* promoter is somewhat unique among σ^{70} - dependent promoters in that transcription begins with a cysteine (Walker et al., 2004). This residue is normally a poor initiator of transcription and as a result the RNA polymerase holoenzyme binds very weakly with the *fis* promoter (Walker et al., 2004). When cellular concentrations of cysteine are low, there is very little transcription from the promoter but as CTPs increase in the cell, so does gene expression from the *fis* promoter (Walker et al., 2004).

As expected from the pattern of Fis concentration in the cell, there is a negative relationship between the intracellular level of RpoS and Fis during stationary phase growth (Cróinín & Dorman, 2007). Fis in fact is able to mediate expression from σ^{S} - dependent genes by binding to a Fis-specific site upstream of σ^{S} promoter regions and blocking RpoS activity during exponential growth (Hirsch & Elliot, 2005).

Fis, as its name suggests, is also essential for the ability of *Salmonella* to switch flagellar types. There are two types of flagellar filaments, FljB and FliC, which are both transcribed from class 3 promoters. Flagellar switching is achieved by inversion of a promoter region. When expression occurs from this promoter, a type B filament is produced and a repressor of type C is created. When the inversion occurs, the repressor of type C is not produced and type C filaments are made (Aldridge et al., 2006). Hin (for H invertase) and Fis are both required for proper inversion (Bruist et al., 1987). Hin seems to mediate the inversion while Fis ensures the appropriate alignment of the inverted DNA (Bruist et al., 1987).

In having two different types of filaments available for use, *Salmonella* is able to evade the host immune system. FliC is a well-studied target of the immune system (Cummings et al., 2005). As bacteria migrate through the small intestine and into the rest of the host, FliC expression is suppressed or switched for FljB expression to avoid detection by T cells (Cummings et al., 2005). Once past the initial site of infection, T cells are no longer able to recognize the pathogen (Cummings et al., 2005).

Finally, the relatedness of alternate sigma factors and pathogenicity can ensure that certain genes are not expressed at the wrong time. The gene *hilA* which is responsible for the regulation of SPI-1 genes is found in the same operon as FliA, the alternate sigma factor for flagellar filament assembly (Lucas et al., 2000). This proximity within the genome allows for the simultaneous control of both mobility and invasion properties, and ensures the likely co-inheritance of the regulatory elements.

9. Conclusion

Differential gene expression through the use of alternate sigma factors is one of numerous regulatory methods available to *Salmonella* to avoid destruction by its host's immune system or sanitation processes and to thrive in a variety of environments. Control through sigma factors intersects control exerted by other regulatory pathways to ensure a highly controllable pattern of gene expression. The full capacity of *Salmonella* to change rapidly and accurately to respond to environmental conditions is still not well understood. Genes that are under the most types of regulatory control are typically the most important in virulence (McDermott et al., 2011) and it is clear that not only are sigma factors highly controlled themselves at the level of transcription and translation, but they are interconnected in a complex web.

From a medical standpoint, rendering *Salmonella* essentially commensal by knocking out various genes for sigma factors may be an area of interest in creating vaccines. *Salmonella* mutants with one or more nonfunctional copies of genes for alternate sigma factors show significantly attenuated growth across hosts and especially in macrophages, which seems to be the most essential characteristic of *Salmonella's* ability to evade the host immune system. Understanding how sigma factors protect the integrity of the bacteria and testing the limits of this protection may provide insight into the development of new sanitation processes that eliminate more of the bacteria and prevent spread.

10. Acknowledgment

This work was supported, in part, by an IRIG-CEG grant from the office of the Executive Vice President for Research at the University of Louisville.

11. References

Aiba, A. & Mizobuchi, K. (1989). Nucleotide Sequence Analysis of Genes *purH* and *purD* Involved in the *de Novo* Purine Nucleotide Biosynthesis in *Escherichia coli*. *Journal of Biological Chemistry*, Vol.264, No.35, (December 1989), pp. 21239-21246, ISSN 0021-9258.

Aldridge, P.D.; Wu, C.; Gnerer, J.; Karlinsey, J.E.; Hughes, K.T.; & Sachs, M.S. (2006). Regulatory protein that inhibits both synthesis and use of the target protein controls flagellar phase variation in *Salmonella enterica*. *Proceedings of the National Academy of Sciences*, Vol.103, No.30, (July 2006), pp. 11340-11345, ISSN 0027-8424

Alpuche-Aranda, C.M.; Racoosin, E.L.; Swanson, J.A.; & Miller, S.I. (1994). *Salmonella* Stimulate Macrophage Macropinocytosis and Persist within Spacious Phagosomes. *Journal of Experimental Medicine*. Vol.179, No.2, (February 1994), pp. 601-608, ISSN 0022-1007

Audia, J.P. & Foster, J.W. (2003) Acid Shock Accumulation of Sigma S in *Salmonella enterica* Involves Increased Translation, Not Regulated Degradation. *Journal of Molecular Microbiology and Biotechnology*. Vol.5, No.1, (March 2003), pp. 17-28, ISSN 1464-1801

Bang, I.S.; Frye, J.G.; McClelland, M.; Velayudhan, J.; & Fang, F.C. (2005) Alternative sigma factor interactions in *Salmonella*: σ^E and σ^H promote antioxidant defenses by enhancing σ^S levels. *Molecular Microbiology*. Vol.56, No.3, (March 2005), pp. 811-823, ISSN 1365-2958

Barchiesi, J.; Espariz, M.; Checa, S.K.; & Soncini, F.C. (2009) Downregulation of RpoN-controlled genes protects *Salmonella* cells from killing by the cationic antimicrobial peptide polymyxin B. *FEMS Microbiol Letters*. Vol.291, No.1, (February 2009) pp. 73-79, ISSN 0378-1097

Barrios, H.; Valderrama, B.; & Morett, E. (1999) Compilation and analysis of σ^{54} – dependent promoter sequences. *Nucleic Acid Research*. Vol.27, No.22, (November 1999), pp. 4305-4313, ISSN 0305-1048

Baumler, A.J.; Kusters, J.G.; Stojiljkovic, I.; & Heffron, F. (1994), *Salmonella* Typhimurium Loci Involved in Survival within Macrophages. *Infection and Immunology*, Vol.62, No.5, (May 1994), pp. 1623-1630, ISSN 0019-9567

Bittner, M.: Saldías, S.: Altamirano, F.; Valvano, M.A., & Cantreras, I. (2004). RpoS and RpoN are involved in the growth-dependent regulation of *rfaH* transcription and O antigen expression in *Salmonella enterica* serovar typhi. *Microbial Pathogenesis*, Vol.36, No.1, (January 2004), pp. 19-24, ISSN 0882-4010

Bonifield, H.R. & Hughes, K.T. (2003). Flagellar Phase Variation in *Salmonella enterica* Is Mediated by a Posttranscriptional Control Mechanism. *Journal of Bacteriology,* Vol.185, No.12, (June 2003), pp. 3567-3574, ISSN 0021-9193.

Brown, K.L. & Hughes, K.T. (1995) The role of anti-sigma factors in gene regulation. *Molecular Microbiology,* Vol.16, No.3, (May 1995), pp. 397-404, ISSN 0950-382X

Brown, L. & Elliot, T. (1996). Efficient Translation of the RpoS Sigma Factor in *Salmonella* Typhimurium Requires Host Factor I, an RNA-Binding Protein Encoded by the *hfq* Gene. *Journal of Bacteriology* Vol.178, No.13, (July 1996), pp. 3763-3770, ISSN 0021-9193

Brown, L. & Elliot, T. (1997). Mutations that Increase Expression of the *rpoS* Gene and Decrease Its Dependence on *hfq* Function in *Salmonella* Typhimurium. *Journal of Bacteriology,* Vol.179, No.3, (February 1997), pp. 656-662, ISSN 0021-9193

Bruist, M.F.; Glasgow, A.C.; & Johnson, R.C. (1987). Fis binding to the recombinational enhancer of the Hin DNA inversion system. *Genes and Development,* Vol.1, No.8, (October 1987), pp. 762-772, ISSN 0890-9369

Buck, M. & Cannon, W. (1992). Specific binding of the transcription factor sigma-54 to promoter DNA. *Nature,* Vol.358, No.6385, (July 1992) pp. 422-424, ISSN 0028-0836

Buck, M.; Gallegos, M.T.; Studholme, D.J.; Guo, Y.; & Gralla, J.D. (2000). The Bacterial Enhancer-Dependent σ^{54} (σ^{N}) Transcription Factor. *Journal of Bacteriology,* Vol.182, No.15, (August 2000), pp. 4129-4136, ISSN 0021-9193

Bueno, S.M.; Riedel, C.A.; Carreño & Kalergis, A.M. (2010). Virulence Mechanisms Displayed by *Salmonella* to Impair Dendritic Cell Function. *Current Medical Chemistry,* Vol.17, No.12, (April 2010), pp. 1156-1166, ISSN 0929-8673

Burgess, R.R. & Travers, A.A. (1969). Factor Stimulating Transcription by RNA Polymerase. *Nature,* Vol.221, No.5175, (January 1969), pp. 43-46, ISSN 0028-0836

Burton, Z.F.; Gross, C.A.; Watanabe, K.K.; & Burgess, R.R (1983). The Operon That Encodes the Sigma Subunit of RNA Polymerase Also Encodes Ribosomal Protein S21 and DNA Primase in E. coli K12. *Cell,* Vol.32, No.2, (February 1983), pp. 335-349, ISSN 0092-8674

Cabeza, M.L.; Aguirre, A.; Soncini, F.C.; & Véscovi, E.G. (2007). Induction of RpoS Degradation by the Two-Component System Regulator RstA in *Salmonella enterica. Journal of Bacteriology,* Vol.189, No.20, (October 2007), pp. 7335-7342, ISSN 0021-9193

Chadsey, M.S.; Karlinsey, J.E.; & Hughes, K.T. (1998). The flagellar anti-σ factor FlgM actively dissociates *Salmonella* Typhimurium σ^{28} RNA polymerase holoenzyme. *Genes and Development,* Vol.12, No.19, (October 1998), pp. 3123–3136, ISSN 0890-9369

Chen, L.M.; Hobbie, S.; & Galán, J.E. (1996). Requirement of CDC42 of Salmonella-induced cytoskeletal and nuclear responses. *Science,* Vol.274, No.5295, (December 1996), pp. 2115-2118, ISSN 0036-8075

Chilcott, G.S. & Hughes, K.T. (2000). Coupling of Flagellar Gene Expression to Flagellar Assembly in *Salmonella enterica* Serovar Typhimurium and *Escherichia coli. Microbiology and Molecular Biology Review,* Vol.64, No.4, (December 2000), pp. 694-708, ISSN 1092-2172.

Cirillo, D.M.; Valdivia, R.H.; Monack, D.M.; & Falkow, S. (1998). Macrophage-dependent induction of the *Salmonella* pathogenicity island 2 type III secretion system and its role in intracellular survival. *Molecular Microbiology,* Vol.30, No.1, (October 1998), pp. 175-188, ISSN 0950-382X

Conlin, C.A. & Miller, C.G. (2000). *opdA*, a *Salmonella enterica* Serovar Typhimurium Gene Encoding a Protease, Is Part of an Operon Regulated by Heat Shock. *Journal of Bacteriology,* Vol.182, No.2, (January 2000), pp. 518-521, ISSN 0021-9193

Coornaert, A.; Lu, A.; Mandin, P.; Spring, M.; Gottesman, S.; & Guillier, M. (2010). MicA sRNA links the PhoP regulon to cell envelope stress. *Molecular Microbiology,* Vol.76, No.2, (April 2010), pp. 467-479, ISSN 0950-382X

Cróinín, T.Ó. & Dorman, C.J. (2007). Expression of the Fis protein is sustained in late-exponential- and stationary-phase cultures of *Salmonella enterica* serovar Typhimurium grown in the absence of aeration. *Molecular Microbiology,* Vol.66, No.1, (2007), pp. 237-251, ISSN 0950-382X

Cummings, L.A.; Rassoulian Barrett, S.L; Wilkerson, W.D.; Fellnerova, I.; & Cookson, B.T. (2005). FliC-Specific CD4+ T Cell Responses are Restricted by Bacterial Regulation of Antigent Expression. *Journal of Immunology,* Vol.174, No.12, (June 2005), pp. 7929-7938, ISSN 0022-1767

Cunning, C. & Elliot, T. (1999). RpoS Synthesis is Growth Rate Regulated in *Salmonella* Typhimurium, but Its Turnover Is Not Dependent on Acetyl Phosphate Synthesis on PTS Function. *Journal of Bacteriology,* Vol.181, No.16, (August 1999), pp. 4853-4862, ISSN 0021-9193

De Las Peñas, A.; Connolly, L.; & Gross, A.C. (1997) The σ^E –mediated response to extracytoplasmic stress in *Escherichia coli* is transduced by RseA and RseB, two negative regulators of σ^E . *Molecular Microbiology,* Vol.24, No.2, (April 1997), pp. 373-385, ISSN 0950-382X

Dodd, C.E.R. & Aldsworth, T.G. (2002). The importance of RpoS in the survival of bacteria through food processing. *International Journal of Food Microbiology,* Vol.74, No.3, (April 2002), pp. 189-194, ISSN 0168-1605

Dombroski, A.J.; Walter, W.A.; & Gross, C.A. (1993). Amino-terminal amino acids modulate sigma-factor DNA-binding activity. *Genes and Development,* Vol.7, No.12A, (December 1993), pp. 2446-2455, ISSN 0890-9369

Dombroski, A.J.; Walter, W.A.; Record, M.T.; Siegele, D.A.; & Gross, C.A. (1992). Polypeptides Containing Highly Conserved Regions of Transcription Initiation Factor σ^{70} Exhibit Specificity of Binding to Promoter DNA. *Cell,* Vol.70, No.3, (August 1992), pp. 501-512, ISSN 0092-8674

Dougan, G.; John, V.; Palmer, S.; & Mastroeni, P. (2011). Immunity to salmonellosis. *Immunology Reviews,* Vol.240, No.1, (March 2011), pp. 196-210, ISSN 0105-2896

Du, H.; Sheng, X.; Zhang, H.; Zou, X.; Ni, B.; Xu, S.; Zhu, Z.; Xu, H.; & Huang, X. (2011). RpoE may Promote Flagellar Gene Expression in *Salmonella enterica* Serovar Typhi Under Hyperosmotic Stress. *Current Microbiology,* Vol.62, No.2, (February 2011), pp.492-500, ISSN 0343-8651

Dunkley, K.D.; Callaway, T.R.; Chalova, V.I.; Anderson, R.C.; Kundinger, M.M.; Dunkley, C.S.; Nisbet, D.J.; & Ricke, S.C. (2008). Growth and genetic responses of *Salmonella* Typhimurium to pH-shifts in an anaerobic continuous culture. *Anaerobe,* Vol.14, No.1, (February 2008), pp. 35-42, ISSN 1075-9964

Eriksson, S.; Lucchini, S.; Thompson, A.; Rhen, M.; & Hinton, J.C.D. (2003). Unravelling the biology of macrophage infection by gene expression profiling of intracellular

Salmonella enterica. Molecular Microbiology, Vol.47, No.1, (2003), pp. 103-118, ISSN 0950-382X

Fang, F.C.; Libby, S.J.; Buchmeier, N.A.; Loewen, P.C.; Switala, J.; Harwood, J; & Guiney, D.G. (1992). The alternative σ factor KatF (RpoS) regulates *Salmonella* virulence. *Proceedings of the National Acadmey of Sciences USA,* Vol.89, No.24, (December 1992), pp. 11978-11982, ISSN 0027-8424

Fang, F.C.; Chen, C.Y.; Guiney, D.G.; & Xu, Y. (1996). Identification of σ^S – Regulated Genes in *Salmonella* Typhimurium: Complementary Regulatory Interactions between σ^S and Cyclic AMP Receptor Protein. *Journal of Bacteriology,* Vol.178, No. 17, (September 1996), pp. 5112-5120, ISSN 0021-9193

Fang, F.C. (2005). Sigma Cascades in Prokaryotic Regulatory Networks. *Proceedings of the National Academy of Sciences,* Vol.102, (2005), pp. 4933-4934, ISSN 0027-8424

Farewell, A.; Kvint, K.; & Nyström, T. (1998) Negative regulation by RpoS: a case of sigma factor competition. *Molecular Microbiology,* Vol.29, No.4, (August 1998), pp. 1039-1051, ISSN 0950-382X

Francis, C.L.; Starnbach, M.N.; & Falkow, S. (1992). Morphological and cytoskeletal changes in epithelial cells occur immediately upon interaction with *Salmonella* Typhimurium grown under low-oxygen conditions. *Molecular Microbiology,* Vol.6, No. 21, (November 1992), pp. 3077-3087, ISSN 0950-382X

Fu, Y. & Galán, J.E. (1999). A *Salmonella* protein antagonizes Rac-1 and Cdc42 to mediate host-cell recovery after bacterial invasion. *Nature,* Vol.401, No.6750, (September 1999), pp. 293-297, ISSN 0028-0836

Galán, J.E. (1996). Molecular and Cellular Bases of *Salmonella* Entry into Host Cells. *Bacterial Invasiveness,* Vol.209, (1996), pp. 43-60, ISSN 0070-217X

Guiney, D.G.; Libby, S.; Fang, F.C.; Krause, M.; & Fierer, J. (1995). Growth-phase regulation of plasmid virulence genes in *Salmonella. Trends in Microbiology,* Vol.3, No.7, (July 1995), pp. 275-279, ISSN 0966-842X

Hansen-Wester, I. & Hensen, M. (2001). Salmonella pathogenicity islands encoding type III secretion systems. *Microbes and Infection,* Vol.3, No.7, (June 2001), pp. 549-559, ISSN 1286-4579

Helmann, J.D. & Chamberlin, M.J. (1987). DNA sequence analysis suggests that expression of flagellar and chemotaxis genes in *Escherichia coli* and *Salmonella Typhimurium* is controlled by an alternate σ factor. *Proceedings of the National Academy of Sciences USA,* Vol.84, No.18, (September 1987), pp. 6422-6424, ISSN 0027-8424

Hensel, M.; Shea, J.E.; Waterman, S.R.; Mundy, R.; Nikolaus, R.; Banks, G.; Vazquez-Torres, A.; Gleeson, C.; Fang, F.C.; & Holden, D.W. (1998). Genes encoding putative effector proteins of the type III secretion system of *Salmonella* pathogenicity island 2 are required for bacterial virulence and proliferation in macrophages. *Molecular Microbiology,* Vol.30, No.1, (October 1998), pp. 163-174, ISSN 0950-382X

Hirsch, M. & Elliot, T. (2005). Fis Regulates Transcriptional Induction of RpoS in *Salmonella enterica. Journal of Bacteriology,* Vol.187, No.5, (March 2005), pp. 1568-1580, ISSN 0021-9193

Hughes, K.T.; Gillen, K.L.; Semon, M.J.; & Karlinsey, J.E. (1993). Sensing Structural Intermediates in Bacterial Flagellar Assembly by Export of a Negative Regulator. *Science,* Vol.262, No.5137, (November 1993), pp. 1277-1280, ISSN 0036-8075

Ibanez-Ruiz, M.; Robbe-Saule, V.; Hermant, D.; Labrude, S.; and Norel, F. (2000). Identification of RpoS (σ^S)-regulated Genes in *Salmonella enterica* Serovar Typhimurium. *Journal of Bacteriology,* Vol.182, No.20, (October 2000), pp. 5749-5756, ISSN 0021-9193

Ikebe, T.; Iyoda, S.; & Kutsukake, K. (1999). Structure and expression of the *fliA* operon of *Salmonella* Typhimurium. *Microbiology,* Vol.145, No.6, (June 1999), pp. 1389-1396, ISSN 1350-0872

Ishihama, A. (1993). Protein-Protein Communication with the Transcription Apparatus. *Journal of Bacteriology,* Vol.175, No.9, (May 1993), pp. 2483-2489, ISSN 0021-9193

Jishage, M., & Ishihama,A. (1995). Regulation of RNA Polymerase Sigma Subunits Synthesis in *Escherichia coli:* Intracellular Levels of σ^{70} and σ^{38}. *Journal of Bacteriology,* Vol.177, No.23, (December 1995), pp. 6832-6835, ISSN 0021-9193

Jones, A.M.; Goodwill, A.; & Elliot, T. (2006). Limited Role for the DsrA and RprA Regulatory RNAs in *rpoS* Regulation in *Salmonella enterica. Journal of Bacteriology,* Vol.188, No.14, (July 2006), pp. 5077-5088, ISSN 0021-9193

Jones, B.D.; Ghori, N.; & Falkow, S. (1994). *Salmonella* Typhimurium Initiates Murine Infection by Penetrating and Destroying the Specialized Epithelial M Cells of the Peyer's Patches. *Journal of Experimental Medicine,* Vol.180, No.9, (Septemeber 1994), pp. 15-23, ISSN 0019-9567

Karlinsey, J.E.; Tanaka, S.; Bettenworth, V.; Yamaguchi, S.; Boos, W.; Aizawa, S.I.; & Hughes, K.T. (2000). Completion of the hook-basal body complex of the *Salmonella* Typhimurium flagellum is coupled to FlgM secretion and *fliC* transcription. *Molecular Microbiology,* Vol.37, No.5, (2000), pp. 1220-1231, ISSN 0950-382X

Karlinsey, J.E. & Hughes, K.T. (2006) Genetic Transplantation: *Salmonella enterica* Serovar Typhimurium as a Host to Study Sigma Factor and Anti-Sigma Factor Interactions in Genetically Intractable Systems. *Journal of Bacteriology,* Vol.188, No.1, (January 2006), pp. 103-114, ISSN 0021-9193

Kenyon, W. J.; Thomas, S.M.; Johson, E.; Pallen, M.J.; & Spector, M.P. (2005). Shifts from glucose to certain secondary carbon-sources result in activation of the extracytoplasmic function sigma factor σ^E in *Salmonella enterica* serovar Typhimurium. *Microbiology,* Vol.151, No.7, (July 2005), pp. 2373-2383, ISSN 1350-0872

Khan, A.Q.; Zhao, L.; Hirose, K.; Miyake, M.; Li, T.; Hashimoto, Y.; Kawamura, Y.; & Ezaki, T. (1998). *Salmonella typhi rpoS* mutant is less cytotoxic than the parent strain but survives inside resting THP-1 macrophages. *FEMS Microbiology Letters,* Vol.161, No.1, (April 1998), pp. 201-208, ISSN 0378-1097

Kilstrup, M.; Jessing, S.G.; Wichmand-Jørgensen, S.B.; Madsen, M.; & Nilsson, D. (1998). Activation Control of *pur* Gene Expression in *Lactococcus lactis*a; Proposal for a Consensus Activator Binding Sequence Based on Deletion Analysis and Site-Directed Mutagenesis of *purC* and *purD* Promoter Regions. *Journal of Bacteriology,* Vol.180, No.15, (August 1998), pp. 3900-3906, ISSN 0021-9193

Komitopoulou, E.; Bainton, N.J.; & Adams, M.R. (2004). Oxidation-reduction potential regulates RpoS levels in *Salmonella* Typhimurium. *Journal of Applied Microbiology,* Vol.96, No.2, (February 2004), pp. 271-278, ISSN 1384-5072

Kowarz, L.; Coynault, C.; Robbe-Saule, V.; & Norel, F. (1994). The *Salmonella* Typhimurium *katF* (*rpoS*) Gene: Cloning, Nucleotide Sequence, and Regulation of *spvR* and *spvABCD* Virulence Plasmid Genes. *Journal of Bacteriology,* Vol.176, No.22, (November 1994), pp. 6852-6860, ISSN 0021-9193

Kutsukake, K. & Iino, T. 1994. Role of the FliA-FlgM Regulatory System on Transcriptional Control of the Flagellar Regulon and Flagellar Formation in *Salmonella* Typhimurium. *Journal of Bacteriology,* Vol.176, No.12, (June 1994), pp. 3598-3605, ISSN 0021-9193

Kutsukake, K.; Iyoda, S.; Ohnishi, K.; & Iino, T. (1994). Genetic and molecular analysis of the interaction between the flagellum-specific and anti-sigma factors in *Salmonella* Typhimurium. *Journal of Environmental Microbiology,* Vol.13, No.19, (October 1994), pp. 4568-4576, ISSN 0261-4189

Lara-Tejero, M. & Galán, J.E. (2009). *Salmonella enterica* Serovar Typhimurium Pathogenicity Island 1-Encoded Type III Secretion System Translocases Mediate Intimate Attachement to Nonphagocytic Cells. *Infection and Immunology,* Vol.77, No.1, (July 2009), pp. 2635-2642, ISSN 0019-9567

Lawhon, S.D.; Maurer, R.; Suyemoto, M.; & Altier, C. (2002). Intestinal short-chain fatty acids alter *Salmonella* Typhimurium invasion gene expression and virulence though BarA/SirA. *Molecular Microbiology,* Vol.46, No.5 (2002), pp. 1451-1464, ISSN 0950-382X

Lee, H.Y.; Cho, S.A.; Lee, I.S.; Park, J.H.; Seok, S.H.; Bae, M.W.; Kim, D.J.; Lee, S.H.; Hur, S.J.; Ban, S.J.; Lee, Y.K.; Han, Y.K.; Cho, Y.K.; & Park, J.H. (2007). Evaluation of *phoP* and *rpoS* mutants of *Salmonella enterica* serovar Typhi as attenuated vaccine candidates: virulence and protective immune responses in intranasally immunized mice. *FEMS Immunology Med Microbiol,* Vol.51, No.2, (2007), pp. 310-318, ISSN 0928-8244

Liu, X. & Matsumura, P. (1994). The FlhD/FlhC Complex, a Transcriptional Activator of the *Escherichia coli* Flagellar Class II Operons. *Journal of Bacteriology,* Vol.176, No.23, (December 1994), pp. 7345-7351, ISSN 0021-9193

Liu, X.; Fukita, N.; Ishihama, A.; & Matsumara, P. (1995). The C-Terminal region of the α Subunit of *Escherichia coli* RNA Polymerase is Required for Transcriptional Activation of the Flagellar Level II Operons by the FlhD/FlhC Complex. *Journal of Bacteriology,* Vol.177, No.17, (September 1995), pp. 5186-5188, ISSN 0021-9193

Löber, S.; Jäckel, D.; Kaiser, N.; & Hensel, M. (2006). Regulation of *Salmonella* pathogenicity island 2 genes by independent environmental signals. *International Journal of Medical Microbiology,* Vol.296, No.7, (Novemeber 2006), pp. 435-447, ISSN 1438-4221

Lucas, R.L.; Lostroh, C.P.; DiRusso, C.C.; Spector, M.P.; Wanner, B.L.; & Lee, C.A. (2000). Multiple Factors Independently Regulate *hila* and Invasion Gene Expression in *Salmonella enterica* Serovar Typhimurium. *Journal of Bacteriology,* Vol.182, No.7, (April 2000), pp. 1872-1882, ISSN 0021-9193

Lucchini, S.; McDermott, P.; Thompson, A.; & Hinton, J.C.D. (2009). The H-NS-like protein StpA represses the RpoS (σ^{38}) regulon during exponential growth of *Salmonella* Typhimurium. *Molecular Microbiology,* Vol.74, No.5, (December 2009), pp. 1169-1186, ISSN 0950-382X

Majdalani, N.; Chen, S.; Murron, J.; St John, K.; & Gottesman, S. (2001). Regulation of RpoS by a novel small RNA: the characterization of RprA. *Molecular Microbiology,* Vol.39, No.5, (March 2001), pp. 1382-1394, ISSN 0950-382X

Mallik, P.; Pratt, T.S.; Beach, M.B.; Bradley, M.D.; Undamatla, J.; & Osuna, R. (2004). Growth Phase-Dependent Regulation and Stringent Control of *fis* are Conserved Processes in Enteric Bacteria and Involve a Single Promoter (*fis* P) in *Escherichia coli*. *Journal of Bacteriology*, Vol.186, No.1, (January 2004), pp. 122-135, ISSN 0021-9193

Matsui, M.; Takaya, A.; & Yamamoto, T. (2008). σ^{38} – Mediated Negative Regulation of *Salmonella* Pathogenicity Island 1 Expression. *Journal of Bacteriology*, Vol.190, No.20, (October 2008), pp. 6636-6645, ISSN 0021-9193

McDermott, J.E.; Yoon, H.; Nakayasu, E.S.; Metz, T.O.; Hyduke, D.R.; Kidawi, A.S.; Palsson, B.O.; Adkins, J.N.; & Heffron, F. (2011). Technologies and approaches to elucidate and model the virulence program of *Salmonella*. *Frontiers in Microbiology*, Vol.2, No.121, (June 2011), pp.1-14., ISSN 1664-302X

McMeechan, A.; Robers, M.; Cogan, T.A.; Jørgensen, F.; Stevenson, A.; Lewis, C.; Rowley, G.; & Humphrey, T.J. (2007). Role of the alternative sigma factors σ^E and σ^S in survival of *Salmonella enterica* serovar Typhimurium during starvation, refrigeration, and osmotic shock. *Microbiology*, Vol.153, No.1, (January 2007), pp. 263-269, ISSN 1350-0872

Minagawa, S.; Ogasawara, H.; Kato, A.; Yamamoto, K.; Eguchi, Y.; Oshima, T.; Mori, H.; Ishihama, A.; & Utsumi, R. (2003). Identification and Molecular Characterization of the Mg^{2+} Stimulon of *Escherichia coli*. *Journal of Bacteriology*, Vol.185, No.13, (July 2003), pp. 3696-3702, ISSN 0021-9193

Monsieurs, P.; De keersmaecker, S.; Navarre, W.W.; Bader, M.W.; De Smet, F.; McClelland, M.; Fang, F.C.; De Moor, B.; Vanderleyden, J.; & Marchal, K. (2005) Comparison of the PhoPQ Regulon in *Escherichia coli* and *Salmonella* Typhimurium. Vol. 60, No. 4 (April 2005), pp. 462-474, ISSN 0022-2844.

Morett, E. & Segovia, L. (1993). The σ^{54} Bacterial Enhancer-Binding Protein Family: Mechanism of Action and Phylogenetic Relationship of Their Functional Domains. *Journal of Bacteriology*, Vol.175, No.19, (October 1993), pp. 6067-6074, ISSN 0021-9193

Muller, C.; Bang, I.S.; Velayudhan, J.; Karlinsey, J.; Paperfort, K.; Vogel, J.; & Fang, F.C. (2009). Acid stress activation of the σ^E stress response in *Salmonella enterica* serovar Typhimurium. *Molecular Microbiology*, Vol.71, No.5, (2009), pp. 1228-1238, ISSN 0950-382X

Mutalik, V.K.: Nonaka, G.; Ades, S.E.; Rhodius, V.A.; & Gross, C.A. (2009). Promoter Strength Properties of the Complete Sigma E Regulon on *Escherichia coli* and *Salmonella enterica*. *Journal of Bacteriology*, Vol.191, No.23 (December 2009), pp. 7279-7287, ISSN 0021-9193

O'Neal, C.R.; Gabriel, W.M.; Turk, A.K.; Libby, S.J.; Fang, F.C.; & Spector, M. (1994). RpoS Is Necessary for Both Positive and Negative Regulation of Starvation Survival Genes during Phosphate, Carbon, and Nitrogen Starvation in *Salmonella* Typhimurium. *Journal of Bacteriology*, Vol.176, No.15, (August 1994), pp. 4610-4616, ISSN 0021-9193

Ohl, M.E. & Miller, S.I. (2001). *Salmonella*: A Model for Bacteria Pathogenesis. *Annual Review of Medicine*, Vol.52, (2001), pp. 259-274, ISSN 0066-4219.

Ohnishi, K.; Katsukake, K.; Suzuki, H.; & Iino, T. (1990). Gene *fliA* encodes an alternative sigma factor specific for flagellar operons in *Salmonella* Typhimurium. *Molecular and General Genetics*, Vol.221, No.2, (April 1990), pp. 139-147, ISSN 0026-8925

Osborne, S.E. & Coombes, B.K. (2009). RpoE fine tunes expression of a subset of SsrB-regulated virulence factors in *Salmonella enterica* serovar Typhimurium. *BMC Microbiololgy*, Vol.9, No.1, (March 2009), pp. 1-10, ISSN 1471-2180

Papenfort, K.; Pfeiffer, V.; Mika, F.; Lucchini, S.; Hinton, J.C.D.; & Vogel, J. (2006). σ^E – dependent small RNAs of *Salmonella* respond to membrane stress of accelerating global omp mRNA decay. *Molecular Microbiology,* Vol.62, No.6, (2006), pp. 1674-1688, ISSN 0950-382X

Rakjumari, K. & Gowrishankar, J. (2001). In Vivo Expression from the RpoS-Dependent P1 Promoter of the Osmotically Regulated *proU* Operon in *Escherichia coli* and *Salmonella enterica* Serovar Typhimurium: Acivation by *rho* and *hns* Mutations and by Cold Stress. *Journal of Bacteriology,* Vol.183, No.22, (November 2001), pp. 6543-6550, ISSN 0021-9193

Rhodius, V.A.; Suh, W.C.; Nonaka, G.; West, J, & Gross, C.A. (2006) Conserved and variable functions of the σ^E-stress response in related genomes. *PLoS Biology,* Vol.4, No.1, (January 2006), pp. e2, ISSN 1544-9173

Robbe-Saule, V.; Lopes, M.D.; Kolb, A.; & Norel, F. (2007). Physiological Effects of Crl in *Salmonella* Are Modulated by σ^S Level and Promoter Specificity. *Journal of Bacteriology,* Vol.189, No.8, (April 2007), pp. 2976-2987, ISSN 0021-9193

Römling, U.; Sierralta, W.D.; Eriksson, K., & Normark, S. (1998). Multicellular and aggregative behavior of *Salmonella* Typhimurium strains is controlled by mutations in the *agfD* promoter. *Molecular Microbiology,* Vol.28, No.2, (April 1998), pp. 249-264, ISSN 0950-382X

Scaife, J.G.; Heilig, J.S.; Rowen, L.; & Calendar, R. (1979). Gene for the RNA polymerase σ subunit mapped in *Salmonella* Typhimurium and *Escherichia coli* by cloning and deletion. *Proceedings of the National Academy of Sciences USA,* Vol.76, No.12, (December 1979), pp. 6510-6514, ISSN 0027-8424

Shea, J.E.; Hensel, M.; Gleeson, C.; & Holden, D.W. (1996). Identification of a virulence locus encoding a secondy type III secretion system in *Salmonella* Typhimurium. *Proceedings of the National Academy of Sciences USA,* Vol.93, No.6, (March 1996), pp. 2593-2597, ISSN 0027-8424

Sittka, A.; Pfeiffer, V.; Tedin, K; & Vogel, J. (2007). The RNA chaperone Hfq is essential for the virulence of *Salmonella* Typhimurium. *Molecular Microbiology,* Vol.63, No.1, (2007), pp. 193-217, ISSN 0950-382X

Slauch, J.; Taylor, R.; & Maloy, S. (1997). Survival in a cruel world: how *Vibrio cholera* and *Salmonella* respond to an unwilling host. *Genes and Development,* Vol.11, No.14, (July 1997), pp. 1761-1774, 0890-9369

Steele-Mortimer, O.; Brumell, J.H.; Knodler, L.A.; Méresse, S.; Lopez, A.; & Finlay, B.B. (2002). The invasion-associated type III associated secretion system of *Salmonella enterica* serovar Typhimurium is necessary for intracellular proliferation and vacuole biogenesis in epithelial cells. *Cell Microbiology,* Vol.4, No.1, (January 2002), pp. 43-54, ISSN 1462-5814

Studholme, D.J. (2002). Enhancer-Dependent Trancription in *Salmonella enterica* Typhimurium: New Members of the σ^N Regulon Inferred from Protein Sequence Homology and Predicted Promoter Sites. *Journal of Molecular Microbiology and Biotechnology,* Vol.4, No.4, (July 2002), pp. 367-374, ISSN 1462-5814

Sutton, A.; Buencamino, R.; & Eisenstark, A. (2000). *rpoS* Mutants in Archival Cultures of *Salmonella enterica* Serovar Typhimurium. *Journal of Bacteriology,* Vol.182, No.16, (August 2000), pp. 4375-4379, ISSN 0021-9193

Testerman, T.L.; Vasquez-Torres, A.; Xu, T.; Jones-Carson, J.; Libby, S.J.; & Fang, F.C. (2002). The alternative sigma factor σ^E controls antioxidant defences required for *Salmonella* virulence and stationary-phase survival. *Molecular Microbiology,* Vol.43, No.5, (2002), pp. 771-782, ISSN 0950-382X

Tobar, J.A.; Carreño, L.J.; Bueno, S.M.; González, P.A.; Mora, J.E.; Quezada, S.A.; & Kalergis, A.M. (2006). Virulent *Salmonella enterica* Serovar Typhimurium Evades Adaptive Immunity by Preventing Dendritic Cells from Activating T Cells. *Infection and Immunity,* Vol.74, No.11, (November 2006), pp. 6438-6448, ISSN 0019-9567

Tu, X.; Latifi, T.; Bougdour, A.; Gottesman, S.; & Groisman, E.A. (2006). The PhoP/PhoQ two-component system stabilizes the alternative sigma factor RpoS in *Salmonella enterica. Proceedings of the National Academy of Sciences,* Vol.103, No.36, (September 2006), pp. 13503-13508, ISSN 0027-8424

Waldminghaus, T.; Heldrick, J.; Brantl, S.; & Narberhaus, F. (2007). FourU: a novel type of RNA thermometer in *Salmonella. Molecular Microbiology,* Vol.65, No.2, (2007), pp. 413-424, ISSN 0950-382X

Walker, K.A.; Atkins, C.L.; & Osuna, R. (1999). Functional Determinants of the *Escherichia coli fis* Promoter: Role of -35, -10, and Transcription Initiation Regions in the Response to Stringent Control and Growth Phase-Dependent Regulation. *Journal of Bacteriology,* Vol.181, No.4, (February 1999), pp. 1269-1280, ISSN 0021-9193

Walker, K.A.; Mallik, P.; Pratt, T.S.; & Osuna, R. (2004). The *Escherichia coli fis* Promoter is Regulated by Changes in the Levels of Its Transcription Initiation Nucleotide CTP. *Journal of Biological Chemistry,* Vol.279, No.49, (December 2004), pp. 50818-50828, ISSN 0021-9258

Webb, C.; Moreno, M.; Wilmes-Riesenberg, M.; Curtis III, R.; & Foster, J.W. (1999). Effects of DksA and ClpP protease on sigma S production and virulence in *Salmonella* Typhimurium. *Molecular Microbiology,* Vol.34, No.1, (October 1999), pp. 112-123, ISSN 0950-382X

Wood, L.F.; Leech, A.J.; & Ohman, D.E. (2006). Cell wall-inhibitory antibiotics activate the alginate biosynthesis operon in *Pseudomonas aeruginosa*: roles of σ^{22} (AlgT) and the AlgW and Prc proteases. *Molecular Microbiology,* Vol.62, No.2, (2006), pp. 412-426, ISSN 0950-382X

Wozniak, C.E.; Chevance, F.F.V.; & Hughes, K.T. (2010). Multiple Promoters Contribute to Swarming and the Coordination of Transcription with Flagellar Assembly in *Salmonella. Journal of Bacteriology,* Vol.192, No.18, (September 2010), pp. 4752-4762, ISSN 0021-9193

Yokoseki, T.; Iino, T.; & Kutsukake, K. (1996). Negative Regulation of FliD, FliS, and FliT of the Export of the Flagellum-Specfic Anti-Sigma Factor, FlgM, in *Salmonella* Typhimurium. *Journal of Bacteriology,* Vol.178, No.3, (February 1996), pp. 899-901, ISSN 0021-9193

19

Assembly and Activation of the MotA/B Proton Channel Complex of the Proton-Driven Flagellar Motor of *Salmonella enterica*

Yusuke V. Morimoto and Tohru Minamino
Osaka University
Japan

1. Introduction

Salmonella enterica can swim by rotating multiple flagella, which arise randomly over the cell surface (Fig. 1A). The flagellum consists of at least three parts: the basal body, the hook, and the filament. The basal body is embedded within the cell membranes and acts as a bi-directional rotary motor powered by an electrochemical potential gradient of protons across the cytoplasmic membrane (Fig. 1B, C). The hook and filament extend outwards in the cell exterior. The filament acts as a helical propeller. The hook exists between the basal body and filament and functions as a universal joint to smoothly transmit torque produced by the motor to the filament. When the motors rotate in counterclockwise direction, the cells can swim smoothly. By quick reversal rotation of the motor to clockwise direction, the cells tumble and change their swimming direction to move toward more favorable environments (Fig. 2) (Berg, 2003; Blair, 2003; Minamino et al., 2008).

In *Salmonella enterica,* five flagellar proteins, MotA, MotB, FliG, FliM and FliN, are responsible for torque generation. Two integral membrane proteins, MotA and MotB, form the stator complex of the motor, which functions as a proton-conducting channel to convert an inwardly directed flux of protons through the proton channel into the mechanical work required for motor rotation. Two highly conserved residues, Pro-173 in MotA and Asp-33 in MotB, are involved in the energy coupling mechanism. FliG, FliM and FliN form the C-ring on the cytoplasmic face of the MS ring and are responsible not only for torque generation but also for switching the direction of motor rotation (Berg, 2003; Blair, 2003; Minamino et al., 2008). Torque is generated by sequential electrostatic interactions between MotA and FliG. A high-resolution observation of flagellar motor rotation has revealed a fine stepping motion with 26 steps per revolution, which corresponds to that of FliG subunits in the C-ring (Sowa et al., 2005; Nakamura et al., 2010). The proton conductivity of the MotA/B proton channel complex is proposed to be suppressed by a plug segment of MotB when the MotA/B complex is not assembled around the basal body (Hosking et al., 2006; Morimoto et al., 2010a). Although a low-resolution structure of the entire basal body containing the stator complexes has been visualized in situ by electron cryotomography (Fig. 3A) (Murphy et al., 2006; Liu et al., 2009; Kudryashev et al., 2010), the stators are missing in highly purified flagellar basal bodies presumably due to highly dynamic interactions between the stator and its binding partners in the basal body (Fig. 3B) (Thomas et al., 2001, 2006). In this chapter, we describe our current understanding of how the stator complex is installed into the motor, how its proton conductivity is activated, and how the proton flow through the proton channel is coupled with torque generation.

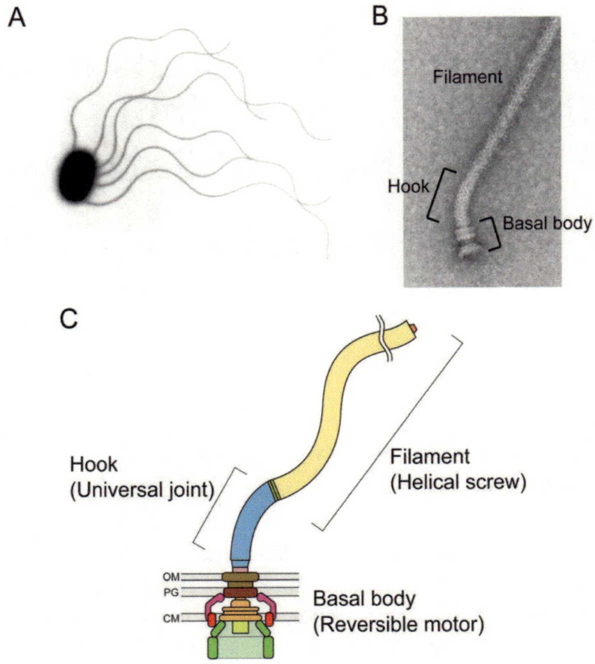

Fig. 1. Bacterial flagella
(A) Electron micrograph of *Salmonella enterica*. Six flagella arise randomly over the cell surface. (B) Electron micrograph of the purified flagellum. (C) Schematic diagrams of the flagellum. The flagellum consists of at least three parts: the basal body, which acts as a reversible rotary motor; the hook, which functions as a universal joint; and the filament, which acts as a helical screw. OM, outer membrane; PG, peptidoglycan layer; CM, cytoplasmic membrane.

Typical swimming pattern of *Salmonella* cells. The cells can swim smoothly when the motors rotate in counterclockwise (CCW) direction, resulting in the formation of a flagellar bundle that produces the thrust. By quick reversal rotation of the motor to clockwise (CW) direction, the bundle is disrupted so that bacteria can tumble and change their swimming direction.

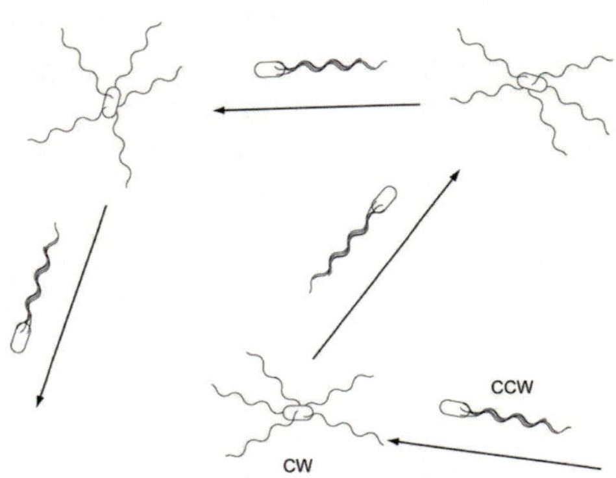

Fig. 2. Bacterial behavior

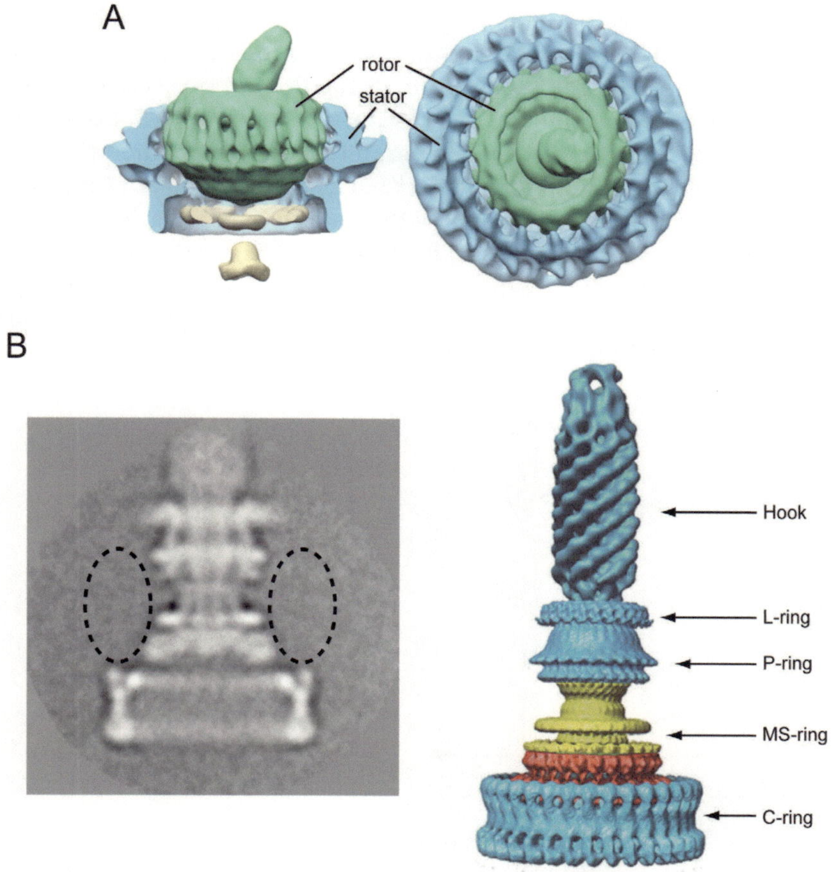

Fig. 3. Structure of bacterial flagellar motor
(A) The entire structure of the *Borrelia burgdorferi* flagellar motor visualized by electron cryotomography. The segmented structure was color coded as follows: rotor, green; C-ring and stator, blue; protein export apparatus, gray (Liu et al., 2009). (B) Three-dimensional (3D) structure of the flagellar basal body isolated from *Salmonella enterica* (Thomas et al., 2006). Left panel: electron cryomicroscopic image of frozen-hydrated hook-basal body in the side view. Right panel: 3D density map of the basal body reconstructed from frozen-hydrated particle images. Dashed circles indicate putative positions of the stator complexes in the motor.

2. MotA/B stator complex acts as a transmembrane proton channel

MotA and MotB are cytoplasmic membrane proteins and form a complex consisting of four copies of MotA and two copies of MotB (Kojima and Blair, 2004). It has been estimated that there are at least 11 copies of the MotA/B complex around the flagellar basal body (Reid et al., 2006). Since MotB has a potential peptidoglycan-binding motif in its C-terminal periplasmic domain (De Mot and Vanderleyden, 1994), the MotA/B complex is postulated to be anchored to the peptidoglycan (PG) layer to act as the stator of the motor. The MotA/B complex forms a transmembrane proton channel that couples an inward-directed proton translocation to torque generation (Blair and Berg, 1990). However, the molecular mechanism of energy coupling between proton influx and flagellar motor rotation remains unknown.

The torque-speed relationship of the flagellar motor has been well characterized (Fig. 4)(Chen and Berg, 2000a, b). As the load is decreased, torque decreases gradually up to a certain speed called the knee point and then falls rapidly to zero. The rotation rate of the proton-driven flagellar motor under a given load is proportional to a proton motive force across the cytoplasmic membrane over the entire range of observation (Gabel and Berg, 2003). The plateau torque at high load is dependent on the number of stators while the motor speed near zero load is independent of the stator number (Fig. 4A) (Ryu et al., 2000; Yuan and Berg, 2008). In the high-torque, low-speed regime, both temperature and solvent-isotope effects are small, while those effects are large in the low-torque, high-speed regime. This suggests that the steep decline of torque at high speed is due to a limit in the rate of proton transfer (Fig. 4B) (Chen and Berg, 2000a, b).

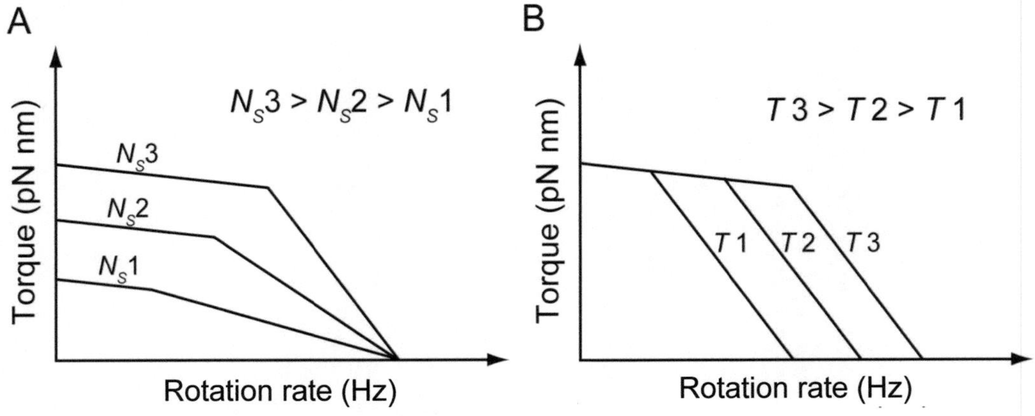

Fig. 4. Torque-speed curve of the bacterial flagellar motor
(A) Effect of the number of functional stators in a motor on the torque-speed relationship. The torque at high load is dependent on the number of stators. The motor speed near zero load is independent of the functional stator number. (Ryu et al., 2000) (B) Effect of temperature on the torque-speed curve. In the low-speed regime, torque is insensitive to changes in temperature. In the high-speed regime, motor speed decreases markedly when temperature is decreased (Chen et al., 2000a).

2.1 Arrangement of transmembrane segments of the MotA/B complex

MotA consists of four transmembrane spans (TMs), two short periplasmic loops and two extensive cytoplasmic regions. MotB consists of an N-terminal cytoplasmic region, one TM and a large periplasmic region containing a putative peptidoglycan-binding motif (Fig. 5A). The four MotA subunits in the stator complex are positioned with their TM3 and TM4 segments adjacent to the dimer of MotB-TM located at the center and their TM1 and TM2 segments in outer positions (Fig. 5B) (Braun et al., 2004). Two conserved charged residues, Arg-90 and Glu-98, in the cytoplasmic loop between TM2 and TM3 are involved in electrostatic interactions with charged residues in the C-terminal domain of FliG to produce torque (Zhou and Blair, 1997; Zhou et al., 1998a). A conserved proline residue of MotA, Pro-173 and Pro-222, are thought to be involved in conformational changes of the stator complex that couple proton influx with torque generation (Braun et al., 1999; Nakamura et al., 2009b). The absolutely conserved and functionally critical aspartic acid residue, Asp-33 of MotB is located near the cytoplasmic end of its TM and is postulated to be a proton-binding site (Sharp et al., 1995; Togashi et al., 1997; Zhou et al., 1998b; Che et al., 2008; Morimoto et al., 2010a). MotB exists as a dimer in the stator complex and these aspartic acid residues are positioned on the surface of the MotB-TM dimer facing MotA-TMs, suggesting that the stator complex is likely to have two proton-conducting pathways (Fig. 5B) (Braun and Blair, 2001). Both protonation and deprotonation of this aspartic acid residue cause conformational changes of the cytoplasmic loop of MotA, which may drive flagellar motor rotation (Kojima and Blair, 2001; Che et al., 2008).

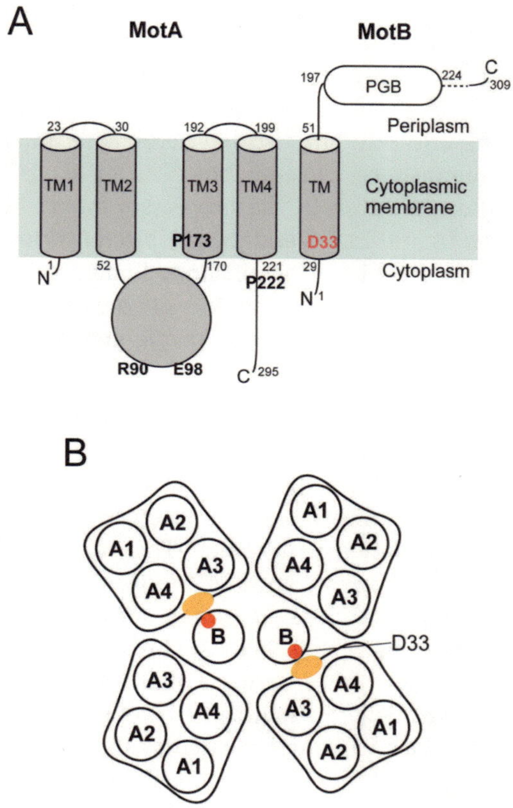

Fig. 5. Topology of MotA and MotB
(A) Cartoon representing the domain organization of MotA and MotB. *Salmonella* MotA and MotB consist of 295 and 309 amino acid residues, respectively. MotA has four transmembrane segments (TM1-TM4), two short periplasmic loops and two large cytoplasmic regions. MotB has an N-terminal cytoplasmic region, one transmembrane segment and a large periplasmic domain containing a putative peptidoglycan-binding motif (PGB) (Braun et al., 1999, 2004; Kojima et al., 2004). Arg-90 and Glu-98 of MotA are required for electrostatic interactions with FliG. Pro-173 and Pro-222 of MotA are proposed to be responsible for conformational changes of the stator complex that couple proton influx with torque generation. Asp-33 in MotB is postulated to play an important role in proton translocation. (B) Arrangement of transmembrane segments of the MotA/B complex, which consists of 4 copies of MotA and 2 copies of MotB. The view is from the periplasmic side of the membrane. The complex has two proton conducting pathway shown by orange ellipsoids. (Braun et al., 2004).

2.2 Asp-33 of MotB and Pro-173 of MotA are responsible for energy coupling between proton flow and motor rotation

Asp-33 of MotB is a highly conserved and protonatable residue, and is believed to be involved in the proton-relay mechanism (Sharp et al., 1995; Togashi et al., 1997; Zhou et al., 1998b). An increase in the intracellular proton concentration suppresses or even abolishes the flagellar motor function. This suggests that a decrease in the intracellular pH presumably interferes with proton dissociation from Asp-33 to the cytoplasm, thereby slowing the torque generation reaction cycle of the motor (Minamino et al., 2003; Nakamura et al., 2009a). Therefore, it seems likely that both protonation and deprotonation of this Asp play key roles in the torque generation cycle. A D33E mutation in MotB causes ca. 40% reduction in stall torque and a sharp decline in the torque-speed curve with an apparent maximal rotation rate of ca. 20 Hz. This suggests that the D33E mutation not only reduces the proton conductivity significantly but also interferes with an actual torque generation step by the stator-rotor interactions considerably (Che et al., 2008). The stall torque is recovered nearly to the wild-type levels by the suppressor mutations in the transmembrane helices TM2 and TM3 of MotA and in TM and the periplasmic domain of MotB. In contrast, high-speed rotation under low load is still significantly limited even in the presence of these suppressor mutations. These suggest that the second-site mutations recover energy coupling of an inward-directed proton translocation with torque generation but not the maximum proton conductivity (Che et al., 2008).

Pro-173 is highly conserved among MotA orthologs. Since point mutations at Pro-173 affect not only motor function but also proton flow through the MotA/B complex, this prolyl residue seems to play a critical role in the proton-relay mechanism (Braun et al., 2004). *E. coli* *motA*(P173C)/*motB*(D32C) double mutant strain gives a high yield of disulfide-linked MotA/B heterodimers upon oxidation with iodine. This suggests that Pro-173 of MotA is positioned in the proton channel near Asp-32 of MotB, which corresponds to Asp-33 in *Salmonella* MotB (Braun et al., 2004). The *Salmonella motA*(P173A) mutant produces stall torque at wild-type levels (Nakamura et al., 2009b). However, the P173A mutation causes a sharp decline in the torque-speed curve with a maximum rotation rate of ca. 25 Hz (Nakamura et al., 2009b). These suggest that the P173A mutation reduces the maximum proton conductivity of the MotA/B complex but not the efficiency of energy coupling between proton translocation and torque generation. Since Pro-173 of MotA is likely to be very close to Asp-33 of MotB in the MotA/B complex structure (Braun et al., 2004), and because Pro is known to induce a kink in α-helix, its replacement with Ala would relax the conformational strain of the MotA/B complex, resulting in a change in protein dynamics to slow down the rates of conformational changes that switch the exposure of Asp-33 to the outside or the inside of the cell. Therefore, Pro-173 is proposed to play an important role in facilitating the resetting of the position of Asp-33 relative to the proton pathway in the conformational change between the two distinct states to facilitate proton translocation when the motor spins at high speed (Nakamura et al., 2009b).

2.3 Role of conserved charged residues in MotA in stator assembly around the motor

Over-expression of MotA inhibits motility of wild-type cells. Neither cell growth, flagellar formation, nor proton motive force across the cytoplasmic membrane is affected by overproduced MotA. However, stall torque is significantly reduced. Since the stall torque is dependent on the number of functional stators in the motor (Fig. 4), this suggests that MotA occupies the stator-binding sites of the motor and reduces the number of functional stators (Morimoto et al., 2010b). In agreement with this, fluorescent spots of MotA-mCherry have been observed at the same position as those of GFP-FliG even in the absence of MotB (Fig. 6) (Morimoto et al., 2010b). Thus, MotA alone can be installed into a motor.

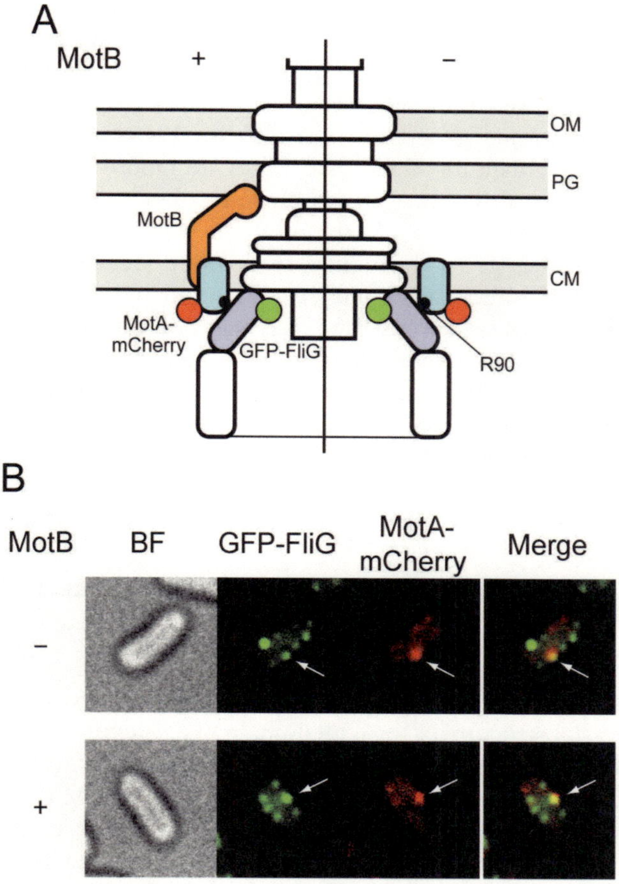

Fig. 6. Co-localization of GFP-FliG and MotA-mCherry
(A) Cartoon representing the basal body and positions of GFP-FliG and MotA-mCherry in the presence (+) or absence (-) of MotB. (B) Bright-field (BF) and fluorescence images of GFP-FliG and MotA-mCherry observed by fluorescence microscopy. The fluorescence images of GFP-FliG (green) and MotA-mCherry (red) are merged in the right panel. (Morimoto et al., 2010b).

Two charged residues of MotA, Arg-90 and Glu-98, are involved in electrostatic interactions with charged residues of FliG for torque generation (Zhou & Blair, 1997; Zhou et al., 1998a). The *motA*(R90E) and *motA*(E98K) alleles are recessive and hence do not exert a negative dominance when their expression levels were the same as those of wild-type cells (Zhou & Blair, 1997; Morimoto et al., 2010b). Interestingly, however, an increase in the expression level of the MotA(R90E)/B complex by more than 10-fold allows 70% of the cells to swim in liquid media (Morimoto et al., 2010b). In agreement with this, the R90E mutation markedly decreases the number and intensity of fluorescent spots of GFP-MotB. Since the loss-of-function phenotype of the *motA*(R90E) and *motA*(E98K) alleles are considerably suppressed by the *fliG*(D289K) and *fliG*(R281V) mutations, respectively (Zhou et al., 1998a), this suggests that the interactions between MotA Arg-90 and FliG Asp-289 and between MotA Glu-98 and FliG Arg-281 are critical not only for torque generation but also for the assembly of the stators into the motor (Morimoto et al., 2010b).

Polar localization of the PomA/B complex of *Vibrio alginolyticus*, which are homologs of the MotA/B complex and acts as the stator of the motor fueled by the sodium motive force across the cytoplasmic membrane, is greatly affected by changes in the external concentration of sodium ions (Fukuoka et al., 2009). This suggests that sodium ions are required not only for torque generation but also for the efficient assembly process of PomA/B. In contrast, neither the D33N nor D33A mutation in *Salmonella* MotB, which abolishes the proton flow through a proton channel, affects stator assembly around the motor, indicating that stator assembly in the proton-driven motor is not dependent on the proton conductivity of the MotA/B complex. In addition, depletion of the proton motive force across the cytoplasmic membrane by a protonophore, carbonyl cyanide *m*-chlorophenylhydrazone does not abolish the subcellular localization of the stator labeled with GFP, indicating that the stators remain to exist around the rotor even in the absence of the proton motive force. This is supported by the finding that the stator actually switches its functional state between the active and inactive ones without detaching from the rotor completely when PMF is largely reduced (Nakamura et al., 2010). Therefore, it is much likely that the assembly of the *Salmonella* MotA/B complex into the motor is not obligatorily linked to the process of the proton translocation through the proton channel of the MotA/B complex.

2.4 MotB$_C$ controls the proton channel activity during stator assembly

The periplasmic domain of MotB (MotB$_C$) consisting of residues 78 through 309 Kojima et al., 2008 contains a putative peptidoglycan-binding (PGB) motif, which shows sequence similarity to other Omp-like proteins (Fig. 7A) (De Mot and Vanderleyden, 1994). Interestingly, the crystal structure of the core domain of *Salmonella* MotB$_C$, which consists of residues 99 through 276 has a typical OmpA-like structure, and shows considerable structural similarities to the C-terminal regions of PAL and RmpM (Fig. 7A) (Kojima et al., 2009). Mutations in the PGB motif of MotB significantly impair motility, indicating that anchoring MotA/B complex to the PG layer is critical for the motor function. Stator resurrection experiments have shown that abrupt drops in the rotation rate occur frequently even in steadily rotating motors (Block and Berg, 1984; Blair and Berg, 1988; Sowa et al., 2005). Consistently, fluorescent photo-bleaching studies of GFP-fused MotB have shown a rapid exchange and turnover of the stator complexes between the membrane pool and the basal body (Leake et al., 2006). These results suggest that the association between MotA/B and its target site on the basal body are highly dynamic.

MotB$_C$ forms homo-dimer in solution (Fig. 7B) (Kojima et al., 2008, 2009). Over-expression of MotB$_C$ inihibits motility of wild-type cells when expressed in the periplasm. An in-frame deletion of resiudes 197-210 not only inhibits dimerization of MotB$_C$ but also significantly reduces its inhibitory effect on wild-type motility. These results suggest that dimerization of MotB$_C$ is responsible for the proper targeting and stable anchoring of the MotA/B complex to the putative stator binding sites of the basal body (Kojima et al., 2008). Recently, site-directed disulfide crosslinking experiments have shown an interaction between MotB$_C$ and the P ring of the basal body (Hizukuri et al., 2010).

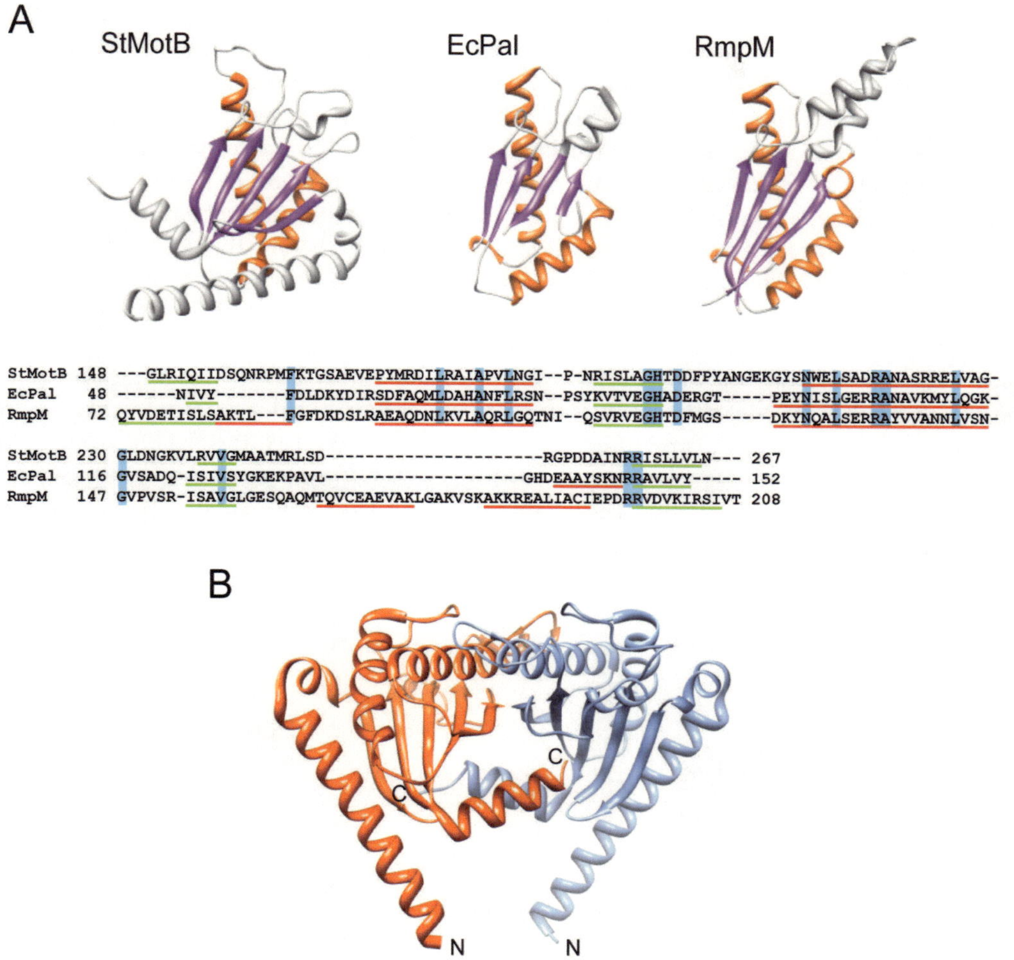

Fig. 7. Crystal structure of the C-terminal domain of MotB
(A) Comparison of various OmpA-like domains. Cα ribbon diagrams of three OmpA-like domains and their structure-based sequence alignment. StMotB, *Salmonella typhimurium* $MotB_{C2}$ (2zvy); EcPal, *Escherichia coli* Pal (1oap); RmpM, the C-terminal domain of RmpM from *Neisseria meningitidis* (1r1m). Conserved secondary structural elements are colored: orange, α-helix; purple, β-strand. Residues highlighted in light blue in the aligned sequences are conserved in these three proteins. Regions of secondary structures are indicated below the corresponding sequences: red line, α-helix; green line, β-strand. (B) Cα ribbon representations of the $MotB_{C2}$ dimer. The two subunits are shown in blue and orange. (Kojima et al., 2009)

Cell growth is not impaired significantly by over-expression of the *E. coli* MotA/B complex (Stolz and Berg, 1994). In contrast, the cell growth is severely impaired by co-expression of MotA with a MotB-TetA chimera protein, in which the first 60 residues of MotB are fused to a 50 residue sequence encoded by an open reading frame in the *tetA* gene (Blair and Berg, 1990). Since the replacement of Asp-32 to other residues in the MotB-TetA chimera protein has been shown to suppress proton leakage caused by co-overproduction of MotA with the

MotB-TetA chimera protein. Therefore, it has been suggested that the proton conductivity of the MotA/B complex is suppressed prior to stator assembly around a motor. An in-frame deletion of residues 51-70 or 52-71 within the periplasmic domain of *E. coli* MotB or *Salmonella* MotB, respectively, a region, which is highly conserved among the MotB orthologs, causes considerable proton leakage, thereby arresting cell growth (Hosking et al., 2006; Morimoto et al., 2010a). This suggests that the deleted region of MotB acts as a plug segment that inserts into a proton channel within the cytoplasmic membrane to prevent from premature proton translocation through the channel before the association with a motor and that upon stator assembly in the motor, the plug leaves the channel, allowing the stator to conduct protons (Fig. 8). Interestingly, however, cell growth is not significantly impaired by in-frame deletion of residues 51-100 in *Salmonella* MotB, which contains the plug segment (Muramoto and Macnab, 1998; Kojima et al., 2009). This indicates that a proton channel of the MotA/B(Δ51-100) complex is not formed prior to its assembly around the rotor although the plug is missing. The introduction of the L119P or L119E substitution into MotB(Δ51-100) causes growth impairment due to significant proton leakage (Kojima et al., 2009; Morimoto et al., 2010a). Therefore, it is likely that some other region within the periplasmic domain of MotB also regulates proper formation of the proton channel during stator assembly.

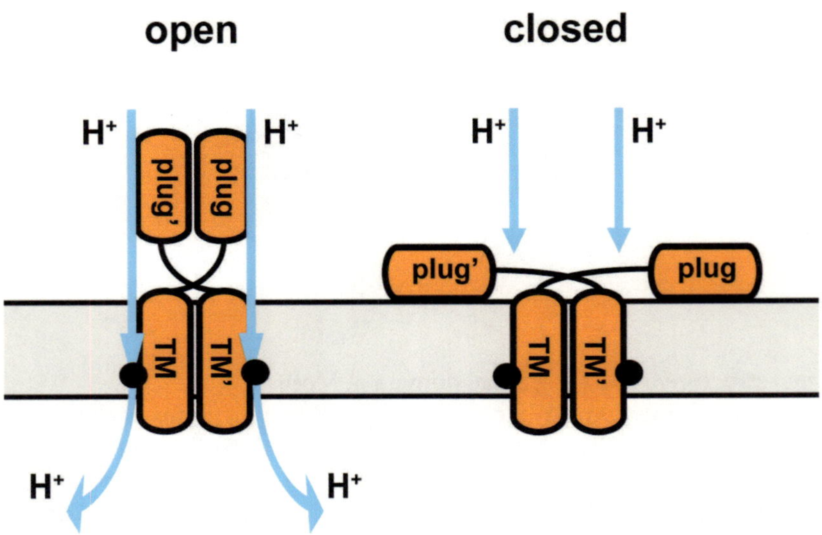

Fig. 8. Schematic diagram of the plug region of MotB

Cartoon representing the position of the plug in the open and closed states of the MotA/B proton channel. Only the MotB TMs and plugs are shown, in a view parallel with the plane of the cytoplasmic membrane. Asp-33 in MotB is shown as a black dot. Blue arrows indicate the proton flow through proton channels. In the open state, the plugs leave the membrane and associate with each other via their hydrophobic faces to hold the proton channel open. In the closed state, the plugs insert into the cell membrane parallel with its periplasmic face and interfere with channel formation (Hosking et al., 2006).

MotB(Δ51-100) is still functional, indicating that MotB(Δ51-100) can form a functional stator complex along with MotA (Muramoto and Macnab, 1998). Since the distance between the surface of the hydrophobic core layer of the cytoplasmic membrane and that of the PG layer is about 100 Å, and the crystal structure of the core domain of $MotB_C$ is only about 50 Å tall, the crystal structure of the core domain of *Salmonella* $MotB_C$ is so small that MotB(Δ51-100) cannot reach the PG layer if connected directly to the transmembrane helix by the deletion of residues 51-100. Therefore, a large conformational change would be required for the PGB sites on the top surface of $MotB_C$ to reach the PG layer. Since a specific interaction between a cytoplasmic loop between TM-2 and TM-3 in MotA and FliG is required for stator assembly around a rotor of the motor, it is possible that the interaction between MotA and FliG may trigger conformational changes in $MotB_C$ that open the proton channel and allow the stator to be anchored to the PG layer (Fig. 9).

MotA and MotB are colored blue and orange, respectively. Arg-90 of MotA, which is required for stator assembly into the motor, is shown as a black dot. An interaction between MotA and FliG may trigger conformational changes in $MotB_C$ that open the proton channel and allow the stator to be anchored to the PG layer (Kojima et al., 2009; Morimoto et al., 2010b).

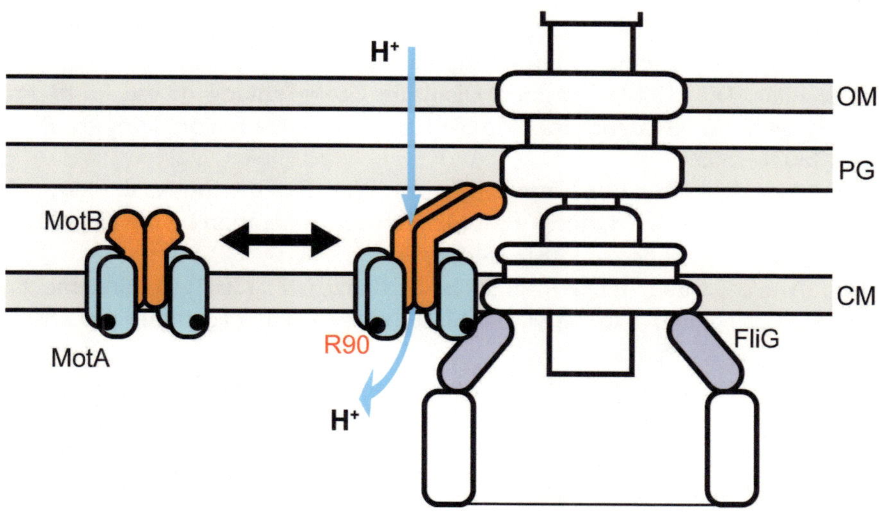

Fig. 9. Model for stator assembly into the motor

3. Conclusion

The MotA/B complex, which is composed of four copies of MotA and two copies of MotB, acts as a proton channel to couple proton flow to torque generation. The crystal structure of the C-terminal periplasmic domain of MotB ($MotB_C$) shows significant structure similarities to other PGB domains such as the C-terminal regions of PAL and RmpM, suggesting that an association of $MotB_C$ with the PG layer anchors the MotA/B complex to be the stator around the rotor. Interestingly, the MotA/B complex does not always associate with a motor during flagellar motor rotation, suggesting that the association of the MotA/B complex to its target sites on the basal body is highly dynamic. A plug segment in the periplasmic domain of MotB prevents the proton channel from leaking protons into the cytoplasm when the MotA/B complex is not assembled into the motor. An electrostatic interaction between MotA and FliG is required not only for the efficient assembly of the MotA/B complexes around the rotor but also for the proton channel formation to conducts protons coupled with torque generation.

4. Acknowledgment

We acknowledge K. Namba for continuous support and encouragement and N. Kami-ike and Y-S. Che and S. Nakamura for helpful discussions. Y.V.M. is a research fellow of the Japan Society for the Promotion of Science. This work has been supported in part by Grants-in-Aid for Scientific Research from the Ministry of Education, Culture, Sports, Science and Technology of Japan to Y.V.M. and T.M.

5. References

Berg, H.C. (2003) The rotary motor of bacterial flagella. *Annu Rev Biochem* 72: 19–54.

Blair, D.F., & Berg, H.C. (1988) Restoration of torque in defective flagellar motors. *Science* 242: 1678–1681.

Blair, D.F., & Berg, H.C. (1990) The MotA protein of *E. coli* is a proton-conducting component of the flagellar motor. *Cell* 60: 439–449.

Blair, D. F. (2003) Flagellar movement driven by proton translocation. *FEBS Lett* 545: 86–95.

Block, S.M., & Berg, H.C. (1984) Successive incorporation of force-generating units in the bacterial rotary motor. *Nature* 309: 470–472.

Braun, T. & Blair, D.F. (2001) Targeted Disulfide Cross-Linking of the MotB Protein of *Escherichia coli*: Evidence for Two H+ Channels in the Stator Complex. *Biochemistry* 40: 13051–13059.

Braun, T., Poulson, S., Gully, J.B., Empey, J.C., Van Way, S., Putnam, A., & Blair, D.F. (1999) Function of proline residues of MotA in torque generation by the flagellar motor of Escherichia coli. *J Bacteriol* 181: 3542–3551.

Braun, T.F., Al-Mawasawi, L.Q., Kojima, S. & Blair, D.F. (2004) Arrangement of core membrane segments in the MotA/MotB protein-channel complex of *Escherichia coli*. *Biochemistry* 43: 35–45.

Che, Y-S., Nakamura, S., Kojima S., Kami-ike, N., Namba, K. & Minamino, T. (2008) Suppressor analysis of the MotB(D33E) mutation to probe the bacterial flagellar motor dynamics coupled with proton translocation. *J Bacteriol* 190: 6660–6667.

Chen, X. & Berg, H. C. (2000a) Torque-speed relationship of the flagellar motor of *Escherichia coli*. *Biophys J* 78: 1036–1041.

Chen, X. & Berg, H. C. (2000b) Solvent-isotope and pH effects on flagellar rotation in *Escherichia coli*. *Biophys J* 78: 2280–2284.

De Mot, R. & Vanderleyden, J. (1994) The C-terminal sequence conservation between OmpA-related outer membrane proteins and MotB suggests a common function in both gram-positive and gram-negative bacteria, possibly in the interaction of these domains with peptidoglycan. *Mol Microbiol* 12: 333–334.

DeRosier, D. (2006) Bacterial Flagellum: Visualizing the Complete Machine In Situ. *Current Biology* 16: 928–930.

Fukuoka, H., Wada, T., Kojima, S., Ishijima, A. & Homma M. (2009) Sodium-dependent dynamic assembly of membrane complexes in sodium-driven flagellar motors. *Mol Microbiol* 71: 825–835.

Gabel, C.V. & Berg, H.C. (2003) The speed of the flagellar rotary motor of *Escherichia coli* varies linearly with protonmotive force. *Proc Natl Acad Sci USA* 100: 8748–8751.

Hizukuri, Y., Kojima, S. & Homma, M. (2010) Disulfide cross-linking between the stator and the bearing components in the bacterial flagellar motor. *J Biochem* 148: 309–318.

Hosking, E.R., Vogt, C., Bakker, E.P. & Manson, M.D. (2006) The *Escherichia coli* MotAB proton channel unplugged. *J Mol Biol* 364: 921-937.

Kihara, M. & Macnab, R.M. (1981) Cytoplasmic pH mediates pH taxis and weak-acid repellent taxis of bacteria. *J Bacteriol* 145: 1209-1221.

Kojima, S. & Blair, D.F. (2001) Conformational change in the stator of the bacterial flagellar motor. *Biochemistry* 40: 13041-13050.

Kojima, S. & Blair, D.F. (2004) Solubilization and purification of the MotA/MotB complex of *Escherichia coli*. *Biochemistry* 43: 26-34.

Kojima, S., Furukawa, Y., Matsunami, H., Minamino, T. & Namba, K. (2008) Characterization of the periplasmic domain of MotB and implications for its role in the stator assembly of the bacterial flagellar motor. *J Bacteriol* 190: 2259-2266.

Kojima, S., Imada, K., Sakuma, M., Sudo, Y., Kojima, C., Minamino, T., Homma, M. & Namba, K. (2009) Stator assembly and activation mechanism of the flagellar motor by the periplasmic region of MotB. *Mol Microbiol* 73: 710-718.

Kudryashev, M., Cyrklaff, M., Wallich, R., Baumeister, W. & Frischknecht, F. (2010) Distinct in situ structures of the Borrelia flagellar motor. *J Struct Biol* 169:54-61.

Leake, M.C., Chandler, J.H., Wadhams, G.H., Bai, F., Berry, R.M. & Armitage, J.P. (2006) Stoichiometry and turnover in single, functioning membrane protein complexes. *Nature* 443: 355-358.

Liu, J., Lin, T., Botkin, D.J., McCrum, E., Winkler, H. & Norris, S.J. (2009) Intact Flagellar Motor of Borrelia burgdorferi Revealed by Cryo-Electron Tomography: Evidence for Stator Ring Curvature and Rotor/C-Ring Assembly Flexion. *J Bacteriol* 191: 5026-5036.

Minamino, T., Imae, Y., Oosawa, F., Kobayashi, Y. & Oosawa, K. (2003) Effect of intracellular pH on the rotational speed of bacterial flagellar motors. *J Bacteriol* 185: 1190-1194.

Minamino, T., Imada, K. & Namba, K. (2008) Molecular motors of the bacterial flagella. *Curr Opin Struct Biol* 18:693-701.

Morimoto, Y.V., Che, Y-.S., Minamino, T. & Namba, K. (2010a) Proton-conductivity assay of plugged and unplugged MotA/B proton channel by cytoplasmic pHluorin expressed in *Salmonella*. *FEBS lett* 584: 1268-1272.

Morimoto, Y.V., Nakamura, S., Kami-ike, N., Namba, K. & Minamino, T. (2010b) Charged residues in the cytoplasmic loop of MotA are required for stator assembly into the bacterial flagellar motor. *Mol Microbiol* 78: 1117-1129

Muramoto, K. & Macnab, R.M. (1998) Deletion analysis of MotA and MotB, components of the force-generating unit in the flagellar motor of *Salmonella*. *Mol Microbiol* 29: 1191-202.

Murphy, G.E., Leadbetter, J.R. & Jensen, G.J. (2006) In situ structure of the complete Treponema primitia flagellar motor. *Nature* 442: 1062-1064.

Nakamura, S., Kami-ike, N., Yokota, P.J., Kudo, S., Minamino, T. & Namba, K. (2009a) Effect of intracellular pH on the torque-speed relationship of bacterial proton-driven flagellar motor. *J Mol Biol* 386: 332-338.

Nakamura, S., Morimoto, Y.V., Kami-ike, N., Minamino, T. & Namba, K. (2009b) Role of a conserved prolyl residue (Pro-173) of MotA in the mechanochemical reaction cycle of the proton-driven flagellar motor of Salmonella. *J Mol Biol* 393: 300-307.

Nakamura, S., Kami-ike, N., Yokota, J.P., Minamino, T. & Namba, K. (2010) Evidence for symmetry in the elementary process of bidirectional torque generation by the bacterial flagellar motor. *Proc Natl Acad Sci USA* 107: 17616-17620.

Reid, S.W., Leake, M.C., Chandler, J.H., Lo, C.J., Armitage, J.P. & Berry, R.M. (2006) The maximum number of torque-generating units in the flagellar motor of *Escherichia coli* is at least 11. *Proc Natl Acad Sci USA* 103: 8066–8071.

Ryu, W.S., Berry, R.M. & Berg, H.C. (2000) Torque-generating units of the flagellar motor of *Escherichia coli* have a high duty ratio. *Nature* 403: 444–447.

Sharp, L.L. Zhou, J. & Blair, D.F. (1995) Tryptophan-scanning mutagenesis of MotB, an integral membrane protein essential for flagellar rotation in *Escherichia coli*, *Biochemistry* 34, 9166–9171.

Sowa, Y., Rowe, A.D., Leake, M.C., Yakushi, T., Homma, M., Ishijima, A. & Berry, R.M. (2005) Direct observation of steps in rotation of the bacterial flagellar motor. *Nature* 437: 916–919.

Stolz, B. & Berg, H.C. (1991) Evidence for interactions between MotA and MotB, torque-generating elements of the flagellar motor of *Escherichia coli*. *J Bacteriol* 173: 7033–7037.

Thomas, D., Morgan, D.G. & DeRosier, D.J. (2001) Structures of bacterial flagellar motors from two FliF-FliG gene fusion mutants. *J Bacteriol* 183: 6404–6412.

Thomas, D.R., Francis, N.R., Chen, X. & DeRosier, D.J. (2006) The three-dimensional structure of the flagellar rotor from a clockwise-locked mutant of *Salmonella enterica* serovar Typhimurium. *J Bacteriol* 188: 7039–7048.

Togashi, F., Yamaguchi, S., Kihara M., Aizawa, S.-I. & Macnab, R.M. (1997) An extreme clockwise switch bias mutation in *fliG* of *Salmonella typhimurium* and its suppression by slow-motile mutations in *motA* and *motB*. *J Bacteriol* 179: 2994–3003.

Yuan, J., & Berg, H.C. (2008) Resurrection of the flagellar rotary motor near zero load. *Proc Natl Acad Sci USA* 105: 1182–1185.

Zhou, J. & Blair, D.F. (1997) Residues of the cytoplasmic domain of MotA essential for torque generation in the bacterial flagellar motor. *J Mol Biol* 273: 428–439.

Zhou, J., Lloyd, S. A. & Blair, D.F. (1998a) Electrostatic interactions between rotor and stator in the bacterial flagellar motor. *Proc Natl Acad Sci USA* 95: 6436–6441.

Zhou, J., Sharp, L.L., Tang, H.L., Lloyd, S.A. & Blair, D.F. (1998b) Function of protonatable residues in the flagellar motor of *Escherichia coli*: a critical role for Asp32 of MotB. *J Bacteriol* 180: 2729–2735.

20

Molecular Armory of *S.* Typhi: Deciphering the Putative Arsenal of Our Enemy

Chantal G. Forest and France Daigle
Department of Microbiology & Immunology/University of Montreal
Canada

1. Introduction

The outer surface of bacteria is the first to interact with host components, such as the immune system, the extracellular matrix or cells. The bacterial Gram-negative cell wall is complex and composed of an inner membrane (IM), a periplasmic space and a thin peptidoglycan layer, all surrounded by an outer membrane (OM). The OM is a bilayered structure consisting mainly of phospholipids, proteins and lipopolysaccharide (LPS) and serves as an impermeable barrier to prevent the escape of periplasmic molecules but also acts as a barrier for entry of external molecules. *Salmonella enterica* comprises more than 2500 serovars, based on three major antigens located at the cell surface: O antigen, capsule and flagella. All serovars are highly conserved genetically but have different host ranges and cause different diseases. In humans, *Salmonella* infection causes gastroenteritis, often associated with serovars Typhimurium and Enteritidis or typhoid-like disease, which is associated with serovars Typhi and Paratyphi. *S.* Typhi strains belong to serogroup D1 with the antigenic formula O:9,12; Vi+; H-d. These strains are human-restricted and besides asymptomatic carriers, no environmental reservoir is known.

S. Typhi is a monomorphic bacterium, showing very little genetic diversity (Kidgell et al., 2002) and up to 5% of its annotated coding sequences are pseudogenes (Holt et al., 2009; Parkhill et al., 2001). Genome degradation may be responsible for its host specificity; however the *S.* Typhi genome may harbour specific genes for its systemic dispersion and survival. *S.* Typhi remains a major public health problem in developing countries. Antimicrobial resistance has become a problem in endemic regions, and it is becoming imperative to develop new vaccine strategies or discover new antimicrobial targets to combat this microorganism. Bacterial surface proteins may correspond to these targets by being immunogenic or essential for virulence. Most virulence factors are usually located within genomic locations called *Salmonella* Pathogenicity Islands (SPIs) and are tightly regulated by global regulators such as PhoP-PhoQ, RcsDBC, OmpR-EnvZ and RpoS. This review will focus on molecules localized at the outer membrane of *S.* Typhi and their role in pathogenesis. A complete analysis of adhesive molecules, such as the 12 fimbrial systems, curli, type IVB pilus, autotransporters and afimbrial adhesins will be presented. We will also discuss the importance of polysaccharides such as the Vi capsule and LPS. Furthermore, the complex surface structures generated by secretion systems, such as type three secretion systems (T3SS), flagella and T6SS that are so important for invasion, intracellular survival and to highjack the host defence system will be discussed. Finally, methods used to inhibit these adhesive structures will be described.

2. Fimbrial adhesins

Fimbriae (also called pili) are proteinaceous structures that can be observed as filaments anchored on the bacterial cell surface. These structures can mediate crucial interactions during host infection like adherence, invasion or biofilm formation, and are classified according to their mechanism of assembly. Most of the fimbriae present in *S*. Typhi genome are assembled by the chaperone/usher pathway, but there are also one representative of the nucleation/precipitation pathway (*csg*) and one type IVB pilus. This section will briefly describe each mechanism of expression and the current knowledge related to *S*. Typhi and their putative roles.

2.1 Mechanisms of fimbrial assembly

2.1.1 The chaperone/usher pathway

Twelve fimbrial systems detected in *S*. Typhi belong to the chaperone/usher pathway (CUP) assembly class (Fig. 1). A classic fimbrial operon usually harbours at least four different genes. The filaments are composed of major and minor fimbrial subunits assembled by the cooperative work of the chaperone and the usher. After translocation by

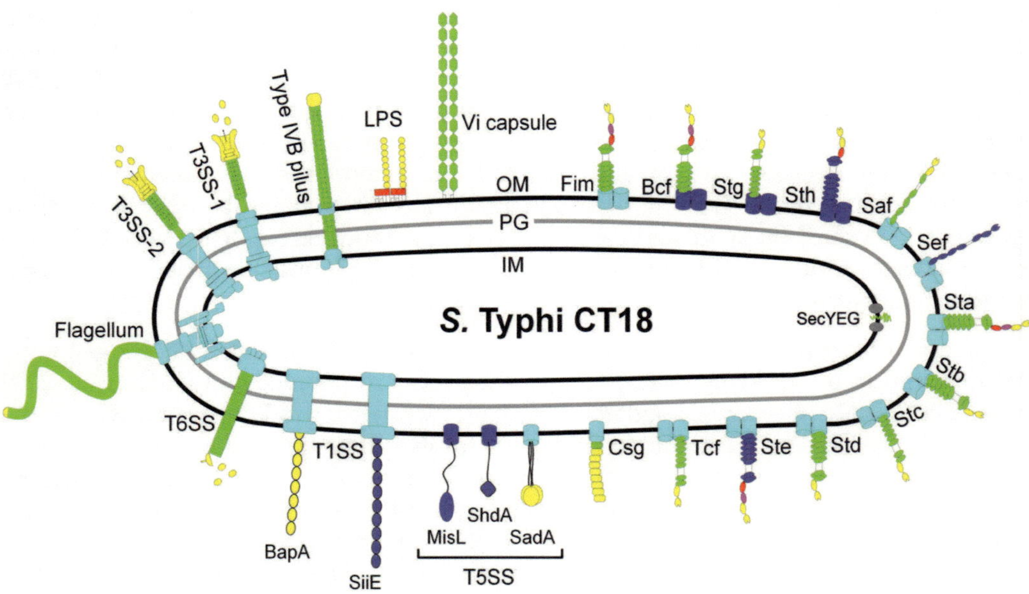

Fig. 1. Schematic representation of the important surface structures identified in *S*. Typhi CT18. Adhesive components are shown in yellow, membrane components are cyan and pseudogenes are shown in blue (pseudogenes of the T6SS are not shown). The twelve representatives of the CUP are grouped in fimbrial clades and are drawn according to previous observations (Salih et al., 2008) or based on their homologues found in *E. coli* K-12 (Korea et al., 2011). STY0405 putative autotransporter, STY0351 adhesin, and PagC which are known to be implicated in virulence were omitted from the drawing, as well as STY1980 (MAM7). IM stands for inner membrane, PG for peptidoglycan and OM for outer membrane.

the Sec general secretory pathway, the periplasmic chaperone protects the subunits and brings them to the OM usher, which specifically translocates subunits to the cell surface. Fimbrial biogenesis by the CUP pathway is a self-energized process catalyzed by both the usher and the presence of high-energy intermediates in the folding of the chaperone-subunit complexes (Jacob-Dubuisson et al., 1994; Nishiyama et al., 2008; Sauer et al., 2002; Zavialov et al., 2002). Classification based upon sequence homology between the different ushers (Nuccio & Bäumler, 2007) revealed members in the γ1- (*bcf, fim, stg, sth*), γ3- (*saf, sef*), γ4- (*sta, stb, stc*), π- (*std, ste*) and the α-fimbrial clades (*tcf*) in *S.* Typhi (Fig. 1).

2.1.2 Nucleation/precipitation pathway

The thin aggregative fimbriae, also known as curli or TAFI, encoded by the *csgDEFG csgABC* gene cluster belongs to this class of adhesin. The first steps of biogenesis are similar to the CUP : after translocation by the Sec pathway, CsgA and CsgB fimbrial subunits are secreted by the CsgG outer membrane protein at the bacterial cell surface. The major difference between curli and CUP lies in its extracellular fiber growth assembly (Hammar et al., 1996). After secretion of the CsgB subunit, CsgA precipitates, polymerizes on CsgB and adopts an insoluble structure related to amyloid fibers (Hammar et al., 1996).

2.1.3 Type IVB pili

One of the most studied adhesive structures of *S.* Typhi is the type IVB pilus encoded by the *pil* operon located on SPI-7. Although type IV pili also produce long and flexible structures on the bacterial cell surface, their mechanism of assembly strongly differs from the CUP and curli pathways as it requires many structural proteins and is an ATP-dependent process. First, PilS prepilins are translocated through the IM into the periplasm and a specific prepilin peptidase cleaves the N-terminal signal peptide (reviewed in Craig & Li, 2008). An integral IM protein mobilizes a specific ATPase from the cytoplasm which drives pilus assembly. An oligomeric channel called the secretin found in the OM allows the exit of the pilus at the cell surface of the bacteria. ATP hydrolysis moves the pilus out in the secretin pore allowing the recruitment of new prepilin subunits. Unlike CUP and Csg fimbriae, Type IV pili are still connected to the IM of the bacteria and can be retracted rapidly inside the bacteria.

2.2 Roles of fimbrial adhesins during typhoid fever

In most studies, *Salmonella* fimbriae are involved during intestinal colonization (Althouse et al., 2003; Chessa et al., 2009; Weening et al., 2005), or in biofilm formation (Boddicker et al., 2002; Ledeboer et al., 2006), although they can also be used during the systemic phase (Edwards et al., 2000; Lawley et al., 2006). Interestingly, each serovar of *Salmonella enterica* harbours a unique combination of fimbrial operons, probably to avoid cross-immunity between two serovars infecting the same host (Norris & Bäumler, 1999; Nuccio et al., 2011). As *S.* Typhi infects only humans, little is known regarding the conditions of expression or the implication of each fimbrial adhesin during the course of infection. While some clues may be found in the literature, there is still much work to be done. Three fimbrial systems are clustered within pathogenic islands: *tcf* (Typhi colonizing factor) and *saf* (*Salmonella* atypical fimbriae) are found within SPI-6, while *sef* is in SPI-10 (Sabbagh et al., 2010).

Proteins expressed during infection were detected in blood of patients with typhoid fever (Charles et al., 2010; Harris et al., 2006; Hu et al., 2009). Interestingly, six proteins related to fimbrial adhesins led to the formation of antibodies after typhoid fever (TcfB, StbD, CsgG, CsgF, CsgE and BcfD). Since three proteins belonging to the thin aggregative fimbriae were identified, it suggests a strong production *in vivo* as well as an important role during infection. Csg implication during attachment to surfaces, bacterial autoaggregation and in biofilm formation is well known for *S.* Typhimurium and *E. coli* (Jonas et al., 2007). Nevertheless, a clear characterization of *csg* is needed for *S.* Typhi as there seem to be variations in expression between the different isolates (Römling et al., 2003; White et al., 2006). In *S.* Typhi, a strong expression of *csg* and *saf* fimbrial operons was observed inside human macrophages (Faucher et al., 2006).

The *bcf, sef, ste, stg* and *sth* fimbrial systems harbour pseudogenes that might disrupt the production of the corresponding fimbriae (Townsend et al., 2001). However, deletion of *stg* leads to reduced adhesion on epithelial cells as well as enhancement of the phagocytosis rate by macrophages (Forest et al., 2007). Furthermore, the presence of antibodies directed against BcfD is intriguing since the *bcfC* usher harbours two premature stop codons (Parkhill et al., 2001). The Bcf, Stb, Stc, Std and Sth fimbrial systems are required for the intestinal persistence of *S.* Typhimurium in mice, but their roles during the pathogenesis of *S.* Typhi still need to be evaluated (Weening et al., 2005). Sta and Tcf do not seem to be used for adhesion or invasion of non-polarized human epithelial cells while both are expressed at high NaCl concentrations (Bishop et al., 2008). Since these two fimbriae are found almost exclusively in the genome of serovars causing typhoid fever, they might be involved during the systemic phase or for the chronic carrier state (Nuccio et al., 2011). Although roles for Saf (Carnell et al., 2007; Lawley et al., 2006), Sef (Edwards et al., 2000) and Std fimbriae (Chessa et al., 2008; Weening et al., 2005) have been observed in other serovars of *Salmonella*, their true implication during typhoid fever needs to be investigated.

Type 1 fimbriae encoded by the *fim* operon are the best studied fimbrial adhesins and are frequently found in enteric bacteria. Fim are characterized by their mannose-sensitive binding properties, but their cell tropism seems to vary greatly between species and even between different strains of the same serovar (Thankavel et al., 1999). In *S.* Typhi, most clinical strains are fimbriated (*fim*+) and afimbriated strains are less adhesive and invasive than the fimbriated ones (Duguid et al., 1966; Satta et al., 1993). The ability of type 1 fimbriae to agglutinate yeast is abolished when the Vi capsule is expressed (Miyake et al., 1998). In *S.* Typhimurium, Fim appears to be the only fimbrial adhesin expressed in Luria-Bertani (LB) broth as confirmed by electron microscopy and flow cytometry (Duguid et al., 1966; Humphries et al., 2003). In *S.* Typhi, a complete deletion of *fim* also showed no evident fimbrial structures on the cell surface of the bacteria after growth in LB broth (Fig. 2).

Type IVB pili interact with the cystic fibrosis transmembrane conductance regulator (CFTR), a receptor upregulated and actively used by *S.* Typhi for its interaction with human epithelial cells (Lyczak & Pier, 2002; Pier et al., 1998; Tsui et al., 2003). These pili can also mediate bacterial self-association in conditions found in the intestinal tract, probably by enhancing binding efficiency prior to cell invasion (Morris et al., 2003a; Morris et al., 2003b). A direct correlation was observed between the level of surface-exposed CFTR and the efficiency of invasion of *S.* Typhi through the intestinal barrier (Pier et al., 1998). This specific interaction can be blocked by the addition of prepilin pre-PilS in the cell culture medium or with monoclonal antibodies specific to the first extracellular domain of CFTR

(Pier et al., 1998; Zhang et al., 2000). A piliated strain also adheres and invades human monocytes in a greater extent than a non-piliated strain and its expression can also increase IL-6 and NF-kappa B production in human monocytes by activating protein kinase C (Pan et al., 2005; F. Wang et al., 2005). Only a few other serovars, such as *S.* Paratyphi B and C, *S.* Heidelberg and *S. bongori* possess the genetic information coding for type IVB pili (Nuccio et al., 2011). Other functions could potentially be found in future studies as Type IV pili are also implicated in a variety of processes like biofilm formation, immune escape, DNA uptake and phage transduction in other pathogenic bacteria (reviewed in Craig & Li, 2008). These pili can also act as pistons, retracting subunits into the bacteria while it is still attached to a surface in a mechanism called "twitching motility" providing flagella-independent motility (reviewed in Mattick, 2002).

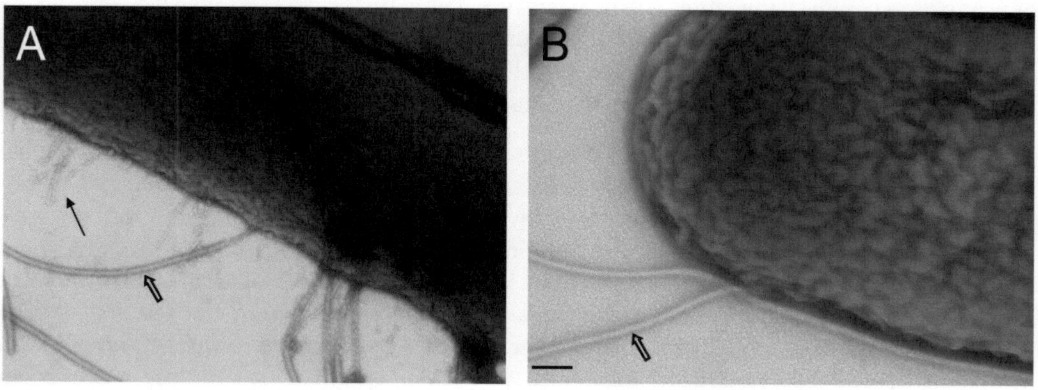

Fig. 2. Surface observation of *S.* Typhi grown in LB broth by transmission electron microscopy. After negative staining with phosphotungstate 1%, fimbriae were observed at the cell surface of the wild-type ISP1820 strain (A), while no structure was observed when *fim* was deleted (B). Black arrow shows fimbria and the open arrows indicate flagella. Black bar = 100 nm.

No genes related to fimbrial operons were found after a screening for mutants with a competitive disadvantage in humanized mice engrafted with hematopoietic stem cells (Libby et al., 2010). This result strongly suggests that fimbrial operons are mostly required during interaction with human epithelial cells, such as intestinal and gallbladder cells, that are absent from this mice model. Moreover, functional redundancy is often observed for fimbrial adhesins making it hard to evaluate their true contribution by single mutations. In order to understand the specific role played by each fimbrial system, our laboratory is currently creating a *S.* Typhi strain with deletions of all its fimbrial adhesins. This strain will greatly help to evaluate the global contribution of each fimbrial adhesins during association with eukaryotic cells.

3. Non fimbrial adhesins

3.1 Type 1 secretion systems

In *Salmonella*, some important surface structures are expressed by different mechanisms and can be classified as non fimbrial adhesins. In *S.* Typhi, there are two examples of adhesins secreted by a type I secretion system (T1SS) : SiiE and BapA. In T1SS, the secreted proteins directly pass through a channel formed between the IM and OM of the bacteria by the recognition of a signal at the C-terminus (China & Goffaux, 1999 as cited in Main-Hester et al., 2008). SPI-4, present in all *Salmonella* strains, encodes a T1SS responsible for the secretion of SiiE, the largest protein found in *Salmonella* (595 kDa) (Latasa et al., 2005; Main-Hester et al., 2008). Its cell surface expression requires the IM ATPase SiiF, the periplasmic adaptor SiiD and an outer membrane channel formed by SiiC (Gerlach et al., 2007). This adhesion system acts in a coordinated way with the T3SS of SPI-1 and is involved during the intestinal phase of infection (Gerlach et al., 2008). Previously annotated as two distinct ORFs in *S.* Typhi (STY4458-4459) (Parkhill et al., 2001), *siiE* harbours a premature stop codon probably rendering this large adhesin non-functional (Main-Hester et al., 2008; Morgan et al., 2004). An immunoblot done with antibodies directed against SiiE (STY4458) demonstrated the absence of production of SiiE in the whole cell proteins of *S.* Typhi further suggesting a lack of function in this serovar (Main-Hester et al., 2008). However, a transposon insertion in STY4458 showed a reduced competitive fitness in humanized mice, suggesting SiiE functionality and an uncharacterized role during interaction with hematopoietic cells (Libby et al., 2010).

A second T1SS is clustered within SPI-9 and secretes another large repetitive protein called BapA (**b**iofilm-**a**ssociated **p**rotein) due to its similarity with BapA of *Staphylococcus aureus*. Well described in *S.* Enteritidis, BapA is involved in bacterial autoaggregation strongly inducing biofilm formation and is also required during the interaction with the intestinal mucosa (Latasa et al., 2005). Its expression is under the control of CsgD, an important regulator also coordinating curli fimbriae and cellulose production needed for biofilm production (Jonas et al., 2007). Again, solving the components required for biofilm formation by *S.* Typhi is crucial since *bcsC* (STY4184), essential for cellulose and biofilm production, is a pseudogene (Parkhill et al., 2001; Zogaj et al., 2001).

3.2 Type 5 secretion systems

Autotransported adhesins can be monomeric or trimeric and are considered as type 5 secretion systems. *S.* Typhi harbours two monomeric examples of autotransported adhesins, *shdA* (STY2755) found in the CS54 island and *misL* (STY4030) clustered in SPI-3, as well as one representative of a trimeric autotransporter called *sadA* (STY4105). An N-terminal signal sequence allows their translocation into the periplasm by the Sec general secretory pathway, then a β-domain found at the C-terminal end of the protein adopts a β-barrel conformation in the OM allowing secretion of the passenger domain into the extracellular space (reviewed in Nishimura et al., 2010). ShdA is widely distributed in *S. enterica* subspecies I and appears to be produced during typhoid fever despite the presence of a frameshifting sequence (Harris et al., 2006; Parkhill et al., 2001). Interestingly, ShdA and MisL can bind fibronectin in other serovars of *Salmonella* and are both considered as pseudogenes in *S.* Typhi (Dorsey et al., 2005; Kingsley et al., 2002). SadA harbours homology to the trimeric autotransporter adhesin YadA of *Yersinia enterocolitica*, a highly repetitive fibrous surface protein (Grosskinsky et al., 2007). YaiU (STY0405) encodes a fourth putative autotransported adhesin with no known role except that antibodies against the protein are produced during a typhoid fever (Harris et al., 2006).

3.3 Other adhesins

Besides fimbrial and afimbrial adhesins, other surface-exposed proteins can act as adhesins and mediate crucial roles during typhoid fever. One of the most hydrophobic proteins encoded in the *S*. Typhi chromosome, STY0351, was recently characterized in detail and might be used as a potential vaccine target. This cell-surface protein is a novel adhesin directly involved in the pathogenesis of *S*. Typhi by conferring strong binding to the laminin extracellular matrix (Ghosh et al., 2011) and is positively regulated by the PhoP-PhoQ two-component system (Charles et al., 2009). It also possesses high immunogenic properties and STY0351-specific antibodies confer protection in a mouse model (Charles et al., 2010; Ghosh et al., 2011). PagC is another surface-exposed protein activated by the PhoP-PhoQ system that is produced and actively recognised by antibodies from patients having previously suffered from typhoid fever (Charles et al., 2010; Harris et al., 2006). Previously associated with survival within macrophages (Miller et al., 1989), PagC possesses serum resistance activity (Nishio et al., 2005) and can promote OM vesicle release in *S*. Typhimurium (Kitagawa et al., 2010), but none of these roles are confirmed yet for *S*. Typhi.

Multivalent adhesion molecules (MAM) are outer membrane proteins harbouring 6 or 7 mammalian cell entry domains and are widely found in pathogenic Gram-negative bacteria (Krachler et al., 2011). MAM mediates early interactions with different cell types by providing protein as well as lipid interactions with fibronectin and phosphatidic acid (Krachler et al., 2011). The specificity for certain cell types is thought to be provided by the other adhesins clustered throughout the genome of the bacteria. In *S*. Typhi, BLASTP analysis revealed that STY1980 harbours about 96% homology with MAM7 of the EPEC strain *E. coli* O127:H6 (Altschul et al., 1990) and could be implicated during the primary interactions with the intestinal mucosa.

4. Capsule and LPS

S. Typhi produces a group 1 exopolysaccharide known as the Vi antigen. Thus, *S*. Typhi is one of the few *Salmonella* serovars that get shielded by an extracellular polysaccharide layer constituting the Vi capsule. The Vi polysaccharide is a linear homopolymer of α(1→4)-2-acetamido-3-*O*-acetyl-2-deoxy-α-D-galacturonic acid (Heyns et al., 1959) and constitutes the major component of an injectable conjugated vaccine presently used against typhoid fever world-wide (World Health Organization, 2003). Vi has been involved in pathogenicity by evading the host innate immune system as it protects bacteria from phagocytosis and complement-mediated killing (Kossack et al., 1981). The *in vitro* masking of the OAg by the Vi antigen has been known for a long time (Felix & Pitt, 1934 as cited in Robbins & Robbins, 1984), prevents recognition by TLR-4, and limited C3 deposition to the cell surface (Looney & Steigbigel, 1986), which will lead to reduced clearance of the bacteria (Wilson et al., 2011). Vi is preferentially expressed at low osmolarity and early during infection of human macrophages or mice and will be downregulated with the progression of infection (Daigle et al., 2001; Faucher et al., 2006; Janis et al., 2011). The expression of Vi reduces invasion, probably by limiting the access of the T3SS-1 (Arricau et al., 1998; L. Zhao et al., 2001) or by masking other adhesion molecules including Fim. Vi is also important for surviving in macrophages (Hirose et al., 1997). Vi is tightly regulated by its own activator TviA (Hashimoto et al., 1996; Virlogeux et al., 1996), the two-component system OmpR-EnvZ (Pickard et al., 1994), the Rcs system (Arricau et al., 1998; Virlogeux et al., 1996) and repressed by RpoS (Santander et al., 2007).

Lipopolysaccharide (LPS) is the principal component of the outer membrane of Gram-negative bacteria and a major virulence determinant of many pathogens (Raetz & Whitfield,

2002). It is a glycolipid consisting in three structural regions covalently linked: (i) lipid A, also known as endotoxin, a hydrophobic anchor composed of acyl chains linked to phosphorylated *N*-acetylglucosamine; (ii) the inner and outer core composed of conserved oligosaccharides and; (iii) a variable polysaccharide chain or OAg. *Salmonella* OAg exhibits extensive composition and structural variation and has been divided into 46 O serogroups (Popoff et al., 2001). The O9 antigen of *S.* Typhi is characterized by the presence of a tyvelose residue. In response to acidified macrophage phagosomes, genes activated by the PhoP-PhoQ and PmrA-PmrB systems can modify the global structure of LPS and protect *Salmonella* from being killed by the immune system, notably by antimicrobial peptides (reviewed in Gunn, 2008). Heterogeneity in the length of the OAg repeats has been observed (P. Reeves, 1993) and is important for serum resistance and interaction with host cells (Bravo et al., 2011; Hoare et al., 2006; Hölzer et al., 2009). The *S.* Typhi OAg is essential for serum resistance but is not required for cell invasion (Hoare et al., 2006). Internalization of *S.* Typhi by epithelial cells involves the LPS core (Hoare et al., 2006) which acts as a ligand for CFTR (Lyczak et al., 2001; Pier et al., 1998). The *S.* Typhi LPS core is involved in intracellular replication in macrophages (unpublished data), as observed with *S.* Typhimurium (Nagy et al., 2006; Zenk et al., 2009). *S.* Typhi does not have a bimodal distribution of OAg as it cannot produce very long OAg, consisting of more than 100 repeats of OAg units, because the major regulator Wzz (FepE) is non functional (Raetz & Whitfield, 2002). LPS biosynthesis involves many genes located in different clusters on the chromosome and may be controlled through several regulatory systems (P.R. Reeves et al., 1996). In *S.* Typhi, OAg expression is regulated by RfaH under the control of sigma factor RpoN (Bittner et al., 2002).

5. Secretion systems

5.1 Type 3 secretion systems

S. enterica harbours two distinct type 3 secretion systems (T3SSs) located on SPI-1 (T3SS-1) and SPI-2 (T3SS-2) that are crucial to its virulence along with a flagellar apparatus. T3SSs are complex molecular machines built from more than 20 different proteins, forming a structure similar to a molecular syringe (Kubori et al., 1998, Kimbrough & Miller, 2000 as cited in Sanowar et al., 2010). IM and OM rings are connected by a channel called the needle complex. These structures can inject many protein effectors directly from the bacterial cytoplasm to the cytoplasm of the eukaryotic cells, allowing a direct manipulation of host cellular pathways. The injection process is energized by specific cytoplasmic ATPase and direct contact with the eukaryotic cells is needed in order to activate secretion. Although T3SS are surface-exposed molecules, the lack of specific antibodies against the T3SS in the sera of convalescent patients of typhoid fever (Charles et al., 2010; Harris et al., 2006; Hu et al., 2009) might be a consequence of their tight regulation.

5.1.1 T3SS-1

In order to cause a systemic infection, *Salmonella* must first cross the intestinal epithelial barrier. Conditions found in the intestine, such as low oxygen tension and high osmolarity, are known to induce T3SS-1 of *Salmonella* by the HilA central regulator (Bajaj et al., 1996, Galán & Curtiss, 1990 and Jones & Falkow, 1994 as cited in Altier, 2005). Injection of effectors secreted by the T3SS-1 mediates the invasion of non-phagocytic epithelial cells by *Salmonella* (Galán & Curtiss, 1989; Galán, 1999). Effectors interact with the actin cytoskeleton and induce membrane ruffles around the bacteria allowing its internalisation into epithelial cells. In *S.* Typhi, the contribution of the T3SS-1 during invasion of epithelial cells was confirmed with *invA*, *sipEBCDA* or *iagAB* (*hilAB*) mutants (Galán & Curtiss, 1991; Hermant et al., 1995; Miras et al., 1995). The T3SS-1 of *S.* Typhi may also play a role during the systemic phase of the infection (Haraga et al., 2008; Libby et al., 2010).

5.1.2 T3SS-2

After reaching the epithelial submucosa, *Salmonella* encounters and enters immune system cells like macrophages, dendritic cells and neutrophils. The intracellular environment of these cells promotes induction of the T3SS-2, which is regulated by the SsrA-SsrB two-component regulatory system. Inside cells, bacteria are found in a SCV (*Salmonella*-containing vacuole) and inject T3SS-2 effectors to modify the SCV, alter host pathways and promote intracellular survival (Brumell et al., 2001; Waterman & Holden, 2003; Yu et al., 2004). Although *S.* Typhimurium absolutely requires the T3SS-2 for its intramacrophage survival (Cirillo et al., 1998; Hensel et al., 1998), a complete deletion of this system does not impair survival of *S.* Typhi in human macrophages (Forest et al., 2010). Nevertheless, *S.* Typhi T3SS-2 might be required for survival in other immune cells, as a mutant harbouring a transposon insertion in *ssrB* is disadvantaged in a humanized mouse model (Libby et al., 2010).

5.1.3 Flagella

The flagellar apparatus constitutes a third T3SS that is under the control of a highly organized transcriptional hierarchy involving three promoter classes with *flhDC* being the first activator (Kutsukake et al., 1990 and Karlinsey et al., 2000 as cited in Chevance & Hughes, 2008). In *Salmonella*, each cell harbours 6-8 peritrichous flagella built from more than 25 different proteins (Harshey, 2011). The final structure is composed of a basal body, including a stationary and a moving rotor, an external hook and the filament comprised of flagellin (Harshey, 2011). Secretion of flagellin subunits and motility processes are powered by the proton motive force (Minamino & Namba, 2008 and Paul et al., 2008 as cited in Chevance & Hughes, 2008). Subspecies I, II, IIIa and IV of *Salmonella enterica* are considered biphasic since they can alternatively express FliC or FljB major flagellar subunits in a mechanism known as phase variation (Lederberg & Iino, 1956; Simon et al., 1980). Most *S.* Typhi strains do not possess the *fljB* locus and are monophasic, but some isolates contain a 27 kb linear plasmid harbouring the *fljB*:z66 encoding for a novel flagellin (S. Baker et al., 2007; Frankel et al., 1989). Flagella normally contribute to the virulence through motility and chemotaxis (Macnab, 1999), but can also be implicated during biofilm formation (Crawford et al., 2010a). Flagellin can be detected by TLR-5 present at the cell surface of monocytes, dendritic cells and epithelial cells inducing proinflammatory and adaptive immune responses. In *S.* Typhi, TviA directly downregulates flagellar expression thereby avoiding its early recognition by the intestinal mucosa (Winter et al., 2008). Flagellar genes are involved in survival within macrophages or during the systemic phase of infection (Bäumler et al., 1994; Chan et al., 2005; Klumpp & Fuchs, 2007; Libby et al., 2010; Y. Zhao et al., 2002). Nevertheless, the real contribution of the flagellar apparatus is hard to evaluate since expression of the T3SS-1 is co-regulated with the flagella (Eichelberg & Galán, 2000; Saini et al., 2010). Interestingly, patients harbouring antibodies directed against flagella had uncomplicated typhoid fever, while prevalence of anti-OMP (outer membrane proteins) antibodies was associated with increased ileal perforation rates (Nambiar et al., 2009).

5.2 Type 6 secretion systems

Type 6 secretion systems are newly-discovered structures present in about 25% of sequenced Gram-negative bacterial genomes (Boyer et al., 2009). In *S. enterica* subsp. I, T6SS can be identified within SPI-6 (*S.* Typhi), SPI-19, SPI-20 or SPI-21 (Blondel et al., 2009). T6SS are contractile injection machinery harbouring strong similarities to the tail sheath and spike of bacteriophages (Bönemann et al., 2010). These tubular structures can penetrate eukaryotic as well as prokaryotic membranes in a cell-contact dependant way in order to inject protein effectors. T6SS are often required within phagocytic cells (Ma et al., 2009; Pukatzki et al., 2009), but they can also be implicated in biofilm formation (Aschtgen et al., 2008; Enos-Berlage et al., 2005), colonization of the gastrointestinal tract (Blondel et al., 2010), quorum sensing (Weber et al., 2009) as well as in the delivery of toxins to other cells (Hood et al., 2010). Although *S.* Typhi harbours a pseudogene in a key component of its T6SS, the system is functional and its presence corresponds to an enhanced cytotoxicity toward epithelial cells (M. Wang et al., 2011). T6SS expression is regulated by RcsB, PmrA and Hfq (M. Wang et al., 2011). Its contribution during the interaction with hematopoietic cells should be further studied since a transposon insertion in two genes encoded within SPI-6 showed a competitive disadvantage in humanized mice (Libby et al., 2010).

Surface structure	Role in virulence	Observed for S. Typhi	Observed in other serovars
Bcf and Stb	Seroconversion	Harris 2006; Hu 2009	
	Intestinal persistence in mice		Weening 2005
Fim	Binds to mannose, adhesion and invasion of epithelial cells	Satta 1993	Althouse 2003
	Biofilm		Boddicker 2002
Stg	Adhesion to epithelial cells	Forest 2007	
Sth	Long-term infection of mice		Lawley 2006
Saf	Intestinal colonization of swine		Carnell 2007
	Long-term infection of mice		Lawley 2006
Sef	Interaction with macrophages		Edwards 2000
Stc	Intestinal persistence in mice		Weening 2005
Std	Binds to α(1,2)fucose		Chessa 2009
	Intestinal persistence in mice		Weening 2005
Tcf and YaiU	Seroconversion	Harris 2006	
Csg	Seroconversion	Harris 2006	
	Biofilm		Ledeboer 2006
SiiE	Adhesion to apical side of epithelial cells		Gerlach 2008
	Colonization of the gastrointestinal tract		Blondel 2010
BapA	Interaction with intestinal mucosa, bacterial autoaggregation and biofilm		Latasa 2005
ShdA	Seroconversion	Harris 2006	
	Binds to fibronectin		Kingsley 2002
MisL	Intestinal colonization, binds to fibronectin		Dorsey 2005

Surface structure	Role in virulence	Observed for *S.* Typhi	Observed in other serovars
Type IVB pili	Binds to CFTR, cellular invasion Bacterial self-association	Pan 2005; Pier 1998 Morris 2003b	Morris 2003a
STY0351	Seroconversion Cell adhesion and binds to laminin	Charles 2010 Ghosh 2011	
PagC	Seroconversion Survival within macrophages Serum resistance OM vesicle release	Charles 2010; Harris 2006	Miller 1989 Nishio 2005 Kitagawa 2010
Vi Capsule	Host immune system evasion Intramacrophage survival	Kossack 1981; Looney, 1986; Wilson 2011 Hirose 1997	
LPS	Binds to CFTR Antimicrobial peptides resistance Serum resistance Intramacrophage survival	Lyczak 2001 Baker 1999 Hoare 2006 Unpublished data	Gunn 2008 Bravo 2008 Nagy 2006
T3SS-1	Effectors secretion and invasion of eukaryotic cells	Galán 1991; Hermant 1995	Galán 1989, 1999
T3SS-2	Effectors secretion and intramacrophage survival		Cirillo 1998; Hensel 1998
Flagella	Motility and chemotaxis Intramacrophage survival Biofilm formation	Liu 1988 Unpublished data	Macnab 1999 Bäumler 1994 Crawford 2010a
T6SS	Colonization of the gastrointestinal tract		Blondel 2010

Table 1. *S.* Typhi surface structures considered in this review and their roles in virulence.

6. Future perspectives

The multidrug-resistance observed for *S.* Typhi strains is of great concern since the total number of cases has increased during the last decade (Crump et al., 2004; Pang et al., 1998). There are two crucial lines of defence that should be improved in order to win the combat against typhoid fever : prevention and treatment. The best vaccine would be safe, given in a single dose, offering an efficient and long lasting immunity and remain stable at room temperature. Next generation vaccines have been recently tested in human trials (reviewed in Lindow et al., 2011). The expression of surface structures is tightly coordinated to avoid recognition by the immune system. Nevertheless, we have some clues regarding the structures recognized during typhoid fever (Charles et al., 2010; Harris et al., 2006; Hu et al., 2009). Since antibodies promote killing of *S.* Typhi (Lindow et al., 2011), a good approach to improve the efficiency of vaccines might be to create an avirulent strain expressing its immunogenic structures on inducible promoters inside antigen presenting cells (S. Wang et al., 2011).

Another strategy in the fight against *S.* Typhi should be the identification and treatment of the 1-5% infected individuals who become asymptomatic carriers (Crawford et al., 2010b; Parry et al., 2002). This task is complicated as antibiotherapy is often unsuccessful to remove biofilms found in the gallbladder, especially on gallstones, and surgical removal of the gallbladder is usually required but expensive (Crawford et al., 2010b; Prouty et al., 2002) Hence, efforts should be taken to understand the specific structures required for biofilm formation by *S.* Typhi in order to develop therapies to eliminate typhoid carriage.

Novel strategies are being developed to target surface structures implicated in bacterial pathogenesis as potential treatments (reviewed in Lynch & Wiener-Kronish, 2008). For example, pilicides are small compounds preventing interactions between the OM usher and chaperone-subunits complexes of type 1 pili, hence interfering with fimbrial biogenesis (Pinkner et al., 2006). Since most surface structures of *Salmonella* are expressed by the CUP, targeting the fimbrial ushers might be a useful method to eliminate colonisation and avoid the resulting antimicrobial resistance. Moreover, curlicides are able to interfere with CsgA polymerization as well as type 1 fimbrial biogenesis resulting in the blocking of biofilm accumulation (Cegelski et al., 2009). Similarly, small-molecule inhibitors and inactivating antibodies can target binding or translocation of effectors by T3SS (Hudson et al., 2007; Neely et al., 2005; Nordfelth et al., 2005; Swietnicki et al., 2011). Targeting the capsule or LPS biosynthetic pathways might be a good approach to fight against *S.* Typhi since there is no corresponding enzyme in its human host (Cipolla et al., 2010; Goller & Seed, 2010).

Finally, understanding the role and function of *S.* Typhi surface proteins is primordial as these molecules are the first ones to directly interact with host components or cells, leading to a possibility for the development of new strategies to fight typhoid (see Table 1).

7. Acknowledgments

This work was supported by the Canadian Natural Sciences and Engineering Research Council (NSERC) grant number 251114-06. C.G.F. was supported by scholarships from NSERC. We are grateful to Dr. George Szatmari for editing of the manuscript.

8. References

Althouse, C., Patterson, S., Fedorka-Cray, P. & Isaacson, R. E. (2003). Type 1 fimbriae of *Salmonella enterica* serovar Typhimurium bind to enterocytes and contribute to colonization of swine *in vivo*. *Infection and Immunity*, Vol. 71, No. 11, pp. 6446-6452, ISSN 0019-9567

Altier, C. (2005). Genetic and environmental control of *Salmonella* invasion. *Journal of Microbiology*, Vol. 43 Spec No, pp. 85-92, ISSN 1225-8873

Altschul, S. F., Gish, W., Miller, W., Myers, E. W. & Lipman, D. J. (1990). Basic local alignment search tool. *Journal of Molecular Biology*, Vol. 215, No. 3, pp. 403-410, ISSN 0022-2836

Arricau, N., Hermant, D., Waxin, H., Ecobichon, C., Duffey, P. S. & Popoff, M. Y. (1998). The RcsB-RcsC regulatory system of *Salmonella typhi* differentially modulates the expression of invasion proteins, flagellin and Vi antigen in response to osmolarity. *Molecular Microbiology*, Vol. 29, No. 3, pp. 835-850, ISSN 0950-382X

Aschtgen, M. S., Bernard, C. S., De Bentzmann, S., Lloubès, R. & Cascales, E. (2008). SciN is an outer membrane lipoprotein required for type VI secretion in enteroaggregative *Escherichia coli*. *Journal of Bacteriology*, Vol. 190, No. 22, pp. 7523-7531, ISSN 1098-5530

Bajaj, V., Lucas, R. L., Hwang, C. & Lee, C. A. (1996). Co-ordinate regulation of *Salmonella typhimurium* invasion genes by environmental and regulatory factors is mediated by control of *hilA* expression. *Molecular Microbiology*, Vol. 22, No. 4, pp. 703-714, ISSN 0950-382X

Baker, S., Hardy, J., Sanderson, K. E., Quail, M., Goodhead, I., Kingsley, R. A., Parkhill, J., Stocker, B. & Dougan, G. (2007). A novel linear plasmid mediates flagellar variation in *Salmonella* Typhi. *PLoS Pathogens*, Vol. 3, No. 5, p. e59, ISSN 1553-7374

Baker, S. J., Gunn, J. S. & Morona, R. (1999). The *Salmonella typhi* melittin resistance gene *pqaB* affects intracellular growth in PMA-differentiated U937 cells, polymyxin B resistance and lipopolysaccharide. *Microbiology*, Vol. 145, No. 2, pp. 367-378, ISSN 1350-0872

Bäumler, A. J., Kusters, J. G., Stojiljkovic, I. & Heffron, F. (1994). *Salmonella typhimurium* loci involved in survival within macrophages. *Infection and Immunity*, Vol. 62, No. 5, pp. 1623-1630, ISSN 0019-9567

Bishop, A., House, D., Perkins, T., Baker, S., Kingsley, R. A. & Dougan, G. (2008). Interaction of *Salmonella enterica* serovar Typhi with cultured epithelial cells: roles of surface structures in adhesion and invasion. *Microbiology*, Vol. 154, No. 7, pp. 1914-1926, ISSN 1350-0872

Bittner, M., Saldías, S., Estévez, C., Zaldívar, M., Marolda, C. L., Valvano, M. A. & Contreras, I. (2002). O-antigen expression in *Salmonella enterica* serovar Typhi is regulated by nitrogen availability through RpoN-mediated transcriptional control of the *rfaH* gene. *Microbiology*, Vol. 148, No. 12, pp. 3789-3799, ISSN 1350-0872

Blondel, C. J., Jiménez, J. C., Contreras, I. & Santiviago, C. A. (2009). Comparative genomic analysis uncovers 3 novel loci encoding type six secretion systems differentially distributed in *Salmonella* serotypes. *BMC Genomics*, Vol. 10, p. 354, ISSN 1471-2164

Blondel, C. J., Yang, H. J., Castro, B., Chiang, S., Toro, C. S., Zaldívar, M., Contreras, I., Andrews-Polymenis, H. L. & Santiviago, C. A. (2010). Contribution of the type VI secretion system encoded in SPI-19 to chicken colonization by *Salmonella enterica* serotypes Gallinarum and Enteritidis. *PLoS One*, Vol. 5, No. 7, p. e11724, ISSN 1932-6203

Boddicker, J. D., Ledeboer, N. A., Jagnow, J., Jones, B. D. & Clegg, S. (2002). Differential binding to and biofilm formation on, HEp-2 cells by *Salmonella enterica* serovar Typhimurium is dependent upon allelic variation in the *fimH* gene of the *fim* gene cluster. *Molecular Microbiology*, Vol. 45, No. 5, pp. 1255-1265, ISSN 0950-382X

Bönemann, G., Pietrosiuk, A. & Mogk, A. (2010). Tubules and donuts: a type VI secretion story. *Molecular Microbiology*, Vol. 76, No. 4, pp. 815-821, ISSN 1365-2958

Boyer, F., Fichant, G., Berthod, J., Vandenbrouck, Y. & Attree, I. (2009). Dissecting the bacterial type VI secretion system by a genome wide *in silico* analysis: what can be learned from available microbial genomic resources? *BMC Genomics*, Vol. 10, p. 104, ISSN 1471-2164

Bravo, D., Silva, C., Carter, J. A., Hoare, A., Alvarez, S. A., Blondel, C. J., Zaldivar, M., Valvano, M. A. & Contreras, I. (2008). Growth-phase regulation of lipopolysaccharide O-antigen chain length influences serum resistance in serovars of *Salmonella*. *Journal of Medical Microbiology*, Vol. 57, No. 8, pp. 938-946, ISSN 0022-2615

Bravo, D., Hoare, A., Silipo, A., Valenzuela, C., Salinas, C., Alvarez, S. A., Molinaro, A., Valvano, M. A. & Contreras, I. (2011). Different sugar residues of the lipopolysaccharide outer core are required for early interactions of *Salmonella enterica* serovars Typhi and Typhimurium with epithelial cells. *Microbial Pathogenesis*, Vol. 50, No. 2, pp. 70-80, ISSN 1096-1208

Brumell, J. H., Rosenberger, C. M., Gotto, G. T., Marcus, S. L. & Finlay, B. B. (2001). SifA permits survival and replication of *Salmonella typhimurium* in murine macrophages. *Cellular Microbiology*, Vol. 3, No. 2, pp. 75-84, ISSN 1462-5814

Carnell, S. C., Bowen, A., Morgan, E., Maskell, D. J., Wallis, T. S. & Stevens, M. P. (2007). Role in virulence and protective efficacy in pigs of *Salmonella enterica* serovar Typhimurium secreted components identified by signature-tagged mutagenesis. *Microbiology*, Vol. 153, No. 6, pp. 1940-1952, ISSN 1350-0872

Cegelski, L., Pinkner, J. S., Hammer, N. D. & other authors. (2009). Small-molecule inhibitors target *Escherichia coli* amyloid biogenesis and biofilm formation. *Nature Chemical Biology*, Vol. 5, No. 12, pp. 913-919, ISSN 1552-4469

Chan, K., Kim, C. C. & Falkow, S. (2005). Microarray-based detection of *Salmonella enterica* serovar Typhimurium transposon mutants that cannot survive in macrophages and mice. *Infection and Immunity*, Vol. 73, No. 9, pp. 5438-5449, ISSN 0019-9567

Charles, R. C., Harris, J. B., Chase, M. R. & other authors. (2009). Comparative proteomic analysis of the PhoP regulon in *Salmonella enterica* serovar Typhi versus Typhimurium. *PLoS One*, Vol. 4, No. 9, p. e6994, ISSN 1932-6203

Charles, R. C., Sheikh, A., Krastins, B. & other authors. (2010). Characterization of anti-*Salmonella enterica* serotype Typhi antibody responses in bacteremic Bangladeshi patients by an immunoaffinity proteomics-based technology. *Clinical and Vaccine Immunology*, Vol. 17, No. 8, pp. 1188-1195, ISSN 1556-679X

Chessa, D., Winter, M. G., Nuccio, S. P., Tükel, C. & Bäumler, A. J. (2008). RosE represses Std fimbrial expression in *Salmonella enterica* serotype Typhimurium. *Molecular Microbiology*, Vol. 68, No. 3, pp. 573-587, ISSN 1365-2958

Chessa, D., Winter, M. G., Jakomin, M. & Bäumler, A. J. (2009). *Salmonella enterica* serotype Typhimurium Std fimbriae bind terminal alpha(1,2)fucose residues in the cecal mucosa. *Molecular Microbiology*, Vol. 71, No. 4, pp. 864-875, ISSN 1365-2958

Chevance, F. F. & Hughes, K. T. (2008). Coordinating assembly of a bacterial macromolecular machine. *Nature Reviews Microbiology*, Vol. 6, No. 6, pp. 455-465, ISSN 1740-1534

China, B. & Goffaux, F. (1999). Secretion of virulence factors by *Escherichia coli*. *Veterinary Research*, Vol. 30, No. 2-3, pp. 181-202, ISSN 0928-4249

Cipolla, L., Gabrielli, L., Bini, D., Russo, L. & Shaikh, N. (2010). Kdo: a critical monosaccharide for bacteria viability. *Natural Product Reports*, Vol. 27, No. 11, pp. 1618-1629, ISSN 1460-4752

Cirillo, D. M., Valdivia, R. H., Monack, D. M. & Falkow, S. (1998). Macrophage-dependent induction of the *Salmonella* pathogenicity island 2 type III secretion system and its role in intracellular survival. *Molecular Microbiology*, Vol. 30, No. 1, pp. 175-188, ISSN 0950-382X

Craig, L. & Li, J. (2008). Type IV pili: paradoxes in form and function. *Current Opinion in Structural Biology*, Vol. 18, No. 2, pp. 267-277, ISSN 0959-440X

Crawford, R. W., Reeve, K. E. & Gunn, J. S. (2010a). Flagellated but not hyperfimbriated *Salmonella enterica* serovar Typhimurium attaches to and forms biofilms on cholesterol-coated surfaces. *Journal of Bacteriology*, Vol. 192, No. 12, pp. 2981-2990, ISSN 1098-5530

Crawford, R. W., Rosales-Reyes, R., Ramírez-Aguilar, M. e. L., Chapa-Azuela, O., Alpuche-Aranda, C. & Gunn, J. S. (2010b). Gallstones play a significant role in *Salmonella* spp. gallbladder colonization and carriage. *Proceedings of the National Academy of Sciences of the United States of America*, Vol. 107, No. 9, pp. 4353-4358, ISSN 1091-6490

Crump, J. A., Luby, S. P. & Mintz, E. D. (2004). The global burden of typhoid fever. *Bulletin of the World Health Organization*, Vol. 82, No. 5, pp. 346-353, ISSN 0042-9686

Daigle, F., Graham, J. E. & Curtiss III, R. (2001). Identification of *Salmonella typhi* genes expressed within macrophages by selective capture of transcribed sequences (SCOTS). *Molecular Microbiology*, Vol. 41, No. 5, pp. 1211-1222, ISSN 0950-382X

Dorsey, C. W., Laarakker, M. C., Humphries, A. D., Weening, E. H. & Bäumler, A. J. (2005). *Salmonella enterica* serotype Typhimurium MisL is an intestinal colonization factor that binds fibronectin. *Molecular Microbiology*, Vol. 57, No. 1, pp. 196-211, ISSN 0950-382X

Duguid, J. P., Anderson, E. S. & Campbell, I. (1966). Fimbriae and adhesive properties in Salmonellae. *Journal of Pathology and Bacteriology*, Vol. 92, No. 1, pp. 107-138, ISSN 0368-3494

Edwards, R. A., Schifferli, D. M. & Maloy, S. R. (2000). A role for *Salmonella* fimbriae in intraperitoneal infections. *Proceedings of the National Academy of Sciences of the United States of America*, Vol. 97, No. 3, pp. 1258-1262, ISSN 0027-8424

Eichelberg, K. & Galán, J. E. (2000). The flagellar sigma factor FliA (sigma(28)) regulates the expression of *Salmonella* genes associated with the centisome 63 type III secretion system. *Infection and Immunity*, Vol. 68, No. 5, pp. 2735-2743, ISSN 0019-9567

Enos-Berlage, J. L., Guvener, Z. T., Keenan, C. E. & McCarter, L. L. (2005). Genetic determinants of biofilm development of opaque and translucent *Vibrio parahaemolyticus*. *Molecular Microbiology*, Vol. 55, No. 4, pp. 1160-1182, ISSN 0950-382X

Faucher, S. P., Porwollik, S., Dozois, C. M., McClelland, M. & Daigle, F. (2006). Transcriptome of *Salmonella enterica* serovar Typhi within macrophages revealed through the selective capture of transcribed sequences. *Proceedings of the National Academy of Sciences of the United States of America*, Vol. 103, No. 6, pp. 1906-1911, ISSN 0027-8424

Felix, A. & Pitt, R. M. (1934). A new antigen of *B. typhosus*. *The Lancet*, Vol. 224, No. 5787, pp. 186-191, ISSN 0140-6736

Forest, C., Faucher, S. P., Poirier, K., Houle, S., Dozois, C. M. & Daigle, F. (2007). Contribution of the *stg* fimbrial operon of *Salmonella enterica* serovar Typhi during interaction with human cells. *Infection and Immunity*, Vol. 75, No. 11, pp. 5264-5271, ISSN 0019-9567

Forest, C. G., Ferraro, E., Sabbagh, S. C. & Daigle, F. (2010). Intracellular survival of *Salmonella enterica* serovar Typhi in human macrophages is independent of *Salmonella* pathogenicity island (SPI)-2. *Microbiology*, Vol. 156, No. 12, pp. 3689-3698, ISSN 1465-2080

Frankel, G., Newton, S. M., Schoolnik, G. K. & Stocker, B. A. (1989). Intragenic recombination in a flagellin gene: characterization of the H1-j gene of *Salmonella typhi*. *EMBO Journal*, Vol. 8, No. 10, pp. 3149-3152, ISSN 0261-4189

Galán, J. E. & Curtiss III, R. (1989). Cloning and molecular characterization of genes whose products allow *Salmonella typhimurium* to penetrate tissue culture cells. *Proceedings of the National Academy of Sciences of the United States of America*, Vol. 86, No. 16, pp. 6383-6387, ISSN 0027-8424

Galán, J. E. & Curtiss III, R. (1990). Expression of *Salmonella typhimurium* genes required for invasion is regulated by changes in DNA supercoiling. *Infection and Immunity*, Vol. 58, No. 6, pp. 1879-1885, ISSN 0019-9567

Galán, J. E. & Curtiss III, R. (1991). Distribution of the *invA*, *-B*, *-C*, and *-D* genes of *Salmonella typhimurium* among other *Salmonella* serovars: *invA* mutants of *Salmonella typhi* are deficient for entry into mammalian cells. *Infection and Immunity*, Vol. 59, No. 9, pp. 2901-2908, ISSN 0019-9567

Galán, J. E. (1999). Interaction of *Salmonella* with host cells through the centisome 63 type III secretion system. *Current Opinion in Microbiology*, Vol. 2, No. 1, pp. 46-50, ISSN 1369-5274

Gerlach, R. G., Jäckel, D., Stecher, B., Wagner, C., Lupas, A., Hardt, W. D. & Hensel, M. (2007). *Salmonella* Pathogenicity Island 4 encodes a giant non-fimbrial adhesin and the cognate type 1 secretion system. *Cellular Microbiology*, Vol. 9, No. 7, pp. 1834-1850, ISSN 1462-5814

Gerlach, R. G., Cláudio, N., Rohde, M., Jäckel, D., Wagner, C. & Hensel, M. (2008). Cooperation of *Salmonella* pathogenicity islands 1 and 4 is required to breach epithelial barriers. *Cellular Microbiology*, Vol. 10, No. 11, pp. 2364-2376, ISSN 1462-5822

Ghosh, S., Chakraborty, K., Nagaraja, T., Basak, S., Koley, H., Dutta, S., Mitra, U. & Das, S. (2011). An adhesion protein of *Salmonella enterica* serovar Typhi is required for pathogenesis and potential target for vaccine development. *Proceedings of the National Academy of Sciences of the United States of America*, Vol. 108, No. 8, pp. 3348-3353, ISSN 1091-6490

Goller, C. C. & Seed, P. C. (2010). High-throughput identification of chemical inhibitors of *E. coli* Group 2 capsule biogenesis as anti-virulence agents. *PLoS One*, Vol. 5, No. 7, p. e11642, ISSN 1932-6203

Grosskinsky, U., Schütz, M., Fritz, M., Schmid, Y., Lamparter, M. C., Szczesny, P., Lupas, A. N., Autenrieth, I. B. & Linke, D. (2007). A conserved glycine residue of trimeric autotransporter domains plays a key role in *Yersinia* adhesin A autotransport. *Journal of Bacteriology*, Vol. 189, No. 24, pp. 9011-9019, ISSN 1098-5530

Gunn, J. S. (2008). The *Salmonella* PmrAB regulon: lipopolysaccharide modifications, antimicrobial peptide resistance and more. *Trends in Microbiology*, Vol. 16, No. 6, pp. 284-290, ISSN 0966-842X

Hammar, M., Bian, Z. & Normark, S. (1996). Nucleator-dependent intercellular assembly of adhesive curli organelles in *Escherichia coli*. *Proceedings of the National Academy of Sciences of the United States of America*, Vol. 93, No. 13, pp. 6562-6566, ISSN 0027-8424

Haraga, A., Ohlson, M. B. & Miller, S. I. (2008). Salmonellae interplay with host cells. *Nature Reviews Microbiology*, Vol. 6, No. 1, pp. 53-66, ISSN 1740-1534

Harris, J. B., Baresch-Bernal, A., Rollins, S. M. & other authors. (2006). Identification of *in vivo*-induced bacterial protein antigens during human infection with *Salmonella enterica* serovar Typhi. *Infection and Immunity*, Vol. 74, No. 9, pp. 5161-5168, ISSN 0019-9567

Harshey, R. M. (2011). New insights into the role and formation of flagella in *Salmonella*, In: *Salmonella: from genome to function*, S. Porwollik (Ed.), pp. 163-186, Caister Academic Press, ISBN 978-1-904455-73-8, Norfolk

Hashimoto, Y., Khan, A. Q. & Ezaki, T. (1996). Positive autoregulation of *vipR* expression in ViaB region-encoded Vi antigen of *Salmonella typhi*. *Journal of Bacteriology*, Vol. 178, No. 5, pp. 1430-1436, ISSN 0021-9193

Hensel, M., Shea, J. E., Waterman, S. R. & other authors. (1998). Genes encoding putative effector proteins of the type III secretion system of *Salmonella* pathogenicity island 2 are required for bacterial virulence and proliferation in macrophages. *Molecular Microbiology*, Vol. 30, No. 1, pp. 163-174, ISSN 0950-382X

Hermant, D., Ménard, R., Arricau, N., Parsot, C. & Popoff, M. Y. (1995). Functional conservation of the *Salmonella* and *Shigella* effectors of entry into epithelial cells. *Molecular Microbiology*, Vol. 17, No. 4, pp. 781-789, ISSN 0950-382X

Heyns, K., Kiessling, G., Lindenberg, W., Paulsen, H. & Webster, M. E. (1959). D-Galaktosaminuornsaure (2-amino-2-desoxy-D-galakturonsaure) als Baustein des Vi-Antigens. *Chemische Berichte*, Vol. 92, No. 10, pp. 2435-2437, ISSN 1099-0682

Hirose, K., Ezaki, T., Miyake, M., Li, T., Khan, A. Q., Kawamura, Y., Yokoyama, H. & Takami, T. (1997). Survival of Vi-capsulated and Vi-deleted *Salmonella typhi* strains in cultured macrophage expressing different levels of CD14 antigen. *FEMS Microbiology Letters*, Vol. 147, No. 2, pp. 259-265, ISSN 0378-1097

Hoare, A., Bittner, M., Carter, J., Alvarez, S., Zaldívar, M., Bravo, D., Valvano, M. A. & Contreras, I. (2006). The outer core lipopolysaccharide of *Salmonella enterica* serovar Typhi is required for bacterial entry into epithelial cells. *Infection and Immunity*, Vol. 74, No. 3, pp. 1555-1564, ISSN 0019-9567

Holt, K. E., Thomson, N. R., Wain, J. & other authors. (2009). Pseudogene accumulation in the evolutionary histories of *Salmonella enterica* serovars Paratyphi A and Typhi. *BMC Genomics*, Vol. 10, p. 36, ISSN 1471-2164

Hölzer, S. U., Schlumberger, M. C., Jäckel, D. & Hensel, M. (2009). Effect of the O-antigen length of lipopolysaccharide on the functions of Type III secretion systems in *Salmonella enterica*. *Infection and Immunity*, Vol. 77, No. 12, pp. 5458-5470, ISSN 1098-5522

Hood, R. D., Singh, P., Hsu, F. & other authors. (2010). A type VI secretion system of *Pseudomonas aeruginosa* targets a toxin to bacteria. *Cell Host Microbe*, Vol. 7, No. 1, pp. 25-37, ISSN 1934-6069

Hu, Y., Cong, Y., Li, S., Rao, X., Wang, G. & Hu, F. (2009). Identification of *in vivo* induced protein antigens of *Salmonella enterica* serovar Typhi during human infection. *Science in China Series C, Life Sciences*, Vol. 52, No. 10, pp. 942-948, ISSN 1862-2798

Hudson, D. L., Layton, A. N., Field, T. R., Bowen, A. J., Wolf-Watz, H., Elofsson, M., Stevens, M. P. & Galyov, E. E. (2007). Inhibition of type III secretion in *Salmonella enterica* serovar Typhimurium by small-molecule inhibitors. *Antimicrobial Agents and Chemotherapy*, Vol. 51, No. 7, pp. 2631-2635, ISSN 0066-4804

Humphries, A. D., Raffatellu, M., Winter, S. & other authors. (2003). The use of flow cytometry to detect expression of subunits encoded by 11 *Salmonella enterica* serotype Typhimurium fimbrial operons. *Molecular Microbiology*, Vol. 48, No. 5, pp. 1357-1376, ISSN 0950-382X

Jacob-Dubuisson, F., Striker, R. & Hultgren, S. J. (1994). Chaperone-assisted self-assembly of pili independent of cellular energy. *Journal of Biological Chemistry*, Vol. 269, No. 17, pp. 12447-12455, ISSN 0021-9258

Janis, C., Grant, A. J., McKinley, T. J., Morgan, F. J., John, V. F., Houghton, J., Kingsley, R. A., Dougan, G. & Mastroeni, P. (2011). *In vivo* regulation of the Vi antigen in *Salmonella* and induction of immune responses with an *in vivo*-inducible promoter. *Infection and Immunity*, Vol. 79, No. 6, pp. 2481-2488, ISSN 1098-5522

Jonas, K., Tomenius, H., Kader, A., Normark, S., Römling, U., Belova, L. M. & Melefors, O. (2007). Roles of curli, cellulose and BapA in *Salmonella* biofilm morphology studied by atomic force microscopy. *BMC Microbiology*, Vol. 7, p. 70, ISSN 1471-2180

Jones, B. D. & Falkow, S. (1994). Identification and characterization of a *Salmonella typhimurium* oxygen-regulated gene required for bacterial internalization. *Infection and Immunity*, Vol. 62, No. 9, pp. 3745-3752, ISSN 0019-9567

Karlinsey, J. E., Tanaka, S., Bettenworth, V., Yamaguchi, S., Boos, W., Aizawa, S. I. & Hughes, K. T. (2000). Completion of the hook-basal body complex of the *Salmonella typhimurium* flagellum is coupled to FlgM secretion and *fliC* transcription. *Molecular Microbiology*, Vol. 37, No. 5, pp. 1220-1231, ISSN 0950-382X

Kidgell, C., Reichard, U., Wain, J., Linz, B., Torpdahl, M., Dougan, G. & Achtman, M. (2002). *Salmonella typhi*, the causative agent of typhoid fever, is approximately 50,000 years old. *Infection, genetic and evolution*, Vol. 2, No. 1, pp. 39-45, ISSN 1567-1348

Kimbrough, T. & Miller, S. (2000). Contribution of *Salmonella typhimurium* type III secretion components to needle complex formation. *Proceedings of the National Academy of Sciences of the United States of America*, Vol. 97, No. 20, pp. 11008-11013, ISSN 0027-8424

Kingsley, R. A., Santos, R. L., Keestra, A. M., Adams, L. G. & Bäumler, A. J. (2002). *Salmonella enterica* serotype Typhimurium ShdA is an outer membrane fibronectin-binding protein that is expressed in the intestine. *Molecular Microbiology*, Vol. 43, No. 4, pp. 895-905, ISSN 0950-382X

Kitagawa, R., Takaya, A., Ohya, M., Mizunoe, Y., Takade, A., Yoshida, S., Isogai, E. & Yamamoto, T. (2010). Biogenesis of *Salmonella enterica* serovar Typhimurium membrane vesicles provoked by induction of PagC. *Journal of Bacteriology*, Vol. 192, No. 21, pp. 5645-5656, ISSN 1098-5530

Klumpp, J. & Fuchs, T. M. (2007). Identification of novel genes in genomic islands that contribute to *Salmonella typhimurium* replication in macrophages. *Microbiology*, Vol. 153, No. 4, pp. 1207-1220, ISSN 1350-0872

Korea, C. G., Ghigo, J. M. & Beloin, C. (2011). The sweet connection: Solving the riddle of multiple sugar-binding fimbrial adhesins in *Escherichia coli*: Multiple *E. coli* fimbriae form a versatile arsenal of sugar-binding lectins potentially involved in surface-colonisation and tissue tropism. *Bioessays*, Vol. 33, No. 4, pp. 300-311, ISSN 1521-1878

Kossack, R. E., Guerrant, R. L., Densen, P., Schadelin, J. & Mandell, G. L. (1981). Diminished neutrophil oxidative metabolism after phagocytosis of virulent *Salmonella typhi*. *Infection and Immunity*, Vol. 31, No. 2, pp. 674-678, ISSN 0019-9567

Krachler, A. M., Ham, H. & Orth, K. (2011). Outer membrane adhesion factor multivalent adhesion molecule 7 initiates host cell binding during infection by Gram-negative pathogens. *Proceedings of the National Academy of Sciences of the United States of America*, Vol. 108, No. 28, pp. 11614-11619, ISSN 1091-6490

Kubori, T., Matsushima, Y., Nakamura, D., Uralil, J., Lara-Tejero, M., Sukhan, A., Galan, J. E. & Aizawa, S. I. (1998). Supramolecular structure of the *Salmonella typhimurium* type III protein secretion system. *Science*, Vol. 280, No. 5363, pp. 602-605, ISSN 0036-8075

Kutsukake, K., Ohya, Y. & Iino, T. (1990). Transcriptional analysis of the flagellar regulon of *Salmonella typhimurium*. *Journal of Bacteriology*, Vol. 172, No. 2, pp. 741-747, ISSN 0021-9193

Latasa, C., Roux, A., Toledo-Arana, A., Ghigo, J. M., Gamazo, C., Penadés, J. R. & Lasa, I. (2005). BapA, a large secreted protein required for biofilm formation and host colonization of *Salmonella enterica* serovar Enteritidis. *Molecular Microbiology*, Vol. 58, No. 5, pp. 1322-1339, ISSN 0950-382X

Lawley, T. D., Chan, K., Thompson, L. J., Kim, C. C., Govoni, G. R. & Monack, D. M. (2006). Genome-wide screen for *Salmonella* genes required for long-term systemic infection of the mouse. *PLoS Pathogens*, Vol. 2, No. 2, p. e11, ISSN 1553-7374

Ledeboer, N. A., Frye, J. G., McClelland, M. & Jones, B. D. (2006). *Salmonella enterica* serovar Typhimurium requires the Lpf, Pef, and Tafi fimbriae for biofilm formation on HEp-2 tissue culture cells and chicken intestinal epithelium. *Infection and Immunity*, Vol. 74, No. 6, pp. 3156-3169, ISSN 0019-9567

Lederberg, J. & Iino, T. (1956). Phase Variation in *Salmonella*. *Genetics*, Vol. 41, No. 5, pp. 743-757, ISSN 0016-6731

Libby, S. J., Brehm, M. A., Greiner, D. L. & other authors. (2010). Humanized nonobese diabetic-scid IL2rgammanull mice are susceptible to lethal *Salmonella* Typhi infection. *Proceedings of the National Academy of Sciences of the United States of America*, Vol. 107, No. 35, pp. 15589-15594, ISSN 1091-6490

Lindow, J. C., Fimlaid, K. A., Bunn, J. Y. & Kirkpatrick, B. D. (2011). Antibodies in Action: Role of Human Opsonins in Killing *Salmonella enterica* Serovar Typhi. *Infection and Immunity*, Vol. 79, No. 8, pp. 3188-3194, ISSN 1098-5522

Liu, S. L., Ezaki, T., Miura, H., Matsui, K. & Yabuuchi, E. (1988). Intact motility as a *Salmonella typhi* invasion-related factor. *Infection and Immunity*, Vol. 56, No. 8, pp. 1967-1973, ISSN 0019-9567

Looney, R. J. & Steigbigel, R. T. (1986). Role of the Vi antigen of *Salmonella typhi* in resistance to host defense *in vitro*. *Journal of Laboratory and Clinical Medicine*, Vol. 108, No. 5, pp. 506-516, ISSN 0022-2143

Lyczak, J. B., Zaidi, T. S., Grout, M., Bittner, M., Contreras, I. & Pier, G. B. (2001). Epithelial cell contact-induced alterations in *Salmonella enterica* serovar Typhi lipopolysaccharide are critical for bacterial internalization. *Cellular Microbiology*, Vol. 3, No. 11, pp. 763-772, ISSN 1462-5814

Lyczak, J. B. & Pier, G. B. (2002). *Salmonella enterica* serovar Typhi modulates cell surface expression of its receptor, the cystic fibrosis transmembrane conductance regulator, on the intestinal epithelium. *Infection and Immunity*, Vol. 70, No. 11, pp. 6416-6423, ISSN 0019-9567

Lynch, S. V. & Wiener-Kronish, J. P. (2008). Novel strategies to combat bacterial virulence. *Current Opinion in Critical Care*, Vol. 14, No. 5, pp. 593-599, ISSN 1531-7072

Ma, A. T., McAuley, S., Pukatzki, S. & Mekalanos, J. J. (2009). Translocation of a *Vibrio cholerae* type VI secretion effector requires bacterial endocytosis by host cells. *Cell Host Microbe*, Vol. 5, No. 3, pp. 234-243, ISSN 1934-6069

Macnab, R. M. (1999). The bacterial flagellum: reversible rotary propellor and type III export apparatus. *Journal of Bacteriology*, Vol. 181, No. 23, pp. 7149-7153, ISSN 0021-9193

Main-Hester, K. L., Colpitts, K. M., Thomas, G. A., Fang, F. C. & Libby, S. J. (2008). Coordinate regulation of *Salmonella* pathogenicity island 1 (SPI1) and SPI4 in

Salmonella enterica serovar Typhimurium. *Infection and Immunity*, Vol. 76, No. 3, pp. 1024-1035, ISSN 1098-5522

Mattick, J. S. (2002). Type IV pili and twitching motility. *Annual Review of Microbiology*, Vol. 56, pp. 289-314, ISSN 0066-4227

Miller, S. I., Kukral, A. M. & Mekalanos, J. J. (1989). A two-component regulatory system (*phoP phoQ*) controls *Salmonella typhimurium* virulence. *Proceedings of the National Academy of Sciences of the United States of America*, Vol. 86, No. 13, pp. 5054-5058, ISSN 0027-8424

Minamino, T. & Namba, K. (2008). Distinct roles of the FliI ATPase and proton motive force in bacterial flagellar protein export. *Nature*, Vol. 451, No. 7177, pp. 485-488, ISSN 1476-4687

Miras, I., Hermant, D., Arricau, N. & Popoff, M. Y. (1995). Nucleotide sequence of *iagA* and *iagB* genes involved in invasion of HeLa cells by *Salmonella enterica* subsp. *enterica* ser. Typhi. *Research in Microbiology*, Vol. 146, No. 1, pp. 17-20, ISSN 0923-2508

Miyake, M., Zhao, L., Ezaki, T. & other authors. (1998). Vi-deficient and nonfimbriated mutants of *Salmonella typhi* agglutinate human blood type antigens and are hyperinvasive. *FEMS Microbiology Letters*, Vol. 161, No. 1, pp. 75-82, ISSN 0378-1097

Morgan, E., Campbell, J. D., Rowe, S. C., Bispham, J., Stevens, M. P., Bowen, A. J., Barrow, P. A., Maskell, D. J. & Wallis, T. S. (2004). Identification of host-specific colonization factors of *Salmonella enterica* serovar Typhimurium. *Molecular Microbiology*, Vol. 54, No. 4, pp. 994-1010, ISSN 0950-382X

Morris, C., Tam, C. K., Wallis, T. S., Jones, P. W. & Hackett, J. (2003a). *Salmonella enterica* serovar Dublin strains which are Vi antigen-positive use type IVB pili for bacterial self-association and human intestinal cell entry. *Microbial Pathogenesis*, Vol. 35, No. 6, pp. 279-284, ISSN 0882-4010

Morris, C., Yip, C. M., Tsui, I. S., Wong, D. K. & Hackett, J. (2003b). The shufflon of *Salmonella enterica* serovar Typhi regulates type IVB pilus-mediated bacterial self-association. *Infection and Immunity*, Vol. 71, No. 3, pp. 1141-1146, ISSN 0019-9567

Nagy, G., Danino, V., Dobrindt, U., Pallen, M., Chaudhuri, R., Emödy, L., Hinton, J. C. & Hacker, J. (2006). Down-regulation of key virulence factors makes the *Salmonella enterica* serovar Typhimurium *rfaH* mutant a promising live-attenuated vaccine candidate. *Infection and Immunity*, Vol. 74, No. 10, pp. 5914-5925, ISSN 0019-9567

Nambiar, M., Harish, B. N., Mangilal, V., Pai, D. & Parija, S. C. (2009). Immunoblot analysis of sera in uncomplicated typhoid fever & with typhoid ileal perforation. *Indian Journal of Medical Research*, Vol. 129, No. 4, pp. 432-437, ISSN 0971-5916

Neely, A. N., Holder, I. A., Wiener-Kronish, J. P. & Sawa, T. (2005). Passive anti-PcrV treatment protects burned mice against *Pseudomonas aeruginosa* challenge. *Burns*, Vol. 31, No. 2, pp. 153-158, ISSN 0305-4179

Nishimura, K., Tajima, N., Yoon, Y. H., Park, S. Y. & Tame, J. R. (2010). Autotransporter passenger proteins: virulence factors with common structural themes. *Journal of Molecular Medicine*, Vol. 88, No. 5, pp. 451-458, ISSN 1432-1440

Nishio, M., Okada, N., Miki, T., Haneda, T. & Danbara, H. (2005). Identification of the outer-membrane protein PagC required for the serum resistance phenotype in *Salmonella enterica* serovar Choleraesuis. *Microbiology*, Vol. 151, No. 3, pp. 863-873, ISSN 1350-0872

Nishiyama, M., Ishikawa, T., Rechsteiner, H. & Glockshuber, R. (2008). Reconstitution of pilus assembly reveals a bacterial outer membrane catalyst. *Science*, Vol. 320, No. 5874, pp. 376-379, ISSN 1095-9203

Nordfelth, R., Kauppi, A. M., Norberg, H. A., Wolf-Watz, H. & Elofsson, M. (2005). Small-molecule inhibitors specifically targeting type III secretion. *Infection and Immunity*, Vol. 73, No. 5, pp. 3104-3114, ISSN 0019-9567

Norris, T. & Bäumler, A. (1999). Phase variation of the *lpf* operon is a mechanism to evade cross-immunity between *Salmonella* serotypes. *Proceedings of the National Academy of Sciences of the United States of America*, Vol. 96, No. 23, pp. 13393-13398, ISSN 0027-8424

Nuccio, S. P. & Bäumler, A. J. (2007). Evolution of the chaperone/usher assembly pathway: fimbrial classification goes Greek. *Microbiology and Molecular Biology Reviews*, Vol. 71, No. 4, pp. 551-575, ISSN 1092-2172

Nuccio, S. P., Thomson, N. R., Fookes, M. C. & Baümler, A. J. (2011). Fimbrial signature arrangements in *Salmonella* In: *Salmonella: from genome to function*, S. Porwollick (Ed.), pp. 149-161, Caister Academic Press, ISBN 978-1-904455-73-8, Norfolk

Pan, Q., Zhang, X. L., Wu, H. Y., He, P. W., Wang, F., Zhang, M. S., Hu, J. M., Xia, B. & Wu, J. (2005). Aptamers that preferentially bind type IVB pili and inhibit human monocytic-cell invasion by *Salmonella enterica* serovar Typhi. *Antimicrobial Agents and Chemotherapy*, Vol. 49, No. 10, pp. 4052-4060, ISSN 0066-4804

Pang, T., Levine, M. M., Ivanoff, B., Wain, J. & Finlay, B. B. (1998). Typhoid fever--important issues still remain. *Trends in Microbiology*, Vol. 6, No. 4, pp. 131-133, ISSN 0966-842X

Parkhill, J., Dougan, G., James, K. D. & other authors. (2001). Complete genome sequence of a multiple drug resistant *Salmonella enterica* serovar Typhi CT18. *Nature*, Vol. 413, No. 6858, pp. 848-852, ISSN 0028-0836

Parry, C. M., Hien, T. T., Dougan, G., White, N. J. & Farrar, J. J. (2002). Typhoid fever. *New England Journal of Medicine*, Vol. 347, No. 22, pp. 1770-1782, ISSN 1533-4406

Paul, K., Erhardt, M., Hirano, T., Blair, D. F. & Hughes, K. T. (2008). Energy source of flagellar type III secretion. *Nature*, Vol. 451, No. 7177, pp. 489-492, ISSN 1476-4687

Pickard, D., Li, J., Roberts, M., Maskell, D., Hone, D., Levine, M., Dougan, G. & Chatfield, S. (1994). Characterization of defined *ompR* mutants of *Salmonella typhi*: *ompR* is involved in the regulation of Vi polysaccharide expression. *Infection and Immunity*, Vol. 62, No. 9, pp. 3984-3993, ISSN 0019-9567

Pier, G. B., Grout, M., Zaidi, T., Meluleni, G., Mueschenborn, S. S., Banting, G., Ratcliff, R., Evans, M. J. & Colledge, W. H. (1998). *Salmonella typhi* uses CFTR to enter intestinal epithelial cells. *Nature*, Vol. 393, No. 6680, pp. 79-82, ISSN 0028-0836

Pinkner, J. S., Remaut, H., Buelens, F. & other authors. (2006). Rationally designed small compounds inhibit pilus biogenesis in uropathogenic bacteria. *Proceedings of the National Academy of Sciences of the United States of America*, Vol. 103, No. 47, pp. 17897-17902, ISSN 0027-8424

Popoff, M. Y., Bockemühl, J., Brenner, F. W. & Gheesling, L. L. (2001). Supplement 2000 (no. 44) to the Kauffmann-White scheme. *Research in Microbiology*, Vol. 152, No. 10, pp. 907-909, ISSN 0923-2508

Prouty, A. M., Schwesinger, W. H. & Gunn, J. S. (2002). Biofilm formation and interaction with the surfaces of gallstones by *Salmonella* spp. *Infection and Immunity*, Vol. 70, No. 5, pp. 2640-2649, ISSN 0019-9567

Pukatzki, S., McAuley, S. B. & Miyata, S. T. (2009). The type VI secretion system: translocation of effectors and effector-domains. *Current Opinion in Microbiology*, Vol. 12, No. 1, pp. 11-17, ISSN 1879-0364

Raetz, C. R. & Whitfield, C. (2002). Lipopolysaccharide endotoxins. *Annual Review of Biochemistry*, Vol. 71, pp. 635-700, ISSN 0066-4154

Reeves, P. (1993). Evolution of *Salmonella* O antigen variation by interspecific gene transfer on a large scale. *Trends in Genetics*, Vol. 9, No. 1, pp. 17-22, ISSN 0168-9525

Reeves, P. R., Hobbs, M., Valvano, M. A. & other authors. (1996). Bacterial polysaccharide synthesis and gene nomenclature. *Trends in Microbiology*, Vol. 4, No. 12, pp. 495-503, ISSN 0966-842X

Robbins, J. D. & Robbins, J. B. (1984). Reexamination of the protective role of the capsular polysaccharide (Vi antigen) of *Salmonella typhi*. *Journal of Infectious Diseases*, Vol. 150, No. 3, pp. 436-449, ISSN 0022-1899

Römling, U., Bokranz, W., Rabsch, W., Zogaj, X., Nimtz, M. & Tschäpe, H. (2003). Occurrence and regulation of the multicellular morphotype in *Salmonella* serovars important in human disease. *International Journal of Medical Microbiology*, Vol. 293, No. 4, pp. 273-285, ISSN 1438-4221

Sabbagh, S. C., Forest, C. G., Lepage, C., Leclerc, J. M. & Daigle, F. (2010). So similar, yet so different: uncovering distinctive features in the genomes of *Salmonella enterica* serovars Typhimurium and Typhi. *FEMS Microbiology Letters*, Vol. 305, No. 1, pp. 1-13, ISSN 1574-6968

Saini, S., Slauch, J. M., Aldridge, P. D. & Rao, C. V. (2010). Role of cross talk in regulating the dynamic expression of the flagellar *Salmonella* pathogenicity island 1 and type 1 fimbrial genes. *Journal of Bacteriology*, Vol. 192, No. 21, pp. 5767-5777, ISSN 1098-5530

Salih, O., Remaut, H., Waksman, G. & Orlova, E. V. (2008). Structural analysis of the Saf pilus by electron microscopy and image processing. *Journal of Molecular Biology*, Vol. 379, No. 1, pp. 174-187, ISSN 1089-8638

Sanowar, S., Singh, P., Pfuetzner, R. A. & other authors. (2010). Interactions of the transmembrane polymeric rings of the *Salmonella enterica* serovar Typhimurium type III secretion system. *MBio*, Vol. 1, No. 3, ISSN 2150-7511

Santander, J., Wanda, S. Y., Nickerson, C. A. & Curtiss III, R. (2007). Role of RpoS in fine-tuning the synthesis of Vi capsular polysaccharide in *Salmonella enterica* serotype Typhi. *Infection and Immunity*, Vol. 75, No. 3, pp. 1382-1392, ISSN 0019-9567

Satta, G., Ingianni, L., Muscas, P., Rossolini, A. & Pompei, R. (1993). The pathogenicity determinants of *Salmonella typhi*: potential role of fimbrial structures, In: *Biology of Salmonella*, F. Cabello, C. Hormaeche, P. Mastroeni & L. Bonina (Eds.), pp. 83-90, Plenum Press, ISBN 0306444925, New York

Sauer, F. G., Pinkner, J. S., Waksman, G. & Hultgren, S. J. (2002). Chaperone priming of pilus subunits facilitates a topological transition that drives fiber formation. *Cell*, Vol. 111, No. 4, pp. 543-551, ISSN 0092-8674

Simon, M., Zieg, J., Silverman, M., Mandel, G. & Doolittle, R. (1980). Phase variation: evolution of a controlling element. *Science*, Vol. 209, No. 4463, pp. 1370-1374, ISSN 0036-8075

Swietnicki, W., Carmany, D., Retford, M., Guelta, M., Dorsey, R., Bozue, J., Lee, M. S. & Olson, M. A. (2011). Identification of small-molecule inhibitors of *Yersinia pestis* Type III secretion system YscN ATPase. *PLoS One*, Vol. 6, No. 5, p. e19716, ISSN 1932-6203

Thankavel, K., Shah, A. H., Cohen, M. S., Ikeda, T., Lorenz, R. G., Curtiss III, R. & Abraham, S. N. (1999). Molecular basis for the enterocyte tropism exhibited by *Salmonella typhimurium* type 1 fimbriae. *Journal of Biological Chemistry*, Vol. 274, No. 9, pp. 5797-5809, ISSN 0021-9258

Townsend, S. M., Kramer, N. E., Edwards, R. & other authors. (2001). *Salmonella enterica* serovar Typhi possesses a unique repertoire of fimbrial gene sequences. *Infection and Immunity*, Vol. 69, No. 5, pp. 2894-2901, ISSN 0019-9567

Tsui, I. S., Yip, C. M., Hackett, J. & Morris, C. (2003). The type IVB pili of *Salmonella enterica* serovar Typhi bind to the cystic fibrosis transmembrane conductance regulator. *Infection and Immunity*, Vol. 71, No. 10, pp. 6049-6050, ISSN 0019-9567

Virlogeux, I., Waxin, H., Ecobichon, C., Lee, J. O. & Popoff, M. Y. (1996). Characterization of the *rcsA* and *rcsB* genes from *Salmonella typhi*: *rcsB* through *tviA* is involved in regulation of Vi antigen synthesis. *Journal of Bacteriology*, Vol. 178, No. 6, pp. 1691-1698, ISSN 0021-9193

Wang, F., Zhang, X. L., Zhou, Y., Ye, L., Qi, Z. & Wu, J. (2005). Type IVB piliated *Salmonella typhi* enhance IL-6 and NF-kappaB production in human monocytic THP-1 cells through activation of protein kinase C. *Immunobiology*, Vol. 210, No. 5, pp. 283-293, ISSN 0171-2985

Wang, M., Luo, Z., Du, H., Xu, S., Ni, B., Zhang, H., Sheng, X., Xu, H. & Huang, X. (2011). Molecular Characterization of a Functional Type VI Secretion System in *Salmonella enterica* serovar Typhi. *Current Microbiology*, Vol. 63, No. 1, pp. 22-31, ISSN 1432-0991

Wang, S., Li, Y., Shi, H., Sun, W., Roland, K. L. & Curtiss III, R. (2011). Comparison of a regulated delayed antigen synthesis system with *in vivo*-inducible promoters for antigen delivery by live attenuated *Salmonella* vaccines. *Infection and Immunity*, Vol. 79, No. 2, pp. 937-949, ISSN 1098-5522

Waterman, S. R. & Holden, D. W. (2003). Functions and effectors of the *Salmonella* pathogenicity island 2 type III secretion system. *Cellular Microbiology*, Vol. 5, No. 8, pp. 501-511, ISSN 1462-5814

Weber, B., Hasic, M., Chen, C., Wai, S. N. & Milton, D. L. (2009). Type VI secretion modulates quorum sensing and stress response in *Vibrio anguillarum*. *Environmental Microbiology*, Vol. 11, No. 12, pp. 3018-3028, ISSN 1462-2920

Weening, E. H., Barker, J. D., Laarakker, M. C., Humphries, A. D., Tsolis, R. M. & Bäumler, A. J. (2005). The *Salmonella enterica* serotype Typhimurium *lpf, bcf, stb, stc, std,* and *sth* fimbrial operons are required for intestinal persistence in mice. *Infection and Immunity*, Vol. 73, No. 6, pp. 3358-3366, ISSN 0019-9567

White, A. P., Gibson, D. L., Kim, W., Kay, W. W. & Surette, M. G. (2006). Thin aggregative fimbriae and cellulose enhance long-term survival and persistence of *Salmonella*. *Journal of Bacteriology*, Vol. 188, No. 9, pp. 3219-3227, ISSN 0021-9193

Wilson, R. P., Winter, S. E., Spees, A. M. & other authors. (2011). The Vi capsular polysaccharide prevents complement receptor 3-mediated clearance of *Salmonella enterica* serotype Typhi. *Infection and Immunity*, Vol. 79, No. 2, pp. 830-837, ISSN 1098-5522

Winter, S. E., Raffatellu, M., Wilson, R. P., Rüssmann, H. & Bäumler, A. J. (2008). The *Salmonella enterica* serotype Typhi regulator TviA reduces interleukin-8 production in intestinal epithelial cells by repressing flagellin secretion. *Cellular Microbiology*, Vol. 10, No. 1, pp. 247-261, ISSN 1462-5822

World Health Organization, Department of Vaccines and Biologicals. (May 2003). *Background document: the diagnosis, prevention and treatment of typhoid fever*. Geneva, Switzerland, pp. 1-38. Available from www.who.int/entity/vaccine_research/documents/en/typhoid_diagnosis.pdf.

Yu, X. J., Liu, M. & Holden, D. W. (2004). SsaM and SpiC interact and regulate secretion of *Salmonella* pathogenicity island 2 type III secretion system effectors and translocators. *Molecular Microbiology*, Vol. 54, No. 3, pp. 604-619, ISSN 0950-382X

Zavialov, A. V., Kersley, J., Korpela, T., Zav'yalov, V. P., MacIntyre, S. & Knight, S. D. (2002). Donor strand complementation mechanism in the biogenesis of non-pilus systems. *Molecular Microbiology*, Vol. 45, No. 4, pp. 983-995, ISSN 0950-382X

Zenk, S. F., Jantsch, J. & Hensel, M. (2009). Role of *Salmonella enterica* lipopolysaccharide in activation of dendritic cell functions and bacterial containment. *Journal of Immunology*, Vol. 183, No. 4, pp. 2697-2707, ISSN 1550-6606

Zhang, X. L., Tsui, I. S., Yip, C. M., Fung, A. W., Wong, D. K., Dai, X., Yang, Y., Hackett, J. & Morris, C. (2000). *Salmonella enterica* serovar Typhi uses type IVB pili to enter human intestinal epithelial cells. *Infection and Immunity*, Vol. 68, No. 6, pp. 3067-3073, ISSN 0019-9567

Zhao, L., Ezak, T., Li, Z. Y., Kawamura, Y., Hirose, K. & Watanabe, H. (2001). Vi-Suppressed wild strain *Salmonella typhi* cultured in high osmolarity is hyperinvasive toward epithelial cells and destructive of Peyer's patches. *Microbiology and Immunology*, Vol. 45, No. 2, pp. 149-158, ISSN 0385-5600

Zhao, Y., Jansen, R., Gaastra, W., Arkesteijn, G., van der Zeijst, B. A. & van Putten, J. P. (2002). Identification of genes affecting *Salmonella enterica* serovar Enteritidis infection of chicken macrophages. *Infection and Immunity*, Vol. 70, No. 9, pp. 5319-5321, ISSN 0019-9567

Zogaj, X., Nimtz, M., Rohde, M., Bokranz, W. & Römling, U. (2001). The multicellular morphotypes of *Salmonella typhimurium* and *Escherichia coli* produce cellulose as the second component of the extracellular matrix. *Molecular Microbiology*, Vol. 39, No. 6, pp. 1452-1463, ISSN 0950-382X

Molecular Diagnosis of Enteric Fever: Progress and Perspectives

Liqing Zhou, Thomas Darton, Claire Waddington and Andrew J. Pollard
University of Oxford
United Kingdom

1. Introduction

Enteric fever is a severe systemic Gram-negative bacterial infection caused by several serovars of *Salmonella enterica* subspecies *enterica*, including *S.* Typhi and *S.* Paratyphi serotypes A (most commonly), B and C. It is characterised by high fever and a myriad of other non-specific features, including abdominal pain and constipation, headache, myalgia and arthralgia, cough, lymphadenopathy and rash. *S.* Typhi, the human-specific causative agent of typhoid fever, is thought to account for an estimated 21 million new cases and 216,000 deaths every year (Crump et al., 2004). *S.* Typhi is generally transmitted in food and water contaminated with faeces from those excreting bacteria, either during the acute illness or during chronic asymptomatic carriage, although infection of health-care or laboratory workers through poor hygiene practices or accidental exposure is also described. Transmission in regions with adequate sanitation and sewage facilities is uncommon as, in general, a relatively high inoculum is required to survive the gastric acid environment and cause infection. Enteric fever is therefore most common in resource-poor settings where the provision of clean drinking water and sewage disposal facilities is inadequate. South and Central Asia, Africa and South and Central America are considered endemic for this disease and particularly high incidence rates are found in the Indian sub-continent and South-east Asia, with rates exceeding 100 per 100,000 population per year (Bhan et al., 2005). In other countries typhoid fever remains an important consideration for travellers both pre- and post-travel (Levine et al., 1982; Ackers et al., 2000; Bhan et al., 2005).

The accurate and rapid clinical diagnosis of enteric fever in these regions is obfuscated by the range of other common fever-causing infections including malaria, dengue fever, leptospirosis, melioidosis and the rickettsioses. Accurate diagnosis to differentiate typhoid fever from these conditions is often difficult, both in the clinic and in the laboratory, but is imperative for effective treatment selection. Even in highly-resourced western countries, physicians often start typhoid treatment empirically whilst awaiting confirmation of the diagnosis. Treatment decisions are further complicated by the increasing prevalence of antibiotic resistance amongst clinical isolates due to plasmid-mediated multidrug resistance (in particular the gyrA gene mutation, conferring variable fluoroquinolone resistance in both *S.* Typhi and *S.* Paratyphi A (Chau et al., 2007)) and the potential for extended-spectrum β-lactamase (ESBL) and carbapenemase-producing strains (Al Naiemi et al., 2008; Pokharel et al., 2006; Nordmann et al., 2008). Rates of illness caused by *S.* Parathyphi and non–typhoidal *Salmonella* are increasing in many endemic areas further complicating accurate laboratory testing (Ochiai et al., 2005; Palit et al., 2006).

It has long been accepted that vaccines represent the most cost effective approach to control typhoid infection, especially in the era of widespread and increasing antibiotic resistance (Parry et al., 2002; Whitaker et al., 2009). However, few countries have taken up routine typhoid immunization, partially due to uncertainty on disease burden and vaccine effectiveness. The development of cheap and reliable enteric fever diagnostics would play a key role in more accurately defining the scale of the problem and thus facilitating both long-term disease control and individual patient treatment (Baker et al., 2010). A combination of accurate diagnosis, effective vaccination and directed treatment could ultimately lead to the eradication of this human-restricted infection if appropriately implemented. Here we review the current means available for enteric fever diagnosis and the progress being made in improving molecular diagnostics in particular.

2. Clinical diagnosis of enteric fever

Enteric fever may affect individuals of any age; recently it has been shown to affect a much higher proportion of children aged less than 5 years than previously thought, causing a similar range of signs and symptoms to those seen in adults (Sinha et al., 1999). Immunosuppressed individuals, those with reduced gastric acid production, biliary and urinary tract abnormalities, haemoglobinpathies and other concomitant infectious diseases (including malaria and schistosomiasis) are at higher risk of acquiring infection and at risk of developing more severe or disseminated disease (Gotuzzo et al., 1991; Khosla et al., 1993; Mathai et al., 1995; Bhan et al., 2002; Crawford et al., 2010).

The clinical presentation of typhoid fever is notoriously variable, ranging from non-specific fever symptoms to fulminant Gram-negative sepsis with multisystem disease. The incubation period is classically 10 to 14 days although can range from 5 to 21 days. Early evidence suggested that as well as asymptomatic carriers, some individuals are capable of remaining asymptomatic and afebrile despite demonstrable bacteraemia (Snyder et al., 1963). The incubation period is likely to be directly proportional to the inoculum ingested and the cell-mediated immune response of the individual infected, although precise correlates of protection have yet to be determined (Sztein, 2007).

In the early days following infection, individuals may develop diarrhoea and abdominal discomfort. Diarrhoea is thought to be more common in certain geographic areas and in individuals with HIV/AIDS and in children less than 1 year of age (Butler et al., 1991). After a variable asymptomatic duration, individuals may develop constipation (10-38%), abdominal pain (30-40%), headache (often a dull frontal aching, 62%) and fever (Stuart & Pollen, 1946; Clark et al., 2010). Various studies have shown that fever is present in from 75 to 100% of microbiologically-confirmed cases on presentation (Stuart & Pullen, 1946; Butler et al., 1991; Clark et al., 2010); it classically starts low and increases in a saw-toothed pattern, often to between 39 and 40°C by the second week (see figure 1).

The spectrum of symptoms experienced is highly varied, and therefore the diagnosis may be missed particularly in areas where other febrile illnesses, such as malaria, tuberculosis or dengue, are common. Other presentations may include a more 'food poisoning' type illness with diarrhoea and vomiting or a predominantly respiratory presentation with symptoms including cough and audible crackles on chest auscultation. Other clinical findings of note include a relative bradycardia (Faget's sign, which occurs in less than 50% of patients), hepatosplenomegaly (20 to 50%) and Rose spots (up to 25%), which are classically described as salmon pink evanescent maculopapular spots seen towards the end of the first week of illness on the trunk, and from which *S.* Typhi may be cultured if biopsied (Parry et al., 2002; World Health Organization, 2003).

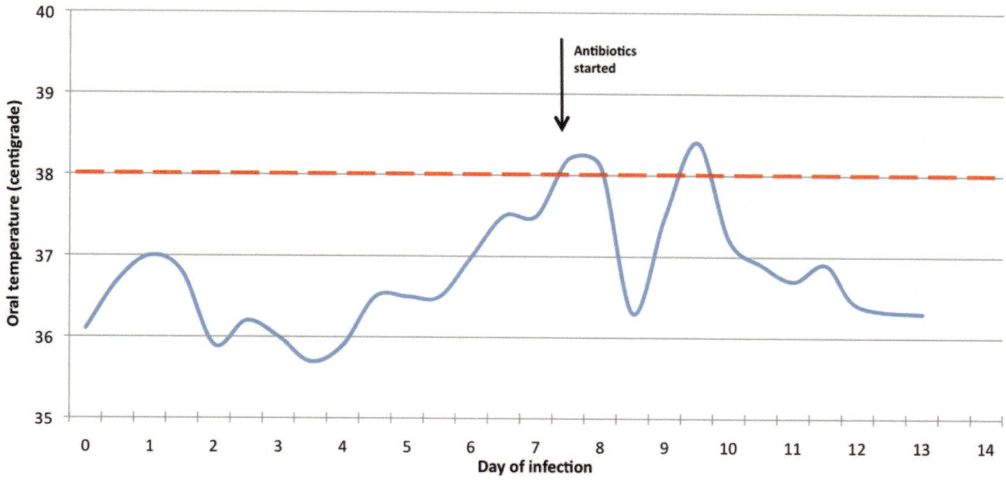

Fig. 1. The variation of oral temperature during typhoid infection

Presentation of neonatal typhoid fever resulting from vertical transmission during late pregnancy is usually within 3 days of delivery; signs including fever, vomiting, diarrhoea, and abdominal distension (Bhan et al., 2005). Significant hepatomegaly and jaundice and seizures can occur (Butler et al., 1991). Typhoid fever typically presents as a milder or atypical illness, often as a severe pneumonia, in children younger than 5 years (Mahle & Levine, 1993). The rate of severe complications is lower than in older age-groups (Mahle & Levine, 1993; Chiu & Lin, 1999; Sinha et al., 1999; Bhan et al., 2005).

Duration of illness before therapy, choice of antimicrobial therapy, strain virulence, inoculum size, previous exposure or vaccination, and other host factors such as HLA type, AIDS or other immune suppression, antacid consumption or concomittant *H. pylori* infection (Bhan et al., 2002) affect severity of the disease. Depending on the clinical resources available, approximately 10–15% of patients may develop more severe disease charaterised by the development of abdominal complications (Bhan et al., 2005). Gastrointestinal bleeding, intestinal perforation and typhoid encephalopathy are the commonest complications (Ali et al., 1997; Parry et al., 2002; World Health Organization, 2003; Bhan et al., 2005). The more details of clinical features of typhoid complications are described in the Seminar by Bhan et al. (Bhan et al., 2005).

Traditionally, the clinical features of paratyphoid fever were thought to be similar or milder than those of typhoid fever. With increasing incidence and more data now available, studies have started to demonstrate an equivalent or even increased rate of complications with paratyphoid infections (Ekdahl et al., 2005; Meltzer et al., 2005; Vollaard et al., 2005; Maskey et al., 2006; Woods et al., 2006). *S.* Paratyphi A, B or C may present with either systemic (Lee et al., 2000; Rajagopal et al., 2002; Mohanty et al., 2003) or localised infection (Fangtham et al., 2008). A relapse rate of 8% has been reported with *S.* Paratyphi A which is increasing in incidence throughout Southeast Asia (Ochiai et al., 2005; Woods et al., 2006; Fangtham et al., 2008) and may be associated with higher rates of complicated disease and outbreaks of infection (Khan et al., 2007; Pandit et al., 2008; Patel et al., 2010). *S.* Paratyphi A and B may present with a non-specific *Salmonella* gastroenteritis with diarrhoea being a predominant symptom (Thisyakorn et al., 1987; Yang et al., 2010). Gastrointestinal symptoms are usually not present with *S.* Paratyphi C infection but there have been cases with systemic complications such as septicaemia and arthritis (Lang et al., 1992).

3. Laboratory diagnosis of enteric fever

Current widely used methods for the diagnosis of individuals with enteric fever include bacterial culture, microscopy and serological assays, specifically the Widal test, which have been recently reviewed by Bhan et al. (2005), Bhutta (2006), Kundu et al. (2006), Wain & Hosoglu (2008) and Parry et al. (2011). Molecular diagnostics of enteric fever, in particular nucleic acid amplification by polymerase chain reaction (PCR), have been growing rapidly in last decade although they are confined within the research setting.

3.1 Bacterial culture

Accurate diagnosis of enteric fever requires isolation (or detection) of the causative organism, preferably from a sterile site (World Health Organization, 2003). Even though an array of specimens including whole blood, bone marrow, stool, duodenal fluid, urine and skin (Rose spots) (Gilman et al., 1975; Vallenas et al., 1985; Hoffman et al., 1986; Rubin et al., 1990) have historically been shown to harbor cultivable bacteria, blood is the most common specimen submitted for culture of *S.* Typhi (Parry et al., 2002; Wain and Hosoglu 2008). Between 45 and 70% of patients with typhoid fever may be diagnosed by blood culture (World Health Organization, 2003; Wain et al., 2001, 2008). The sensitivity of culture from blood is dependent on a variety of factors including the volume of blood taken (and its ratio to enrichment broth), pre-treatment with antibiotics and delay in transportation of the sample to the laboratory (Wain et al., 2008). As the number of circulating bacteria may be extremely low and predominantly intracellular (over 50% in one study (Wain et al., 2001)), any of these variables may significantly affect the growth and therefore the isolation rate. Use of selective media such as ox bile broth may increase this rate, as, while selective for bile resistant organisms, it inhibits some of the bactericidal activity of blood and is capable of releasing intracellular bacteria (Coleman & Buxton, 1907; Kaye et al., 1966; Wain et al., 2008). Research performed in our laboratory has also confirmed that bile (as ox bile soy tryptone broth) causes selective lysis of mammalian cells whilst leaving bacterial cells intact and capable of unhindered growth in culture (Zhou & Pollard, 2010). Whilst useful for research settings, selective culture of blood in bile-containing media outside of highly endemic regions is unhelpful in the general microbiology laboratory although alternative additives such as saponin have also been investigated (Murray et al., 1991; Wain & Hosoglu 2008; Wain et al., 2008).

Although it is thought that a significant inoculum is required to cause typhoid fever, in those with enhanced susceptibility, ingestion of even a small number of *S.* Typhi organisms may be sufficient to cause infection. Previous studies using a typhoid challenge model in healthy adult volunteers demonstrated that as few as 10^5 organisms were capable of causing disease following gastric acid suppression using milk (Glynn et al., 1995). In ongoing challenge studies, we have demonstrated that as few as 700 colony forming units (CFU) of non-attenuated live *S.* Typhi may cause clinical illness after gastric acid suppression using sodium bicarbonate. That very low numbers of *S.* Typhi are found circulating in the bloodstream at onset of symptoms in most typhoid cases is therefore not surprising; in 81 patients diagnosed with typhoid fever, a median level of 0.3 (IQR, 0.1-10) bacteria per millilitre of blood was found (Wain et al., 2001). Therefore, one of the key issues in typhoid diagnostics is how to detect the extremely low level bacteraemia present in a sick patient. Even using modern PCR and related diagnostics, current studies often still employ a pre-culture stage in order to try and maximise the organism detection rate (Nga et al., 2010; Zhou & Pollard, 2010).

Bone marrow harbors over 10 times as many organisms per unit volume than in the blood (Wain et al., 2008). Aside from the degree of patient discomfort involved, bone marrow aspiration and culture may therefore represent a useful addition to blood culture if appropriate facilities exist, particularly in patients who have been heavily antibiotic exposed (Wain et al., 2001) or who are being investigated for haematological conditions or pyrexia of unknown origin simultaneously (Volk et al., 1998).

Stool specimens are commonly collected during the diagnostic work-up of patients with typhoid infection, but there may be difficulty in obtaining specimens due to constipation when rectal swabs are a less good alternative. Stool should be cultured in selenite enrichment broth to maximise the culture yield (Moriñigo et al., 1993) for which standard selenite F medium appears at least as effective as selenite supplemented with mannitol (selenite M) (Wain et al., 2008). The results of a positive stool culture need to be interpreted in light of the clinical condition of the patient to exclude healthy carriers (such as `Typhoid Mary') (Soper, 1939). Stool cultures obtained from acutely ill patients may become positive before blood cultures, immediately preceeding either the primary or secondary bacteraemic phase, and their sensitivity increases with the quantity obtained (Personal observations; Wain et al., 2008). Stool cultures are therefore a useful aid to diagnosis and to guide public health prevention activities in certain settings.

Rose spot skin biopsies (Gilman et al., 1975; Wain et al., 1998) and urine samples may also be used for culturing *S.* Typhi, the latter being culture positive in approximately 7% of confirmed cases (Gilman et al., 1975). Duodenal contents obtained using a duodenal string test or aspiration may be more useful for culture identification of causative organisms, but the procedures required are often poorly tolerated, particularly by young children (Vallenas et al., 1985).

Most diagnoses of enteric fever are still made by blood culture followed by microbiological identification. However, blood culture, whilst considered "routine" in most resource-rich settings, is expensive, requiring specialist facilities and personnel, and time-consuming, taking at least 2 to 5 days for organism growth and positive identification.

3.2 Serological tests

Several serological tests have been developed in order to detect the presence of either *S.* Typhi antigens or the antibody response to it. The classic Widal test, a tube agglutination test developed by Widal F. in 1896 (Widal et al., 1896), detects the presence of agglutinating antibodies in the serum of infected/exposed patients against lipopolysaccharide (LPS; O) and flagella (H) antigens of *S.* Typhi (Olopoenia & King, 2000; World Health Organization, 2003). These antibodies present at 6 to 8 days and 10 to 12 days respectively, following infection; a 4-fold rise in either of these antibodies between acute and convalescent sera is diagnostic (World Health Organization, 2003). The test is only moderately specific for typhoid infection; however, studies from several areas, predominantly endemic for typhoid infection, demonstrate a significant variation in assay performance particularly when using a single Widal test result to make a typhoid fever diagnosis. Reasons for false-positive test results may include previous vaccination or exposure to natural infection, cross-reactivity with epitopes from other enterobacteriaceae or concomittant infections including malaria, typhus and other causes of bacteraemia (Reynolda et al., 1970; Levine et al., 1978; Olopoenia & King, 2000; House et al., 2001; World Health Organization, 2003; Omuse et al., 2010). Likewise, false-negative tests are also seen which may be due to previous antibiotic exposure or other medical conditions capable of reducing the antibody response generated. Widal tests are relatively inexpensive however, particularly in comparison to bacterial culture methods, and are therefore still widely used (Bakr et al., 2011) and are possibly of more benefit in non-endemic settings (Levine et al., 1978; Chew et al., 1992).

Much effort has been put into improving on the classic Widal test over the last twenty years specifically in order to improve the speed and reliability of serological testing (Bhutta & Mansurali, 1999; House et al., 2001; Gasem et al., 2002; Hatta et al., 2002; Jesudason et al., 2002; Olsen et al., 2004; Tam et al., 2008; Fadeel et al., 2011). Several of these assays have subsequently become commerically available; Typhidot® (Malaysian Biodiagnostic Research SDN BHD, Malaysia) and TUBEX assays (IDL Bideh, Solletuna, Sweden) are discussed in further detail below.

Typhidot® is a dot enzyme-linked immunosorbent assay capable of detecting both IgM and IgG antibodies against a *S.* Typhi-specific 50kDa outer membrane protein (OMP) (Ismail et al., 1991; Choo et al., 1994, 1999). OMP dotted onto a nitrocellulose strip is probed with test sera and developed using peroxidase-conjugated antihuman IgM/IgG antibodies and a substrate for colour development (Choo et al., 1994; Kawano et al., 2007).

TUBEX-TF® is an inhibition binding assay that detects the presence of the O9 component of *S.* Typhi LPS. Binding of *S.* Typhi LPS (O9) antibody-coated indicator to *S.* Typhi LPS (antigen)-coated magnetic particles is inhibited by patient sera containing anti-O9 antibodies, which results in a quantitative red-blue colour change (Lim et al., 1998; Oracz et al., 2003). Elevated levels of anti-O9 IgM antibodies together with typical clinical symptoms of typhoid fever probably indicates acute infection with *S.* Typhi (Tam & Lim, 2003; Feleszko et al., 2004; Tam et al., 2008). Subsequent modification of the antigens used has resulted in a similar test for paratyphoid fever which has demonstrated early promise (Tam et al., 2008).

In clinical studies involving small cohorts of hospitalized patients, both the Typhidot and TUBEX tests have demonstrated good performance in clinically suspected typhoid fever cases in comparison to the Widal test, particularly in early infection (Bhutta & Mansurali, 1999; House et al., 2001; Jesudason et al., 2002; Olsen et al., 2004; Begum et al., 2009; Narayanappa et al., 2010). In larger studies both in Asia and Africa, the new generation serological tests have compared less favourably (Dutta et al., 2006; Ley et al., 2011). Data from a large community-based surveillance study in Calcutta from 6697 patients with fever for 3 or more days demonstrated that, using a cut-off of fever for >5 days, the Widal test was more sensitive overall than the other two tests (Widal sensitivity 67%, specificity 85%, PPV 75%, NPV 79%; Typhidot 59%, 75%, 89% and 33%; Tubex 55%, 81%, 72% and 66%)(Dutta et al., 2006). The Widal test was also significantly cheaper but took longer to produce a result. One concern raised by the authors was that there was relatively poor standardisation of the kit reagents in the two newer tests and this may have had an effect due to the large number of tests performed.

More recently, the Dri-Dot Latex agglutination and IgM lateral flow assays have been developed by KIT Biomedical Research, Royal Tropical Institute, The Netherlands, and are simple to use for diagnosis of enteric fever. The validation study of the Dri-Dot Latex agglutination and IgM lateral flow assays for the diagnosis of typhoid fever, carried out in patients with clinically diagnosed typhoid fever in an Egyptian population, has demonstrated that the sensitivity and specificity were 71.4% and 86.3% for the Dri-Dot, and 80% and 71.4% for IgM Lateral Flow assay, respectively. A major limitation of these serologic tests is the limited sensitivity at the early stage of the disease. The sensitivity of these assays was increased to 84.3% when both tests were performed in parallel but the specificity decreased to 70.5%. Given that these assays are rapid and provide easy-to-interpret results, they may be useful for diagnosis of enteric fever in typhoid-endemic countries (Nakhla et al.,2011; Smith et al., 2011).

In summary, although several alternatives exist for diagnosing typhoid serologically, to-date the newer tests have not improved greatly on the performance of a test that is over a century old. With newer techniques for antigen discovery becoming available and an increasing amount of data being collected regarding the immune response to typhoid and paratyphoid infection, rapid and more effective diagnostic serological tests for typhoid infection are likely to become available in the near future.

3.3 Molecular diagnosis of enteric fever

Detecting the presence of *S.* Typhi in clinical samples using highly sensitive molecular techniques is not a recent development. In the 1980s, Rubin et al. designed and used a DNA probe cloned from *Citrobacter freundii* which has similar Vi antigen to *S.* Typhi for detection of *S.* Typhi and demonstrated 99% specificity and sensitivity using lactose-negative colonies or previously identified bacteria from febrile patients in Peru and in Indonesia (Rubin et al., 1988). As a direct diagnostic method however, the DNA probe method cannot detect less than 500 bacteria per ml of blood; patients with typhoid generally have fewer than 15 *S.* Typhi bacteria per ml (Watson, 1955; Wain et al., 1998). The DNA probe method was refined in a further study (Rubin et al., 1989), in which blood samples (and other specimens including bone marrow aspirates) were taken from patients presenting with febrile symptoms and concentrated by centrifugation using a DuPont Isolator tube, followed by overnight incubation of the bacteria on nylon filters. This modification allowed the detection of *S.* Typhi in 42% (13/32) of samples from patients with culture-confirmed typhoid fever using the equivalent of 2.5 ml of blood, compared with 53% (17/33) of these patients by culture of 8 ml peripheral blood. Additionally the probe detected 4 of 47 patients from whom *S.* Typhi was not isolated by culture, suggesting superior sensitivity could be achieved.

These early studies supported the introduction and development of further nucleic acid amplification tests to enable the rapid detection of very small numbers of bacterial components, thus providing new tools for sensitive and specific detection, identification and subsequently resistance testing of microorganisms starting from non-cultured sample material. Aside from the significant time saving over standard culture methods and the ability to detect much smaller number of bacteria, as with other organisms, nucleic acid amplification overcomes the issue of non-culturable or dead material, as is often seen with previous antibiotic treatment (Darton et al., 2009; Ho et al., 2009; Rello et al., 2009). After the early studies using DNA probes and hybridization techniques attention was turned to the use of polymerase chain reaction (PCR) methods for the detection of both *S.* Typhi and *S.* Paratyphi A for diagnosis of enteric fever.

3.3.1 Gene targets of PCR based assays for diagnosis of enteric fever

Generally any genomic sequences specific for *S.* Typhi or Paratyphi can be used as the PCR targets, and are easily available from the published DNA data bases. The widely researched targets for *S.* Typhi PCR-based assays include the *S.* Typhi flagellin gene *fliC-d* (Song et al., 1993; Hague et al., 1999, 2001; Kumar et al., 2002; Prakash et al., 2005; Ambati et al., 2007; Hatta & Smits 2007; Nandagopal et al., 2010; Nath et al., 2010), the *viaB* region encoding the Vi antigen of *S.* Typhi (Hashimoto et al., 1995), the *Salmonella* invasion gene *invA* (Cocolin et al., 1998), *hilA* gene encoding a transcription factor of *S.* Typhi (Sánchez-Jiménez & Cardona-Castro, 2004), Vi polysaccharide export ATP-binding protein *vexC* gene (Farrell et al., 2005), ST5 gene (Aziah et al., 2007), an iron-regulated gene *iroB* (Bäumler et al., 1997), 5S-23S spacer region (Zhu et al., 1996), and a heat shock protein *groEL* gene (Nair et al., 2002).

Other gene targets are also used in multiplex PCR assays, including the tyvelose epimerase gene (*tyv*; previously *rfbE*), *fliC-d*, *fliC-a* and the paratose synthase gene (*prt*; previously *rfbS*) (Hirose et al., 2002; Ali et al., 2009), *invA*, *viaB*, *fliC-d* and *prt* (Kumar et al., 2006), the outer membrane protein C (*ompC*), the putative regulatory protein gene STY4220, the intergenic region (SSPAI) between SSPA1723a and SSPA1724 in serovar Paratyphi A, and *stgA* (a fimbrial subunit protein) in serovar Typhi (Ngan et al., 2010), *stkF* (a putative fimbrial protein), *spa2473*, *spa2539*, *hsdM* (DNA methyltransferase) of *S.* Paratyphi (Ou et al., 2007).

Both *S.* Typhi and *S.* Paratyphi A have extremely limited genetic diversity within their populations and between 1 and 3% of the gene content of the *S.* Typhi and *S.* Paratyphi A genomes are unique (Roumagnac et al., 2006). This may aid DNA test specificity over other Gram-negative organisms. Further genomic exploration of both *S.* Typhi and *S.* Paratyphi A will identify new and better targets and then lead to novel nucleic acid based tests.

3.3.2 Sensitivity and specificity of PCR based assays for diagnosis of enteric fever

PCR-based tests for detecting the causative pathogens of enteric fever have developed rapidly over the last decade; however questions regarding the clinical utility and standardization of tests remain. Key to these issues is the array of methodologies used and variable sensitivities and specificities found. Song et al. (1993) was the first to apply PCR for detection of *S.* Typhi in clinical samples in an attempt to overcome the need for a pre-incubation or concentration step. Two pairs of oligonucleotide primers were designed to amplify the Hd flagella gene (*fliC-d*) of *S.* Typhi by nested PCR. This nested PCR had a minimum detection limit of 10 bacteria as determined by dilutions of DNA from *S.* Typhi and proved highly sensitive and specific using both laboratory and clinical samples. *S.* Typhi DNA was detected in 11 of 12 clinical specimens from patients with confirmed typhoid fever, whereas 10 blood specimens from patients with other febrile disease were all negative. Furthermore, this nested PCR also detected *S.* Typhi DNA from blood samples of 4 patients with suspected typhoid fever on the basis of clinical features but with negative cultures. Since then, many studies on the use of the nested PCR for detection of *S.* Typhi and diagnosis of typhoid fever have been published (Hague et al., 1999, 2001; Kumar et al., 2002; Prakash et al. 2005; Ambati et al., 2007; Hatta & Smits, 2007; Nath et al., 2010; Nandagopal et al., 2010). A nested PCR method was also developed using the *viaB* gene target, but its use in clinical diagnosis of enteric fever remains to be tested even though it demonstrated good sensitivity and specificity in tests performed on DNA samples isolated from clinical bacterial isolates (Hashimoto et al., 1995).

The nested PCR approach significantly improved the detection rate compared to that of blood culture and the Widal test; however its limitations include the longer time taken to perform and the more contaminations in comparison to a conventional PCR assay. Massi et al. utilized just one pair of primers ST1 and ST4 that Song et al. (1993) used for PCR detection of *S.* Typhi, and demonstrated that this single round PCR was also specific and could detect as little as 2-3 copies of *S.* Typhi DNA as determined by serial dilution of genomic DNA from *S.* Typhi (Massi et al., 2003). Using this conventional PCR method, genomic *S.* Typhi DNA was detected in 46 of 73 blood samples collected from patients with clinically suspected typhoid fever who had fever within 3 days of hospitalized admission, and who received no prior antibiotic treatment. PCR compared favourably (63% positivity amongst the clinically suspected cases) to blood culture (13.7%) and the Widal test (35.6%), using these 73 samples. The time taken for PCR analysis of each sample was less than 12 h, rather than 16 h for the nested PCR (Song et al., 1993) and between 3 to 5 days for blood culture.

Conventional PCR generally detects amplification using an agarose gel, which has limitations in sensitivity and speed. Cocolin et al. developed a PCR-microtitre plate hybridization technique for detection of *S.* Typhi *invA* by PCR, and demonstrated enhanced sensitivity and faster availability of results in comparison to a standard agarose gel electrophoresis approach (Cocolin et al., 1998). Other PCR assays were also researched on different gene targets in order to find a rapid and sensitive detection of *S.* Typhi in clinical specimens (Zhu et al., 1996; Bäumler et al., 1997; Nair et al., 2002; Sánchez-Jiménez & Cardona-Castro, 2004; Farrell et al., 2005; Nizami et al., 2006; Aziah et al., 2007).

Real-time PCR (RT-PCR), which is generally detected by measuring a fluorescent signal and has several advantages over conventional PCR has recently been explored, yet not exhaustively, for detection of both *S.* Typhi and *S.* Paratyphi A. Massi et al. applied TaqMan-based real-time PCR (TaqMan assay) to the quantification of *S.* Typhi in the blood of patients suspected of having typhoid fever by targeting the *S.* Typhi flagellin gene in genomic DNAs isolated from blood samples (Massi et al., 2005). Of 55 blood samples taken from suspected typhoid fever patients, eight blood samples with a positive blood culture had *S.* Typhi loads ranging from 1.01×10^3 to 4.35×10^4 copies/ml blood, and from 47 blood samples with negative blood culture, there were 40 (85.1%) TaqMan assay-positive samples with loads ranging from 3.9 to 9.9×10^2 copies/ml blood. In their study, the TaqMan assay detected more than 10^3 copies/ml blood of *S.* Typhi in all of the blood culture-positive samples, whereas less than 10^3 copies/ml blood of *S.* Typhi were detected in the blood culture-negative samples. This suggests that a TaqMan assay may be useful for assessing *S.* Typhi loads, especially in cases of suspected typhoid fever with negative results from the standard blood culture test.

Farrell et al. developed broad-range (Pan) *Salmonella* and *S.* Typhi specific real-time PCR assays using LightCycler (Roche Diagnostics, Indianapolis, IN). Using direct stool samples the pan-*Salmonella* assay was validated with 96% (53/55) sensitivity and 96% (49/51) specificity. However, the *S.* Typhi-specific PCR assay was not sufficiently validated due to the low incidence of *S.* Typhi infections in the test region (Farrel et al., 2005).

All these studies demonstrated that the sensitivity and specificity of PCR assays was significantly better compared to that of blood culture and/or the Widal test, and some selected evaluation studies of these tests are summarized in Table 1.

Test used	Target gene	Samples (n) tested		Blood culture	PCR	Widal test	Reference
nested PCR	*fliC-d*	suspected	16	12BC+ 4BC-	11/12BC+ 4/4BC-		Song et al. 1993
		control	10 febrile		0/10		
nested PCR	*fliC-d*	suspected	55	8BC+ 47BC-	8/8BC+ 24/47BC-	6/8BC+ 23/47BC-	Hague et al. 2001
		control	20 nonfebrile		0/20	9/20	
nested PCR	*fliC-d*	suspected	40	20BC+ 20BC-	20/20BC+ 12/20BC-		Kumar et al. 2002
		control	None				
nested PCR	*fliC-d*	suspected	63	17BC+ 46BC-	17/17BC+ 36/46BC-	12/17BC+ 4/46BC-	Prakash et al. 2005
		Control	25 nonfebrile		0/25	1/25	
nested PCR	*fliC-d*	suspected	119	68BC+ 51BC-	67/68BC+ 26/51BC-	34/68BC+ 11/51BC-	Hatta & Smiths 2007
		control	12 febrile		0/12	4/12	
nested PCR	*fliC-d*	suspected	42	14BC+ 38BC-	14/14BC+ 29/38BC-	7/14BC+ 19/38BC-	Ambati et al. 2007
		control	11 febrile 8 nonfebrile		0/11 0/8	2/11 0/8	
nested PCR	*fliC-d*	suspected	291	6BC+ 285BC-	6/6BC+ 8/285BC-		Nandagopal et al. 2010
		control	10 febrile		0/10		
PCR	*viaB*	suspected	203	26 BC+ 177BC-	10/26BC+ 12/177BC-		Nizami et al. 2006
		control	None				
PCR	*hilA*	suspected	37	34BC+ 3BC-	34/34BC+ 3/3BC-		Sánchez-Jiménez & Cardona-Castro 2004
		control	35 infected with other pathogens 150 healthy volunteers		0/35 0/150		

Test used	Target gene	Samples (n) tested		Blood culture	PCR	Widal test	Reference
PCR	*fliC-d*	suspected	82	28BC+	59/82		Haque et al. 1999
		control	20 nonfebrile		0/20		
PCR	*fliC-d*	suspected	73	10BC+ 63BC-	10/10BC+ 36/63BC-	10/10BC+ 16/63BC-	Massi et al. 2003
		Control	None				
PCR	ST-50	suspected	33BC+ broths		29/33		Aziah et al. 2007
		control	40BC- broths		0/40		
PCR	*fliC-d*	suspected	820	78BC+ 742BC-	73/78BC+ 95/742BC-		Chaudhry et al. 2010
		control	None				
RT-PCR	*fliC-d*	suspected	55	8BC+ 47BC-	8/8BC+ 40/47BC-		Massi et al. 2005
		control	26 nonfebrile		0/26		

BC: Blood culture; BC+: Blood culture positive; BC-: Blood culture negative

Table 1. The results of selected studies on the sensitivity and specificity of PCR, blood culture and Widal test on blood samples from patients with suspected enteric fever

3.3.3 Multiplex PCR detection for *S.* Typhi and *S.* Paratyphi

Classically *S.* Typhi has been considered as the major cause of enteric fever; however, in recent years *S.* Paratyphi and Vi-negative variants of *S.* Typhi have emerged rapidly (Wain et al., 2005; Dong et al., 2010). *S.* Paratyphi A is a causative agent of paratyphoid fever and has become a major cause of enteric fever in Asia. For example, more than 80% of enteric fever outbreaks have been caused by *S.* Paratyphi since 1998, three years after Vi polysaccharide typhoid fever vaccine was introduced in Guangxi province China (Dong et al., 2010). The largest one (495 episodes), which occurred in 2004 in Luocheng County, was caused by a contaminated water supply system. *S.* Paratyphi has been the predominant cause of enteric fever in Guangxi province China since 1999 (Dong et al., 2010). Studies from India and Nepal also suggested that paratyphoid fever caused by *S.* Paratyphi A can contribute up to half of all cases of enteric fever in some settings (Ochiai et al., 2005; Woods et al., 2006). PCR tests using *S.* Typhi specific primers appear to be sensitive to detect typhoid fever, but cannot detect paratyphoid fever. Recent developments in multiplex PCR methods have addressed the issue of paratyphoid as well as typhoid fever diagnosis.

Hirose et al. developed a complex PCR using the primers for O, H, and Vi antigen genes, *tyv* (*rfbE*), *prt* (*rfbS*), *fliC-d*, *fliC-a*, and *viaB*, for the rapid identification of *S.* Typhi and *S.* Paratyphi A. This assay was able to accurately identify and distinguish *S.* Typhi and *S.* Paratyphi A from laboratory isolates; however, its clinical use was not assessed (Hirose et al., 2002). Similarly, Levy et al. developed a multiplex PCR to identify *Salmonella* serogroups A, B and D, and Vi-positive strains. Blinded testing of 664 Malian and Chilean *Salmonella* blood isolates demonstrated 100% sensitivity and specificity; again clinical utility was not assessed (Levy et al. 2008). Kumar et al. explored another set of target genes including those responsible for invasion (*invA*), O (*prt*), H (*fliC-d*) and Vi (*viaB*) antigen genes in a multiplex PCR, and demonstrated accurate identification of laboratory isolates and 100% detection probability when a cell suspension of 10^4 CFU/ml (500 CFU per reaction) was used. *S.* Typhi bacteria were artificially inoculated into water and food (milk and meat rinse) samples and detected by the multiplex PCR after overnight pre-enrichment in buffered peptone water. No *Salmonella* bacteria could be detected from water samples collected from the field by the multiplex PCR or standard culture method (Kumar et al., 2006).

Using the same target genes as Hirose et al. (Hirose et al., 2002), Ali et al. further optimised the primers and applied the nested multiplex PCR directly to clinical blood specimens for diagnosis. Of 42 multiplex PCR-positive blood samples, they showed that 26, 9, and 2 were Vi-positive *S.* Typhi, Vi-negative *S.* Typhi and *S.* Paratyphi A, respectively, and five patients had a mixed infection. Tests with several common pathogens confirmed that the assay was specific (Ali et al., 2009).

The analysis of the genome of *S.* Paratyphi led Ou et al. to identify four gene targets (*stkF, spa2473, spa2539* and *hsdM)* which were used to develop a highly discriminatory multiplex PCR assay (Ou et al., 2007). A valuation study using spiked blood and stool samples demonstrated that the sensitivity of the discriminatory multiplex PCR was 1 x 10^5 CFU/ml and 2 x 10^5 CFU/ml, respectively, and however, the sensitivity can be increased to 1 x 10^4 CFU/ml and 2 x 10^3 CFU/ml after 5 h culture enrichment (Teh et al., 2008). Nagarajan et al. have further improved upon the existing PCR-based diagnostic technique by using one pair of primers that is unique to *S.* Typhi and *S.* Paratyphi A, corresponding to the STY0312 gene in *S.* Typhi and its homolog SPA2476 in *S.* Paratyphi A, and another pair that amplifies the region in *S.* Typhi CT18 and *S.* Typhi Ty2 corresponding to the region between genes STY0313 to STY0316 but which is absent in *S.* Paratyphi A. The possibility of a false-negative result arising due to mutation in hypervariable genes has been reduced by targeting a gene unique to typhoidal *Salmonella* serovars as a diagnostic marker. This set of primers can also differentiate between *S.* Typhi CT18, *S.* Typhi Ty2, and *S.* Paratyphi A, which have stable deletions in this specific locus. The PCR assay designed in this study has a sensitivity of 95% compared to the Widal test which has a sensitivity of only 63% (Nagarajan et al., 2009). Ngan et al. developed another multiplex PCR format in which the outer membrane protein C (*ompC*) was used for detection of members of the *Salmonella* genus, the putative regulatory protein gene STY4220 for the presence of either *S.* Typhi or *S.* Paratyphi A, and the intergenic region (SSPAI) between SSPA1723a and SSPA1724 in serovar Paratyphi A and a fimbrial subunit protein (*stgA*) in serovar Typhi for differentiation between *S.* Typhi and *S.* Paratyphi. This multiplex PCR was evaluated using 124 clinical and reference *Salmonella* serovars and both *S.* Typhi and *S.* Paratyphi A were detected at 100% specificity and sensitivity. This multiplex PCR reaction can detect approximately 1 pg of *Salmonella* genomic DNA. When tested on 8 h enriched spiked blood samples of serovars Typhi and Paratyphi A, the sensitivity was estimated at 4.5 x 10^4 - 5.5 x 10^4 CFU/ml, with similar detection levels observed for spiked fecal samples (Ngan et al., 2010).

Recently Nga et al. used a novel multiplex three colour real-time PCR assay to detect specific target sequences in the genomes of *S.* Typhi and *S.* Paratyphi A. The assay was validated and demonstrated a high level of specificity and reproducibility under experimental conditions with the DNA extracted from blood and bone marrow samples from culture positive and negative enteric fever patients. All bone marrow samples tested were positive for *Salmonella*; however, the sensitivity on blood samples was limited. The assay demonstrated an overall specificity of 100% (75/75) and sensitivity of 53.9% (69/128) on biological samples. The data on the PCR detection limit suggested that PCR performed directly on blood samples may be an unsuitable methodology and a potentially unachievable target for the routine diagnosis of enteric fever because the bacterial load of *S.* Typhi in peripheral blood is low, often below the limit of detection by culture and, consequently, below detection by PCR (Nga et al., 2010).

3.3.4 Novel blood culture PCR system and application in human challenge study

An alternative strategy to increase the sensitivity and specificity of PCR is PCR amplification on the blood culture after a short period of incubation. We have recently developed a fast and highly sensitive blood culture PCR method for detection of *Salmonella* serovar Typhi (Zhou & Pollard, 2010). The method uses an optimised ox bile tryptone soy broth for blood culture with subsequent PCR assay in an attempt to reduce the turn-around time for diagnosis and increase diagnostic sensitivity. By using a 5-hour incubation, 3 CFU of *S.* Typhi cells could mutliply over about 10 generations. This was assessed by a time-course experiment, the results of which were published (Zhou & Pollard, 2010) and are cited here in Table 2.

Incubation time (hour)	CFU[a]	*filC-d* amplicons[b]
0	3	---
1	4	---
2	17	----
3	105	+++
4	209	+++
5	4461	+++

*Three bacteria of *Salmonella* serovar Typhi were incubated in the tryptone soy broth containing 2.4% ox bile and 20% blood. [a] The mean of three independent experiments; [b] *Salmonella* serovar Typhi *fliC-d* amplicons resulting from PCR using the DNA templates prepared from three independent cultures.

Table 2. The growth and PCR detection of *S.* Typhi in ox bile tryptone soy broth blood culture*.

The sensitivity of this blood culture-PCR method was equivalent to 0.75 CFU per millilitre of blood which is similar to the level of clinical typhoid samples which regular PCR cannot detect. The whole blood culture PCR assay takes less than 8 hours to complete rather than several days for conventional blood culture. This novel blood culture PCR method is superior in speed and sensitivity to both conventional blood culture and PCR assays. Its use in clinical diagnosis may allow early detection of the causative organism and facilitate initiation of prompt treatment among patients with typhoid fever. The recent use of this novel culture PCR method to our ongoing human typhoid challenge studies has proved that the advantage of combining culture and PCR amplification is an increase in the speed of a positive confirmatory diagnosis, even though it is unlikely to produce a greater level of sensitivity than that of traditional culture alone. However, practical clinical use in diagnosing enteric fever of this culture PCR system remains to be proved, in particular, using blood samples with antibiotic pre-treatment.

4. Future perspectives

Blood culture has some distinct advantage over other diagnostic methods, such as the combination of bacterial identification with antibiotic susceptibility, and an unquestioned role in providing epidemiological data; however, it has many problems related to its relatively long turnaround time and low sensitivity, especially in patients receiving antibiotic treatment. Detection of bacterial DNA in whole blood by PCR assay is the methodology most able to substantially decrease the turnaround time without bias from the inhibitory effect of antibiotics, yet the published PCR assays for diagnosis of enteric fever are in limited use. Further investigation to develop rapid and reliable diagnostics for enteric fever are urgently needed.

One of the limiting factors in the use of current PCR methodology in clinical diagnosis of enteric fever is the low number of bacteria circulating in the blood of enteric fever patients. Advancement in the use of PCR would require the capture and amplification of a smaller number of bacteria (maybe even a single organism) in blood or other bodily fluids. Such a task is not insurmountable but it will be a challenge to make it cost effective (Baker et al., 2010). An alternative approach to increase the PCR assay sensitivity and specificity is to remove the interfering human genomic DNA present in the samples. To achieve this, selective lysis of human genomic DNA with external nuclease may be usful, as proven in pathogen identification in patients with sepsis (Horz et al., 2008; Handschur et al., 2009). Removal of dominant human genomic DNA causes enrichment of bacterial DNA, thus improving sensitivity and specificity of PCR assays. Using *S.* Typhi spiked blood samples, we have demonstrated that this approach can increase the sensitivity of PCR assays by more than 1,000 fold (unpublished result). However, a field trial with clinical typhoid specimens is needed to confirm the laboratory findings. Reverse transcription PCR may be another choice to detect such a low number of bacteria in typhoid patient blood as the higher number of copies of mRNA for a specific gene target could increase the PCR assay sensitivity. The *fliC* of *S.* Typhi was used as target in the reverse transcription-multiplex PCR assay for simultaneous detection of *Escherichia coli* O157:H7, *Vibrio cholerae* O1 and *S.* Typhi (Morin et al., 2004).

The study on host specific responses to enteric fever may identify signatures of host-pathogen interactions with *S.* Typhi, which will form the basis of development of new molecular diagnostics for enteric fever. Activation of host specific genes or pathways during infection could be identified using DNA microarrays; a physiological signature or metabolic product associated with typhoid could be studied with mass spectrometry or other proteomic technologies. For example, surface-enhanced laser desorption/ionization time-of-flight (SELDI-TOF) mass spectroscopy has been used in identifying SARS protein biomarkers (Mazzulli et al., 2005). All these new technological approaches may add insight into proteins as biomarkers of typhoid infection, and potentially result in a new generation of novel molecular diagnostics for enteric fever.

Enteric fever is endemic in resource poor countries, and development in new technologies should focus on how these can be applied to location with limited resources. Efforts are being made to simplify typhoid PCR assays using pre-prepared and freeze-dried regents (Aziah et al., 2007). However, new PCR technologies, such as isothermal PCR, are of particularly practical use in the diagnosis of enteric fever, as these methods allow for the possibility of developing less-complicated and less-expensive machinery than is necessary for conventional PCR. Several isothermal PCR technologies have been developed (Gill & Ghaemi, 2008), including strand displacement amplification (SDA) (Walker et al., 1992), loop-mediated amplification (LAMP) (Notomi et al., 2000), and helicase-dependent amplification (HDA) (Vincent et al., 2004). Recently, Francois et al. have examined the robustness of LAMP for bacterial diagnostic applications using *S.* Typhi as the target organism (Francois et al., 2011), and demonstrated that LAMP is more sensitive than conventional qPCR and is also a very robust, innovative and powerful molecular diagnostic method. However, SDA, HDA and/or other isothermal amplification methods could be more advantageous over LAMP in multiplex amplifications. The recent surge in paratyphoid disease makes it necessary to develop new diagnostics for detection of both S. Typhi and Paratyphi. Another advantage of isothermal PCR is its potential for use in resource poor or point-of-care settings.

In summary, advancement in genomics and proteomics will further our understanding of molecular pathogenesis of enteric fever, and eventually lead to identification of new targets which could form the basis for new molecular diagnostics. With progress in new technologies, we expect that a new generation of fast and sensitive molecular diagnostics for enteric fever will be developed in the near future.

5. Acknowledgments

LZ and TD are funded by a grant from the Wellcome Trust, UK and CW is funded by the UK National Institute for Health Research (NIHR) Oxford Biomedical Research Centre.

6. References

Ackers, M.L.; Puhr, N.D.; Tauxe, R.V. & Mintz, E.D. (2000). Laboratory-based surveillance of *Salmonella* serotype Typhi infections in the United States: antimicrobial resistance on the rise. JAMA. 2000 May 24-31;283(20):2668-73.

Albaqali, A.; Ghuloom, A.; Al Arrayed, A.; Al Ajami, A.; Shome, D.K.; Jamsheer, A.; Al Mahroos, H.; Jelacic, S.; Tarr, P.I.; Kaplan, B.S. & Dhiman, R.K. (2003). Hemolytic uremic syndrome in association with typhoid fever. Am J Kidney Dis. 2003 Mar; 41(3):709-13.

Ali, A.; Haque, A.; Haque, A.; Sarwar, Y.; Mohsin, M.; Bashir, S. & Tariq, A. (2009). Multiplex PCR for differential diagnosis of emerging typhoidal pathogens directly from blood samples. Epidemiol Infect. 2009 Jan;137(1):102-7.

Al Naiemi, N.; Zwart, B.; Rijnsburger, M.C.; Roosendaal, R.; Debets-Ossenkopp, Y.J.; Mulder, J.A.; Fijen, C.A.; Maten, W.; Vandenbroucke-Grauls, C.M. & Savelkoul, P.H. (2008). Extended-spectrum-beta-lactamase production in a *Salmonella enterica* serotype Typhi strain from the Philippines. J Clin Microbiol. 2008 Aug;46(8):2794-5.

Ambati, S.R.; Nath, G. & Das, B.K. (2007). Diagnosis of typhoid fever by polymerase chain reaction. Indian J Pediatr. 2007 Oct;74(10):909-13.

Aziah, I.; Ravichandran, M. & Ismail, A. (2007). Amplification of ST50 gene using dry-reagent-based polymerase chain reaction for the detection of *Salmonella* Typhi. Diagn Microbiol Infect Dis. 2007 Dec;59(4):373-7.

Baker, S.; Favorov, M. & Dougan, G. (2010). Searching for the elusive typhoid diagnostic. BMC Infect Dis. 2010 Mar 5;10:45.

Balasubramanian, S.; Shivbalan, S. & Miranda, P.K. (2003). Pseudotumour cerebri as an unusual manifestation of typhoid. Ann Trop Paediatr. 2003; 23: 223–24.

Bakr, W.M.; El Attar, L.A.; Ashour, M.S. & El Toukhy, A.M. (2011). The dilemma of widal test - which brand to use? a study of four different widal brands: a cross sectional comparative study. Ann Clin Microbiol Antimicrob. 2011 Feb 8;10:7.

Bäumler, A.J.; Heffron, F. & Reissbrodt, R. (1997). Rapid detection of *Salmonella enterica* with primers specific for iroB. J Clin Microbiol. 1997 May;35(5):1224-30.

Begum, Z.; Hossain, M.A.; Musa, A.K.; Shamsuzzaman, A.K.; Mahmud, M.C.; Ahsan, M.M.; Sumona, A.A.; Ahmed, S.; Jahan, N.A.; Alam, M. & Begum, A. (2009). Comparison between DOT EIA IgM and Widal Test as early diagnosis of typhoid fever. Mymensingh Med J. 2009 Jan;18(1):13-7.

Bhan, M.K.; Bahl, R. & Bhatnagar, S. (2005). Typhoid and paratyphoid fever. Lancet. 2005 Aug 27-Sep 2;366(9487):749-62.

Bhan, M.K.; Bahl, R.; Sazawal, S.; Sinha, A.; Kumar, R.; Mahalanabis, D. & Clemens, J.D. (2002). Association between *Helicobacter pylori* infection and increased risk of typhoid fever. J Infect Dis. 2002 Dec 15;186(12):1857-60.

Bhutta, Z. A. (2006). Current concepts in the diagnosis and treatment of typhoid fever. BMJ. 2006 Jul 8;333(7558):78-82.

Bhutta, Z.A. & Mansurali, N. (1999). Rapid serologic diagnosis of pediatric typhoid fever in an endemic area: a prospective comparative evaluation of two dot-enzyme immunoassays and the Widal test. Am J Trop Med Hyg. 1999 Oct;61(4):654-7.

Butler, T.; Islam, A.; Kabir, I. & Jones, P.K. (1991). Patterns of morbidity and mortality in typhoid fever dependent on age and gender: review of 552 hospitalized patients with diarrhea. Rev Infect Dis. 1991 Jan-Feb;13(1):85-90.

Chaudhry, R.; Chandel, D.S.; Verma, N.; Singh, N.; Singh, P. & Dey, A.B. (2010). Rapid diagnosis of typhoid fever by an in-house flagellin PCR. J Med Microbiol. 2010 Nov;59(Pt 11):1391-3.

Chau, T.T.; Campbell, J.I.; Galindo, C.M.; Van Minh Hoang, N.; Diep, T.S.; Nga, T.T.; Van Vinh Chau, N.; Tuan, P.Q.; Page, A.L.; Ochiai, R.L.; Schultsz, C.; Wain, J.; Bhutta, Z.A.; Parry, C.M.; Bhattacharya, S.K.; Dutta, S.; Agtini, M.; Dong, B.; Honghui, Y.; Anh, D.D.; Canh do, G.; Naheed, A.; Albert, M.J.; Phetsouvanh, R.; Newton, P.N.; Basnyat, B.; Arjyal, A.; La, T.T.; Rang, N.N.; Phuong le, T.; Van Be Bay, P.; von Seidlein, L.; Dougan, G.; Clemens, J.D.; Vinh, H.; Hien, T.T.; Chinh, N.T.; Acosta, C.J.; Farrar, J. & Dolecek, C. (2007). Antimicrobial drug resistance of *Salmonella enterica* serovar Typhi in asia and molecular mechanism of reduced susceptibility to the fluoroquinolones. Antimicrob Agents Chemother. 2007 Dec;51(12):4315-23.

Chew, S.K.; Cruz, M.S. & Lim, Y.S. (1992). Monteiro EH. Diagnostic value of the Widal test for typhoid fever in Singapore. J Trop Med Hyg. 1992 Aug;95(4):288-91.

Chiu, C.H. & Lin, T.Y. (1999). Typhoid fever in children. Lancet. 1999 Dec 4;354(9194):2001-2.

Choo, K.E.; Davis, T.M.; Ismail, A.; Tuan Ibrahim, T.A. & Ghazali, W.N. (1999). Rapid and reliable serological diagnosis of enteric fever: comparative sensitivity and specificity of Typhidot and Typhidot-M tests in febrile Malaysian children. Acta Trop. 1999 Mar 15;72(2):175-83.

Choo, K.E.; Oppenheimer, S.J.; Ismail, A.B. & Ong, K.H. (1994). Rapid serodiagnosisof typhoid feverby dot enzyme immunoassay in an endemic area. Clin Infect Dis. 1994 Jul;19(1):172-6.

Clark, T.W.; Daneshvar, C.; Pareek, M.; Perera, N. & Stephenson, I. (2010). Enteric fever in a UK regional infectious diseases unit: a 10 year retrospective review. J Infect. 2010 Feb;60(2):91-8.

Cocolin, L.; Manzano, M.; Astori, G.; Botta, G.A; Cantoni, C. & Comi, G. (1998). A highly sensitive and fast non-radioactive method for the detection of polymerase chain reaction products from *Salmonella* serovars, such as *Salmonella* Typhi, in blood specimens. FEMS Immunol Med Microbiol. 1998 Nov;22(3):233-9.

Coleman, W. &. Buxton, B.H. (1907). The bacteriology of the blood in typhoid fever. Amer J Med Sci. 1907;133:896-903.

Crawford, R.W.; Rosales-Reyes, R.; Ramírez-Aguilar Mde, L.; Chapa-Azuela, O.; Alpuche-Aranda, C. & Gunn, J.S. (2010). Gallstones play a significant role in *Salmonella* spp. gallbladder colonization and carriage. Proc Natl Acad Sci U S A. 2010 Mar 2;107(9):4353-8.

Crump, J.A.; Luby, S.P. & Mintz, E.D. (2004). The global burden of typhoid fever. Bull World Health Organ. 2004 May;82(5):346-53.

Darton, T.; Guiver, M.; Naylor, S.; Jack, D.L.; Kaczmarski, E.B.; Borrow, R. & Read, R.C. (2009). Severity of meningococcal disease associated with genomic bacterial load. Clin Infect Dis. 2009 Mar 1;48(5):587-94.

Datta, V.; Sahare, P. & Chaturved, P. (2004). Guillain-Barre syndrome as a complication of enteric fever. J Indian Med Assoc. 2004 Mar;102(3):172-3.

Dong, B.Q.; Yang, J.; Wang, X.Y.; Gong, J.; von Seidlein, L.; Wang, M.L.; Lin, M.; Liao, H.Z.; Ochiai, R.L.; Xu, Z.Y.; Jodar, L. & Clemens, J.D. (2010). Trends and disease burden of enteric fever in Guangxi province, China, 1994-2004. Bull World Health Organ. 2010 Sep 1;88(9):689-96.

Dutta, S.; Sur, D.; Manna, B.; Sen, B.; Deb, A.K.; Deen, J.L.; Wain, J.; Von Seidlein, L.; Ochiai, L.; Clemens, J.D. & Kumar, B.hattacharya, S. (2006). Evaluation of new-generation serologic tests for the diagnosis of typhoid fever: data from a community-based surveillance in Calcutta, India. Diagn Microbiol Infect Dis. 2006 Dec;56(4):359-65.

Meltzer, E.; Sadik, C. & Schwartz, E. (2005). Enteric fever in Israeli travelers: a nationwide study. J Travel Med. 2005 Sep-Oct;12(5):275-81.

Maskey, A.P.; Day, J.N.; Phung, Q.T.; Thwaites, G.E.; Campbell, J.I.; Zimmerman, M.; Farrar, J.J. & Basnyat, B. (2006). *Salmonella enterica* serovar Paratyphi A and S. enterica serovar Typhi cause indistinguishable clinical syndromes in Kathmandu, Nepal. Clin Infect Dis. 2006 May 1;42(9):1247-53.

Ekdahl, K.; De Jong, B. & Andersson, Y. (2005). Risk of travel-associated typhoid and paratyphoid fevers in various regions. J Travel Med. 2005 Jul-Aug;12(4):197-204.

Fadeel, M.A.; House, B.L.; Wasfy, M.M.; Klena, J.D.; Habashy, E.E.; Said, M.M.; Maksoud, M.A.; Rahman, B.A. & Pimentel, G. (2011). Evaluation of a newly developed ELISA against Widal, TUBEX-TF and Typhidot for typhoid fever surveillance. J Infect Dev Ctries. 2011 Mar 21;5(3):169-75.

Fangtham, M. & Wilde, H. (2008). Emergence of *Salmonella Paratyphi A* as a Major Cause of Enteric Fever: Need for Early Detection, Preventive Measures, and Effective Vaccines. J Travel Med. 2008 Sep-Oct;15(5):344-50.

Farrell, J.J.; Doyle, L.J.; Addison, R.M.; Reller, L.B.; Hall, G.S. & Procop, G.W. (2005). Broad-range (pan) *Salmonella* and *Salmonella* serotype Typhi-specific real-time PCR assays: potential tools for the clinical microbiologist. Am J Clin Pathol. 2005 Mar;123(3):339-45.

Feleszko, W.; Maksymiuk, J.; Oracz, G.; Golicka, D. & Szajewska, H. (2004). The TUBEX typhoid test detects current *Salmonella* infections. J Immunol Methods. 2004 Feb 1;285(1):137-8.

Francois, P.; Tangomo, M.; Hibbs, J.; Bonetti, E.J.; Boehme, C.C.; Notomi, T.; Perkins, M.D. & Schrenzel, J. (2011). Robustness of a loop-mediated isothermal amplification reaction for diagnostic applications. FEMS Immunol Med Microbiol. 2011 Jun;62(1):41-8.

Gasem, M.H.; Smits, H.L.; Goris, M.G. & Dolmans, W.M. (2002). Evaluation of a simple and rapid dipstick assay for the diagnosis of typhoid fever in Indonesia. J Med Microbiol. 2002 Feb;51(2):173-7.

Gill, P. & Ghaemi, A. (2008). Nucleic acid isothermal amplification technologies: a review. Nucleosides Nucleotides Nucleic Acids. 2008 Mar;27(3):224-43.

Gilman, R.H.; Terminel, M.; Levine, M.M.; Hernandez-Mendoza, P. & Hornick, R.B. (1975). Relative efficacy of blood, urine, rectal swab, bone-marrow, and rose-spot cultures for recovery of *Salmonella* Typhi in typhoid fever. Lancet. 1975 May 31;1(7918):1211-3.

Glynn, J.R.; Hornick, R.B.; Levine, M.M.& Bradley, D.J. (1995). Infecting dose and severity of typhoid: analysis of volunteer data and examination of the influence of the definition of illness used. Epidemiol Infect. 1995 Aug;115(1):23-30.

Gotuzzo, E.; Frisancho, O.; Sanchez, J.; Liendo, G.; Carrillo, C.; Black, R.E. & Morris, J.G. Jr. (1991). Association between the acquired immunodeficiency syndrome and infection with *Salmonella* Typhi or *Salmonella* paratyphi in an endemic typhoid area. Arch Intern Med. 1991 Feb;151(2):381-2.

Handschur, M.; Karlic, H.; Hertel, C.; Hertel, C.; Pfeilstöcker, M. & Haslberger, A.G. (2009). Preanalytic removal of human DNA eliminates false signals in general 16S rDNA PCR monitoring of bacterial pathogens in blood. Comp Immunol Microbiol Infect Dis. 2009 May;32(3):207-19.

Haque, A.; Ahmed, J.; & Qureshi, J.A. (1999). Early detection of typhoid by polymerase chain reaction. Ann Saudi Med. 1999 Jul-Aug;19(4):337-40.

Haque, A.; Ahmed, N.; Peerzada, A.; Raza, A.; Bashir, S. & Abbas, G. (2001). Utility of PCR in diagnosis of problematic cases of typhoid. Jpn J Infect Dis. 2001 Dec;54(6):237-9.

Hashimoto, Y.; Itho, Y.; Fujinaga, Y.; Khan, A.Q.; Sultana, F.; Miyake, M.; Hirose, K.; Yamamoto, H. & Ezaki, T. (1995). Development of nested PCR based on the ViaB sequence to detect *Salmonella* Typhi. J Clin Microbiol. 1995 Nov;33(11):3082.

Hatta, M. & Smits, H.L. (2007). Detection of *Salmonella* Typhi by nested polymerase chain reaction in blood, urine, and stool samples. Am J Trop Med Hyg. 2007 Jan;76(1):139-43.

Hatta, M.; Goris, M.G.; Heerkens, E.; Gooskens, J. & Smits, H.L. (2002). Simple dipstick assay for the detection of *Salmonella* Typhi-specific IgM antibodies and the evolution of the immune response in patients with typhoid fever. Am J Trop Med Hyg. 2002 Apr;66(4):416-21.

Hirose, K.; Itoh, K.; Nakajima, H.; Kurazono, T.; Yamaguchi, M.; Moriya, K.; Ezaki, T.; Kawamura, Y.; Tamura, K. & Watanabe, H. (2002). Selective amplification of tyv (rfbE), prt (rfbS), viaB, and fliC genes by multiplex PCR for identification of *Salmonella enterica* serovars Typhi and Paratyphi A. J Clin Microbiol. 2002 Feb;40(2):633-6.

Hoffman, S.L.; Edman, D.C.; Punjabi, N.H.; Lesmana, M.; Cholid, A., Sundah, S. & Harahap, J. (1986). Bone marrow aspirate culture superior to streptokinase clot culture and 8 ml 1:10 blood-to-broth ratio blood culture for diagnosis of typhoid fever. Am J Trop Med Hyg. 1986 Jul;35(4):836-9.

Horz, H.P.; Scheer, S.; Huenger, F.; Vianna, M.E. & Conrads, G. (2008). Selective isolation of bacterial DNA from human clinical specimens. J Microbiol Methods. 2008 Jan;72(1):98-102.

Ho, Y.C.; Chang, S.C.; Lin, S.R. & Wang, W.K. (2009). High levels of mecA DNA detected by a quantitative real-time PCR assay are associated with mortality in patients with methicillin-resistant *Staphylococcus aureus* bacteremia. J Clin Microbiol. 2009 May;47(5):1443-51.

House, D.; Wain, J.; Ho, V.A.; Diep, T.S.; Chinh, N.T., Bay, P.V.; Vinh, H.; Duc, M.; Parry, C.M.; Dougan, G.; White, N.J. Hien, T.T. & Farrar, J.J. (2001). Serology of typhoid fever in an area of endemicity and its relevance to diagnosis. J Clin Microbiol. 2001 Mar;39(3):1002-7.

Ismail, A.; Kader, Z.S. & Ong, K.H. (1991). Dot enzyme immunosorbent assay for the serodiagnosis of typhoid fever. Southeast Asian J Trop Med Public Health. 1991 Dec;22(4):563-6.

Jesudason, M.; Esther, E. & Mathai, E. (2002). Typhidot test to detect IgG & IgM antibodies in typhoid fever. Indian J Med Res. 2002 Aug;116:70-2.

Kawano, R.L.; Leano, S.A. & Agdamag, D.M. (2007). Comparison of serological test kits for diagnosis of typhoid fever in the Philippines. J Clin Microbiol. 2007 Jan;45(1):246-7.

Kaye, D.; Palmieri, M. & Rocha, H. (1966). Effect of bile on the action of blood against *Salmonella*. J Bacteriol. 1966 Mar;91(3):945-52.

Khosla, S.N.; Jain, N. & Khosla, A. (1993). Gastric acid secretion in typhoid fever. Postgrad Med J. 1993 Feb;69(808):121-3.

Kumar, A.; Arora, V.; Bashamboo, A. & Ali, S. (2002). Detection of *Salmonella* Typhi by polymerase chain reaction: implications in diagnosis of typhoid fever. Infect Genet Evol. 2002 Dec;2(2):107-10.

Kumar, S.; Balakrishna, K. & Batra, H.V. Detection of *Salmonella enterica* serovar Typhi (*S.* Typhi) by selective amplification of invA, viaB, fliC-d and prt genes by polymerase chain reaction in mutiplex format. Lett Appl Microbiol. 2006 Feb;42(2):149-54.

Kundu, R.; Ganguly, N., Ghosh, T.K.; Yewale, V.N.; Shah, R.C. & Shah, N.K. (2006). IAP Task Force. IAP Task Force Report: diagnosis of enteric fever in children. Indian Pediatr. 2006 Oct;43(10):875-83.

Lang, R.; Maayan, M.C.; Lidor, C.; Savin, H.; Kolman, S. & Lishner, M. (1992). *Salmonella* Paratyphi C osteomyelitis: report of two separate episodes 17 years apart. Scand J Infect Dis. 1992; 24: 793–96.

Lee, W.S.; Puthucheary, S.D. & Parasakthi, N. (2000). Extra-intestinal nontyphoidal *Salmonella* infections in children. Ann Trop Paediatr. 2000; 20: 125–29.

Levine, M.M.; Black, R.E. & Lanata, C. (1982). Precise estimation of the numbers of chronic carriers of *Salmonella* Typhi in Santiago, Chile, an endemic area. J Infect Dis. 1982 Dec;146(6):724-6.

Levine, M.M.; Grados, O.; Gilman, R.H.; Woodward, W.E.; Solis-Plaza, R. & Waldman, W. (1978). Diagnostic value of the Widal test in areas endemic for typhoid fever. Am J Trop Med Hyg. 1978 Jul;27(4):795-800.

Levy, H.; Diallo, S.; Tennant, S.M.; Livio, S.; Sow, S.O.; Tapia, M.; Fields, P.I.; Mikoleit, M.; Tamboura, B.; Kotloff, K.L.; Lagos, R.; Nataro, J.P.; Galen, J.E. & Levine, M.M. (2008). PCR method to identify *Salmonella enterica* serovars Typhi, Paratyphi A, and

Paratyphi B among *Salmonella* Isolates from the blood of patients with clinical enteric fever. J Clin Microbiol. 2008 May;46(5):1861-6.

Ley, B.; Thriemer, K.; Ame, S.M.; Mtove, G.M.; von Seidlein, L.; Amos, B.; Hendriksen, I.C.; Mwambuli, A.; Shoo, A.; Kim, D.R.; Ochiai, L.R.; Favorov, M.; Clemens, J.D.; Wilfing, H.; Deen, J.L. & Ali, S.M. (2011). Assessment and comparative analysis of a rapid diagnostic test (Tubex®) for the diagnosis oftyphoid fever among hospitalized children in rural Tanzania. BMC Infect Dis. 2011 May 24;11:147.

Lim, P.L.; Tam, F.C.; Cheong, Y.M. & Jegathesan, M. (1998). One-step 2-minute test to detect typhoid-specific antibodies based on particle separation in tubes. J Clin Microbiol1998;36:2271-8.

Mahle, W.T. & Levine, M.M. (1993). *Salmonella* Typhi infection in children younger than five years of age. Pediatr Infect Dis J. 1993Aug;12(8):627-31.

Maskey, A.P.; Day, J.N.; Phung, Q.T.; Thwaites, G.E.; Campbell, J.I.; Zimmerman, M. Farrar, J.J. & Basnyat, B. (2006). *Salmonella enterica* serovar Paratyphi A and *S. enterica* serovar Typhi cause indistinguishable clinical syndromes in Kathmandu, Nepal. Clin Infect Dis. 2006; 42:1247–1253.

Massi, M. N.; Shirakawa, T.; Gotoh, A.; Bishnu, A.; Hatta, M. & Kawabata, M. (2003). Rapid diagnosis of typhoid fever by PCR assay using one pair of primers from flagellin gene of *Salmonella* Typhi. J Infect Chemother. 2003 Sep;9(3):233-7.

Massi, M.N.; Shirakawa, T.; Gotoh, A.; Bishnu, A.; Hatta, M. & Kawabata, M. (2005). Quantitative detection of *Salmonella enterica* serovar Typhi from blood of suspected typhoid fever patients by real-time PCR. Int J Med Microbiol. 2005 Jun;295(2):117-20.

Mathai, E.; John, T.J.; Rani, M.; Mathai, D.; Chacko, N.; Nath, V. & Cherian, A.M. (1995). Significance of *Salmonella* Typhi bacteriuria. J Clin Microbiol. 1995 Jul;33(7):1791-2.

Mazzulli, T.; Low, D.E. & Poutanen SM. (2005). Proteomics and severe acute respiratory syndrome (SARS): emerging technology meets emerging pathogen. Clin Chem. 2005 Jan;51(1):6-7.

Meltzer, E.; Sadik, C. & Schwartz, E. (2005). Enteric fever in Israeli travelers: a nationwide study. J Travel Med 2005; 12:275–281.

Mohanty, S.; Bakshi, S., Gupta, A.K.; Kapil, A.; Arya, L.S. & Das, B.K. (2003). Venousthrombosis associated with *Salmonella*: report of a case and review of literature. Indian J Med Sci. 2003; 57: 199–203.

Morin, N.J.; Gong, Z. & Li, X.F. (2004). Reverse transcription-multiplex PCR assay for simultaneous detection of Escherichia coli O157:H7, Vibrio cholerae O1, and *Salmonella* Typhi. Clin Chem. 2004 Nov;50(11):2037-44.

Moriñigo, M.A.; Muñoz, M.A.; Martinez-Manzanares, E.; Sánchez, J.M. & Borrego, J.J. (1993). Laboratory study of several enrichment broths for the detection of *Salmonella* spp. particularly in relation to water samples. J Appl Bacteriol. 1993 Mar;74(3):330-5.

Murray, P.R.; Spizzo, A.W. & Niles, A.C. (1991). Clinical comparison of the recoveries of bloodstream pathogens in Septi-Chek brain heart infusion broth with saponin, Septi-Chek tryptic soy broth, and the isolator lysis-centrifugation system. J Clin Microbiol. 1991 May;29(5):901-5.

Nagarajan, A.G.; Karnam, G.; Lahiri, A.; Allam, U.S. & Chakravortty, D. (2009). Reliable means of diagnosis and serovar determination of blood-borne *Salmonella* strains: quick PCR amplification of unique genomic loci by novel primer sets. J Clin Microbiol. 2009 Aug;47(8):2435-41.

Nair, S.; Lin, T.K.; Pang, T. & Altwegg, M. (2002). Characterization of *Salmonella* serovars by PCR-single-strand conformation polymorphism analysis. J Clin Microbiol. 2002 Jul;40(7):2346-51.

Nakhla, I.; El Mohammady, H.; Mansour, A.; Klena, J.D.; Hassan, K.; Sultan, Y.; Pastoor, R., Abdoel, T.H. & Smits, H. (2011). Validation of the Dri-Dot Latex agglutination and IgM lateral flow assays for the diagnosis of typhoid fever in an Egyptian population. Diagn Microbiol Infect Dis. 2011 Aug;70(4):435-41.

Nandagopal, B.; Sankar, S.; Lingesan, K.; Appu, K.C.; Padmini, B.; Sridharan, G. & Gopinath, A.K. (2010). Prevalence of *Salmonella* Typhi among patients with febrile illness in rural and peri-urban populations of Vellore district, as determined by nested PCR targeting the flagellin gene. Mol Diagn Ther. 2010 Apr 1;14(2):107-12.

Narayanappa, D.; Sripathi, R.; Jagdishkumar, K. & Rajani, H.S. (2010). Comparative study of dot enzyme immunoassay (Typhidot-M) and Widal test in the diagnosis of typhoid fever.Indian Pediatr. 2010 Apr;47(4):331-3.

Nath, G.; Mauryal, P., Gulati, A.K.; Singh, T.B.; Srivastava, R.; Kumar, K. & Tripathi, S.K. (2010). Comparison of Vi serology and nested PCR in diagnosis of chronic typhoid carriers in two different study populations in typhoid endemic area of India. Southeast Asian J Trop Med Public Health. 2010 May;41(3):636-40.

Ngan, G.J.; Ng, L.M.; Lin, R.T. & Teo, J.W. (2010). Development of a novel multiplex PCR for the detection and differentiation of *Salmonella enterica* serovars Typhi and Paratyphi A. Res Microbiol. 2010 May;161(4):243-8.

Nga, T.V.; Karkey, A.; Dongol, S.; Thuy, H.N.; Dunstan, S.; Holt, K.; Tu le, T.P.; Campbell, J.I.; Chau, T.T.; Chau, N.V.; Arjyal, A.; Koirala, S.; Basnyat, B.; Dolecek, C.; Farrar, J. & Baker, S. (2010). The sensitivity of real-time PCR amplification targeting invasive *Salmonella* serovars in biological specimens. BMC Infect Dis. 2010 May 21;10:125.

Nizami, S.Q.; Bhutta, Z.A.; Siddiqui, A.A. & Lubbad, L. (2006). Enhanced detection rate of typhoid fever in children in a periurban slum in Karachi, Pakistan using polymerase chain reaction technology. Scand J Clin Lab Invest. 2006;66(5):429-36.

Notomi, T.; Okayama, H.; Masubuchi, H.; Yonekawa, T.; Watanabe, K.; Amino, N. & Hase, T. (2000). Loop-mediated isothermal amplification of DNA. Nucleic Acids Res. 2008; 28: e63.

Nordmann, P.; Lartigue, M.F. & Poirel, L. (2008). Beta-lactam induction of ISEcp1B-mediated mobilization of the naturally occurring bla(CTX-M) beta-lactamase gene of Kluyvera ascorbata. FEMS Microbiol Lett. 2008 Nov;288(2):247-9.

Ochiai, R.L. Wang, X.; von Seidlein, L.; Yang, J.; Bhutta, Z.A.; Bhattacharya, S.K.; Agtini, M.; Deen, J.L.; Wain, J.; Kim, D.R.; Ali, M.; Acosta, C.J.; Jodar, L. & Clemens, J.D. (2005). *Salmonella* Paratyphi A rates, Asia. Emerg Infect Dis. 2005 Nov;11(11):1764-6.

Olopoenia, L.A. & King, A.L. (2000). Widal agglutination test - 100 years later: still plagued by controversy. Postgrad Med J. 2000 Feb;76(892):80-4.

Olsen, S.J.; Pruckler, J.; Bibb, W.; Nguyen, T.M.; Tran, M.T. & Nguyen, T.M.; Sivapalasingam, S.; Gupta, A.; Phan, T.P.; Nguyen, T.C.; Nguyen, V.C.; Phung, D.C. & Mintz, E.D. (2004). Evaluation of rapid diagnostic tests for typhoid fever. J Clin Microbiol. 2004 May;42(5):1885-9.

Omuse, G.; Kohli, R. & Revathi, G. (2010). Diagnostic utility of a single Widal test in the diagnosis of typhoid fever at Aga Khan University Hospital (AKUH), Nairobi, Kenya. Trop Doct. 2010 Jan;40(1):43-4.

Oracz, G.; Feleszko, W.; Golicka, D.; Maksymiuk, J.; Klonowska, A. & Szajewska, H. (2003) Rapid diagnosis of acute *Salmonella* gastrointestinal infection. Clin Infect Dis. 2003 Jan 1;36(1):112-5.

Ou, H.Y.; Ju, C.T.; Thong, K.L.; Ahmad, N.; Deng, Z.; Barer, M.R. & Rajakumar, K. (2007). Translational genomics to develop a *Salmonella enterica* serovar Paratyphi A multiplex polymerase chain reaction assay. J Mol Diagn. 2007 Nov;9(5):624-30.

Pandit, A.; Arjyal, A.; Paudyal, B.; Campbell, J.C.; Day, J.N.; Farrar, J.J. & Basnyat, B. (2008). A patient with paratyphoid A fever: an emerging problem in Asia and not always a benign disease. J Travel Med. 2008 Sep-Oct;15(5):364-5.

Palit, A.; Ghosh, S.; Dutta, S.; Sur, D.; Bhattacharya, M.K. & Bhattacharya, S.K. (2006). Increasing prevalence of *Salmonella enterica* serotype Paratyphi-A in patients with enteric fever in a periurban slum setting of Kolkata, India. Int J Environ Health Res. 2006 Dec;16(6):455-9.

Parry, C.M.; Hien, T.T.; Dougan, G.; White, N.J. & Farrar, J.J. (2002).Typhoid fever. N Engl J Med. 2002 Nov 28;347(22):1770-82.

Parry, C.M.; Wijedoru, L.; Arjyal, A. & Baker, S. (2011). The utility of diagnostic tests for enteric fever in endemic locations. Expert Rev Anti Infect Ther. 2011 Jun;9(6):711-25.

Patel, T.A.; Armstrong, M.; Morris-Jones, S.D.; Wright, S.G. & Doherty, T. (2010). Imported enteric fever: case series from the hospital for tropical diseases, London, United Kingdom. Am J Trop Med Hyg. 2010 Jun;82(6):1121-6.

Pokharel, B.M.; Koirala, J.; Dahal, R.K.; Mishra, S.K.; Khadga, P.K. & Tuladhar, N.R. (2006). Multidrug-resistant and extended-spectrum beta-lactamase (ESBL)-producing *Salmonella enterica* (serotypes Typhi and Paratyphi A) from blood isolates in Nepal: surveillance of resistance and a search for newer alternatives. Int J Infect Dis. 2006 Nov;10(6):434-8.

Prakash, P.; Mishra, O.P., Singh, A.K.; Gulati, A.K. & Nath, G. (2005). Evaluation of nested PCR in diagnosis of typhoid fever. J Clin Microbiol. 2005 Jan;43(1):431-2.

Rajagopal, A.; Ramasamy, R.; Mahendran, G. & Thomas, M. (2002). Hepatic abscess complicating paratyphoid infection. Trop Gastroenterol. 2002; 23: 181–82.

Reynolds, D.W.; Carpenter, R.L. & Simon, W.H. (1970). Diagnostic specificity of Widal's reaction for typhoid fever. JAMA. 1970 Dec 21;214(12):2192-3.

Rello, J.; Lisboa, T.; Lujan, M.; Gallego, M.; Kee, C.; Kay, I.; Lopez, D.; Waterer, G.W. & DNA-Neumococo Study Group. (2009).Severity of pneumococcal pneumonia associated with genomic bacterial load. Chest. 2009 Sep;136(3):832-40.

Rubin, F.A.; Kopecko, D.J.; Sack, R.B.; Sudarmono, P.; Yi, A.; Maurta, D.; Meza, R.; Moechtar, M.A.; Edman, D.C. & Hoffman, S.L. (1988). Evaluation of a DNA probe for identifying *Salmonella* Typhi in Peruvian and Indonesian bacterial isolates. J Infect Dis. 1988 May;157(5):1051-3.

Rubin, F.A.; McWhirter, P.D.; Punjabi, N.H.; Lane, E.; Sudarmono, P.; Pulungsih, S.P.; Lesmana, M.; Kumala, S.; Kopecko, D.J. & Hoffman, S.L. (1989). Use of a DNA probe to detect *Salmonella* Typhi in the blood of patients with typhoid fever. J Clin Microbiol. 1989 May;27(5):1112-4.

Rubin, F.A.; McWhirter, P.D.; Burr, D.; Punjabi, N.H.; Lane, E.; Kumala, S.; Sudarmono, P.; Pulungsih, S.P.; Lesmana, M. & Tjaniadi, P. (1990). Rapid diagnosis of typhoid fever through identification of *Salmonella* Typhi within 18 hours of specimen acquisition by culture of the mononuclear cell-platelet fraction of blood. J Clin Microbiol. 1990 Apr;28(4):825-7.

Sánchez-Jiménez, M.M. & Cardona-Castro, N. (2004). Validation of a PCR for diagnosis of typhoid fever and salmonellosis by amplification of the *hil*A gene in clinical samples from Colombian patients. J Med Microbiol. 2004 Sep;53(Pt 9):875-8.

Sinha, A.; Sazawal, S.; Kumar, R.; Sood, S.; Reddaiah, V.P.; Singh, B.; Rao, M.; Naficy, A.; Clemens, J.D. & Bhan, M.K. 1999. Typhoid fever in children aged less than 5 years.Lancet. 1999 Aug 28;354(9180):734-7.

Smith, S.I.; Bamidele, M.; Fowora, M.; Goodluck, H.T.; Omonigbehin, E.A.; Akinsinde, K.A.; Fesobi, T.; Pastoor, R.; Abdoel, T.H. & Smits, H.L. (2011). Application of a point-of-care test for the serodiagnosis of typhoid fever in Nigeria and the need for improved diagnostics. J Infect Dev Ctries. 2011 Jul 27;5(7):520-6.

Snyder, G.E.; Shaps, H.J. & Nelson, M. (2004). Multiple organ dysfunctionsyndrome associated with *Salmonella* Typhi infection. Am J Emerg Med. 2004; 22: 138–39.

Snyder, M.J.; Hornick, R.bB.; Mccrumb, F.R. Jr.; Morse, L.J. & Woodward, T.E. (1963). asymptomatic typhoidal bacteremia in volunteers. antimicrob agents chemother (bethesda). 1963;161:604-7.

Song, J.H.; Cho, H.; Park, M.Y.; Na, D.S.; Moon, H.B. & Pai, C.H. (1993). Detection of Salmonella Typhi in the blood of patients withtyphoid fever by polymerase chain reaction. J Clin Microbiol. 1993 Jun;31(6):1439-43.

Soper, G.A. (1939). The Curious Career of Typhoid Mary. Bull N Y Acad Med. 1939 Oct;15(10):698-712.

Stuart, B.M. & Pullen, R.L. (1946). Typhoid fever: clinical analysis of three hundred and sixty cases. Arch Intern Med. 1946;78:629–661.

Sztein, M.B. (2007). Cell-mediated immunity and antibody responses elicited by attenuated *Salmonella enterica* serovar Typhi strains used as live oral vaccines in humans. Clin Infect Dis. 2007 Jul 15;45 Suppl 1:S15-9.

Tam, F.C. & Lim, P.L. (2003). The TUBEX typhoid test based on particle-inhibition immunoassay detects IgM but not IgG anti-O9 antibodies. J Immunol Methods. 2003 Nov;282(1-2):83-91.

Tam, F.C.; Wang, M.; Dong, B.; Leung, D.T.; Ma, C.H. & Lim, P.L. (2008). New rapid test for paratyphoid a fever: usefulness, cross-detection, and solution. Diagn Microbiol Infect Dis. 2008 Oct;62(2):142-50.

Teh, C.S.; Chua , K.H.; Puthucheary, S.D. & Thong, K.L. (2008). Further evaluation of a multiplex PCR for differentiation of *Salmonella* Paratyphi A from other *Salmonellae*. Jpn J Infect Dis. 2008 Jul;61(4):313-4.

Thisyakorn, U.; Mansuwan, P. & Taylor, D.N. (1987). Typhoid and paratyphoid fever in 192 hospitalized children in Thailand. Am J Dis Child. 1987 Aug;141(8):862-5.

Vallenas, C.; Hernandez, H.; Kay, B.; Black, R. & Gotuzzo, E. (1985). Efficacy of bone marrow, blood, stool and duodenal contents cultures for bacteriologic confirmation of typhoid fever in children. Pediatr Infect Dis. 1985 Sep-Oct;4(5):496-8.

Vincent, M.; Xu, Y. & Kong, H. (2004). Helicase-dependent isothermal DNA amplification. EMBO reports, 2004; 5: 795–800.

Volk, E.E.; Miller, M.L.; Kirkley, B.A. & Washington, J.A. (1998). The diagnostic usefulness of bone marrow cultures in patients with fever of unknown origin. Am J Clin Pathol. 1998 Aug;110(2):150-3.

Vollaard, A.M.; Ali, S.; Widjaja, S.; Asten, H.A.; Visser, L.G.; Surjadi.; C. & van Dissel, J.T. (2005). Identification of typhoid fever and paratyphoid fever cases at presentation in outpatient clinics in Jakarta, Indonesia. Trans R Soc Trop Med Hyg. 2005; 99:440–450.

Wain, J. & Hosoglu, S. (2008). The laboratory diagnosis of enteric fever. *J Infect Dev Ctries.* 2008 Dec 1;2(6):421-5.

Wain, J.; Diep, T.S.; Ho, V.A.; Walsh, A.M.; Nguyen, T.T.; Parry, C.M. & White, N.J. (1989). Quantitation of bacteria in blood of typhoid fever patients and relationship between counts and clinical features, transmissibility, and antibiotic resistance. J Clin Microbiol. 1998 Jun;36(6):1683-7.

Wain, J.; House, D.; Zafar, A.; Baker, S.; Nair, S.; Kidgell, C.; Bhutta, Z.; Dougan, G. & Hasan, R. (2005). Vi antigen expression in *Salmonella enterica* serovar Typhi clinical isolates from Pakistan. J Clin Microbiol. 2005 Mar;43(3):1158-65.

Wain, J.; Pham, B.V.; Ha, V.; Nguyen, N.M.; To, S.D.; Walsh, A.L.; Parry, C.M.; Hasserjian, R.P.; HoHo, V.A.; Tran, T.H.; Farrar, J.; White, N.J. & Day, N.P. (2001). Quantitation of bacteria in bone marrow from patients with typhoid fever: relationship between counts and clinical features. J Clin Microbiol. 2001 Apr;39(4):1571-6.

Wain, J.; To, S.D.; Phan, V.B.B.; Walsh, A.L.; Ha, V.; Nguyen, M.D.; Vo, A.H.; Tran, T.H.; Farrar, J.; White, N.J.; Parry, M. & Day, N.P.J. (2008). Specimens and culture media for the laboratory diagnosis of typhoid fever. *J Infect Dev Ctries.* 2008 Dec 1;2(6):469-74.

Walker, G.T.; Fraiser, M.S.; Schram, J.L.; Little, M.C.; Nadeau, J.G. & Malinowski, D.P. (1992). Strand-displacement amplification-an isothermal, in vitro DNA amplification technique. Nucleic Acids Res. 1992; 20: 1691–1696.

Watson, K. C. (1955). Isolation of *Salmonella* Typhi from the blood stream. J Lab Clin Med. 1955 Jul;46(1):128-34.

Whitaker, J.A.; Franco-Paredes, C.; del Rio, C. & Edupuganti, S. (2009). Rethinking typhoid fever vaccines: implications for travelers and people living in highly endemic areas. J Travel Med. 2009 Jan-Feb;16(1):46-52.

Widal, F.M. (1896). Serodiagnostic de la fiévre typhoide a-propos d'uve modification par MMC Nicolle et al. Halipie. Bull Soc Med Hop Paris, 1896; 13:561–566.

Woods, C.W.; Murdoch, D.R.; Zimmerman, M.D.; Glover, W.A.; Basnyat, B.; Wolf, L.; Belbase, R.H. & Reller, L.B. (2006). Emergence of *Salmonella enterica* serotype Paratyphi A as a major cause of enteric fever in Kathmandu, Nepal.Trans R Soc Trop Med Hyg. 2006 Nov;100(11):1063-7.

World Health Organization. Background document: The diagnosis, treatment and prevention of typhoid fever. WHO/V&B/03.07.Geneva: World Health Organization, 2003.

Yang, H.H.; Gong, J.; Zhang, J.; Wang, M.L,.; Yang, J.; Wu, G.Z,.; Quan, W.L.; Gong, H.M. & Szu, S.C. (2010).An outbreak of *Salmonella* Paratyphi A in a boarding school: a community-acquired enteric fever and carriage investigation. Epidemiol Infect. 2010 Dec;138(12):1765-74.

Zhou, L. & Pollard, A.J. (2010). A fast and highly sensitive blood culture PCR method for clinical detection of *Salmonella enterica* serovar Typhi. Ann Clin Microbiol Antimicrob. 2010 Apr 19;9:14.

Zhu, Q.; Lim, C.K. & Chan, Y.N. (1996). Detection of *Salmonella* Typhi by polymerase chain reaction. J Appl Bacteriol. 1996 Mar;80(3):244-51.

22

Comprehending a Molecular Conundrum: Functional Studies of Ribosomal Protein Mutants from *Salmonella enterica* Serovar Typhimurium

Christina Tobin Kåhrström[1], Dan I. Andersson[1] and Suparna Sanyal[2,*]
[1]*Department of Medical Biochemistry and Microbiology*
[2]*Department of Cell and Molecular Biology*
Uppsala University
Sweden

1. Introduction

Of all the molecules present in the living organism, proteins are the most abundant and are often described as the most fundamental. This is a reasonable assertion, considering the enormous diversity of crucial cellular functions that are performed by proteins, which range from structural support and signal transduction to enzyme catalysis and immune defence. Given the vital nature of their function, efficient and orderly production of proteins is essential for cell fitness and survival.

In every living cell, protein synthesis or translation as it is otherwise known, is performed by complex, dynamic ribonucleoprotein particles known as ribosomes. Conversion of the genetic code into biologically active proteins is an elaborate process that relies on the availability of mRNA template, as well as amino acid substrates that are delivered to the ribosome attached to tRNA molecules. In addition, the ribosome is assisted by a number of protein factors, known as "translation factors", which serve to streamline and accelerate various sub-steps of the process. Having said that, however, all phases of the translation cycle can be performed in the absence of such factors, albeit slow, so the ribosome can be regarded as the core of translation. It manages to manufacture proteins at an incredible speed (up to 20 amino acids per second) and with very few errors (one in every 1,000 - 10,000 codons deciphered) (Kramer & Farabaugh, 2007). In *Escherichia coli (E. coli)*, ribosomes account for up to 50% of the dry mass of the cell and considering their central role in gene expression, it is not surprising that the cell devotes up to 40% of its total energy to ribosome production during rapid growth (Nierhaus, 1991; Nierhaus, 2006). The immensity of the task of the ribosome is adequately reflected in the sophistication of its structure, where the modern ribosome represents one of the largest and most complex cellular machines. Despite substantial progress in terms of genetic, biochemical and structural techniques, designed to delineate the mechanism of action of the ribosome, many aspects of protein synthesis and ribosome function remain to be elucidated.

* Corresponding Author

1.1 Bacterial ribosomes – Structure and function

Ribosomes are universally conserved and are composed of ribosomal RNA (rRNA) and ribosomal proteins (r-proteins) in all organisms. Ribosomal RNA is the major structural component of all cytoplasmic ribosomes, where it accounts for approximately two thirds of the total mass. The remaining third consists of a large number of mostly small, basic ribosomal proteins (r-proteins) that are scattered over the surface of the structure. The simplest ribosome, that of the bacterial cell, totals approximately 2.5 MDa and is over 200 Å in width (Williamson, 2009), establishing it as the largest enzymatic particle in the cell. The number of ribosomes in the cell can reach up to tens of thousands in order to cope with the increased demand for protein synthesis during periods of rapid cell division (Bremer & Dennis, 1996).

All ribosomes consist of two subunits of unequal size. In prokaryotes the smaller of the two subunits is known as the 30S and the larger subunit is known as the 50S, which are named based on their coefficient of sedimentation. The subunits exist as free, separated molecules in the cell cytoplasm when inactive but associate to form a translation-competent 70S ribosome upon the initiation of protein synthesis. The 30S is composed of one strand of 16S rRNA (1,542 nucleotides) and 21 r-proteins. As expected the 50S contains more rRNA (23S and 5S containing 2,904 and 120 nucleotides, respectively) and more protein (33 r-proteins). For many years, the detailed structure of the ribosome was elusive due to limitations of crystallographic techniques, which was compounded by the tremendous size of the particle. However, at the turn of the century, crystallographic images of ribosomal subunits at the atomic level appeared and marked a gigantic leap forward in our understanding of the structural mysteries (Ban et al., 2000; Wimberly et al., 2000). Since then detailed images of

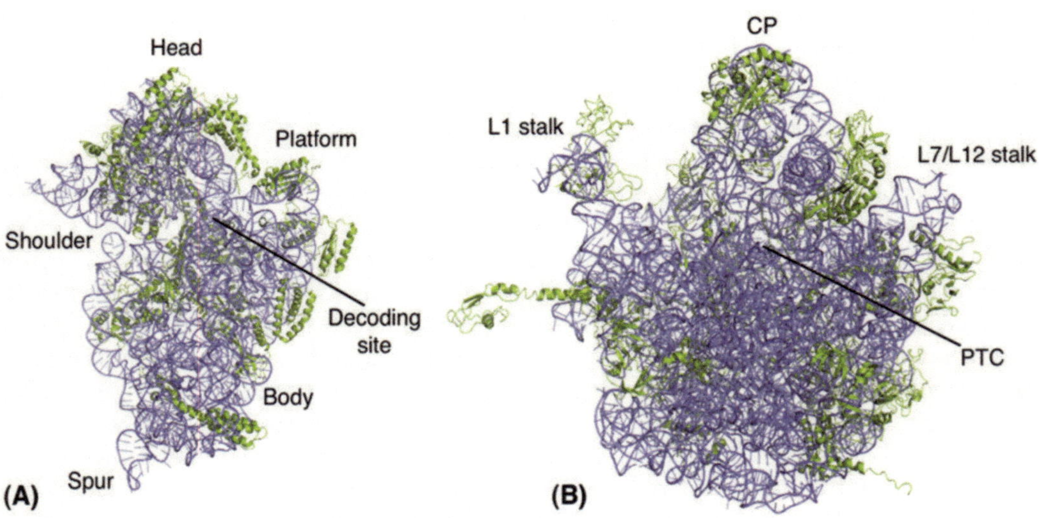

Fig. 1. **High-resolution crystal structures of the ribosomal subunits.** Tertiary structures of the bacterial 30S (A) and 50S (B) viewed from the inter-subunit face. Ribosomal RNA depicted in blue and r-proteins as green ribbons. Abbreviations are as follows: CP, central protuberance; PTC, peptidyl-transferase centre. The image was generated in PyMol (www.pymol.org) from the coordinates of the crystal structure of the *T. thermophilus* ribosome (PDB ID 2J00 & 2J01)(Selmer et al., 2006).

the full ribosome with translation ligands bound have been generated and to date the highest resolution crystal structure available is that of the *Thermus thermophilus (T. thermophilus)* 70S ribosome (Figure 1) (Selmer et al., 2006).

As clearly illustrated by the crystal structure, the two subunits are markedly different in their overall shape. The morphology of each subunit is an inherent feature of the folds adopted by each rRNA species and gives rise to a rigid large subunit and a more flexible small subunit. The 50S is a compact, compressed particle consisting of a hemispherical base with three conspicuous protuberances designated the L1 stalk, the central protuberance (CP) and the L7/L12 stalk (Figure 1B). The two rRNA strands (23S and 5S rRNAs) are highly interlaced to form a dense rRNA mesh. In contrast, the 30S is not only smaller in size, but is also less compact. The four secondary structure domains of the 16S rRNA correlate well to distinct regions of the three dimensional structure such as the head, body and platform (Figure 1A). The r-proteins are spatially dispersed at the periphery and back of the subunits, remote from the main functional sites such as the decoding centre, peptidyl-transferase centre (PTC) and the inter-subunit face. With this realisation, the controversy surrounding the basis of ribosomal enzymatic activity was finally laid to rest since the structures established that the PTC was devoid of protein and the ribosome was quickly recognised as a ribozyme (Nissen et al., 2000). In addition, high-resolution structures of the 30S revealed that decoding was primarily mediated by dynamic rearrangements of the 16S rRNA upon cognate tRNA binding at the ribosomal A-site (Ogle et al., 2003). Together, these studies propelled rRNA into the spotlight, securing its superior position as the major mediator of ribosomal function.

1.2 The ribosome at work

A detailed description of bacterial translation is beyond the scope of this text, however a brief overview is presented to facilitate a clear understanding of the experiments that will be described later. The process can be conceptually divided into four major phases as described below.

1.2.1 Initiation

Initiation begins on the 30S subunit and requires the binding of an mRNA template that carries the blueprint for the protein product. Next, selective and rapid binding of the unique, initiator tRNA (fMet-tRNA^{fMet}) to the 30S subunit takes place. This event is coordinated by the action of three initiation factors (IF1, IF2 and IF3), the principal one being the G-protein factor IF2, forming the 30S preinitiation complex. The 50S subunit is recruited and the initiation factors are released to form what is known as a 70S initiation complex (IC) that is now ready to proceed to the next phase.

1.2.2 Elongation

During elongation, the polypeptide grows as a result of the processive addition of amino acids that are delivered to the 70S ribosome as aminoacyl-tRNAs in a ternary complex with EF-Tu and GTP. Upon acceptance of the cognate substrate, rapid peptidyl transfer occurs. The tRNA-mRNA complex is re-positioned by a distance of exactly one codon to facilitate further addition of aminoacyl-tRNAs and this translocation step is stimulated by GTP hydrolysis on EF-G. Amino-acyl tRNA selection, peptidyl transfer and translocation are repeated until a stop codon appears at the A-site.

1.2.3 Termination

In eubacteria, two release factor proteins (RF1 and RF2) recognize stop codons in a semi-specific manner and activate release of the nascent protein from the P-site tRNA to terminate translation. A third release factor RF-3, removes and recycles RF1 and RF2.

1.2.4 Ribosome recycling

During the final phase, ribosome recycling factor (RRF), in combination with EF-G are required to split the 70S into its subunits. The deacylated tRNA attached to the P-site of the 30S is ejected upon IF3 binding, the 30S can slide along the mRNA to re-initiate translation or the mRNA is also released. This event leaves the ribosome and its factors available to participate in further rounds of translation.

1.3 Ribosomal proteins

Despite the predominance of rRNA, the bacterial ribosome does contain an impressive array of 54 individual r-proteins. In *E. coli* and *Salmonella enterica* serovar Typhimurium, 21 proteins are associated with the small subunit (S proteins) and 33 with the large subunit (L proteins) (Wilson & Nierhaus, 2005). Among eukaryotes, the number of r-proteins increases by approximately 20-30 (Doudna & Rath, 2002). In bacteria, all r-proteins, with the exception of L7/L12, are present as a single copy per ribosome.

The overall abundance of rRNA and its direct involvement in the major tasks of the ribosome (decoding and peptidyl-transfer) have allowed the r-proteins to evade direct scrutiny and their contribution to translation is largely ill-defined. Furthermore, many of these proteins tend to be highly conserved, which forcefully calls our attention to questions regarding their functional roles (Lecompte et al., 2002). In general, they are considered important for the maintenance and stability of the overall structure of the ribosome (Cech, 2000). This assumption is largely due to their extensive contact with rRNA where many of the proteins contain extended projections that insert into the busy network of rRNA helices, prompting the idea that they probably promote or may even facilitate correct folding of the rRNA into its active conformation. However, few studies have directly addressed this issue and we are in the dark regarding the functional roles of most of the proteins. With this in mind, our research has focused on ascertaining the requirement and involvement of particular r-proteins for optimal cell growth and ribosome activity. We have posed the following questions:

1. If rRNA is responsible for the basic function of the ribosome then what, if any, are the selective advantages offered by the r-proteins? In other words, are they all actually necessary for ribosome function?
2. Is it possible to create mutants that completely lack a r-protein and mutants that carry a non-native version of the protein from another species?
3. What are the physiological consequences of such mutations with respect to cell fitness and ribosome function?

4. If such mutations confer fitness costs (i.e. slower growth), is it possible to compensate for such costs?
5. What are the mechanisms of fitness compensation that evolve in response to removal and replacement of r-proteins?

By addressing such questions we are ultimately interested in probing the complexity and robustness of the translation apparatus. To approach some useful answers to these questions, we have used *Salmonella enterica* serovar Typhimurium LT2 (hereafter referred to as *S. typhimurium*) as a model organism and introduced deletions of the genes encoding the r-proteins S20 and L1 and replaced S20, L1 and L17 with orthologous counterparts from close and phylogenetically distant relatives, including the archaeon *Sulfolobus acidocaldarius* and the eukaryote *Saccharomyces cerevisiae*.

2. Using *S. typhimurium* as a model in the ribosome field

E. coli has long served as a model organism for genetic and biochemical studies of bacterial ribosome function. However, due to the co-linearity of their genomes, *S. typhimurium* represents a convenient alternative for such studies and is preferable in our case due to a more favourable and better characterized genetic background for the purposes of genetic suppression studies (McClelland et al., 2001) (see below). Although highly similar in terms of ribosomal gene content, *S. typhimurium* does possess some unique features that are described below.

2.1 Primary sequences of rRNA and r-proteins

In terms of the basic building blocks of the ribosome, rRNA and r-proteins, the genes encoding these components are generally highly conserved between *E. coli* and *S. typhimurium*, a reflection of their close phylogenetic relationship. In both organisms, there are seven independent rRNA operons (*rrnA, rrnB, rrnC, rrnD, rrnE, rrnG* and *rrnH)*, each encoding a single copy of the 16S, 23S and 5S rRNAs. The genes encoding the 16S and 5S rRNAs show strong similarities; however, more variation is detected between the genes encoding the 23S rRNA species (*rrl* genes). In particular, the primary sequences of *rrl* genes in *S. typhimurium* are between 90 and 110 nucleotides longer due to the presence of so-called intervening sequences (IVSs) that are removed during maturation (Burgin et al., 1990). Despite this discrepancy in the length of their primary 23S rRNA sequences, the mature, core sequence in *S. typhimurium* is nearly identical (97%) to that of *E. coli* (Burgin et al., 1990).

In terms of the r-proteins, a high degree of conservation is also observed upon alignment of the amino acid sequences of *S. typhimurium* LT2 proteins and *E. coli* K-12 MG1655 proteins. For the 21 r-proteins associated with the small subunit, a median similarity of 99.2% is detected with an average identity of 98.9% and a standard deviation of 0.9%. Similarly, for the 33 r-proteins associated with the large subunit, the median amino acid identity is 98.9% with an average similarity of 97.7% and a standard deviation of 3.6%. From these calculations, we can conclude that there is slightly more variation in the amino acid sequences of large subunit proteins when comparing the primary sequences of *S. typhimurium* LT2 and *E. coli* K-12 MG1655. However, overall, a high degree of conservation exists, which is not surprising given the close phylogenetic relationship.

2.2 rRNA processing during ribosome biogenesis

During transcription of the rRNA operons, the primary transcripts are processed to mature products by means of RNase cleavage and chemical modification (Kaczanowska & Ryden-Aulin, 2007). The vast majority of studies that have examined these processing events have looked at the *E. coli* system only, however it is expected that *rrn* processing in close relatives such as *S. typhimurium* should be highly similar.

Primary *rrn* transcripts of *E. coli* are initially substrates for the endoribonuclease RNase III that catalyzes separation of the rRNAs into pre-16S (17S), pre-23S and pre-5S (9S) species (Nierhaus, 2006). Final trimming of the 5′ and 3′ ends of each transcript involves a number of exonucleases and occurs in the context of pre-ribosomal particles (Deutscher, 2009). In some genera of bacteria, including *S. typhimurium*, mature 23S rRNA is not fully intact but is fragmented during processing. Experiments have revealed that the fragments arise due to RNase III-mediated removal of intervening sequences (Burgin et al., 1990). Although the resulting fragments of 23S rRNA are not re-ligated they are fully functional. Some heterogeneity exists between the seven copies of 23S rRNA genes in *S. typhimurium* LT2 with regard to the presence of these additional sequences. In the case of *rrlG* and *rrlH*, an insertion of approximately 110 nucleotides is observed in helix-25 (located at nucleotide position 550, approximately) and *rrlA, rrlB, rrlC, rrlD, rrlE* and *rrlH* contain an insertion of approximately 90 nucleotides in helix-45 (located at nucleotide position 1170, approximately). Interestingly, ribosomes of a *S. typhimurium* mutant lacking RNase III remain functional, implying that fragmentation is not required for the activity of *S. typhimurium* ribosomes (Mattatall & Sanderson, 1998). This would also suggest that it is unlikely that these extra sequences evolved to support proper functioning of *S. typhimurium* ribosomes. Their intermittent distribution among diverse genera of bacteria would suggest that they may have been acquired by horizontal gene transfer (Mattatall & Sanderson, 1996).

2.3 Unusual sucrose gradient profile of *Salmonella* ribosomes

Analysis of ribosome function *in vitro* requires the extraction of large quantities of intact ribosomes from the cell using a standard sucrose density ultracentrifugation protocol (Johansson et al., 2008). Typically, this involves preparing a pure cell lysate that is passed through two sucrose cushions to remove cell debris. Ribosomal particles (70S, 50S and 30S) are subsequently separated on a final sucrose gradient (10 – 50%) based on differences in their densities. The standard protocols available are optimised for *E. coli* and pure fractions of each ribosomal particle are easily obtainable. The high degree of similarity between *S. typhimurium* and *E. coli* might, *a priori*, lead one to expect a similar profile when the protocol is applied to *S. typhimurium*. However, in our hands, we have consistently observed a striking difference.

Looking at a typical, large-scale 70S purification profile from *E. coli* K12 strain MRE600 (Figure 2A), clean, distinct peaks are observed for each ribosomal particle, as indicated. In contrast, the 70S peak from wild-type *S. typhimurium* LT2 contains a distinct shoulder (Figure 2B). Upon examination of the protein and rRNA content of the second, smaller peak, we observed that this contains 30S particles only, indicating that the 70S and 50S peaks coincide when ribosomes are prepared from *S. typhimurium* on a large scale. This is a consistent feature of the wild-type strain, as well as all r-protein mutant strains that we have worked with. At the present time, there is no definitive explanation for these observations but the unusual co-migration of 70S and 50S species may be related to 23S rRNA processing differences between the species, or, 70S ribosomes of *S. typhimurium* may be composed of loosely-coupled subunits that require a higher magnesium concentration for stabilization.

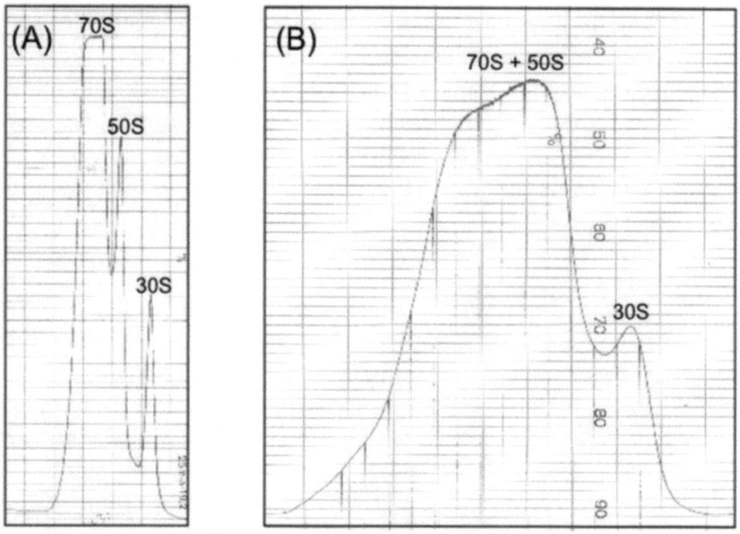

Fig. 2. **Sucrose gradient ultracentrifugation profiles obtained during 70S ribosome purification.** (A) Profile obtained from *E. coli* MRE600 showing three separate peaks for 70S, 50S and 30S particles. (B) Profile obtained from wild-type *S. typhimurium* showing a distinctive shouldered peak containing a mixture of 70S and 50S particles followed by a 30S peak.

2.4 Advantages of using *S. typhimurium* as a model

E. coli is traditionally regarded as the first choice model organism for studies of ribosome function. However, it has recently become clear that the most frequently used K-12 strain has mutations in components that function in translation. Mutations in the genes *prmB* (encoding class-I release factor RF2) and *rpsG* (encoding ribosomal protein S7) represent two well-characterized examples. O' Connor et al. have reported that in all K-12 strains of *E. coli,* RF2 carries a threonine residue at position 246 as opposed to alanine, which is typically found at this position in the majority of bacterial RF2 proteins (O'Connor & Gregory, 2011). In the case of *rpsG,* a point mutation alters its canonical UGA stop codon to a leucine codon (Schaub & Hayes, 2011). Thus, the S7 protein of all K-12 strains carries an extension of 23 amino acids at its C-terminus. This protein is essential and particularly important during 30S assembly. Both of these mutations were identified as being partially responsible for the fitness cost and ribosomal perturbations associated with an *rluD* null mutation.

These studies serve to highlight the importance of using a model organism with a clean genetic background. The presence of underlying, undetected mutations complicates the matter of defining the mechanism and cause of observed phenotypes associated with a mutation of interest due to the unavoidable likelihood of synergistic and epistatic interactions. Our research has concentrated on the effects of r-protein removal and replacement in terms of bacterial fitness and ribosome function with a strong focus on suppression genetics. So, although *E. coli* K-12 is undoubtedly the most well-studied model organism, *S. typhimurium* represents a more suitable and reliable model for the purposes of our studies.

3. Isolation and characterisation of ribosomal protein mutants

The scarcity of studies designed to examine the distinct functional roles of r-proteins, despite their high level of conservation in all three phylogenetic kingdoms, certainly warrants further experimentation aimed at understanding their contributions to cell fitness and ribosome activity. To address this issue, genetically defined *S. typhimurium* mutants were constructed in which the target proteins were either completely removed (S20 and L1) from the chromosome or replaced (S20, L1 and L17) on the chromosome with orthologous counterparts from other species.

3.1 Previous studies of r-protein mutants

The majority of the early research on mutants lacking r-proteins was initiated by the work of Dabbs and colleagues. Beginning in the mid-70s, various antibiotic selection systems were developed for the isolation of *E. coli* mutants with alterations in r-proteins (Dabbs & Wittman, 1976; Dabbs, 1978). Most of the mutants that lacked a r-protein were isolated by chemically mutagenizing antibiotic sensitive cells, selecting for antibiotic dependence followed by selection for reversion of the antibiotic dependent phenotype (Dabbs, 1979). Using such methods, *E. coli* strains were isolated lacking one or more of 16 individual r-proteins (S1, S6, S9, S13, S17, S20, L1, L11, L15, L19, L24, L27, L28, L29, L30 and L33) (Dabbs, 1991). In all of these studies, absence of each protein was only verified on the protein level by means of two-dimensional gel electrophoresis and immunological methods using antibodies specific for each missing protein. The mutants exhibited a conditional lethal phenotype and were varied in terms of growth properties. These studies were certainly pioneering in terms of showing the non-essential nature of certain r-proteins but follow-up studies designed to determine the nature of the fitness costs and ribosomal defects were hampered by the chemical mutagenesis and selection methods used for the isolation of mutants. These strains were subject to mutagenesis on a genome-wide scale and were therefore not fully defined genetically, which creates difficulty in specifically linking the observed phenotypes to absence of the protein. In the past few years, much progress has been made in the techniques used for the manipulation of bacterial genetics (Datsenko & Wanner, 2000; Sharan et al., 2009). These methods have made it possible to introduce precise deletions of targeted genes and a number of research groups have been successful in obtaining r-protein null mutants (Wower et al., 1998; Cukras & Green, 2005; Bubunenko et al., 2007; Korepanov et al., 2007). In a recent work the number of the L7/L12 proteins have been varied by deletion of the binding site of one L7/L12 dimer on the L10 protein (Mandava et al., 2011). The characterisation of such mutants has advanced our current knowledge of the functions of some of the r-proteins; unfortunately, however, these mutants are all limited to the species *E. coli*.

Attempts to produce functionally active hybrid ribosomes harboring non-native r-proteins have previously been undertaken (Liu et al., 1989; Giese & Subramanian, 1991). The majority of these studies only examined functional activity in terms of polysome formation. However, highly divergent proteins such as S18 from rye chloroplast, that shares only 35% amino acid identity with *E. coli* S18, was incorporated into 30-40% of *E. coli* monosomes and polysomes upon expression from a plasmid (Weglohner et al., 1997). The ability of these hybrid ribosomes to form polysomes indicates that they were capable of forming functional complexes, although the extent of their functionality during specific steps of translation was not examined. In the same study, L12 from *Arabidopsis* chloroplasts was also incorporated into ribosomes but these hybrid ribosomes failed to form functional polysomes *in vivo* and were inactive in poly(U)-dependent poly(Phe) synthesis *in vitro*. In another study, the *E. coli* proteins of the GTPase-associated centre (L10, L11 and L7/L12) were replaced with their rat counterparts *in vitro* (Uchiumi et al., 2002). Although incorporated into the *E. coli* ribosome, eukaryotic elongation factors were required to support protein synthesis *in vitro*. So although divergent r-proteins can be assembled into the bacterial ribosome, proteins with defined functions, such as interactions with bacterial specific translation factors, lack function and do not preserve protein synthesis.

3.2 Construction of r-protein mutants

In our studies, mutants of *S. typhimurium* that completely lacked an r-protein, and mutants in which the native r-protein gene was replaced with closely related as well as phylogenetically distant orthologues were created. Due to its simplicity and precision, lambda red recombineering was used for the construction of all mutants (Datsenko & Wanner, 2000). For removal of S20 and L1, a kanamycin resistance cassette was PCR amplified using primers with 50 nucleotide 5' tails homologous to the flanking sequence of the target gene (*rplA* and *rpsT*). Electroporation of the linear DNA product into the cell resulted in substitution of the r-protein gene with the selectable kanamycin resistance cassette to create mutants lacking S20 (Tobin et al., 2010) and L1 (Figure 3A). A similar procedure was used for the generation of S20, L1 and L17 replacement mutants, however in this case the PCR fragment consisted of the open reading frame (ORF) of the orthologous replacement gene and an adjacent kanamycin resistance cassette (Lind et al., 2010). Homologous recombination resulted in replacement of the target r-protein ORF (*rpsT, rplA* and *rplQ*) with its orthologous ORF and the kanamycin resistance cassette (Figure 3B). Congenic wild-type control strains were also constructed and carried the kanamycin cassette adjacent to the native r-protein ORFs. In the case of both types of constructions, the native promoter and terminator sequences were preserved. Using this technique, individual mutants lacking the r-proteins S20 (ΔS20) and L1 (ΔL1) as well as replacement mutants carrying heterologous versions of S20, L1 and L17 were created.

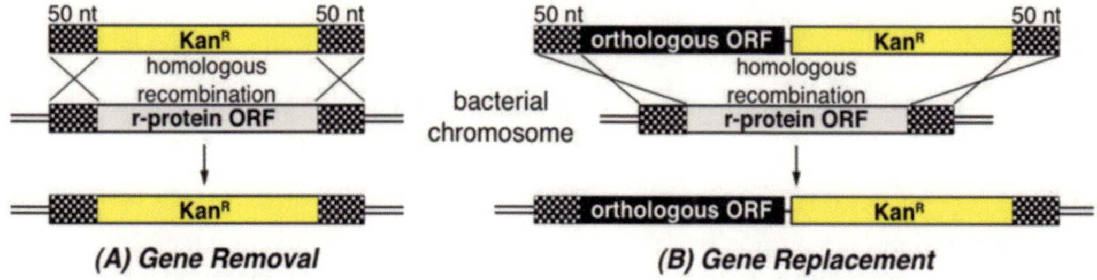

Fig. 3. **Schematic diagram representing the technique employed to generate r-protein mutants.** The recombining fragments in (A) and (B) were designed with 50 nucleotides of homology to the flanking sequences of the r-protein target genes to facilitate homologous recombination and replacement on the chromosome.

3.3 Quantification of fitness costs

In a laboratory setting, determining exponential growth rate is the most straightforward method for assaying fitness. To quantify the physiological effect of r-protein removal and replacement, we measured the doubling time of the wild-type and ribosomal mutant strains using a Bioscreen C analyzer. Relative fitness values were calculated as the growth rate of each mutant normalized to that of the wild-type reference strain used in each experiment (set to 1.0). Although relatively easy to execute, this measurement fails to evaluate fitness over the entire growth cycle and is unable to detect very small differences in fitness (sensitivity of ~ 3%). A more labour intensive method that overcomes such limitations is pair-wise competition experiments where the test strain and wild-type are genetically tagged and compete over many generations (sensitivity of ~ 0.3%). This method was used as a more sensitive fitness parameter in some of our experiments.

3.4 Compensatory evolution

Removal and replacement of highly conserved r-proteins, that function within a central component of the cell, constitute deleterious mutations and confer fitness costs, i.e. slower growth. Because such mutants grow more slowly and therefore produce fewer progeny, they will eventually be out-grown by competitors of higher fitness and eliminated from the population. However, if the mutant can persist in the population, it has the potential to develop further mutations that suppress or compensate the fitness cost of the initial deleterious mutation. Such compensatory mutations (denoted CM) can restore fitness back to the wild-type level and effectively neutralize the deleterious effect of the initial mutation (deletion or replacement of a r-protein). Alternatively, the fitness cost may be only partially relieved by the CM, which increases fitness but not to the extent of wild-type fitness (Figure 4A). Here, we are interested in knowing if and by what mechanisms the fitness costs of L1 removal and S20, L1 and L17 replacement can be compensated. This is not only helpful in the sense that it may provide clues to the functional roles of the proteins, but it also provides a unique opportunity to reveal novel co-operative mechanisms in ribosome function.

The experiment is designed to optimize purifying selection, which reduces genetic diversity so that the population stabilizes on the most favourable (fittest) genotype. During the

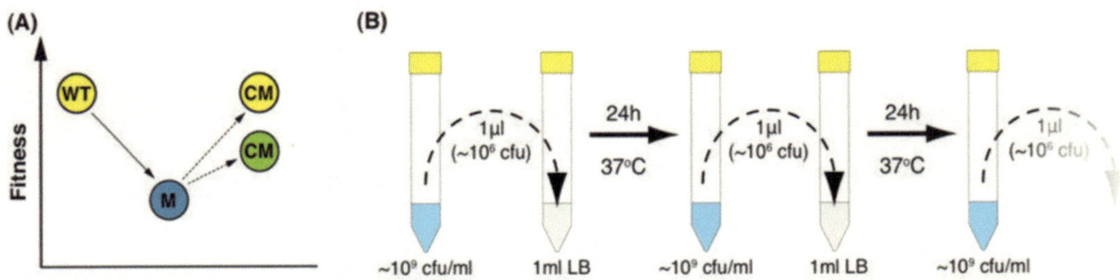

Fig. 4. **Compensatory evolution by serial passage.** (A) Schematic illustration of the principle of compensatory evolution. A deleterious mutation (M) is introduced into a wild-type population (WT) and reduces fitness. Compensatory mutations (CM) that reduce the fitness cost of the initial deleterious mutation can restore fitness completely (yellow) or partially restore fitness (green). (B) Schematic illustration of the serial passage experiment used for the isolation of compensated mutants.

evolutionary process, CMs that reduce the fitness cost conferred by loss or replacement of the r-protein become more common in successive generations. Independent lineages of the mutants are serially passaged in liquid growth medium (LB) for a number of generations. To maintain continuous population growth and to ensure that all genetic variants are represented during the entire evolutionary process, large bottlenecks of ~ 10^6 cells are used (Figure 4B). This experimental design maximises the potential to fix the compensated mutant of highest fitness. When mutants of higher fitness constitute the majority of the population, the experiment is terminated and a single colony is examined for the presence of candidate compensatory mutations that increase fitness. To verify that the identified mutations are responsible for improving fitness, genetic reconstructions are performed and fitness is quantified.

3.5 *In vivo* and *in vitro* analysis of ribosomal function

For a full appreciation of the functional roles of deleted r-proteins, both *in vivo* and *in vitro* techniques were employed to compare the activity of mutant ribosomes with their wild-type counterparts.

3.5.1 *In vivo* system

Synthesis of an easily detectable reporter protein was used here to measure the rate of polypeptide elongation and ribosomal misreading of stop codons and frameshifting. Polypeptide elongation rates of exponentially growing cultures were measured by determining the exact time taken to produce the first detectable β-galactosidase molecule following IPTG induction (Miller, 1992). As *S. typhimurium* does not harbor the *lac* operon, the normal inducible *lac* operon was supplied on an F′ factor and was transferred to strains by means of conjugation. This method was used to determine the rate of polypeptide elongation in the strains lacking r-proteins S20 and L1.

The synthesis of β-galactosidase was also used to determine the frequency of stop codon read-through and frameshifting of an L1-depleted ribosome. In this instance, strains carried an F′ factor in which the *lacI* and *lacZ* genes are fused for constitutive expression of β-galactosidase. However, the ribosome must read-through a premature stop codon (UGA_{189} or UAG_{220}) or a +1 or -1 frameshift in *lacI* to produce an active molecule of the enzyme, the activity of which is detected as described above. A read-through value is calculated based on the amount of enzyme produced by the mutated *lacIZ* construct relative to that produced in a congenic strain harbouring a non-mutated *lacIZ* construct (Bjorkman et al., 1999). A second assay, based on luciferase expression, was also employed to determine if L1 depleted ribosomes were prone to general misreading of sense codons (Kramer & Farabaugh, 2007).

3.5.2 *In vitro* system

The translation cycle is composed of a large number of intermediate sub-steps that proceed extremely fast *in vivo*. Thus, in order to specifically examine defined steps in translation, analysis of ribosome function in a controlled *in vitro* translation system is absolutely necessary. For the characterization of S20- and L1-depleted ribosomes, we have employed a reconstituted cell-free translation system that is optimized to meet *in vivo* expectations in so far as it allows measurement of *in vitro* reactions in the millisecond range (Ehrenberg et al., 1989). Ribosomal particles and all other translation components are prepared to high purity according to standard protocols. Additionally, all experiments are performed in polymix buffer that mimics the pH and complex ionic conditions of the bacterial cell (Pettersson & Kurland, 1980). Using this system, r-protein depleted ribosomes can be accurately compared with their wild-type counterparts in all steps of the translation cycle. Although the system was developed for *E. coli*, it has previously been shown that the system can be applied to ribosomes from *S. typhimurium* (Tubulekas et al., 1991).

4. R-protein deletion mutants

Genetically defined mutants of *S. typhimurium*, lacking individual r-proteins (ΔS20 and ΔL1), represent powerful tools for the analysis of the function of these proteins in the context of translation and can also reveal their potential roles in other cellular processes. Below follows a summary of the fitness costs, compensatory mechanisms and the *in vivo* and *in vitro* analysis of the mutants lacking S20 and L1.

4.1 Removal of S20 and L1 confers substantial fitness costs

Loss of small subunit protein S20 reduced exponential growth rate approximately three-fold relative to the wild-type under standard growth conditions (LB broth at 37°C), corresponding to a relative fitness value of 0.33 (Table 1) (Tobin et al., 2010). Upon deletion of large subunit protein L1, the generation time of the mutant was reduced two-fold compared to wild-type under standard growth conditions (Table 1). This fitness cost was even more pronounced during growth at lower temperatures, indicative of a cold-sensitive phenotype. In the case of both mutants, complete restoration of the wild-type growth rate was observed upon induced expression of the deleted gene from an arabinose-inducible plasmid, verifying that the fitness costs were specifically attributable to loss of each respective protein (Figure 5A and B).

Strain	Growth Temperature	Relative Growth Rate
Wild-Type	n/a	1.0
ΔS20	37°C	0.33
ΔL1	30°C	0.36
ΔL1	37°C	0.52
ΔL1	44°C	0.58

Table 1. **Fitness costs associated with removal of S20 and L1.** The generation time of the wild-type strain is set to 1.0 and is used to normalize the growth rate of each mutant at the temperatures specified.

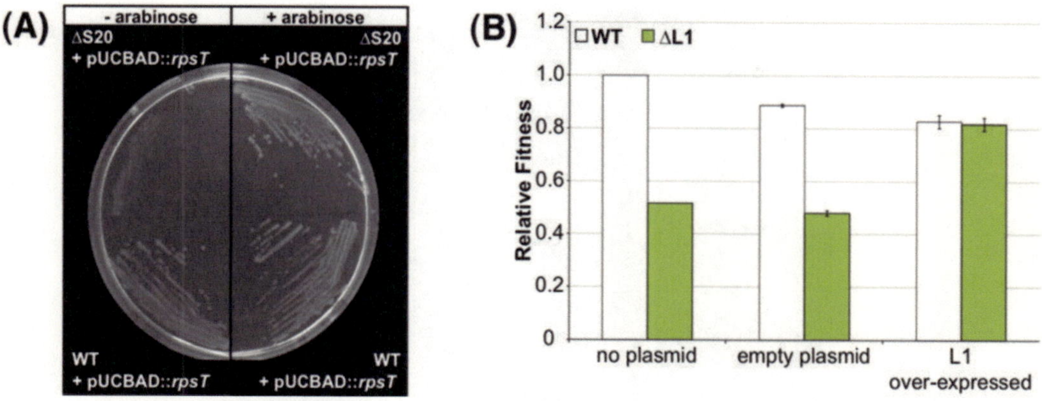

Fig. 5. **Complementation of fitness costs upon induced expression of the deleted r-protein gene from an inducible plasmid.** (A) In the absence of the arabinose inducer, the ΔS20 strain grows very poorly relative to the wild-type (left-hand side of image). In the presence of arabinose, expression of the *rpsT* gene is induced and growth of the mutant matches that of wild-type (right-hand side of image) (Tobin et al., 2010). (B) Growth rates of the ΔL1 mutant relative to the wild-type. In the presence of the arabinose inducer, *rplA* is expressed and fitness of the mutant matches that of wild-type. Error bars represent standard error of the mean.

4.2 Compensatory mutations that mitigate the costs of L1 deletion

Twelve independent lineages of the ΔL1 mutant were evolved for approximately 300 generations to determine if and by what mechanisms compensation could be achieved. Upon isolation of faster-growing mutants, four were chosen at random and subject to whole-genome sequencing to identify candidate compensatory mutations responsible for suppressing the fitness cost associated with loss of L1. A single nucleotide substitution in the *rplB* gene and a small deletion in the *rplS* gene were detected. These mutations resulted in the amino acid substitution E194K in large subunit protein L2 (encoded by *rplB*) and loss of the Leu codon at position 100 of L19 (referred to as *rplS* ΔL100) (Figure 6A). Using a different ΔL1 ancestral strain, the amino acid substitution P102L in the *rplN* gene (encoding large subunit protein L14) was also identified (Figure 6A). Strain reconstructions confirmed that each individual mutation was necessary and sufficient for fitness improvement and all three increased growth rate to a similar extent. In any combination, all three compensatory mutations demonstrated negative epistasis in the ΔL1 background. In the wild-type strain, each individual mutation reduced fitness and this became even more pronounced when the mutations were combined (Figure 6B).

4.3 Phenotypes of previous L1 deletion mutants

Two independent *E. coli* knockout mutants of L1 were previously isolated as spontaneous revertants of chemically mutagenized spectinomycin- and kasugamycin-dependent strains (Dabbs, 1977; Dabbs, 1980). Examination of the activity of ribosomes purified from these strains suggested that absence of L1 reduced the *in vitro* production of polypeptide by 50%, corresponding to an approximate 50% reduction in growth rate (Subramanian & Dabbs, 1980). To probe further into the ribosomal deficiencies, a follow-up study examined the

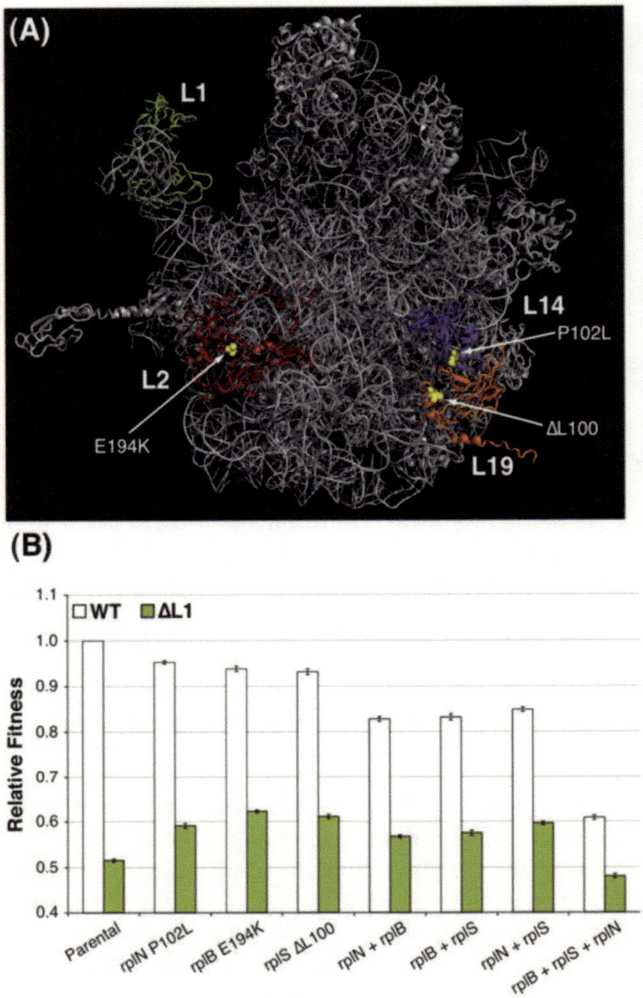

Fig. 6. **Compensation for the fitness costs of L1 deletion.** (A) Crystal structure of the *T. thermophilus* 50S subunit showing the localization of compensatory mutations (yellow spheres) in the r-proteins L2 (red), L14 (purple) and L19 (orange). Position of the L1 protein is shown in green. All other rRNA and protein residues are depicted in grey. The image was created in PyMol (www.pymol.org) using the coordinates of the *T. thermophilus* 50S subunit structure (PDB ID 2J01) (Selmer et al., 2006). (B) Genetic reconstructions and fitness effects of compensatory mutations in the ΔL1 (green bars) and wild-type (white bars) backgrounds. Relative fitness was calculated as the growth rate of each strain as a fraction of the wild-type growth rate. Error bars represent standard error of the mean.

activity of L1-depleted ribosomes using a number of partial reactions. It was found that both the binding of N-acetyl-Phe-tRNA to the P-site and stimulation of EF-G dependent GTP hydrolysis in the presence of tRNA and mRNA were significantly compromised with these ribosomes (Sander, 1983). Another L1 deletion mutant was isolated in an independent study as a spontaneous revertant of a chemically mutagenized erythromycin-dependent strain (Wild, 1988). This strain produced an excess of free ribosomal subunits and fewer 70S ribosomes when the sedimentation profile of ribosomes was examined. In addition, a genetically defined *rplA* deletion strain has been constructed in *E. coli* (Baba et al., 2006), but at the time of writing no details of the phenotype of this mutant are known.

4.3.1 Misreading phenotype

The proposed involvement of L1 in regulating release of the E-site tRNA and the coupling of decoding accuracy at the A-site to occupation of the E-site (Wilson & Nierhaus, 2006) prompted us to investigate the decoding properties of the L1-depleted ribosome. By means of β-galactosidase assays (described in 3.5.1), the level of frameshifting and stop codon readthrough was measured *in vivo*. The only significant difference between the wild-type and mutant was detected with respect to UGA readthrough, which was increased approximately three to five-fold in the case of the ΔL1 mutant, independent of codon context. Misreading of sense codons was also examined although no significant differences were detected, suggesting that L1 plays a minor role, at most, in decoding at the A-site. Furthermore, none of the identified compensatory mutations altered readthrough of UGA in the ΔL1 background.

4.3.2 Polysome analysis

It was previously shown that L1 has RNA chaperone activity (Ameres et al., 2007), so a role for L1 in ribosome biogenesis is possible. To investigate the distribution of different ribosomal particles in the cell, polysome profiles were examined and compared to the profile obtained from wild-type cells (Figure 7). The most striking observation of the mutant

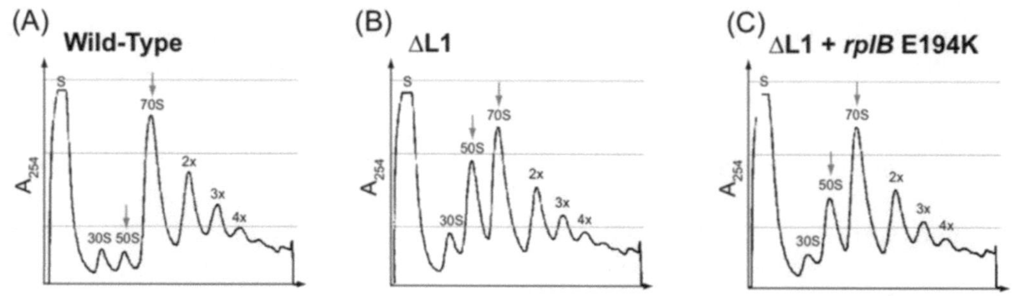

Strain	Peak heights of ribosomal particles relative to sum of all peak heights[a] 30S	50S	70S	2x	3x	4x	Total polysomes[b]	Total 70S particles[c]
Wild-Type	0.08	0.07	0.37	0.22	0.15	0.11	0.48	0.85
ΔL1	0.11	0.23	0.29	0.16	0.11	0.09	0.36	0.65
ΔL1+ *rplB* E194K (CM)	0.09	0.19	0.32	0.18	0.12	0.09	0.39	0.71

Fig. 7. **Polysome profiles obtained following immediate translational arrest in log-phase.** Distribution of ribosomal particles in the wild-type (A), ΔL1 mutant (B) and the ΔL1 mutant with the compensatory mutation (CM) in *rplB* (encoding L2). Each peak corresponds to each different particle as labelled and polysomes are labelled as 2x, 3x and 4x. [a] The table shows average peak heights for each particle relative to the the sum of all peak heights and were based on at least three independent profiles. [b] Total polysomes were calculated as the sum of 2x, 3x and 4x peak heights. [c] Total 70S particles were calculated as the sum of 70S, 2x, 3x and 4x peak heights.

profile (Figure 7B) was the large excess of free 50S subunits, which was increased three-fold compared to the wild-type (Figure 7A). Furthermore, this increase in free subunits was biased specifically towards the 50S as the amount of free 30S was only slightly increased. Thus, removal of L1 leads to an imbalance in formation of the ribosomal subunits. This increase in free subunits occurred at the expense of functional 70S complexes, which were reduced from 0.85 in the wild-type to 0.65 in the mutant. However, the ratio of 70S monosomes to polysomes was the same for the mutant and wild-type, indicating that those 70S ribosomes that were formed could translate as efficiently as the wild-type. Upon overexpression of L1, these anomalies in ribosomal particle partitioning were removed, specifically identifying loss of L1 as the cause of the altered profile. The reduction of 70S complexes as monosomes and polysomes is likely to be responsible for the slow growth rate of the ΔL1 mutant as the translational capacity of the strain is likely to be substantially compromised. Interestingly, the E194K amino acid substitution in L2 conferred a small but reproducible reduction in the proportion of free ribosomal subunits and a consequent increase in the fraction of active 70S complexes (Figure 7C).

4.4 L1 plays a major role in ribosome biogenesis

A number of *in vivo* and *in vitro* methods were used in this study to evaluate the role of L1 in ribosome function. Based on the results of these assays, we propose that large subunit protein L1 is crucial for promoting balanced formation of the ribosomal subunits in *S. typhimurium*. This defect is further supported by the observed cold sensitivity of the ΔL1 mutant, a feature that is often associated with aberrant ribosome biogenesis (Dammel & Noller, 1993; Bubunenko et al., 2006). It is not yet clear why the production of free ribosomal subunits is disproportionate, but a few alternative explanations are feasible. L1 has known RNA chaperone activity so the protein may be directly involved in biogenesis of the small subunit; however, no evidence is currently available to support this suggestion. The effect of L1 deletion on 30S production may be more indirect. It is conceivable that in the absence of L1, 50S subunits are more prone to misassembly than the wild-type. This, in turn, may perturb 30S assembly via sequestering of accessory factors required for the biogenesis of both subunits, for example. Alternatively, if the 30S subunits lack properly assembled association partners, final maturation of the 30S may be impaired and/or the 30S subunits may be more susceptible to the action of degradative RNases as previously suggested (Deutscher, 2009). Although only one of the three confirmed compensatory mutations (*rplB* E194K) displayed a detectable improvement in ribosomal particle partitioning (Figure 7C), the remaining two (*rplN* P102L and *rplS* ΔLeu) occur in proteins directly involved in formation of bridging contacts required for 70S complex formation (Selmer et al., 2006). Thus, it would appear as though these two compensatory mutations may alter subunit interactions and possibly increase 70S production. Furthermore, additional compensatory mutations in the genes *rpsM* (encoding S13 that forms bridges B1a and B1b with the 50S subunit) and *engA* (encoding the 50S biogenesis factor Der) provide more evidence that L1 plays an important role in ribosome biogenesis.

Along with helices 76-78 of the 23S rRNA, L1 occupies a highly mobile region of the 50S subunit known as the L1 stalk. Crystal structures of the 50S and 70S revealed that this stalk can adopt both an "open" and "closed" conformation, suggestive of an underlying functional role in the release of deacylated tRNA from the E-site thereby alluding to a role for this region in the translocation step of polypeptide elongation (Harms et al., 2001; Yusupov et al., 2001). These observations sparked a number of structural-based investigations aimed at investigating L1 stalk dynamics which all indicate that this region is involved in modulating decaylated tRNA transit and release during translocation (Valle et al., 2003; Fei et al., 2008; Munro et al., 2010; Trabuco et al., 2010). Thus, to determine the activity of L1 depleted ribosomes in the elongation step of translation, a number of *in vivo* and *in vitro* assays are currently underway.

4.5 Phenotype of S20 deletion mutant

Knockout mutants of S20 have been isolated previously as antibiotic dependent revertants and as a suppressor of nonsense codons (Dabbs, 1978; Dabbs, 1979; Ryden-Aulin et al., 1993). Both types of mutants displayed initiation defects in terms of initiator tRNA binding (Gotz et al., 1990) and subunit association (Gotz et al., 1989; Ryden-Aulin et al., 1993). In another study, an S20 knockout mutant was obtained as a suppressor of erythromycin dependence and produced precursor 30S particles and fewer 70S complexes, as measured by density ultracentrifugation (Wild, 1988). More recently, the recombineering approach has been used to isolate genetically defined, in-frame deletions of *rpsT* in *E. coli,* but data to describe the phenotypic effects of these deletions is currently unavailable (Baba et al., 2006; Bubunenko et al., 2007).

4.5.1 Polypeptide formation *in vivo*

The rate at which the ΔS20 mutant forms polypeptide *in vivo* was compared to the wild-type strain using the β-galactosidase assay. Similar to the results of the ΔL1 mutant, no defect in the rate of polypeptide chain elongation was detected, however a reproducible reduction in the rate of accumulation of synthesized protein was evident (Tobin et al., 2010). Considering that S20 is a designated 30S subunit protein and given the results of previous studies, we hypothesized that the reduced rate of protein accumulation was likely the result of impaired initiation. A reduction in the frequency of mRNA initiation would directly decrease the number of rounds of translation per mRNA and reduce the yield of protein production. Thus, the activity of S20-depleted 30S subunits were compared to those obtained from the wild-type, using a number of *in vitro* methods designed to measure each distinct step of translation initiation.

4.5.2 Reduced mRNA binding *in vitro*

The rate of template binding was measured using a radioactively labeled mRNA with a strong Shine-Dalgarno (SD) sequence. In both the presence and absence of initiator tRNA and the initiation factors, the rate of mRNA binding to ΔS20 30S subunits was reduced approximately 3.5-fold and maximum binding required 40 minutes compared to only 10 minutes for the wild-type. Since similar rates of mRNA binding were observed with and without the initiation ligands, a primary impairment in mRNA binding could be concluded. Reconstitution with purified S20 restored the wild-type mRNA binding phenotype and established that defective mRNA association was a direct consequence of S20 removal (Figure 8A). In addition, titration of mRNA revealed that a substantial fraction (~ 25%) of the S20-depleted 30S subunits were completely inactive in the binding of mRNA (Figure 8B). Since the rate of fMet-tRNA^{fMet} binding emulated that of mRNA and was therefore used to detect the level of mRNA bound to 30S subunits in this assay, the possibility of unstable initiator tRNA binding could not be entirely excluded as the underlying cause of incomplete ΔS20 30S occupancy with mRNA. Thus the stability of initiator tRNA binding was measured by its rate of dissociation from 30S pre-initiation complexes. The results demonstrated that dissociation of fMet-tRNA^{fMet} occurred at the same rate for the mutant and wild-type. Hence, we could conclude that reduced initiator tRNA binding was a secondary, consequential effect of a primary impairment in mRNA binding (Tobin et al., 2010).

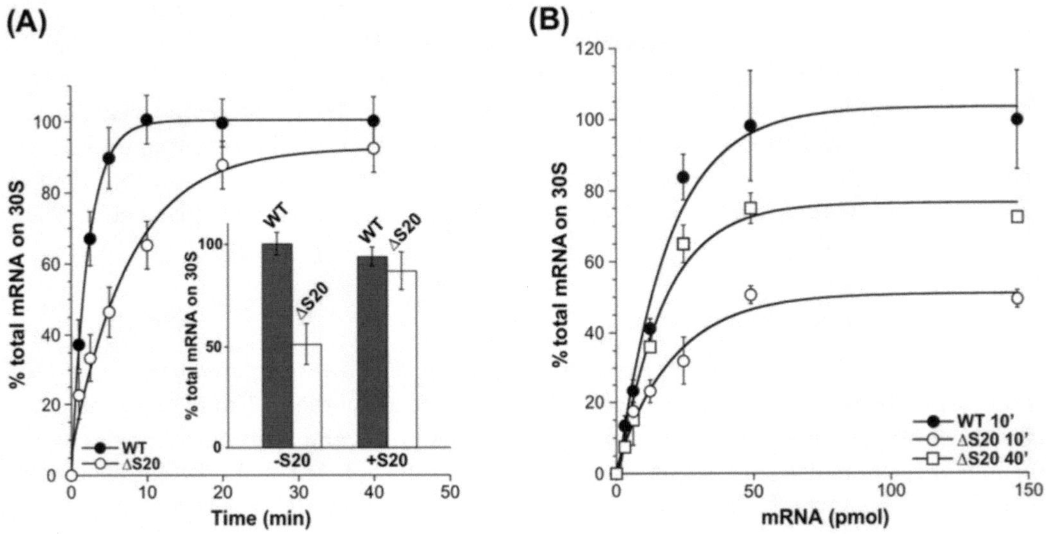

Fig. 8. **Activity of wild-type and S20-depleted 30S subunits in mRNA binding.** (A) The rate of mRNA binding to the mutant 30S subunit is reduced by a factor of approximately 3.5. Upon reconstitution with purified S20 protein, this impairment is removed (insert). (B) Upon titration with mRNA, a considerable fraction of the mutant 30S subunits failed to associate with mRNA. (Tobin et al., 2010)

4.5.3 Defective subunit association

The kinetics of 50S association to wild-type and S20-depleted 30S subunits was also measured in a stopped-flow instrument using light scattering. This assay demonstrated that naked ΔS20 30S subunits were severely impaired in association with wild-type 50S subunits and no improvement was observed when the 50S was added in excess (Figure 9A). However, a pronounced improvement (from ≤ 20% to ~ 40%) in the association capacity of the mutant 30S was observed upon pre-incubation with mRNA, initiator tRNA and the initiation factors. Similar to the results of mRNA binding, subunit association was further improved upon extension of the ΔS20 30S pre-incubation time with initiation components to 40 minutes (Figure 9B) (Tobin et al., 2010).

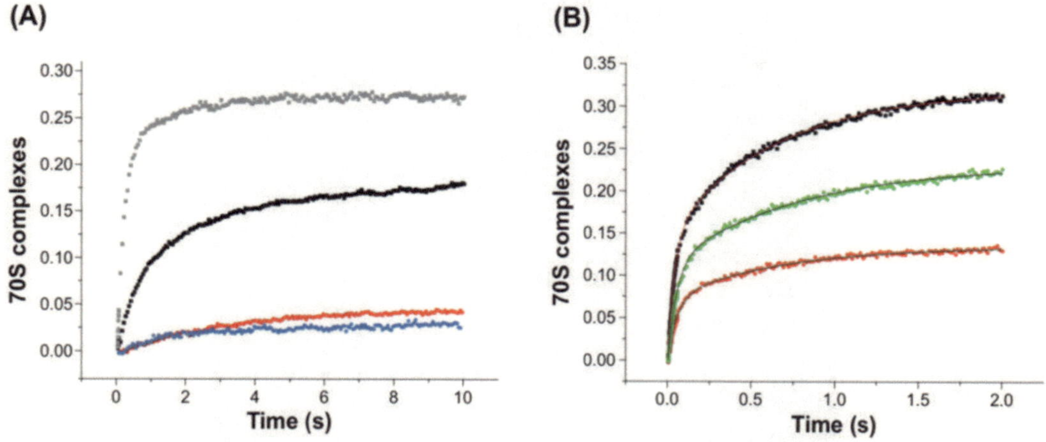

Fig. 9. **Kinetics of subunit association measured by light scattering.** (A) In the absence of the initiation ligands and when the ratio of 30S to 50S is 1:1, very few mutant 70S complexes are formed (red circles) compared to wild-type (black squares). The addition of 5x more 50S to the reaction (wild-type, grey squares; ΔS20, blue circles), did not increase 70S formation in the case of the mutant. (B) Association kinetics in the presence of mRNA, initiator tRNA, IF1 and IF2 following pre-incubation for 10 minutes (wild-type, black squares; ΔS20, red circles) and 40 minutes (ΔS20, green circles). (Tobin et al., 2010)

4.6 S20 is required for correct structural positioning of h44

Defects in the rate and extent of mRNA binding, as well as the poor association capacity of S20-depleted 30S subunits are likely to account for the reduced rate of protein accumulation observed *in vivo* and the prolonged generation time of the ΔS20 mutant. These impairments were puzzling as we could not reconcile them with the topographical location of S20 in mature 30S particles. The protein (Figure 10) is located at the base of the body of the 30S subunit, distal to the mRNA binding channel and subunit interface. However S20 has been shown to interact with helix 44 of the 16S rRNA during 30S assembly and in mature 30S particles (Brodersen et al., 2002; Dutca & Culver, 2008). High-resolution crystal structures have shown that this helix stretches across the entire length of the 30S body and forms part of the A- and P- sites where mRNA binding occurs (Schluenzen et al., 2000) and it also forms many bridging contacts with the 50S subunit (Selmer et al., 2006). Hence, upon removal of S20, h44 most likely adopts a suboptimal structural position that impairs the binding of mRNA and inhibits association with the 50S subunit (Tobin et al., 2010). Since prolonged incubation with the initiation components concealed these defects to some degree, it is likely that these 30S ligands promote a structural rearrangement of h44 that permits more stable binding of mRNA and facilitates docking of the 50S subunit.

5. R-protein replacement mutants

Besides the knowledge that can be gained regarding the essentiality and putative roles of r-proteins by examining genetically defined deletion mutants, r-protein replacement studies offer a unique opportunity to ask some more general questions. Using lambda red recombineering, the ORFs of S20, L1 and L17 were replaced with both closely related and

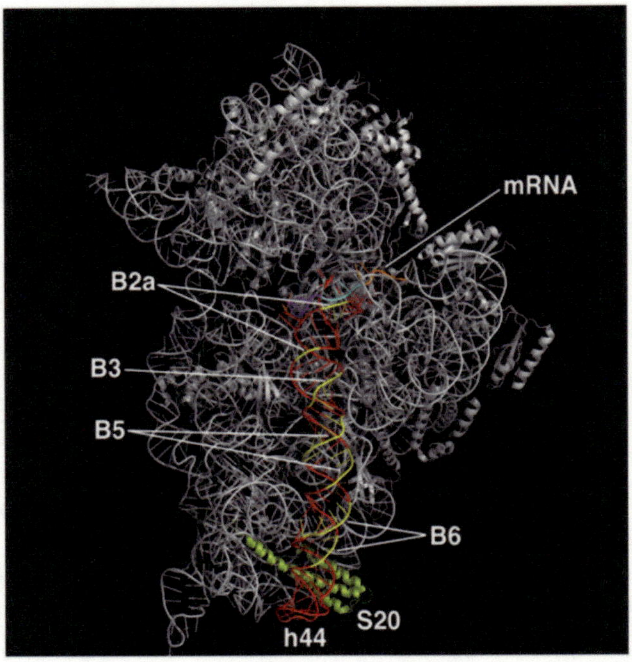

Fig. 10. **Structure of the 30S subunit highlighting the proposed involvement of S20 in mRNA binding and subunit association.** S20 (green ribbon) interacts with and possibly stabilizes h44 (red) in an orientation that is optimized for mRNA (orange; A-site, purple; P-site, cyan) binding and interactions with the 50S subunit (bridges B2a, B3, B5 and B6 depicted in yellow) (Tobin et al., 2010). All other rRNA and protein residues are depicted in grey. The image was created in PyMol (www.pymol.org) from the coordinates of the *T. thermophilus* 30S subunit (PDB ID 2J00) (Selmer et al., 2006).

highly divergent orthologues on the chromosome of *S. typhimurium* (Lind et al., 2010). Such hybrid mutants address fundamental evolutionary questions regarding translational robustness and the plasticity of the *bone fide* ribosomal components. Highly sensitive fitness measurements were performed to directly examine the costs of replacement and to indirectly determine the functional capacity of hybrid ribosomes. In addition, compensatory evolution of replacement mutants with large fitness costs revealed a general mechanism for suppressing loss of functionality when a divergent protein is imported into the ribosome.

5.1 Modest fitness costs upon r-protein replacement

Considering the highly conserved nature of r-proteins and their involvement in one of the key processes of gene expression, their removal was expected to confer substantial reductions in cell fitness. The physiological effects of r-protein replacement however, was more difficult to predict, although it was reasonable to expect relatively weaker fitness costs, even if the non-native protein lacked a high degree of homology to the host protein. The non-native replacement proteins ranged from close relatives, such as those from other proteobacteria *E. coli* and *Klebsiella pneumoniae,* to phylogenetically distant orthologues such as those from the eukaryote *Saccharomyces cerevisiae* and the archaeon *Sulfolobus acidocaldarius* (Lind et al., 2010). Exponential growth rates were measured in four different media where the doubling time of the wild-type strain varied from 20 - 120 minutes and the growth rates of hybrid strains were expressed relative to this (Figure 11A showing L1 replacement mutants only). In the case of the S20 replacement mutants, all strains had higher fitness than the null mutant, irrespective of the growth medium used and even when amino acid identity fell to only 32%. Similarly, the fitness of the majority of L1 replacement mutants was only modestly reduced relative to wild-type, although more substantial costs were evident when the amino acid identity of the homologue reached as low as 20-30% (Figure 11A). Since L17 is an essential r-protein, comparisons to a null mutant were not feasible, however, a substantial fitness reduction relative to the wild-type, was only observed when amino acid identity of the orthologue fell below 50%. Interestingly, higher fitness of certain L17 hybrid mutants relative to wild-type was also evident. A general trend that emerged was a reduction in relative fitness as phylogenetic distance increased, however the costs of replacement for the more homologous proteins were diminutive in comparison to the costs of removal.

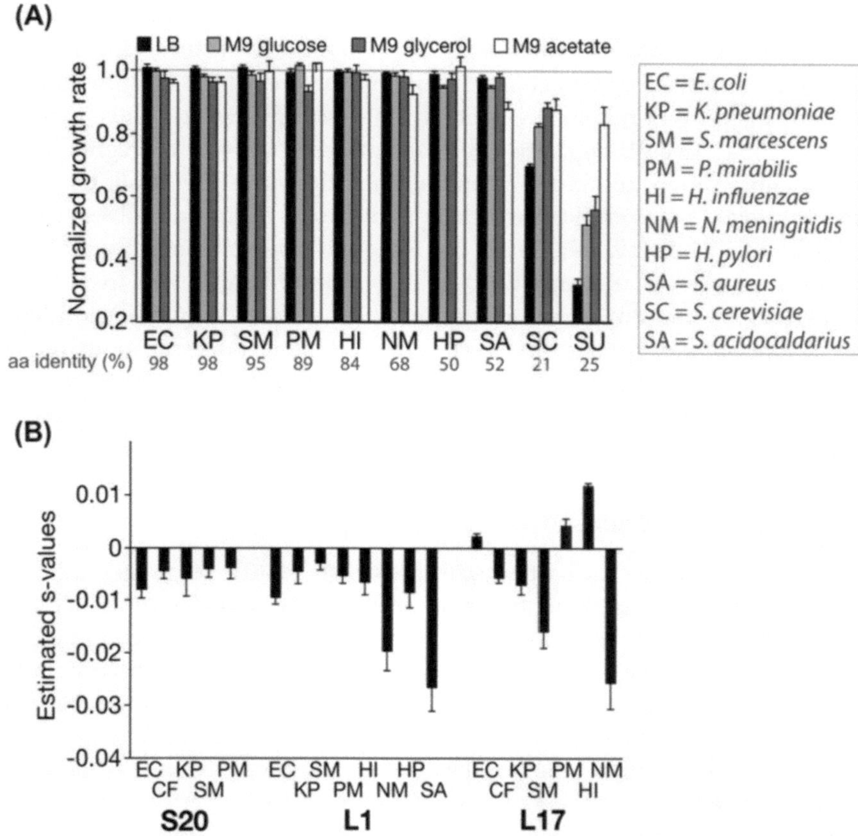

Fig. 11. **Fitness costs associated with replacement of r-proteins.** (A) Exponential growth rates of L1 replacement mutants in LB and minimal M9 medium with glucose, glycerol or acetate as carbon source. The growth rate of each mutant was normalized to that of a congenic wild-type strain in each respective medium (set to 1.0). (B) Selection coefficients associated with non-native S20, L1 and L17 r-proteins, estimated by means of pair-wise competitive growth with a congenic wild-type strain. Error bars in (A) and (B) represent standard error of the mean (SEM).

For those replacement mutants that displayed very small fitness costs as measured by exponential growth, pair-wise competition experiments were performed with the wild-type for a more sensitive estimate of the fitness costs (Lind et al., 2010). Using this method, we found that the majority of transfers were deleterious. In Figure 11B, the selection coefficient associated with each non-native protein is shown, which, in most cases, was less than or equal to -0.01, meaning that most of the imported genes conferred costs of 1% or less. Modelling was also performed to determine if such weak fitness costs represent an effective barrier for fixation of these proteins in nature via horizontal gene transfer. The results suggest that the fixation probability of such modestly counter-selected alleles is virtually nil in large natural populations of bacteria (Lind et al., 2010).

5.2 High functional conservation of r-proteins

Since the rate of bacterial growth is the product of the cellular ribosome concentration, times the rate of ribosome function (Bremer & Dennis, 1996), the fitness assays also provide an indirect measure of the translational capacity of the hybrid ribosomes. Given the generally larger fitness costs associated with complete loss of function in the null mutants, we were certain that the majority of non-native proteins improved fitness and thus appear to be at least semi-functional. Even though the replacement genes were often highly divergent in terms of base composition, codon usage and amino acid identity, overall, the fitness costs were relatively weak and significant reductions in fitness were only observed when the amino acid identity fell below 50% or so. So, although some of these proteins evolved in highly divergent organisms, they appear to function extraordinarily well in their non-native context. For example, L1 from *Helicobacter pylori* only shares 50% amino acid identity with the native *S. typhimurium* protein; the cost of replacement, however, is extremely small (approximately 1%). This clearly demonstrates the robustness of the ribosome and protein synthesis in general, and it also suggests that functional constraints are highly conserved between these proteins.

5.3 Increased dosage rescues suboptimal r-proteins

Those replacement mutants that harboured fitness costs of 10% or greater were subject to compensatory evolution to determine if and by what mechanisms fitness compensation could be achieved. After between 40 – 250 generations of growth, the S20 mutant (carrying the *H. influenzae* orthologue) and the L1 mutant (carrying the *S. cerevisiae* orthologue) showed increased fitness and were examined for an increase in the copy number of the non-native gene by Southern hybridization (Lind et al., 2010). Indeed, a two- to three-fold increase was detected in some of the lineages and corresponded to increased expression of the orthologous protein when Western blots were performed. To verify that overproduction of the non-native protein constitutes a general mechanism of fitness compensation, the orthologous proteins were expressed from an inducible high-copy number plasmid and fitness was measured. Exponential growth rates confirmed that for the majority of replacement mutants, increased dosage of the non-native protein conferred higher fitness (Figure 12). Thus, insufficient expression of the divergent protein (possibly due to unstable mRNA/protein), or a requirement for more of the protein to restore proper ribosome function and/or assembly, are two likely scenarios that could be at least partially accountable for the fitness costs of r-protein replacement. Such imbalances in the stoichiometry of interacting cellular components has previously been suggested to confer deleterious effects (Papp et al., 2003).

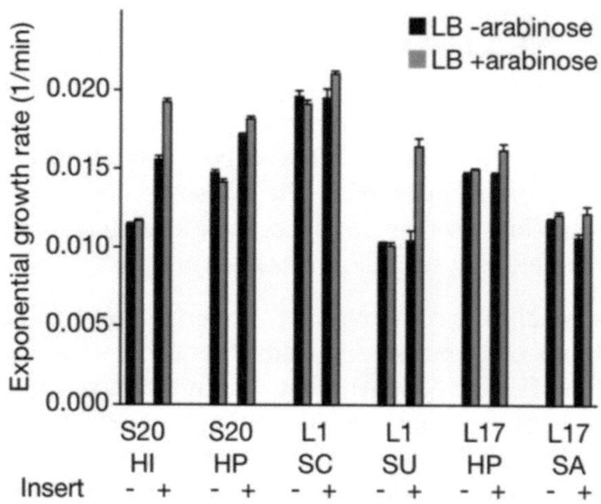

Fig. 12. **Growth compensation of r-protein replacement mutants via increased dosage of the non-native protein.** Exponential growth rates of mutants harbouring the arabinose inducible, high-copy number plasmid with (+) and without (-) the non-native gene. Abbreviations for divergent proteins from each respective species are the same as in Figure 11. Error bars represent SEM.

6. Concluding remarks and future perspectives

The ability to ascribe discrete functional roles to distinct components of the ribosome is essential to improve our understanding of how translation works and is a vital step towards furthering our knowledge of how this magnificent machine has evolved to the complex structure we see today in modern cells. The most fundamental aspect of the studies described herein, is directed towards resolving ribosome complexity to some degree in terms of the selective contributions made by certain r-proteins. The major tasks of the ribosome are RNA-mediated; however, the results of this study highlight the importance of the r-proteins for optimal function. Upon loss of either S20 or L1, we see that the cell is indeed viable; however, the substantial reductions in fitness reflect the requirement of the proteins for maintenance of proper ribosome function. In the case of both deletion mutants, the impairments in function appear to stem from perturbations in the higher order structure of the rRNA, suggesting, that both L1 and S20 are important in stabilizing the overall morphology of the subunits. Upon loss of S20, mRNA binding is severely impaired and association of the mutant 30S species with 50S subunits is drastically reduced. Both of these defects appear to occur as secondary effects caused by a primary disturbance in 16S rRNA structure; namely, distortion of the penultimate helix, h44. Similarly, in the absence of L1, an excess of free 50S subunits is formed in the cell, likely due to subunit misassembly in an L1-depleted environment. Moreover, the majority of compensatory mutations selected as a response to L1 removal were mapped to other r-proteins dispersed at various sites of the small and large subunit, suggesting that they may amend the structural perturbations to some degree. The variation in the topographical distribution of the compensatory mutations also highlights the high degree of co-operativity inherent to the ribosome. Thus, in both cases, it seems that loss of the protein indirectly perturbs protein synthesis via alterations in the overall morphology of the ribosome. Perhaps this is not altogether surprising, considering that both proteins are primary rRNA binders and are thus considered particularly important for initiating global folding of the major rRNA domains. One major strength and unique feature of the studies described herein, is our attempt to explain the observed fitness costs in terms of the costs to ribosome function detected by our *in vitro* system. Unfortunately, very few studies have attempted to bridge the crucial gap between both sets of data. This is a considerable challenge, given the inherent complexity of the ribosome and the enormous level of co-operativity within the structure itself and at the cellular level. It is, however, an essential step towards capturing a complete picture of the mechanism of translation.

In contrast to the substantial costs conferred by r-protein removal, in general, replacement of such proteins with orthologous counterparts from other species had only modest deleterious effects on fitness. This finding implies that the non-native proteins are capable of functioning in their new environment, despite having evolved in divergent species, clearly demonstrating the plasticity and robustness of the translation apparatus. This may suggest conservation in the overall shape of the proteins or at least those residues that interact with the target sites of the ribosome, akin to structural mimics of the native proteins. Overall the results emphasize the superiority of functional requirement over conservation of the primary sequence of amino acids, lending support to the suggestion that the major function of the r-proteins is to maintain the structural integrity of the ribosome.

Future work in this area should concentrate on studies designed to delineate the specific roles of other r-proteins during translation. With a large array of approximately fifty proteins, the task is challenging. However, recent advances in genetic engineering has allowed us to construct precise deletions of various r-proteins, and the replacement approach offers a new avenue for dissecting the roles of essential proteins. By examining the function of hybrid ribosomes *in vitro*, distinct steps of the translation cycle can be evaluated and the contributions made by essential r-proteins could be exposed. The findings of these studies also highlight the usefulness of compensatory evolution in terms of revealing otherwise concealed cooperative mechanisms for partially restoring ribosome function.

7. Acknowledgments

This work was supported by research grants to S.S. and D.A. from the Swedish Research Council and Knut and Alice Wallenberg Stiftelse; to S.S. from Carl Tryggers Stiftelse, Göran Gustafssons Stiftelse and Wenner-Gren Stiftelse.

8. References

Ameres, S. L., Shcherbakov, D., Nikonova, E., Piendl, W., Schroeder, R. and Semrad, K. (2007). RNA chaperone activity of L1 ribosomal proteins: phylogenetic conservation and splicing inhibition. *Nucleic Acids Res*, Vol. 35, No. 11, pp. 3752-3763

Baba, T., Ara, T., Hasegawa, M., Takai, Y., Okumura, Y., Baba, M., Datsenko, K. A., Tomita, M., Wanner, B. L. and Mori, H. (2006). Construction of Escherichia coli K-12 in-frame, single-gene knockout mutants: the Keio collection. *Mol Syst Biol*, Vol. 2, No. pp. 2006 0008

Ban, N., Nissen, P., Hansen, J., Moore, P. B. and Steitz, T. A. (2000). The complete atomic structure of the large ribosomal subunit at 2.4 A resolution. *Science,* Vol. 289, No. 5481, pp. 905-920

Bjorkman, J., Samuelsson, P., Andersson, D. I. and Hughes, D. (1999). Novel ribosomal mutations affecting translational accuracy, antibiotic resistance and virulence of Salmonella typhimurium. *Mol Microbiol,* Vol. 31, No. 1, pp. 53-58

Bremer, H. and Dennis, P. P. (1996). Modulation of Chemical Composition and Other Parameters of the Cell by Growth Rate, In: *Escherichia coli and Salmonella: Cellular and Molecular Biology,* F. C. Neidhart, pp. 1553-1566, ASM Press, Washington D.C.

Brodersen, D. E., Clemons, W. M., Jr., Carter, A. P., Wimberly, B. T. and Ramakrishnan, V. (2002). Crystal structure of the 30 S ribosomal subunit from Thermus thermophilus: structure of the proteins and their interactions with 16 S RNA. *J Mol Biol,* Vol. 316, No. 3, pp. 725-768

Bubunenko, M., Baker, T. and Court, D. L. (2007). Essentiality of ribosomal and transcription antitermination proteins analyzed by systematic gene replacement in Escherichia coli. *J Bacteriol,* Vol. 189, No. 7, pp. 2844-2853

Bubunenko, M., Korepanov, A., Court, D. L., Jagannathan, I., Dickinson, D., Chaudhuri, B. R., Garber, M. B. and Culver, G. M. (2006). 30S ribosomal subunits can be assembled in vivo without primary binding ribosomal protein S15. *RNA,* Vol. 12, No. 7, pp. 1229-1239

Burgin, A. B., Parodos, K., Lane, D. J. and Pace, N. R. (1990). The excision of intervening sequences from Salmonella 23S ribosomal RNA. *Cell,* Vol. 60, No. 3, pp. 405-414

Cech, T. R. (2000). Structural biology. The ribosome is a ribozyme. *Science,* Vol. 289, No. 5481, pp. 878-879

Cukras, A. R. and Green, R. (2005). Multiple effects of S13 in modulating the strength of intersubunit interactions in the ribosome during translation. *J Mol Biol,* Vol. 349, No. 1, pp. 47-59

Dabbs, E. R. (1977). A spectinomycin dependent mutant of Escherichia coli. *Mol Gen Genet,* Vol. 151, No. 3, pp. 261-267

Dabbs, E. R. (1978). Mutational alterations in 50 proteins of the Escherichia coli ribosome. *Mol Gen Genet,* Vol. 165, No. 1, pp. 73-78

Dabbs, E. R. (1979). Selection for Escherichia coli mutants with proteins missing from the ribosome. *J Bacteriol,* Vol. 140, No. 2, pp. 734-737

Dabbs, E. R. (1980). The ribosomal components responsible for kasugamycin dependence, and its suppression, in a mutant of Escherichia coli. *Mol Gen Genet,* Vol. 177, No. 2, pp. 271-276

Dabbs, E. R. (1991). Mutants lacking individual ribosomal proteins as a tool to investigate ribosomal properties. *Biochimie,* Vol. 73, No. 6, pp. 639-645

Dabbs, E. R. and Wittman, H. G. (1976). A strain of Escherichia coli which gives rise to mutations in a large number of ribosomal proteins. *Mol Gen Genet,* Vol. 149, No. 3, pp. 303-309

Dammel, C. S. and Noller, H. F. (1993). A cold-sensitive mutation in 16S rRNA provides evidence for helical switching in ribosome assembly. *Genes Dev,* Vol. 7, No. 4, pp. 660-670

Datsenko, K. A. and Wanner, B. L. (2000). One-step inactivation of chromosomal genes in Escherichia coli K-12 using PCR products. *Proc Natl Acad Sci U S A,* Vol. 97, No. 12, pp. 6640-6645

Deutscher, M. P. (2009). Maturation and degradation of ribosomal RNA in bacteria. *Prog Mol Biol Transl Sci*, Vol. 85, No. pp. 369-391

Doudna, J. A. and Rath, V. L. (2002). Structure and function of the eukaryotic ribosome: the next frontier. *Cell*, Vol. 109, No. 2, pp. 153-156

Dutca, L. M. and Culver, G. M. (2008). Assembly of the 5' and 3' minor domains of 16S ribosomal RNA as monitored by tethered probing from ribosomal protein S20. *J Mol Biol*, Vol. 376, No. 1, pp. 92-108

Ehrenberg, M., Bilgin, N. and Kurland, C. G. (1989). Design and use of a fast and accurate in vitro translation system., In: *Ribosomes and Protein Synthesis: A Practical Approach*, G. Spedding, pp. 101-129, Oxford University Press, New York

Fei, J., Kosuri, P., MacDougall, D. D. and Gonzalez, R. L., Jr. (2008). Coupling of ribosomal L1 stalk and tRNA dynamics during translation elongation. *Mol Cell*, Vol. 30, No. 3, pp. 348-359

Giese, K. and Subramanian, A. R. (1991). Expression and functional assembly into bacterial ribosomes of a nuclear-encoded chloroplast ribosomal protein with a long NH2-terminal extension. *FEBS Lett*, Vol. 288, No. 1-2, pp. 72-76

Gotz, F., Dabbs, E. R. and Gualerzi, C. O. (1990). Escherichia coli 30S mutants lacking protein S20 are defective in translation initiation. *Biochim Biophys Acta*, Vol. 1050, No. 1-3, pp. 93-97

Gotz, F., Fleischer, C., Pon, C. L. and Gualerzi, C. O. (1989). Subunit association defects in Escherichia coli ribosome mutants lacking proteins S20 and L11. *Eur J Biochem*, Vol. 183, No. 1, pp. 19-24

Harms, J., Schluenzen, F., Zarivach, R., Bashan, A., Gat, S., Agmon, I., Bartels, H., Franceschi, F. and Yonath, A. (2001). High resolution structure of the large ribosomal subunit from a mesophilic eubacterium. *Cell*, Vol. 107, No. 5, pp. 679-688

Johansson, M., Bouakaz, E., Lovmar, M. and Ehrenberg, M. (2008). The kinetics of ribosomal peptidyl transfer revisited. *Mol Cell*, Vol. 30, No. 5, pp. 589-598

Kaczanowska, M. and Ryden-Aulin, M. (2007). Ribosome biogenesis and the translation process in Escherichia coli. *Microbiol Mol Biol Rev*, Vol. 71, No. 3, pp. 477-494

Korepanov, A. P., Gongadze, G. M., Garber, M. B., Court, D. L. and Bubunenko, M. G. (2007). Importance of the 5 S rRNA-binding ribosomal proteins for cell viability and translation in Escherichia coli. *J Mol Biol*, Vol. 366, No. 4, pp. 1199-1208

Kramer, E. B. and Farabaugh, P. J. (2007). The frequency of translational misreading errors in E. coli is largely determined by tRNA competition. *RNA*, Vol. 13, No. 1, pp. 87-96

Lecompte, O., Ripp, R., Thierry, J. C., Moras, D. and Poch, O. (2002). Comparative analysis of ribosomal proteins in complete genomes: an example of reductive evolution at the domain scale. *Nucleic Acids Res*, Vol. 30, No. 24, pp. 5382-5390

Lind, P. A., Tobin, C., Berg, O. G., Kurland, C. G. and Andersson, D. I. (2010). Compensatory gene amplification restores fitness after inter-species gene replacements. *Mol Microbiol*, Vol. 75, No. 5, pp. 1078-1089

Liu, X. Q., Gillham, N. W. and Boynton, J. E. (1989). Chloroplast ribosomal protein gene rps12 of Chlamydomonas reinhardtii. Wild-type sequence, mutation to streptomycin resistance and dependence, and function in Escherichia coli. *J Biol Chem*, Vol. 264, No. 27, pp. 16100-16108

Mandava, C. S., Peisker, K., Ederth, J., Kumar, R., Ge, X., Szaflarski, W., and Sanyal, S (2011). Bacterial ribosome requires multiple L12 dimers for efficient initiation and elongation of protein synthesis involving IF2 and EF-G. *Nucleic Acid Research*, doi: 10.1093/nar/gkr1031.

Mattatall, N. R. and Sanderson, K. E. (1996). Salmonella typhimurium LT2 possesses three distinct 23S rRNA intervening sequences. *J Bacteriol*, Vol. 178, No. 8, pp. 2272-2278

Mattatall, N. R. and Sanderson, K. E. (1996). Salmonella typhimurium LT2 possesses three distinct 23S rRNA intervening sequences. *J Bacteriol*, Vol. 178, No. 8, pp. 2272-2278

Mattatall, N. R. and Sanderson, K. E. (1998). RNase III deficient Salmonella typhimurium LT2 contains intervening sequences (IVSs) in its 23S rRNA. *FEMS Microbiol Lett*, Vol. 159, No. 2, pp. 179-185

McClelland, M., Sanderson, K. E., Spieth, J., Clifton, S. W., Latreille, P., Courtney, L., Porwollik, S., Ali, J., Dante, M., Du, F., Hou, S., Layman, D., Leonard, S., Nguyen, C., Scott, K., Holmes, A., Grewal, N., Mulvaney, E., Ryan, E., Sun, H., Florea, L., Miller, W., Stoneking, T., Nhan, M., Waterston, R. and Wilson, R. K. (2001). Complete genome sequence of Salmonella enterica serovar Typhimurium LT2. *Nature*, Vol. 413, No. 6858, pp. 852-856

Miller, J. H. (1992). *A Short Course in Bacterial Genetics*, Cold Spring Harbour Laboratory Press, Cold Spring Harour, New York

Munro, J. B., Altman, R. B., Tung, C. S., Cate, J. H., Sanbonmatsu, K. Y. and Blanchard, S. C. (2010). Spontaneous formation of the unlocked state of the ribosome is a multistep process. *Proc Natl Acad Sci U S A*, Vol. 107, No. 2, pp. 709-714

Nierhaus, K. H. (1991). The assembly of prokaryotic ribosomes. *Biochimie*, Vol. 73, No. 6, pp. 739-755

Nierhaus, K. H. (2006). Bacterial Ribosomes: Assembly, In: *Encyclopedia of Life Sciences*, pp. Pages, John Wiley & Sons Ltd., Retrieved from http://www.els.net/

Nissen, P., Hansen, J., Ban, N., Moore, P. B. and Steitz, T. A. (2000). The structural basis of ribosome activity in peptide bond synthesis. *Science*, Vol. 289, No. 5481, pp. 920-930

O'Connor, M. and Gregory, S. T. (2011). Inactivation of the RluD pseudouridine synthase has minimal effects on growth and ribosome function in wild-type Escherichia coli and Salmonella enterica. *J Bacteriol*, Vol. 193, No. 1, pp. 154-162

Ogle, J. M., Carter, A. P. and Ramakrishnan, V. (2003). Insights into the decoding mechanism from recent ribosome structures. *Trends Biochem Sci*, Vol. 28, No. 5, pp. 259-266

Papp, B., Pal, C. and Hurst, L. D. (2003). Dosage sensitivity and the evolution of gene families in yeast. *Nature*, Vol. 424, No. 6945, pp. 194-197

Pettersson, I. and Kurland, C. G. (1980). Ribosomal protein L7/L12 is required for optimal translation. *Proc Natl Acad Sci U S A*, Vol. 77, No. 7, pp. 4007-4010

Ryden-Aulin, M., Shaoping, Z., Kylsten, P. and Isaksson, L. A. (1993). Ribosome activity and modification of 16S RNA are influenced by deletion of ribosomal protein S20. *Mol Microbiol*, Vol. 7, No. 6, pp. 983-992

Sander, G. (1983). Ribosomal protein L1 from Escherichia coli. Its role in the binding of tRNA to the ribosome and in elongation factor g-dependent gtp hydrolysis. *J Biol Chem*, Vol. 258, No. 16, pp. 10098-10103

Schaub, R. E. and Hayes, C. S. (2011). Deletion of the RluD pseudouridine synthase promotes SsrA peptide tagging of ribosomal protein S7. *Mol Microbiol*, Vol. 79, No. 2, pp. 331-341

Schluenzen, F., Tocilj, A., Zarivach, R., Harms, J., Gluehmann, M., Janell, D., Bashan, A., Bartels, H., Agmon, I., Franceschi, F. and Yonath, A. (2000). Structure of functionally activated small ribosomal subunit at 3.3 angstroms resolution. *Cell*, Vol. 102, No. 5, pp. 615-623

Selmer, M., Dunham, C. M., Murphy, F. V. t., Weixlbaumer, A., Petry, S., Kelley, A. C., Weir, J. R. and Ramakrishnan, V. (2006). Structure of the 70S ribosome complexed with mRNA and tRNA. *Science*, Vol. 313, No. 5795, pp. 1935-1942

Sharan, S. K., Thomason, L. C., Kuznetsov, S. G. and Court, D. L. (2009). Recombineering: a homologous recombination-based method of genetic engineering. *Nat Protoc*, Vol. 4, No. 2, pp. 206-223

Subramanian, A. R. and Dabbs, E. R. (1980). Functional studies on ribosomes lacking protein L1 from mutant Escherichia coli. *Eur J Biochem*, Vol. 112, No. 2, pp. 425-430

Tobin, C., Mandava, C. S., Ehrenberg, M., Andersson, D. I. and Sanyal, S. (2010). Ribosomes lacking protein S20 are defective in mRNA binding and subunit association. *J Mol Biol*, Vol. 397, No. 3, pp. 767-776

Trabuco, L. G., Schreiner, E., Eargle, J., Cornish, P., Ha, T., Luthey-Schulten, Z. and Schulten, K. (2010). The role of L1 stalk-tRNA interaction in the ribosome elongation cycle. *J Mol Biol*, Vol. 402, No. 4, pp. 741-760

Tubulekas, I., Buckingham, R. H. and Hughes, D. (1991). Mutant ribosomes can generate dominant kirromycin resistance. *J Bacteriol*, Vol. 173, No. 12, pp. 3635-3643

Uchiumi, T., Honma, S., Nomura, T., Dabbs, E. R. and Hachimori, A. (2002). Translation elongation by a hybrid ribosome in which proteins at the GTPase center of the Escherichia coli ribosome are replaced with rat counterparts. *J Biol Chem*, Vol. 277, No. 6, pp. 3857-3862

Valle, M., Zavialov, A., Sengupta, J., Rawat, U., Ehrenberg, M. and Frank, J. (2003). Locking and unlocking of ribosomal motions. *Cell*, Vol. 114, No. 1, pp. 123-134

Weglohner, W., Junemann, R., von Knoblauch, K. and Subramanian, A. R. (1997). Different consequences of incorporating chloroplast ribosomal proteins L12 and S18 into the bacterial ribosomes of Escherichia coli. *Eur J Biochem*, Vol. 249, No. 2, pp. 383-392

Wild, D. G. (1988). Reversion from erythromycin dependence in Escherichia coli: strains altered in ribosomal sub-unit association and ribosome assembly. *J Gen Microbiol*, Vol. 134, No. 5, pp. 1251-1263

Williamson, J. R. (2009). The ribosome at atomic resolution. *Cell*, Vol. 139, No. 6, pp. 1041-1043

Wilson, D. N. and Nierhaus, K. H. (2005). Ribosomal proteins in the spotlight. *Crit Rev Biochem Mol Biol*, Vol. 40, No. 5, pp. 243-267

Wilson, D. N. and Nierhaus, K. H. (2006). The E-site story: the importance of maintaining two tRNAs on the ribosome during protein synthesis. *Cell Mol Life Sci*, Vol. 63, No. 23, pp. 2725-2737

Wimberly, B. T., Brodersen, D. E., Clemons, W. M., Jr., Morgan-Warren, R. J., Carter, A. P., Vonrhein, C., Hartsch, T. and Ramakrishnan, V. (2000). Structure of the 30S ribosomal subunit. *Nature*, Vol. 407, No. 6802, pp. 327-339

Wower, I. K., Wower, J. and Zimmermann, R. A. (1998). Ribosomal protein L27 participates in both 50 S subunit assembly and the peptidyl transferase reaction. *J Biol Chem*, Vol. 273, No. 31, pp. 19847-19852

Yusupov, M. M., Yusupova, G. Z., Baucom, A., Lieberman, K., Earnest, T. N., Cate, J. H. and Noller, H. F. (2001). Crystal structure of the ribosome at 5.5 A resolution. *Science*, Vol. 292, No. 5518, pp. 883-896

23

Molecular Technologies for *Salmonella* Detection

Robert S. Tebbs, Lily Y. Wong, Pius Brzoska and Olga V. Petrauskene
Life Technologies, Foster City, CA
USA

1. Introduction

Salmonella has been associated with some of the most devastating foodborne outbreaks in recent history. *Salmonella* outbreaks have been linked to a variety of foods including produce [Alfalfa Sprouts- 2009, 2010, 2011; pistachios-2009; cantaloupes-2008, 2011 etc.], processed foods [peanuts - 2009], and prepared foods [turkey burgers- 2011, Banquet Pot Pies - 2007]. The contamination of commercial shell eggs with *Salmonella* Enteriditis in 2010 led to the recall of over a half a billion eggs, and the contamination of peanut-containing products with *Salmonella* Typhimurium in 2008-2009 led to one of the largest recalls in U.S. history with over 3,900 products being recalled. The Peanut Corporation of America, responsible for the *Salmonella* outbreak in peanuts, was forced into bankruptcy. Multiple lawsuits were filed against Wright County Egg and Hillandale Farms responsible for the *Salmonella* outbreak in eggs. Despite their own internal testing which showed *Salmonella* contamination, these facilities still shipped product. The 2008 outbreak of *Salmonella* in jalapeno peppers resulted in 1442 persons infected with *Salmonella* Saintpaul across 43 states, the District of Columbia, and Canada. Unfortunately, the tomato industry was implicated early in the investigation, which resulted in economic losses to the tomato industry in hundreds of millions of dollars. Because *Salmonella* is widespread in the environment (in such places as chicken houses), vegetable plants and animals (as well as meat samples, eggs etc.), rapid, reliable, and validated pathogen detection methods are needed for use in production facilities, public health labs, as well as in the regulatory and monitoring agencies. To provide comprehensive rapid food testing solutions, all components of a pathogen detection system should be addressed: sample preparation, detection and data analysis.

Fluorescent quantitative real-time PCR is the most sensitive method for detection, monitoring and measurement of pathogen levels. The method also can be used for strain identification based on single-nucleotide polymorphism detection. A key element in designing PCR assays is an algorithm to select primers and probes because they define accuracy - specificity and inclusivity of the PCR tests. The ability to design highly specific assays becomes easier as the number of bacterial genomes added to the public domain increases.

There are a number of sample preparation methods available that are fast and easy for PCR-based pathogen detection using both low throughput (manual) and high throughput (automated) methods.

A multiplex (multi-color) real-time PCR analysis, if designed correctly, provides simultaneous and specific detection of a number of pathogens in the same reaction and can save time and money. In addition to multiplexing, other technologies improve operator experience such as lyophilized configuration and fast cycling format.

Effective data analysis software can significantly improve test workflow as well as accuracy of the presence or absence calls. Software packages can simplify analysis by displaying results graphically to make the system fail-proof even for novice users.

To further characterize detected *Salmonella* species, isolates can be sequenced using modern whole genome sequencing platforms.

2. Genetic methods complement biochemical and phenotypic analyses

Salmonella serotypes are classified by the Kauffmann-White-Schema which is maintained by the WHO and the Collaborating Center for Reference and Research at Institute Pasteur. There are only two species *Salmonella enterica,* which is associated with human infections, and *Salmonella bongori,* which is mainly found in lizards. This schema was based mainly on DNA analysis and bonified by the judiciary of bacterial nomenclature (Center for Disease Control, 2004). Under the schema, there are six subspecies. The serotypes are I: *Salmonella enterica* subsp enterica, II: *Salmonella enterica* subsp. Salamae, III: *Salmonella enterica* subsp. Arizonae, IIIb *Salmonella enteric*a subsp. Diarizonae, IV: *Salmonella enteric*a subsp. Houtenae and VI *Salmonella enterica* susp. Indica. *Salmonella* serotyping is traditionally based on immunoreactive antibodies against the O and H antigens. Different classification schemes based on phylogenetic analyses of 16S and housekeeping genes have been proposed (Boyd et al., 1996; Tindall, 2005).

Classification of bacteria is traditionally based on immunogenic and metabolic behavior. Analysis of bacterial genomes however led to reclassification and debates on the taxonomical classification. For example, Pupo et al. (2000) studied the phylogenetic relations of several housekeeping genes and the O-antigen of species of the genus *Shigella* and concluded that several species of *Shigella* are clusters of *Escherichia coli*.

The nomenclature change in *Salmonella* was subsequently supported by genomic evidence as well. McQuiston et al. (2008) showed that a set of four housekeeping genes supports the *Salmonella* classification, and microarray analysis of the gene homologues in *Salmonella* result in a similar grouping (Porwollik et al., 2002). More recently, whole genome sequencing of *Enterobacter sakazakii* isolates revealed that this group is phylogenetically different from other *Enterobacter* species and was renamed to *Cronobacter sakazakii* (Iversen et al., 2008). The breakout of *Cronobacter* was supported by biochemical and microarray analyses (Healy et al., 2009).

Since the completion of the first bacterial genome of Hemophilus influenza in 1995 (Fleischmann et al., 1995), more than 1000 bacterial genomes have been completely sequenced. Currently, 21 serovars of *Salmonella enterica* subsp. enterica have been sequenced as well as *Salmonella bongori*. Many shotgun sequencing projects are still in progress, and the number of genomes will continue to increase. New metrics for taxonomical evaluation based on complete genomes have been proposed (Kunin et al., 2005). Complete genomic information does not change the phylogeny based on 16S and

MLST substantially (Coenye & Vandamme, 2003), but it allows the study of specific genes present and absent across phylogenetic groups.

3. Sample preparation for real-time PCR detection of *Salmonella*

The successful detection of pathogenic organisms by genetic methods requires microbial lysis to release nucleic acids and efficient removal of inhibitors. Sample preparation can also serve to concentrate nucleic acids for improved sensitivity. Food and environmental samples create unique challenges for sample preparation due to the heterogeneous nature of the different matrices. The method used must account for the type and amount of organism to be lysed, the sample matrix, and the user's needs and limitations (cost, ease-of-use, time-to-results, sample throughput and capacity, and multi-functionality).

Samples that contains inhibitory compounds can lead to partial or complete inhibition of PCR. Food and culture media both contain components that can inhibit PCR (Rosen et al., 1992; Andersen & Omiecinski, 1992; Atmar et al., 1993; Demeke & Adams, 1992; Lofstrom et al., 2004) (for a review, see Wilson, 1997). PCR inhibitors originating from the food samples include humic acid from soil (Tsai & Olson, 1992a; Tsai & Olson, 1992b), proteins and aminoglycans from animal samples such as hemoglobin, lactoferrin and heparin (Al-Soud & Radstrom, 2001), polysaccharides from plant material (Demeke & Adams, 1992; Monteiro et al., 1997), melanin from hair and skin (Eckhart et al., 2000), etc. Media including modified Rappaport broth and phosphate buffered saline can inhibit PCR (Rossen et al., 1992). PCR can also be inhibited by contaminants from the nucleic acid extraction phase including ionic detergents (Weyant et al., 1990), phenol, ethanol, proteinase K, guanidinium, and salts (Al-Soud & Radstrom, 2001).

The control of PCR inhibition can be addressed on several fronts. Inhibitory effects can be minimized by optimizing the PCR mix. Bovine serum albumin (BSA) was shown to reduce PCR inhibition by humic acid (McGregor et al., 1996) and hemoglobin (Al-Soud & Radstrom, 2001), possibly through direct interaction with the inhibitory components such that they cannot interfere with PCR amplification. The single-stranded DNA binding protein from bacteriophage T4 (gp32) also reduced PCR inhibition caused by hemoglobin (Al-Soud & Radstrom, 2001). The addition of Tween® 20 or DMSO reversed PCR inhibition from low concentrations of the polysaccharides dextran sulfate and gum ghatti (Demeke & Adams, 1992). Inhibitors that affect polymerase activity can be partially mitigated by increasing the polymerase concentration. PCR kit manufacturers often develop proprietary formulations to optimize PCR through design of experiment (DOE) studies. For example, Environmental Master Mix version 2 (EMMv2) was developed by Applied Biosystems specifically for complex samples containing potential inhibitory components (Figure 1). PCR inhibition can be monitored using an internal positive control (IPC) (Tebbs et al., 2010). Samples that show no amplification of target and IPC either contain inhibitors or the PCR reaction was improperly prepared. Technical errors are greatly minimized with new lyophilized formulations that only require the addition of sample. Amplification of the internal control gives confidence that a negative result is not due to inhibition. A simple mitigation to inhibited samples is dilution (Tsai & Olson, 1992a; Tsai & Olson, 1992b). For samples in which the target DNA is not the limiting factor, inhibitors can be diluted below their effective threshold to allow for PCR amplification. In addition, efficient DNA extraction following bacterial enrichment removes PCR inhibitors and improves accurate detection.

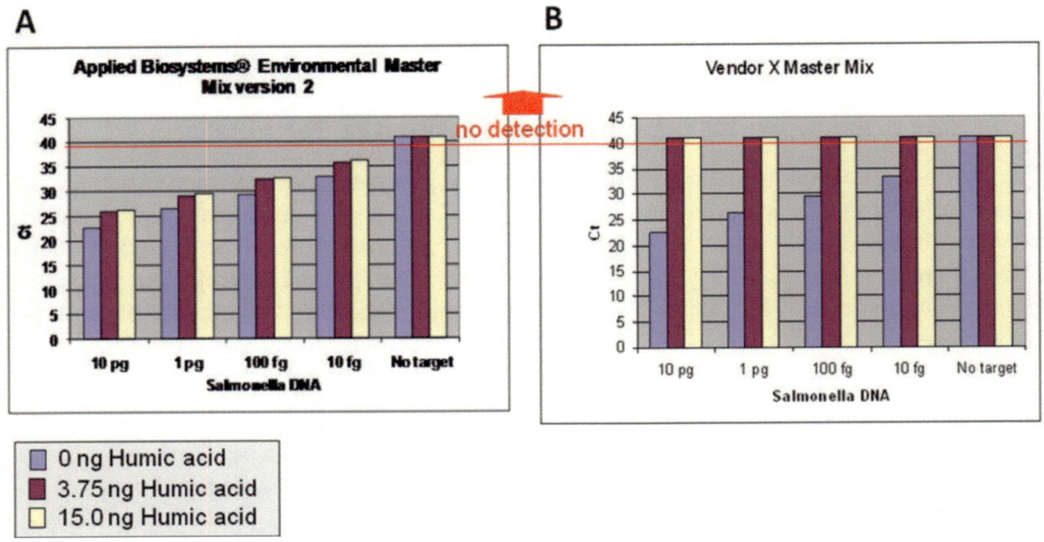

Fig. 1. Real-time PCR Master Mixes can mitigate PCR inhibition. (A) Environmental Master Mix version 2 shows detection of *Salmonella* DNA in the presence of 3.75 ng and 15.0 ng of humic acid. (B) Master mix from another source shows complete inhibition in the presence of the same amount of humic acid. Real-time PCR was performed on the 7500Fast instrument.

Food borne pathogens are usually present in small quantities in food and therefore require enrichment to detect their presence. The United States requires testing for selected pathogens in the nation's food supply. This is true for *Salmonella* species in foods such as ready-to-eat products and whole shell eggs. A standard practice for screening food for regulated pathogens is to mix 25 grams of food with 225 mL of broth (1:9 food to broth ratio). Reference methods are based on traditional culture procedures and typically use a 2-step enrichment procedure, first in non-selective broth (pre-enrichment) and second in selective broth, prior to biochemical and serological characterization. These protocols are designed to detect down to a single viable organism. The pre-enrichment step allows recovery of injured or otherwise weakened *Salmonella*, whereas selective enrichment favors growth of *Salmonella* over background flora that competes with *Salmonella* for available nutrients. The U.S. FDA *Bacteriological Analytical Manual* (BAM) for *Salmonella* pre-enriches in different broths depending on the food matrix (typically lactose broth or tryptic soy broth), followed by selective enrichment in Rappaport-Vassiliadis (RV) medium and tetrathionate (TT) broth (Andrews & Hammack, 2011). Pre-enrichment is for 24 ± 2 h at 35°C, and selective enrichment is for 24 ± 2 h at 42°C for RV and 35°C (food with low microbial load) or 43°C (food with high microbial load) for TT. The U.S. FDA protocol for sampling and detecting *Salmonella* in poultry houses pre-enriches environmental samples in buffered peptone water (24 ± 2 h at 35°C) and then selectively enriches in RV (24 ± 2 h at 42°C) and TT (24 ± 2 h at 43°C) (Food and Drug Administration, 2008). The International Organization for Standardization (ISO) reference method for the detection of *Salmonella* in food (ISO 6579:2002(E)) recommends pre-enrichment in buffered peptone water (other broths are necessary for some food types) for 18 ± 2 h at 37°C followed by selective enrichment in Rappaport-Vassiliadis medium with soya (RVS broth) for 24 ± 3 h at 41.5°C and Muller-Kauffman tetrathionate/novobiocin broth (MKTTn broth) for 24 ± 3 h at 37°C

(ISO 6579:2002 [E]). The enrichment time alone for these traditional culture methods totals 2 days. Following enrichment, the samples are plated to selective agar plates for 24-48 h growth and then transferred to slants for another 24 h growth. Presumptive detection of *Salmonella* is determined in 4 to 5 days (BS plates are left for 48 ± 2 h for BAM method).

Food producers desire faster time-to-results since it provides great cost benefits. The Food and Safety Inspection Service (FSIS) requests all meat and poultry products be held by producers until test result indicate no pathogen is present. The FSIS recently proposed new regulations requiring test results be received before meat and poultry can be shipped, the so called "Test-and Hold" policy (Department of Agriculture, 2011). To the producer, storing product is not only costly but also shortens the product shelf life.

Rapid methods can shorten time-to-results to less than 24 h for *Salmonella*. To be adopted by the food industry, new methods must undergo AOAC validation to demonstrate equivalency to reference culture methods. The AOAC developed the Performance Tested Methods^{SM} (PTM) program for the purpose of certifying commercial test kits (AOAC Research Institute website). Even with AOAC validation demonstrating equivalency, the FDA BAM considers positive results from rapid methods to be presumptive that must either be confirmed by culture or accepted as true positive (negative samples are accepted as true negative). Rapid methods are fast because detection is immediate, but also because enrichment requirements are usually shorter. Most PCR methods only require a single-step enrichment to demonstrate equivalency to reference standards. Well designed PCR assays can detect a single genomic copy of *Salmonella* and thus the limit of detection for PCR is largely determined by sample preparation.

Multiple methods have been used to lyse pathogens including physical, chemical and enzymatic, or combinations of the three (Table 1). Common physical methods include temperature (freeze/thaw or heat), bead-beating, and sonication. Freeze/thaw lysis is a traditional method in which the cellular suspension is transferred between freezing and warm conditions, for example between a dry ice-ethanol bath and a 37°C water bath. During the freeze cycle ice crystals cause cells to expand and rupture. Multiple freeze/thaw cycles are required for efficient lysis which makes the procedure rather lengthy and is usually only associated with "home brew" methods. Microbial cells can also be lysed by heating at 95°C to 100°C. The lysis efficiency of heat is dependent on the microorganism, but is generally poor. Heat is often combined with chemical and/or enzymatic treatment to increase the lysis efficiency which is discussed later. If enzymatic treatment is used, then the heat step serves two functions, it can break open cells and inactivate enzymatic activity. Protease is common for bacterial lysis and if used must be inactivated before adding sample to a PCR mix since proteases will destroy DNA polymerase. Sonication uses high frequency sound waves to create localized regions of low pressure resulting in micro bubbles that rapidly form and implode, ultimately breaking open cells. Bead-beating is another physical method used for breaking open cells. Typically an equal volume of silica or zirconium beads (approximately 0.1 mm diameter) are combined with a sample and mixed on a laboratory vortex. Lysis is complete in 3-5 minutes. Bead-beating has a tendency to generate foam which can be controlled by using anti-foam agents. Bead-beating and sonication can result in greatly fragmented, low molecular weight nucleic acids. However, fragmentation is of minor concern for real-time PCR since assays are designed to amplify small fragments of typically less than 100 base pairs.

Lysis Method	Category	Product	Notes	Test Kit Name	Manufacturer
Bead-Beating/ Chemical/Filter	Manual	DNA		IT 1-2-3™ Sample Purification Kits	Idaho Technology
Chemical	Automated	Lysate	DNA Hybridization	GeneQuence® *Salmonella*	Neogen
Chemical/ Enzyme/ Heat	Simple high throughput	Lysate	2-step enrich (except meat and poultry)	BAX® System PCR Assay *Salmonella*	DuPont Qualicon
Chemical/Heat	Simple	Lysate		PrepSEQ® Rapid Spin Sample Preparation Kit	Life Technologies
Chemical/Heat	Simple	Lysate	2-step enrich	Foodproof® ShortPrep I Kit	BIOTECON Diagnostics
Chemical/Heat	Simple	Lysate		iQ-Check Salmonlla II Easy Extraction I	Bio-Rad
Chemical/Heat	Simple high throughput	Lysate	96-well Deepwell centrifugation	iQ-Check® *Salmonella* II Deepwell protocol	Bio-Rad
Chemical/Heat/ Magnetic beads	Automated	DNA		Foodproof® Magnetic Preparation Kit I	BIOTECON Diagnostics
Chemical/Heat/ Magnetic beads	Semi-automated	DNA/ RNA		PrepSEQ® Nucleic Acid Extraction Kit	Life Technologies
Chemical/Heat/ Filter	Manual	DNA		Foodproof® Sample Preparation Kit	BIOTECON Diagnostics
Chemical/Heat/ Filter	Manual	DNA		Biotest MMB Prep *Salmonella*	Biotest AG
Chemical/Heat/ Filter	Manual	DNA		SureFood® Prep *Salmonella*	Congen Biotechnologie
Sonication/Heat	Automated	DNA		GeneDisc® *Salmonella*	Pall Corp.

Table 1. Sample preparation kits for detecting *Salmonella* by genetic methods. The kits included were chosen from the AOAC Research Institute online website of Performance Tested Methods℠ Validated for detection of *Salmonella* using genetic methods (http://www.aoac.org/testkits/testedmethods.html). Details for sample preparation were obtained from readily available information from company websites and might not be part of the AOAC approved workflow. AES and BioControl have AOAC validation for real-time PCR detection of *Salmonella*, but were omitted from the current list since details of their sample preparation methods were not available on their website.

Many chemicals have been used in cell lysis. The most common chemicals are detergents. Detergents disrupt the lipid bilayer surrounding cells. There are many types of detergents of varying strengths. Ionic detergents such as sodium dodecyl sulfate (SDS) are stronger than nonionic or zwitterionic detergents and are often employed for microbial lysis to extract DNA. In addition to disrupting lipids, SDS has the advantage of denaturing proteins, including DNAse and RNAse, and thus protecting nucleic acid during extraction. Because detergents cannot lyse cell walls, bacteria are often pre-treated with enzymes (proteases or lysozyme) before addition of detergent. Chaotropic salts are also commonly used for bacterial lysis. Guanidinium thocyanate and guanidinium chloride lyse cell membranes by denaturing proteins. Chemicals used in bacterial lysis are by nature hazardous and must be disposed of as hazardous waste.

The use of magnetic particles for sample preparation has increased in recent years. Imunomagnetic separation (IMS) uses metal beads coated with antibodies specific to the target microbe of interest. A magnet can then be used to attract the bead containing the target microbe. The beads can be washed, and the presence of the target organism can be determined by plating onto selective agar, PCR, or other detection methods. Another solution is to use solid phase capture in which antibodies are linked to a solid support. The target microbe can be captured as sample passes across the support. For example, antibodies linked to a pipette tip can capture the target organism by collecting sample with a pipetting device. In theory, the target analyte binds while unwanted material passes through. The analyte can be further purified through a series of wash steps. In practice, antibodies typically show background capture of non-target organisms (Fratamico et al., 2011), and therefore the use of IMS is often combined with a detection method such as PCR or biochemical characterization. Furthermore, the sample matrix (i.e. high fat content) can affect binding of an antibody to its antigenic substrate (Bosilevac et al., 2010; Fitzmaurice, 2006). Both false positive and false negative results have been reported for antibody-based methods. Both immunomagnetic beads and solid support systems have been used in combination with antibodies or phage-binder proteins to capture microbes. Phage-binder proteins are the proteins responsible for phage binding to host bacteria and are very host specific. Both technologies (beads and solid support) have also been used to capture nucleic acids from microbial lysates. Metal beads coated with silica and glass fiber filters are commonly used to capture nucleic acids. DNA binds under conditions of salt and high alcohol, and is eluted with aqueous solutions. Heating the elution buffer can improve recovery by increasing the ability of the nucleic acid to dissolve in solution. The advantage of these systems is increased target concentration and improved target purity without the need for centrifugation and aspiration—methods that are difficult to automate. The use of magnetic beads to capture nucleic acids eliminates the concern associated with antibody specificity since total DNA and RNA can be captured indiscriminately. The same is true for purification columns that bind nucleic acids to silica membranes. The specificity of the assay is determined by the detection method. The binding capacity for nucleic acids can be much higher for magnetic particles compared to that of standard spin columns. The disadvantage with the capture of total nucleic acids is the potential for the capture of large amounts of non-targeted DNA relative to target DNA.

There are ways to simplify sample preparation. How to simplify depends on the needs of the end-user. If obtaining results within an 8-hour work shift is critical, then simplification becomes more challenging. Quick time-to-results requires concentrating the microbe from large sample volumes in combination with efficient microbial lysis and DNA/RNA recovery. To meet this demand sample preparation becomes more complex. Automation can simplify the process, but adds additional costs for equipment. A common practice is to use magnetic particles to capture microbes or microbial nucleic acid since magnetic particles can be easily added to and extracted from an aqueous mixture. Furthermore, procedures using magnetic particles are simple to automate. Instruments can be designed to dispense and aspirate liquids, but instruments that perform these functions are typically more complex.

Increased enrichment times have the advantage of increasing the concentration of the microbe which can greatly simplify sample preparation (Figure 2). Enrichment also dilutes dead cells that could be present in the sample matrix. A 2-step enrichment method (e.g. pre-enrichment followed by selective enrichment) will also dilute the sample matrix which can reduce the impact of inhibitory substances associated with food and environmental samples, thus creating a more consistent sample for sample preparation. Double-enrichment has not found favor in molecular methods that are expected to be rapid. Indeed, PCR is very sensitive and double-enrichment is excessive for most applications. Most food and environmental samples can be enriched overnight (16-18 h) in one broth to allow *Salmonella,* if present, to grow to concentrations that are above the detection limit of PCR even when simple sample preparation methods are used.

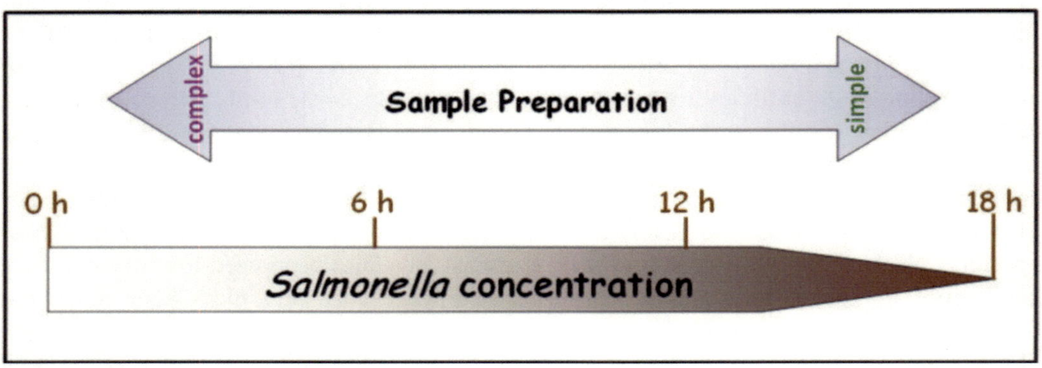

Fig. 2. Increasing *Salmonella* enrichment time can simplify sample preparation. Increased enrichment time increases *Salmonella* concentration requiring less volume and lower efficient sample preparation.

The simplest sample preparation methods dilute enriched samples into a solution that is compatible with the detection method. Indeed, many Gram-negative bacteria are lysed by boiling in water for 10 minutes. Because PCR amplification begins with a denaturation step (typically 95°C for 10 minutes) it is theoretically possible to add diluted sample directly to PCR. However, this doesn't seem to work well for many samples. Some level of lysis prior to adding to the PCR mix improves detection. For example, the addition of a simple 10 minute boiling step prior to setting up a PCR greatly improves detection. It is likely that boiling denatures enzymes and degrades substrates that disrupt the PCR reaction. A simple sample preparation method is shown in Figure 3.

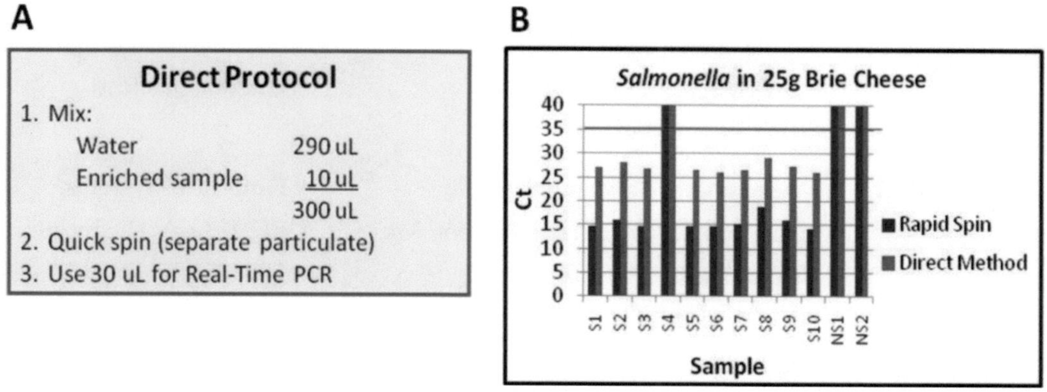

Fig. 3. Simple sample preparation for real-time PCR detection of *Salmonella*. (A) According to the direct protocol, sample is diluted in water and briefly centrifuged for 10 to 15 seconds in a table-top centrifuge. (B) Twenty-five grams of Brie cheese was spiked with 1-3 CFU *Salmonella enterica* serotype Typhimurium (strain Q210) and enriched at 37°C for 16 hours in buffered peptone water. The Direct Method showed a >10 Ct difference compared to the PrepSEQ® Rapid Spin method, but there was 100% correlation for detection of *Salmonella* between the two methods. Sample 4 (S4) which also received the spike gave negative results by both sample preparation methods, demonstrating all samples were spiked with low concentrations of *Salmonella* (i.e. fractional positive spike). Ten Cts correspond to a 1000-fold dilution in available DNA. Samples were analyzed on the 7500 Fast instrument using the MicroSEQ® *Salmonella* spp. Detection Kit.

4. Genetic-based methods for detection of *Salmonella* in foods

Genetic methods involve specific detection of RNA or DNA sequences to determine presence of the pathogen. There are a number of available kits in the market that apply genetic methods for the detection of *Salmonella* (Table 2). The most common genetic detection methods are PCR-based technologies. In the simplest form, conventional PCR involves amplification of a target DNA sequence using primers. The reaction is cycled between denaturing and annealing temperatures and may include a specific temperature for extension. The reaction generates an amplicon which can be detected on an agarose gel when stained with an intercalating dye such as ethidium bromide. The amplicon must be of the expected size for the sample to be called positive.

A DNA-binding dye, such as SYBR® Green, can be added to PCR and monitored by a real-time PCR instrument. SYBR® Green preferentially binds double-stranded DNA resulting in a DNA-Dye complex that shows a unique absorbance and emission spectrum. SYBR® Green dye will detect PCR products as they are amplified. Highly specific primer designs are required to avoid false positives because SYBR® Green dye will bind to all double-stranded DNA including any mis-primed products. Melt curve analysis of the PCR products of SYBR® Green dye reactions can be added to the end of a real-time PCR run to collect melting temperature (Tm) data of the PCR products amplified. This additional layer of data provides another check that the product amplified is of the expected Tm which is indicative of the fragment length. There are numerous examples of SYBR® Green PCR assays used to detect *Salmonella* in food or environmental samples (Nam et al., 2005; Techathuvanan et al., 2011).

Method	Test Kit Name	Manufacturer
PCR/melt curve analysis	BAX® System for *Salmonella*	DuPont Qualicon
Real-time PCR	Assurance GDS® for *Salmonella*	BioControl Systems
	Foodproof® *Salmonella* Detection Kit	BIOTECON Diagnostics
	GeneDisc® *Salmonella*	Pall Corp.
	iQ-Check® *Salmonella* II Kit	Bio-Rad
	MicroSEQ® *Salmonella* spp. Detection Kit	Life Technologies
	Salmonella species LT Test Kit	Idaho Technology
	SureFood® *Salmonella* PLUS V	Congen
DNA hybridization	GeneQuence® *Salmonella*	Neogen
NASBA	Nuclisens EasyQ® Basic Kit*	bioMerieux
LAMP	LoopAmp® DNA or RNA Amplification Kit*	Eiken Chemical Company

* General reagent kit which is not *Salmonella* specific.

Table 2. Commercial kits utilizing genetic methods to detect *Salmonella*.

Using fluorogenic probes with real-time PCR has rapidly become the standard for genetic detection because of its high specificity and sensitivity to detect low copy numbers. Many real-time instrument platforms have the ability to complete a run under one hour because of fast temperature ramping and improvements in master mix chemistries. TaqMan® assay uses target-specific primers and a probe that is labeled with a fluorescent reporter dye on the 5′ end and a quencher dye on the 3′ end (Tebbs et al., 2009; Balachandran et al., 2011). The probe anneals to the target DNA sequence between the two primer sites. As the primer extends during each cycle of the PCR, the 5′ nuclease activity of Taq polymerase displaces the probe from the DNA strand, separating the reporter dye and quencher dye in the process, and fluorescent signal is emitted. An example of a real-time assay which detects *Salmonella* Typhimurium is shown in Figure 4. Details of TaqMan data analysis will be further discussed.

An alternative fluorescent probe is the molecular beacon. The stem-and-loop structure of a molecular beacon probe consists of a target-specific sequence (which forms the loop) and non-target sequences that are complementary at the 5′ and 3′ end of the probe (forming the stem). When the probe is in a closed loop shape with the 5′ and 3′ ends hybridized to one another, the fluorescent reporter dye is quenched. When the molecular beacon probe hybridizes to the amplicon during PCR, the stem-and-loop structure opens, separating the fluorophore from the quencher releasing fluorescence. The application of molecular beacons in *Salmonella* detection in foods has been tested in a variety of food matrices (Bhaqwat et al., 2008; Patel & Bhagwat, 2008; Liming & Bhagwat, 2004).

Another variation of real-time PCR employs Scorpions technology. Scorpions are PCR primers covalently linked to a probe (Carters, et al., 2008). The reporter dye on the probe is prevented from fluorescing by a quencher dye on a separate complementary oligo. Upon primer extension, a probe-binding sequence is created which allows the probe to bind intramolecularly and generate fluorescence.

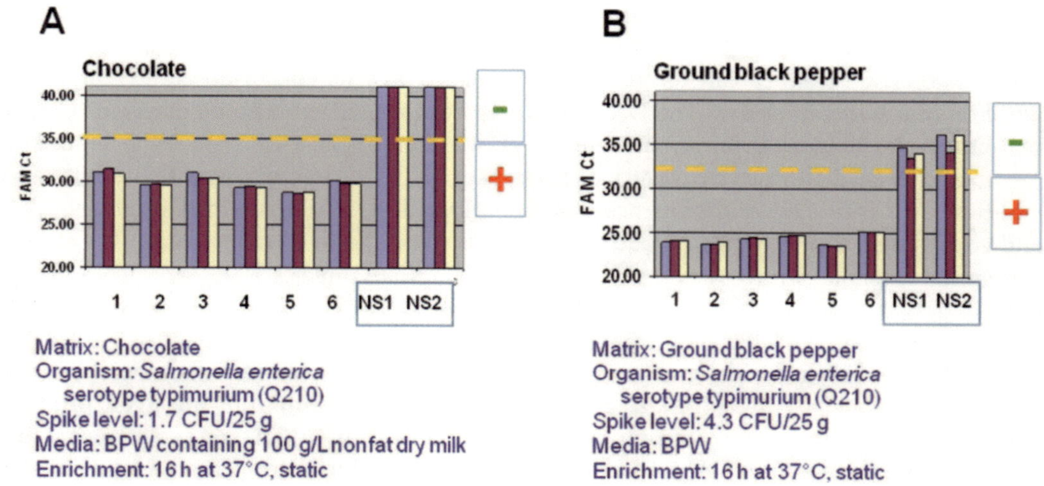

Fig. 4. Real-time PCR detection of *Salmonella.* 25 g of chocolate (A) 25 g of chocolate or (B) 25 g of black paper spiked with *Salmonella* were enriched for 16 hours. Six samples were spiked with 1-5 CFU *Salmonella* and 2 samples were not spiked with *Salmonella* (NS1 and NS2). Samples were prepared by the PrepSEQ® Rapid Spin Sample Preparation kit (in triplicate), and analyzed on the 7500Fast instrument using the MicroSEQ® *Salmonella spp.* Detection Kit.

RNA can also serve as the initial template for PCR for *Salmonella* detection. Detecting *Salmonella* RNA can serve as an indicator of viability of the bacteria (González-Escalona et al., 2009). RNA transcripts are likely present in higher copies than genomic DNA which can increase the sensitivity of the assay. In reverse transcription-PCR (RT-PCR), RNA is first converted to DNA by reverse transcriptase, and then PCR amplification occurs using the newly created DNA strands.

Alternative methods to real-time PCR have also recently emerged. The principle difference of these methods from PCR is that they use different approaches for generating new DNA or RNA with each cycle of amplification. In standard PCR, a denaturation step creates new DNA strands for DNA amplification to occur, theoretically doubling DNA template with each cycle. In contrast, loop-mediated isothermal amplification (LAMP) technology uses auto-cycling strand displacement DNA synthesis to create new DNA template. A *Bst* DNA polymerase large fragment with high strand displacement activity is added to the reaction. There are two general stages of LAMP: generation of template from the input sample and cycling amplification (Tomita et al., 2008). Typically, four primer sets are used to target six independent sequences flanking the target DNA. An inner primer hybridizes to the target DNA and elongates. This is followed by strand displacement which is primed by an outer primer; in this step, the outer primer hybridizes to the target DNA, displacing the newly created single strand DNA. Because each inner primer consists of a 5′ overhang that becomes self-complementary to a sequence as the primer extends, the newly created single strand DNA forms a structure that has loops at each end. This DNA with stem-loop structure is the template of LAMP cycling. During LAMP cycling, the inner primer initiates auto-strand displacement with the template; also, self-priming occurs within the template. In short, the products are multiple stem-loop structures and elongated products containing the target sequence. LAMP reaction occurs at a constant temperature, typically 60-65 °C, and can be carried out in a water bath or heat block. Because a tremendous amount of DNA is formed in the reaction, the reaction by-product magnesium pyrophosphate forms a precipitate. The turbidity can be visible to the naked eye or visualized by UV after the addition of a fluorescent dye. The DNA products from LAMP can also be detected using a real-time turbidimeter. Application of LAMP in detection of *Salmonella* species in foods has previously been demonstrated (Ueda & Kuwabara, 2009). Another alternative method to real-time PCR is nucleic acid sequence-based amplification (NASBA) which amplifies RNA and creates new RNA strands by addition of a promoter site to complementary DNA. The isothermal method, which is typically run at 41 °C, first converts RNA into DNA using reverse transcriptase, then hydrolyzes RNA from the RNA-DNA hybrid using Rnase H. A target-specific primer, with a T7 promoter sequence at its 5′ end, hybridizes to the single-stranded DNA. T7 RNA polymerase binds to the promoter region of the newly created double-stranded DNA to synthesize new RNA templates. Detection of the RNA product from NASBA can be accomplished by DNA hybridization followed by electrochemiluminescence. NASBA has previously been used to detect *Salmonella* Enteritidis in foods (D'Souza & Jaykus, 2003). Although there is no AOAC certified kit specifically for *Salmonella* detection by LAMP or NASBA, there are commercially available kits to perform these types of detection.

DNA hybridization is another useful way to detect target sequences of *Salmonella*. Labeled single-stranded DNA probes are added to a sample to detect either *Salmonella* DNA or RNA sequence. In one form of DNA hybridization, a poly-dA capture probe is added to a lysed sample in a microwell coated with poly-dT to detect *Salmonella*-specific rRNA sequence; simultaneously, a detector probe with a 5′ horse-radish peroxidase (HRP) label is added to detect the same rRNA target (Mozola et al., 2007). Unhybrized probes are washed away, and after addition of a HRP substrate, the hybridization is detected by chemiluminescence. DNA hybridization can also be done using a dot blot format whereby a labeled probe is immobilized on a membrane (Iida et al., 1993).

Genetic technologies such as whole genome sequencing, microarrays, and SNP analysis are useful for identifying and typing *Salmonella*. However, these methods are not yet widely used for routine screening of food samples because they typically require more detailed workflows.

5. Analysis of real-time PCR data

In TaqMan® real-time PCR assay, the fluorescence released by the reporter dye during each cycle increases exponentially until the reaction reaches saturation. The cycle number at which the fluorescent signal first crosses the threshold value is the cycle threshold (C_T). It is dependent on the baseline which is established in the early cycles of the PCR. The threshold value, referred to as delta Rn (normalized reporter signal), can be adjusted by the user. The threshold value should be set above baseline noise in the early cycles of PCR and within the exponential amplification phase for positive samples (Figure 5). Using PCR replicates of positive samples is a useful way to decide upon the appropriate threshold to use for data analysis. The appropriate delta Rn value will be dependent upon the assay and application and, once set, should be used for all samples for consistent analysis. Low C_T values indicate high copy number of the target sequence, while high C_T values indicate low copy number. The typical limit of detection is 10 to 100 copies of purified genomic DNA and 10^3 to 10^4 CFU/mL before sample preparation. Most assays for *Salmonella* detection are typically qualitative, producing data that can be categorized as positive or negative. However, assay runs can be designed to be quantitative. Quantitative real-time assays should be validated and shown to amplify with high efficiency. The linear range for quantitation should be based on the exponential phase of amplification. Unknown samples to be quantitated should be run alongside DNA standards during real-time PCR.

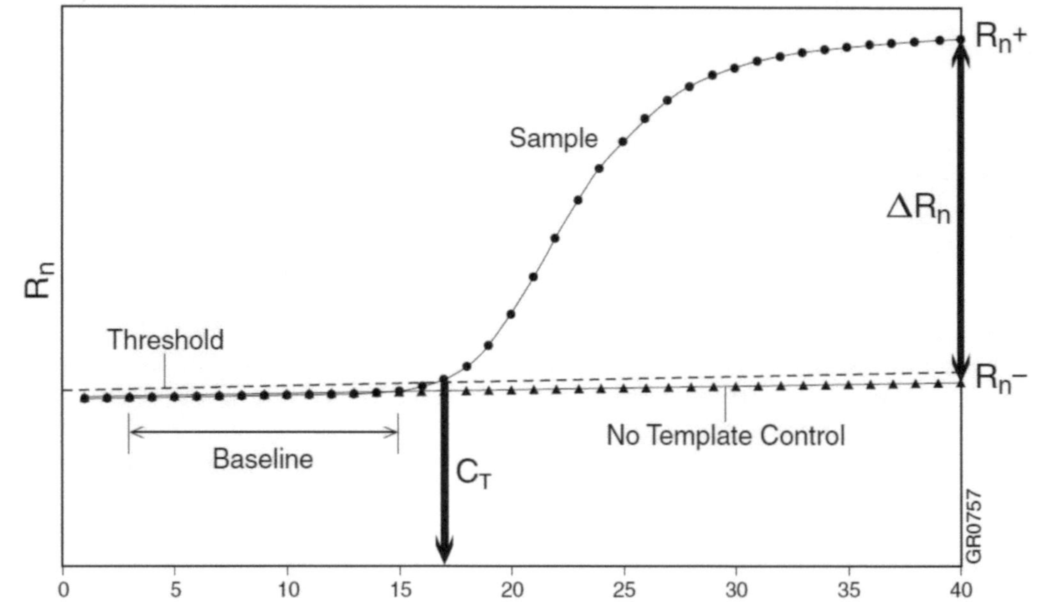

Fig. 5. Demonstration of a TaqMan® amplification curve and parameters. Amplification results in increased fluorescence (Rn). The Ct value reflects the beginning of amplification.

In PCR using SYBR® Green dye, a real-time amplification plot is generated that is similar to a TaqMan® PCR assay. Melt curve analysis (also known as a dissociation curve analysis) is typically added to the end of a SYBR® Green PCR. During the dissociation stage, the instrument increases in temperature over several minutes. For positive samples, SYBR® Green is initially bound to the amplicons. As the double-stranded amplicon dissociates, there is a drop in SYBR® Green fluorescence. The change in fluorescence is plotted against the temperature (Figure 6). Unknown samples should be compared to no-template reactions. Samples that are positive should have product of the expected Tm and, if the assay is well-designed, should not have other products such as primer-dimer or mis-primed products.

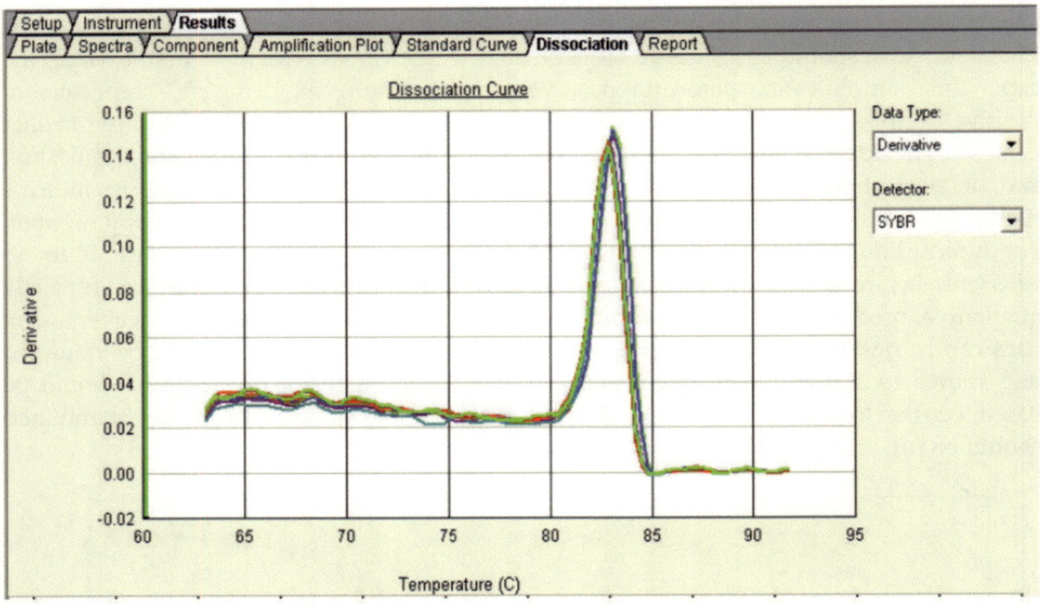

Fig. 6. Derivative of a melting curve from a reaction with SYBR® Green dye reaction. The Tm is determined by the peak of the derivative.

6. Software

Easy-to-use software is an important component of applying genetic methods to detect Salmonella. It is crucial to have accurate, reproducible, and unbiased data interpretation. Results should be clearly stated in convenient formats to the end user. In RapidFinder™ Express Software (Life Technologies) for food pathogen detection, algorithms were developed to interpret real-time PCR data and allow for sensitive detection while avoiding false positive results. Results are stated as positive or negative depending on cutoff values. In cases in which a positive or negative assessment cannot be made (e.g, the internal positive control failed indicating inhibition), a warning assessment is generated along with an explanation (Figure 7).

7. Bioinformatic tools for real-time PCR assays design

Selecting a good genomic target is critical to designing a real-time PCR assay. Appropriate genomic targets have to be sequenced from multiple strains in order to design highly specific primers and probes which cover a set of desired target species (*inclusion set*) and exclude from detecting a set of other bacterial genomes (*exclusion set*). Examples of broadly sequenced bacterial DNA targets are the 16S gene, *gapA, recA, rpoB*, among others. We developed and validated a standard bioinformatics assay design tool to generate primer and probe combinations for real-time PCR pathogen detection. The first step of the design is generation of a target consensus sequence based on multiple sequence alignments of all available target sequences using clustalW algorithm (Larkin et al., 2007). Sequences can be used from all available public databases. At the second step, a set of well described selection criteria (Larkin et al., 2007; Endrizzi et al., 2002; Kramer & Coen, 2000) has to be applied, such as optimal Tm, nucleotide distribution (*e.g.* avoid high GC content and poly-N stretches), absence of cross-hybridization; and amplicon size (optimal size is 60-150 base pairs). This set of rules can be applied to select candidate primer and probe sequences that target a signature nucleic acid sequence in a microbe of interest. A set of optimal assays has to be evaluated, considering criteria of hybridization patterns of the two primers and a TaqMan® probe to the intended target sequence (Endrizzi et al., 2002). At the third step, those assays with the highest specificity are selected. The specificity is determined based on nucleic acid sequence comparisons of the binding sites for the assay primers and probes with genomic sequences from other bacterial species (exclusion set), being sure to include closely related species in the analysis. These genomic sequences have to be from multiple available databases, as well as from additional sequences that can be specifically generated for the design of the TaqMan® detection assays. Based on this sequence comparison, specific primers and probes can be selected. The best primers contain the highest number of mismatches to other non-target bacteria genomes, with mismatches preferentially located at the 3'-prime region of the primers. This minimizes the possibility that an assay will be selected that generates a false-positive signal (Furtado et al., 2004).

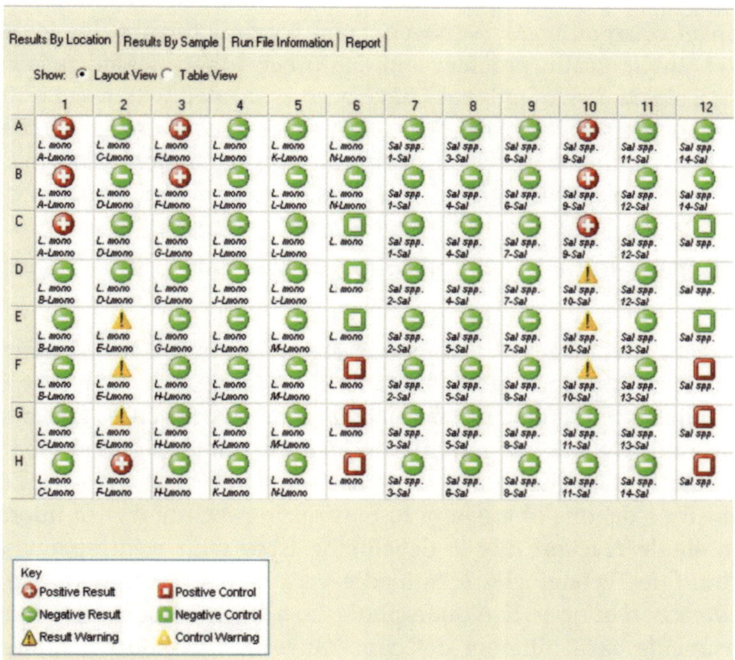

Fig. 7. RapidFinder™ Express Software for food pathogen detection displays positive, negative, and warning assessments for real-time PCR.

Additional DNA targets can be amplified and sequenced. This is often required when inclusion/exclusion testing show non-detection of inclusion strains or unwanted detection of exclusion strains. This requires the design of sequencing primers upstream and downstream of the assay target. It might also be useful to create a specific signature sequence database by sequencing additional samples, which can increase the confidence of specific assay designs. Sequence files can be analyzed using clustalW multiple sequence alignment. The Applied Biosystems® MicroSEQ® ID validated method can be used for sequencing the 16S fragment. Using the 16S gene as a target for specific pathogen detection is challenging because it contains conservative sequences across multiple bacterial species. However, when primers and probes have to detect a broad range of species, families, genus or higher order, the 16S target is ideal or often is the only choice.

Experimental validation of the assay specificity is a critical step in the final assay selection. To test for assay specificity, a panel containing a diverse group of *bacteria* isolates (target and exclusion strains) has to be established and used for experimental validation. The panel must be well characterized by stereotyping or sequence-based bacterial identification (Tanner et al., 2006). Preferably, the panel will contain ATCC type-strains.

8. *Salmonella* detection background

More than 2,400 *Salmonella* serotypes have been reported, all of which are potentially pathogenic. The species *Salmonella* enterica, with its 6 main subspecies is of clinical relevance for humans and is the causative agent of food borne illnesses or salmonellosis. However, for tracking purposes it is often important to have a very specific serotype assay to measure and contain the spread of an outbreak pathogen. Food borne outbreaks due to *Salmonella* have become a major public health problem and can occur either as food poisoning triggered epidemics or as isolated cases. Outbreaks have been associated with raw meats and poultry, eggs, milk and dairy products, seafood, coconut sauces, salad dressings, cocoa, chocolate, and peanuts. The combination of efficient sample preparation protocols and reliable detection of *Salmonella* is a solid path forward for molecular detection methods.

9. Design options: Single-plex, multiplex, degenerate primers and probes & optimization

The most important advantages of real-time PCR are the ability for quantification of target concentration and multiplexing with different dyes per target. Since real-time PCR measures target amplification by monitoring the increase in fluorescence generated by probe degradation, the only limitation to multiplexing within a single reaction tube is the number of fluorophores that can be distinguished by the detection system (i.e. optics and software). From the chemistry side, one of the keys to maximizing the number of fluorogenic signals measured in a single reaction mix is developing dyes with well-separated and narrow emission spectra. Life Technologies identified several dye sets and real-time PCR systems that allow for detection of up to five fluorophores in a single reaction mix. It is important to note that instruments have different detection ranges for monitoring fluorescent energy. Detecting multiple targets can also be achieved through novel engineering designs; an example being the 384-well format Custom TaqMan® Array card that can be used in combination with the Applied Biosystems 7900HT Fast real-time PCR System (Tebbs et al., 2010), and the OpenArray® real-time PCR System. These Systems split a common sample amongst multiple reaction chambers prior to real-time PCR amplification and detection.

Since the 7500Fast real-time PCR system capability allows for measuring five fluorophores in a single reaction mix, it is possible to create real-time reaction applications capable of detecting 5 target organisms in a single tube. However, for high accuracy applications, two of the five channels are often used as system controls. We created a number of applications where one channel is assigned to the internal positive control (IPC) to monitor the presence of PCR inhibitors, and another channel is used to control for well-to-well variation and normalization of fluorescence detection by using a ROX™ dye as a standard dye. Detection of IPC is indicative of a successful PCR amplification. Thus, with the inclusion of two controls, three targets can be detected in a single reaction tube. Each assay target is evaluated independently through the dye assigned to that target. Important considerations when designing multiplex real-time PCR assays include: first, development of several specific working assays for each target to have a choice in a final configuration. Each assay should be tested for quantification efficiency. Second, each assay must be tested against a large panel of microorganisms that include both inclusive and exclusive strains to identify highly specific assays. It is possible to add additional primers and probes containing variant base sequences (degenerate sequences) if some inclusive strains are not detected or weakly detected. Third, fluorogenic dye signals should be balanced by adjusting primer/probe concentrations: it is essential to perform statistics-based DOE (Design of Experiments) studies to optimize primer and probe concentrations for optimal detection of each target species. The final multiplex assay can be further optimized by standard PCR optimization techniques including adjusting magnesium and enzyme concentration, annealing temperature, probe lengths, and instrument settings.

10. Design and validation of existing real-time PCR *Salmonella* assays

Specific assays were designed and tested for detection of (i) *Salmonella* species in food samples, (ii) *Salmonella* Enteriditis in eggs and environmental samples, and (iii) *Salmonella* Typhimurium (Table 3). The selection of the target genes was based on specific applications: whether targeting detection of all *Salmonella* species in one reaction or targeting a specific serotype. Experimental validation is an essential part of molecular assay development. Testing and validation of the complete workflow is a critical element in the acceptance of a detection assay in food safety testing laboratories.

***Salmonella* target organism**	**Gene Target**
Salmonella species	*hilA* gene
Salmonella Enteriditis	*Prot6e* gene
Salmonella Typhimurium	*Target 1/Target 2*

Table 3. Real-time PCR assays for *Salmonella.*

Our *Salmonella* spp. detection assay is a rapid, sensitive real-time PCR test, that, when combined with the automated PrepSEQ® Nucleic Acid extraction method or the manual PrepSEQ® Rapid Spin extraction method, allows the completion of *Salmonella* spp. detection within 18-19 hours, compared to 3-5 days required by for the traditional culture-based methods (Andrews & Hammack, 2011). As described in the previous section, each real-time PCR reaction contains an Internal Positive Control (IPC) that monitors for the presence of inhibitors for reliable negative results. The assay was designed as a complete reaction mix (no target DNA) in a lyophilized format to allow for minimal pipetting steps and addition of maximum sample volume. This workflow allows for robust *Salmonella* detection and creates the possibility of testing composite or pooled samples reliably.

The assay was validated for *Salmonella* detection in different food matrices including a variety of food matrices which were previously associated with food recalls or outbreaks (Carroll, 2009; Cahill et al., 2008; van Cauteren et al., 2009; Munnoch et al., 2009; Reiter et al., 2007): raw ground beef, raw chicken wings, chocolate, raw shrimp, Brie cheese, shell eggs, cantaloupe, black pepper, dry infant formula, and dry pet food. The detection was complemented by two sample preparation protocols for flexible detection work-flow set up: manual Rapid Spin column-based method and high-throughput automated method. The complete workflow was evaluated against the reference ISO 6579 culture confirmation method. Examples for detecting *Salmonella* in "difficult" matrices chocolate and black pepper are shown in Figure 4 (above). The sensitivity and specificity rates for *Salmonella* spp. detection assays were 100%, with no false negative or false positive samples observed with both sample preparation methods. Inclusivity panel contained 100 *Salmonella* strains based on variety of serotypes. Exclusivity panel contained 30 different bacterial isolates, including genetically close microorganisms as well as bacteria that are common organisms in the environment (Balachandran et al., 2011).

A special study was conducted to demonstrate detection of *Salmonella* in peanut butter, as a part of the Emergency Response Validation program, that followed the peanut butter outbreak in the United States in 2009 (Tebbs et al., 2009). The method was evaluated using *S. enterica* ser. Typhimurium ATCC14028 strain and the reference FDA-BAM protocol was used as culture confirmation method. There was complete agreement between the automated PrepSEQ® NA Extraction method and culture confirmation for uninoculated samples (see Table 5 in Tebbs et al., 2009). Also, Chi-square analyses indicated that the proportions of positives for the *Salmonella* spp. detection method and the reference method were not statistically different at the 5% level of significance.

A specific *Salmonella* Typhimurium assay was designed using duplex assay approach: two different assay probes carry different fluorescent dyes. This two-target approach increases confidence calling the test positive: both fluorescent signals should be positive (Figure 8). An example of positive *Salmonella* Typhimurium detection using this two-target assay is presented in Figure 9.

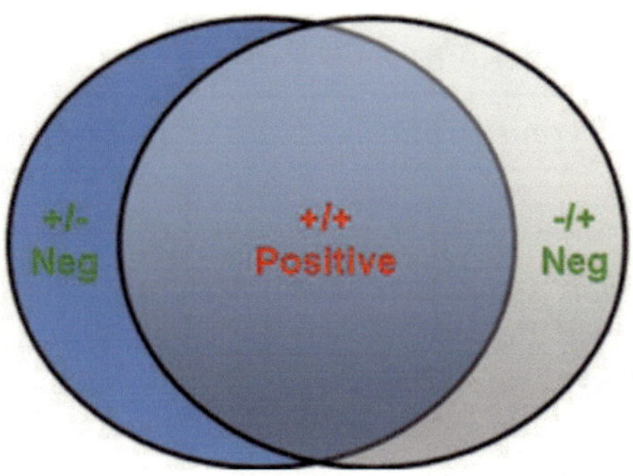

Fig. 8. Diagram representing a duplex real-time PCR assay for detection of *Salmonella* Typhimurium. Each assay detects *S.* Typhimurium plus some non-Typhimurium strains. Because each assay detects a different set of non-Typhimurium strains, only when both assays are positive is the sample positive for *S.* Typhimurium. The assays are labeled with a different fluorophore to be detected independently by real-time PCR.

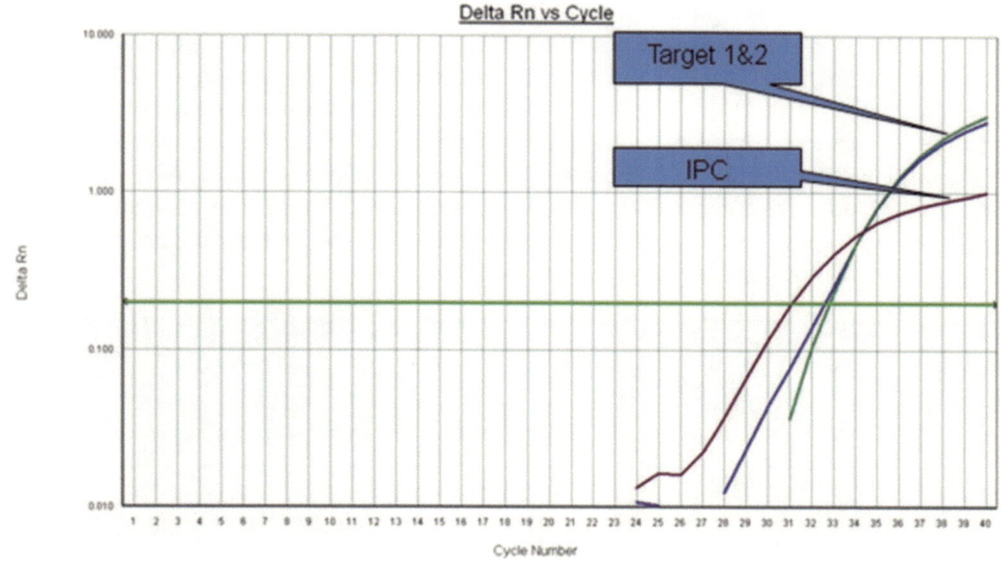

Fig. 9. Example showing positive detection of *Salmonella* Typhimurium with a two-target assay. The assay for target 1 uses FAM™, the assay for target 2 uses VIC®, and the assay for IPC uses NED™. The assay was analyzed on the 7500Fast real-time PCR instrument.

Real-time PCR methods for detecting foodborne pathogens offer the advantages of simplicity and quick time to results compared to traditional culture methods. Our assays demonstrated high accuracy detection of *Salmonella* strains in inclusivity panels, and good discrimination against detection of exclusivity panels.

11. Conclusion

Rapid methods offer great advantages to food producers minimizing risks associated with long hold times during pathogen testing. This is clearly illustrated with requirements for testing whole shell eggs for *Salmonella enterica* serovar Enteritidis (SE). In July of 2009 the U.S. Food and Drug Administration announced The Federal Egg Safety Program, a new regulation that requires routine environmental tests of poultry houses for presence of *Salmonella* Enteritidis (Food and Drug Administration, 2009). If SE is present in the environment, there is a requirement to test eggs prior to their distribution for sale. According to the regulation, 50 egg pools consisting of 20 eggs per pool must be tested every 2 weeks for 8 weeks. The traditional method, designed and approved by the FDA, takes up to ten days to get results (Andrews & Hammack, 2011). According to the FDA approved method, egg pools sit for 4 days at room temperature to allow growth of SE, and then a 25 gram sample is pre-enriched in modified typtic soy broth with ferrous sulfate. The sample is then grown in selective media, then selective agars for presumptive detection, and then confirmed by biochemical and serological methods. The procedure is laborious and expensive. A recently developed real-time PCR assay allows detection of SE in egg pools in less than 27 hours. The TaqMan® *Salmonella* Enteritidis Detection Kit (Life Technologies) enriches egg pool samples for 24 hours, following which the samples are prepped and combined with a PCR reaction mix for detection by real-time PCR. Because sample prep is fully automated, the total hands on time following enrichment is less than one hour. A method comparison study showed that the real-time PCR method was equivalent to the FDA reference method (Table 4). The FDA reported that the real-time PCR kit was equivalent to the FDA BAM Chapter 5, *Salmonella* method for detection of *Salmonella* Enteritidis in accuracy, precision, and sensitivity (FDA website). The Pennsylvania Layer Industry and Penn Ag approved the use of the real-time PCR method as an option for testing of egg and environmental samples without the need for culture confirmation. The trend appears to show increased acceptance of real-time PCR and other fast methods as alternatives to the more cumbersome culture methods.

Inoculation Level	Inoculating Organism	U.S. FDA BAM	TaqMan® Salmonella Enteritidis Method		X^2	Relative Sensitivity	False Negative Rate	False Positive Rate
			Presumed	Confirmed				
Experiment 1								
Control	N/A	0/5	0/5	0/5	-	-	0%	0%
Spike	*S. enterica* ser. Enteritidis ATCC 13076	16/20	16/20	16/20	0	100%	0%	0%
Experiment 2								
Control	N/A	0/5	0/5	0/5	-	-	0%	0%
Spike	*S. enterica* ser. Enteritidis ATCC 13076	11/20	13/20	13/20	0.41	118%	0%	0%

Table 4. Methods comparison showed that the TaqMan® Real-time PCR method was equivalent to the FDA BAM method for detection of *Salmonella* Enteritidis in whole shell eggs. The results from chi-square analysis on two independent experiments indicated no difference between the two methods ($\chi^2 = 0$ and 0.41 for Experiment 1 and Experiment 2, respectively). No false positive or false negative results were observed.

12. References

Al-Soud WA, Radstrom P (2001). Purification and characterization of PCR-inhibitory components in blood cells. *Journal of Clinical Microbiology,* 39(2):485-493.

Andersen MR, Omiecinski CJ (1992). Direct extraction of bacterial plasmids from food for polymerase chain reaction amplification. *Applied and Environmental Microbiology* 58(12):4080-4082.

Andrews WH, HammackT (2011). Bacteriological Analytical Manual, Chapter 5, *Salmonella.* In *U.S. Food and Drug Administration, Bacteriological Analytical Manual Online* (http://www.fda.gov/Food/ScienceResearch/LaboratoryMethods/Bacteriological AnalyticalManualBAM/ucm070149.htm). Accessed July 27, 2011.

AOAC Research Institute website. (http://www.aoac.org/testkits/testkits.html). Accessed July 27, 2011.

Atmar RL, Metcalf TG, Neill FH, Estes MK (1993). Detection of enteric viruses in oysters by using the polymerase chain reaction. *Applied and Environmental Microbiology* 59(2):631-635.

Balachandran P, Cao Y, Wong L, Furtado MR, Petrauskene OV, Tebbs RS (2011). Evaluation of Applied Biosystems MicroSEQ® Real-Time PCR system for detecgtion of *Salmonella* spp. in food: *Performance Tested Method*SM 031001. *Journal of AOAC International,* 94(4):1106-1116.

Bhagwat AA, Patel J, Chua T, Chan A, Cruz SR, Aguilar GA (2008). Detection of *Salmonella* species in foodstuffs. *Methods in Molecular Biology*, 429(II):33-43.

Bolsilevac JM, Kalchayanand N, Schmidt JW, Shackelford SD, Wheeler TL, Koohmaraie M (2010). Inoculation of beef with low concentrations of Escherichia coli O157:H7 and examination of factors that interfere with its detection by culture isolation and rapid methods. *Journal of Food Protection*, 73(12):2180-2188.

Boyd EF, Wang FS, Whittam TS, Selander RK (1996). Molecular genetic relationships of the *salmonellae. Applied and Environmental Microbiology*, 62(3):804–808.

Cahill SM, Wachsmuth IK, Costarrica Mde L, et al (2008). Powdered infant formula as a source of *Salmonella* infection in infants. *Clin Infect Dis.*, 46:268-273.

Carroll C (2009). Corporate Reputation Review 12, 64-82.

Carters R, Ferguson J, Gaut R, Ravetto P, Thelwell N, Whitcombe D (2008). Design and use of scorpions fluorescent signaling molecules. *Methods in Molecular Biology*, 429(II):99-115.

Center for Disease Control (2004). *Salmonella* Annual Summary 2004.

Coenye T, Vandamme P (2003).Extracting phylogenetic information from whole-genome sequencing projects: the lactic acid bacteria as a test case. *Microbiology*, 149(Pt 12):3507–3517

Demeke T, Adams RP (1992). The effects of plant polysaccharides and buffer additives on PCR. *BioTechniques*, 12(3):332-334.

Department of Agriculture (2011). Not applying the mark of inspection pending certain test results. In *Federal Register*, 76(69):19952-19970.

D'Souza, D.H., Jaykus, L.-A. (2003). Nucleic acid sequence based amplification for the rapid and sensitive detection of *Salmonella enterica* from foods. *J Applied Microbiol.* 95, 1343–1350.

Eckhart L, Bach J, Ban J, Tschachler E (2000). Melanin binds reversibly to thermostable DNA polymerase and inhibits its activity. *Biochemical and Biophysical Research Communications*, 271(3):726-730.

Endrizzi K, Fischer J, Klein K, Schwab M, Nussler A, Neuhaus P, Eichelbaum M, Zanger UM (2002). Discriminative quantification of cytochrome P4502D6 and 2D7/8 pseudogene expression by TaqMan real-time reverse transcriptase polymerase chain reaction. *Anal. Biochem.*, 300: 121-131.

Fitzmaurice J (2006). Detection of verotoxin genes VT 1 and VT 2 in Escherichia coli O157:H7 in minced beef using immunocapture and real-time PCR. *Methods in Molecular Biology*, 345:91-96.

Fleischmann RD, Adams MD, White O, Clayton RA, Kirkness EF, Kerlavage AR, Bult CJ, Tomb JF, Dougherty BA, Merrick JM, et al. (1995). Whole-genome random sequencing and assembly of *Haemophilus influenza. Rd. Science*, 269(5223):496-512.

Food and Drug Administration website, Testing methodology for *Salmonella* Enteritidis (SE), (http://www.fda.gov/Food/FoodSafety/Product-SpecificInformation/EggSafety/EggSafetyActionPlan/ucm228796.htm). Accessed July 26, 2011.

Food and Drug Administration (2008). Environmental sampling and detection of *Salmonella* in poultry houses. In *U. S. Food and Drug Administration website* (http://www.fda.gov/Food/ScienceResearch/LaboratoryMethods/ucm114716.htm). Accessed July 27, 2011.

Food and Drug Administration (2009). Prevention of *Salmonella* Enteriditis in Shell Eggs During Production, Storage, and Transportation; Final Rule (July 9, 2009). *Federal Register*, Vol 74 (130): 33030-33101.

Fratamico P, Bagi LK, Cray WC, Narang N, Yan X, Median M, Liu M (2011). Detection by multiplex real-time polymerase chain reaction assays and isolation of shiga toxin-producing *Escherichia coli* serogroups 026, 045, 0103, 0111, 0121, and 0145 in ground beef. *Foodborne Pathogens and Disease*, 8(5):601-607.

Furtado M.R, Petrauskene OV, Livak KJ (2004). Application of Real-Time Quantitative PCR in the Analysis of Gene Expression. In *Horizon Bioscience*. DNA Amplification: Current Technologies and Applications. 131-145.

González-Escalona N, Hammack TS, Russell M, Jacobson AP, De Jesús AJ, Brown EW, Lampel KA (2009). Detection of live *Salmonella* spp. cells in produce by a TaqMan-based quantitative reverse transcriptase real-time PCR targeting invA mRNA. *Applied and Environmental Microbiology*, 75(11):3714-3720.

Healy B, Huynh S, Mullane N, O'Brien S, Iversen C, Lehner A, Stephan R , Parker CT, Fanning S (2009). Microarray-based comparative genomic indexing of the *Cronobacter* genus (*Enterobacter sakazakii*). *International Journal of Food Microbiology*, 136(2):159-164.

Iida K, Abe A, Matsui H, Danbara H, Wakayama S, Kawahara K (1993). Rapid and sensitive method for detection of *Salmonella* strains using a combination of polymerase chain reaction and reverse dot-blot hybridization. *FEMS Microbiol Lett.*, 114(2):167-172.

ISO 6579:2002 (E). *Microbiology of food and animal feeding stuffs - Horizontal method for the detection of Salmonella spp.* (2002) 4th Ed., INTERNATIONAL STANDARD, Geneva, Switzerlan

Iversen C, Mullane N, McCardell B, Tall BD, Lehner A, Fanning S, Stephan R, Joosten H (2008). *Cronobacter* gen. nov., a new genus to accommodate the biogroups of *Enterobacter sakazakii*, and proposal of *Cronobacter sakazakii* gen. nov., comb. nov., *Cronobacter malonaticus* sp. nov., *Cronobacter turicensis* sp. nov., *Cronobacter muytjensii* sp. nov., *Cronobacter dublinensis* sp. nov., *Cronobacter* genomospecies 1, and of three subspecies, *Cronobacter dublinensis* subsp. dublinensis subsp. nov., *Cronobacter dublinensis* subsp. lausannensis subsp. nov. and *Cronobacter dublinensis* subsp. lactaridi subsp. nov. *International Journal of Systematic and Evolutionary Microbiology*, 58(Pt 6):1442-1447.

Kramer MF, and Coen DM (2000). Enzymatic Amplification of DNA by PCR: Standard Procedures and Optimization. In *Current Protocols in Toxicology*. A.3C.1-A.3C.14.

Kunin V, Ahren D, Goldovsky L , Janssen P, Ouzounis CA (2005). Measuring genome conservation across taxa: divided strains and united kingdoms. *Nucleic Acids Research*, 33(2):616-621.

Larkin MA, Blackshields G, Brown NP, Chenna R, McGettigan PA, McWilliam H, Valentin F, Wallace IM, Wilm A, Lopez R, Thompson JD, Gibson TJ, Higgins DG (2007). ClustalW and ClustalX version 2. *Bioinformatics*, 23: 2947-2948.

Liming SH, Bhagwat AA (2004). Application of a molecular beacon-real-time PCR technology to detect *Salmonella* species contaminating fruits and vegetables. *International Journal of Food Microbiology*, 95(2):177-187.

Lofstrom C, Knutsson R, AAxelsson CE, Radstrom P (2004). Rapid and specific detection of *Salmonella* spp. in animal feed samples by PCR and culture enrichment. *Applied and Environmental Microbiology,* 70(1):69-75.

McGregor DP, Forster S, Steven J, Adair J, Leary SE, Leslie DL, Harris WJ, Titball RW (1996). Simultaneous detection of microorganisms in soil suspension based on PCR amplification of bacterial 16S rRNA fragments. *Biotechniques,* 21(3):463-6, 468, 470-1.

McQuiston JR, Herrera-Leon S, Wertheim BC, Doyle J, Fields PI, Tauxe RV, Logsdon JM (2008). Molecular phylogeny of the salmonellae: relationships among *Salmonella* species and subspecies determined from four housekeeping genes and evidence of lateral gene transfer events. *Journal of Bacteriology,* 190(21):7060-1067.

Monteiro L, Bonnesaison D, Vekris A, Petry KG, Bonnet J, Vidal R, Cabrita J, Megraud F (1997). Complex polysaccharides as PCR inhibitors in feces: *Helicobacter pylori* model. *Journal of Clinical Microbiology,* 35(4):995-998.

Mozola MA, Peng X, Wendorf M (2007). Evaluation of the GeneQuence DNA hybridization method in conjunction with 24-hour enrichment protocols for detection of *Salmonella* spp. in select foods: collaborative study. *Journal of AOAC International,* 90(3):738-755.

Munnoch SA, Ward K, Sheridan S, Fitzsimmons GJ, Shadbolt CT, Piispanen JP, Wang Q, Ward TJ, Worgan TL, Oxenford C, Musto JA, McAnulty J, Durrheim DN (2009). A multi-state outbreak of *Salmonella* Saintpaul in Australia associated with cantaloupe consumption. *Epidemiology and Infection,* 137(3):367-374.

Nam HM, Srinivasan V, Gillespie BE, Murinda SE, Oliver SP (2005). Application of SYBR green real-time PCR assay for specific detection of *Salmonella* spp. in dairy farm environmental samples. *International Journal of Food Microbiology,* 102(2):161-71.

Patel JR, Bhagwat AA (2008). Rapid real-time PCR assay for detecting *Salmonella* in raw and ready-to-eat meats. *Acta Vet Hung.,* 56(4):451-8.

Porwollik S, Wong RM McClelland M (2002). Evolutionary genomics of *Salmonella*: gene acquisitions revealed by microarray analysis. *Proceedings of the National Academy of Sciences,* 99(13):8956-8961.

Pupo GM, Lan R, Reeves PR (2000). Multiple independent origins of *Shigella* clones of *Escherichia coli* and convergent evolution of many of their characteristics. *Proceedings of the National Academy of Sciences,* 97:(19)10567-10572.

Reiter MG, Fiorese ML, Moretto G, López MC, Jordano R (2007). Prevalence of *Salmonella* in poultry slaughterhouse. *J. Food Prot.,* 70:1723-1725.

Rossen L, Norskov P, Holmstrom K, Rasmussen OF (1992). Inhibition of PCR by components of food samles, microbial diagnostic assays and DNA-extraction solutions. *International Journal of Food Protection,* 17:37-45.

Tanner MA, Scarpati E, Sharma S, Furtado MR (2006). MicroSeq®: A 16S rRNA Gene Sequencing System for Bacterial Identification. In Volume III of Encyclopedia of Rapid Microbiological Methods. 205-225.

Tebbs RS, Cao YY, Balachandran P, Petrauskene O (2009). TaqMan *Salmonella* enterica Detection Kit. Performance Tested Method 020803. *Journal of AOAC International,* 92(6):1895-901.

Tebbs RS, Liu J-K, Furtado MR, Petrauskene O (2010). Mulitiplex detection of pathogenic organisms using TaqMan real-time PCR. In *Biodetection Technologies, Technical Responses to Biological Threats,* 6th Edition, Knowledge Press, pages 5-13.

Techathuvanan C, D'Souza DH (2011). Optimization of rapid *Salmonella* enterica detection in liquid whole eggs by SYBR green I-Based real-time reverse transcriptase-polymerase chain reaction. *Foodborne Pathogens and Disease*, 8(4):527-534.

Tindall BJ, Grimont PA, Garrity GM, Euzeby JP (2005). Nomenclature and taxonomy of the genus *Salmonella. International Journal of Systematic and Evolutionary Microbiology*, 55(Pt 1):521-524.

Tomita N, Mori Y, Kanda H, Notomi T (2008). Loop-mediated isothermal amplification (LAMP) of gene sequences and simple visual detection of products. *Nat Protoc.* 3(5):877-882.

Tsai Y-L, Olson BH (1992a). Detection of low numbers of bacterial cells in soils and sediments by polymerase chain reaction. *Applied and Environmental Microbiology*, 58(2):754-757.

Tsai Y-L, Olson BH (1992b). Rapid method for separation of bacterial DNA from humic substances in sediments for polymerase chain reaction. *Applied and Environmental Microbiology*, 58(7):2292-2295.

Ueda, S. and Kuwabara, Y. (2009). The rapid detection of *Salmonella* from food samples by loop-mediated isothermal amplification. *Biocontrol Science*. 14(2), 73-76.

van Cauteren D, Jourdan-da Silva N, Weill FX, King L, Brisabois A, Delmas G, Vaillant V, de Valk H (2009). Outbreak of *Salmonella enterica* serotype Muenster infections associated with goat's cheese, France, March 2008. *Eurosurveillance*, 14(31):19290.

Weyant RS, Edmonds P, Swaminathan B (1990). Effect of ionic and nonionic detergents on the *Taq* polymerase. *BioTechniques*, 9(3)308-309.

Wilson IG (1997). Inhibition and facilitation of nucleic acid amplification. *Applied and Environmental Microbiology*, 63(10):3741-3751.